{understanding pharmacology

a physiologic approach }

Leilani Grajeda-Higley, RN, MSA, PhD
San Diego State University
San Diego, California

D1605032

APPLETON & LANGE
Stamford, Connecticut

Copyright © 2000 by Appleton & Lange

All rights reserved. This book, or any parts thereof, may not be used or reproduced in any manner without written permission. For information, address Appleton & Lange, Four Stamford Plaza, PO Box 120041, Stamford, Connecticut 06912-0041.

www.appletonlange.com

99 00 01 02 03/ 10 9 8 7 6 5 4 3 2 1

Prentice Hall International (UK) Limited, *London*
Prentice Hall of Australia Pty. Limited, *Sydney*
Prentice Hall Canada, Inc., *Toronto*
Prentice Hall Hispanoamericana, S.A., *Mexico*
Prentice Hall of India Private Limited, *New Delhi*
Prentice Hall of Japan, Inc., *Tokyo*
Simon & Schuster Asia Pte. Ltd., *Singapore*
Editora Prentice Hall do Brasil Ltda., *Rio de Janeiro*
Prentice Hall, *Upper Saddle River, New Jersey*

Library of Congress Catalog Card Number: 99-073102

Acquisitions Editor: Patricia E. Casey
Development Editor: Elisabeth Church Garofalo
Production Editor: Karen Davis
Art Manager: Eve Siegel
Designer: Mary Skudlarek
Original Art: Leilani Grajeda-Higley
Art Rendering: Daniel J. Knopsnyder

ISBN 0-8385-8136-6
90000
9 780838 581360

PRINTED IN THE UNITED STATES OF AMERICA

For Lorenzo

Contents

INTRODUCTION: *Pharmacology and the Master Systems*

Section I   The Nervous System and Drugs

1   Sodium and Drugs That Affect the Action Potential

2   Drugs That Affect Calcium, Phosphorus, and the Completion of the Action Potential

Section IV The Gastrointestinal Tract and Drugs

19 Drugs That Work in the Intestinal Lumen

Section V Critical Thinking

20 Over the Counter: The Pharmacist Speaks

21 The Nurse Takes Action

Contributors

Ruth N. Grendell, DNSc, RN
Professor of Nursing
Department of Nursing
Point Loma Nazarene University
San Diego, California

Dawn L. Metrisin
Pharmacist and Manager
Longs Drug Stores
La Jolla, California

Reviewers

Vonna Cranston, RN, MS, CNS
Henderson State University
Arkadelphia, Arkansas

Catherine Lazo-Miller, CNS, MS
Legal Nurse Consultant
Hammond, Indiana

John Miller, RN, MN
Formerly Tacoma Community College
Tacoma, Washington

Heather Stephen-Selby, RN, BSN
Seattle Central Community College
Seattle, Washington

Nora M. Tully, RN, EdD
Queensborough Community College
Bayside, New York

Preface

▶ PHARMACOLOGY AND THE STUDENT NURSE

Student nurses often find pharmacology daunting, as do some nurses. The drug names are often long and hard to pronounce. Drug actions can injure or kill the patient. Ordering drugs, administering them, observing the patient's response and/or adverse reactions, responding with therapeutic interventions, and documenting the whole process take up the greatest amount of the nurse's time. The nurse is in the position of ensuring that the order is correct and that the right drug gets to the right patient at the right time, in the right dose, by the right route. In addition, the nurse must be able to teach the patient in plain language about the drug and answer any questions. This is a tremendous responsibility!

On realizing this, student nurses often request more pharmacology. Unfortunately, many of them also find the subject boring. I certainly did—so dry and dull that I declined a request from a teaching colleague to take over her pharmacology class because she was "burned out" with teaching it. But, as an act of friendship, I reconsidered and offered to teach a few of her classes. What an epiphany. As those who love to teach the subject already know, pharmacology isn't dull at all. It's dynamic, in constant flux as science makes new discoveries. All the life sciences come together in pharmacology: anatomy, biology, chemistry, microbiology, physiology, even pathology. Pharmacology tests and challenges the wits and skills of the nurse.

▶ A UNIQUE METHOD OF TEACHING PHARMACOLOGY: A PARADIGM SHIFT

The complexity of the challenge of teaching pharmacology hit me as I was drifting off to sleep after teaching one of those first classes and thinking about how difficult the subject was for students. In a flash of insight I realized that the body speaks three languages: nervous system—using neurotransmitters in the language of neurons and muscle cells; endocrine system—using both neurotransmitters and hormones in gland language; and immune system—using cytokines. Not only is there communication within the systems, but the systems talk to each other. Cells are studded with receptors to obtain information from other cells. Cells keep up a constant barrage of "conversations" with each other to maintain the body at homeostasis.

Medicines simply mimic those three languages. Drug molecules have "shapes" that match the "shape" or structure of the naturally occurring messenger molecule; however, drug molecules may have unintended configurations or shapes that cause them to lock into cell receptors not directly targeted, causing intentional or unintentional side effects.

This new way of looking at pharmacology is a paradigm shift, signaling that once seen this way, the subject will never seem the same again. The science of pharmacology is the accumulation of thousands of years of observations and knowledge. It has built up like a house that has one room added here and another one there. The student is introduced to this maze or labyrinth of modern and ancient information and must make sense of it. The result is a sense of being overwhelmed. But if we take the cell's point of view, pharmacology becomes more easily comprehensible. Cells talk and the nurse must listen.

▶ MAKING THE COMPLEX COMPREHENSIBLE: ILLUSTRATIONS

I began to teach in this modality, then found myself stumped when a student asked for an explanation of the difference between T_3 and T_4 hormones. I gave a tedious, erudite lecture on the subject and watched the students' eyes glaze over. The next week I brought posters I'd illustrated in cartoon form of how the thyroid traps iodine and creates its hormones. Instant understanding. In the weeks that followed I made more posters. The students wouldn't leave the class on their breaks. They stayed to copy the cartoons for their notes. I made information sheets and handed them out. After a couple of years I had quite a stack of information sheets. It looked like a book . . . in a jumbled way. It would take years and many wonderful, intelligent people to turn those notes into the book it became. In the meantime the science kept changing. Old drugs came and went, new drugs were discovered. New uses for old drugs were found.

▶ TEXT LIMITATIONS AND EMPHASIS

To keep the book as compact as possible, not every drug in use in the United States is included. But the most commonly used are. Discussion of drug interactions is not as extensive as it could be. In fact, a whole text could be devoted to the subject of drug interactions and the Master Systems. The book's emphasis is on medications using Master System cell communication to affect therapeutic outcomes. The drug side effects have been listed, not according to frequency, but according to how they affect the three Master Systems. The only classification of a side effect I am not yet satisfied with is that of edema. Edema can occur in any and all three systems, even simultaneously, but usually edema is a response by the kidneys to a perceived drop in blood volume. In other words, edema is typically an endocrine response.

Although the frequency of the appearance of a side effect is vastly important, the student must be alert to even the most infrequent event. Viewing side effects by Master System reveals patterns of how the body is affected holistically, no matter the frequency. For example, although the drug may cause an allergy, an immune system response, the patient may experience itching, a function

of the nervous system. The systems work together. To ignore or deny subjective or objective observations as too infrequent to be possible is to do the patient a disservice, and possibly jeopardize her health.

▶ TEAMWORK

Writing a book takes team work. The editor, Josephine Della Peruta, and Julie Warren, a genius with computers, originally put the notes and illustrations in order. Later, at Appleton & Lange, editors Trish Casey and Kathy Riedell championed the text. Many nursing instructors reviewed the early version of this book favorably and added important suggestions. To my delight, pharmacists have also appreciated the concept of Master System languages, noting it makes possible to understand in minutes what takes them years to learn. Editor Elisabeth Church Garofalo worked closely with me to get the book through production. Ruth Grendell, who has taught pharmacology for some 15 years, wrote the chapter, "The Nurse Takes Action," integrating the Master Systems approach to pharmacology with the nursing arts. Pharmacist Dawn Metrisin took on the task of explaining pharmacokinetics and discussing the interactions of drugs described in "The Nurse Takes Action." She then wrote the chapter "Over the Counter: The Pharmacist Speaks" in which drug metabolism and pharmacokinetics are discussed. Their chapters are in the critical thinking section.

▶ CONCLUSION

I hope that students will find the subject fascinating and that the book will make them safe practitioners of one of nursing's most important responsibilities. I also welcome the criticisms and insights of nursing instructors who value the study of pharmacology and find it as fascinating as I do.

Leilani Grajeda-Higley

Acknowledgments

The following people helped make this book possible either through direct production and help or moral support or both. Thank-you to Trish Casey and Elisabeth Church Garofalo, and Karen Davis at Appleton & Lange for their faith in the project. Thank-you to Al and Marcia Brengle, Dorothy and Harold Higley, Lorenzo Higley, Melinda DeCuir, Ellen Holcomb, Rudy and Lucy Grajeda, and Joyce Bowden, who was the first to tell me, "I believe in you."

Introduction: Pharmacology and the Master Systems

Pharmacology is a dynamic science, a work in progress, a nexus of all the life sciences. It began as an accumulation of observations of how humans responded to the use of roots, leaves, seeds, and the bark of plants. Then, almost 100 years ago, scientists hunched that drugs must somehow act on the surface of body cells. The science of pharmacology has arrived at the present knowledge that cells communicate through the lock-and-key fit of molecules and their receptor sites. The science of pharmacology is delving deeper into the cell, exploring the action of drugs on DNA in target cells.

Cells talk to each other using three distinct languages, and pharmacology mimics what they say and how they say it. With the possible exception of red blood cells, the billions of cells of the three great physiologic systems—the nervous system, which includes muscles; the endocrine system; and the immune system—communicate to maintain the body. Because these three systems, each using specific molecules of communication, control and coordinate all the organs and subsystems within them, they are called Master Systems in this text. Cell language consists of a simple, yet elegant use of molecular shapes. Each system has its own particular messenger molecules. In the nervous system they are called neurotransmitters or neurohormones. The endocrine system uses hormones, and the immune system sends out cytokines. Although each system is basically communicating within itself to oversee and control the actions of cells within the system's organs, its messenger molecules also influence the other systems. For example, brain cells talk to each other with their neurotransmitters, but neurons also come under the influence of sex hormones from the endocrine system. A system can also use messengers from another system for its own purposes; for example, the neuro-

transmitters serotonin and bradykinin are also used in the immune system.

▶ THE MASTER SYSTEMS

Classifying drugs by their molecular languages into the three physiologic or Master Systems, that is, the nervous system, the endocrine system, and the immune system, breaks from the complex, traditional system, which uses more than 25 categories that include a mix of anatomic, disease, therapeutic, drug action, and hormonal headings as well as several physiologic subsystems. However, medications, with few exceptions, can be classified in one of the three physiologic systems. Not only does this concise method of categories simplify learning, it gives the practitioner a single, clearer, holistic picture of the science and practice of pharmacology by using the same method the body uses for its own cell communication. Take, for example, the traditional classification of cardiovascular drugs. Some of those drugs mimic neurotransmitters that act in the central nervous system, but they can affect the heart because heart muscle uses some of the same neurotransmitters. Those readers accustomed to seeing diuretics classified with cardiovascular drugs because they lower blood volume, and thus blood pressure, may be surprised to find them in the endocrine system; however, control of blood volume is clearly a function of the endocrine system. Diuretics work in the endocrine system to decrease the volume a diseased heart must pump. In addition, the endocrine system can cause hypertension, albeit more slowly than the nervous system, by constricting blood vessels, and there are drugs to control this form of hypertension. Anticoagulants, too, are traditionally classified as cardiovascular drugs. But anticoagulants actually counter the clotting function of the immune response. In health

TABLE INTRO–1 Drug Categories by Master System

Nervous System	Endocrine System	Immune System
Drugs affecting the action potential and the electrolytes: sodium, potassium, chloride (includes anesthetics)	Releasing hormones	Antiallergy drugs (intertwine with nervous and endocrine system drugs)
Calcium, phosphorus, and blocking drugs including COPD drugs	Tropic hormones, eg, adrenocorticotropic hormones	Anticoagulants
Drugs for the parasympathetic system: acetylcholine—cholinergics and anticholinergics	Glucocorticoids	Mucolytics
Drugs for the sympathetic system: catecholamines—sympathomimetics and blockers, including cardiovascular drugs, emetics and antiemetics, stimulants, major tranquilizers, antidepressants, muscle relaxants, anesthetics, COPD drugs	Aldosterone	Nonsteroidal antiinflammatories and analgesics
	ACE inhibitors	Antibiotics
	Blood volume expanders	Antifungals
	Diuretics	Antiparasitics
	Antidiuretic hormone	Antivirals
	Oxytocin	Antineoplastics (intertwine with endocrine system drugs)
Serotonin, antidepressants, migraine drugs	Growth hormone	Immunosuppressants
	Somatostatin	Passive immunity agents
Histamine: antihistamines and H_2 blockers	Thyroid hormones	Vaccines
	Parathyroid hormones	
γ-Aminobutyric acid (GABA): sedatives, hypnotics, anticonvulsants, anxiolytics, muscle relaxants, anesthetics	Sex hormones	
Opiates and opiate blockers		

Alimentary Canal

Charcoal

Laxatives

Worming agents

Antacids

Bowel cleansing agents

Vitamins

all three systems work together to maintain balance. In disease all systems are affected. The physiologic approach to drugs in treating disease takes into consideration all three Master Systems and the way the body organizes itself (Table Intro–1).

Like three intertwined trees with one common root, the three systems cannot exist without each other. Inextricably interwoven and connected with one another, the actions of one impact the actions of the others. For example, emotional stress or trauma, a nervous system experience, may disrupt the routine rhythms of the endocrine system. In turn, the endocrine system may respond to the stress with increased glucocorticoid production to make more energy available to handle the stress. Glucocorticoids then suppress the immune response, leaving the individual more vulnerable to disease. Knowledge of these influences is exploited in pharmacology, where, for example, steroids from the endocrine system are essential in treating autoimmune disease or al-lergy by tamping down the immune response to foreign matter.

▶ **THE ALIMENTARY CANAL: AN ALIEN SPACE**

Although the three Master Systems work together, an alien space runs through the core of the body, a place that is neither nervous system, endocrine system, nor immune system. That place is the alimentary canal, truly a waterway that traverses the body. The walls of the alimentary canal are heavily guarded and patrolled by the mobile cells of the immune system to fight off other forms of life vying for the same nutrients or for entry into the body. Muscles of the nervous system propel canal contents, while endocrine hormones determine which proteins, minerals, sugars, and fluids to draw from what we eat or drink. Some drugs used in the alimentary canal simply coat the canal walls or interact with the contents floating in the lumen.

▶ RECEPTORS, VASCULARITY, AND DRUG DISTRIBUTION

Medication molecules may mimic cell language, but they don't "know" where to go to be therapeutic. They drift in the bloodstream attached to little protein carriers. As they leave the protein carriers to which they were bound, they float until they lock into cell receptors with corresponding shapes. Drug distribution depends on blood supply. The more vascular an area is, the more molecules it will receive. As blood levels of the freed-up drug molecules drop, more plasma-bound drug molecules are released from the plasma proteins. And, of course, the plasma proteins have receptors too. Except for red blood cells, all of the billions of cells of the nervous, immune, and endocrine systems are studded with receptors as if they were tiny hams studded with cloves. Cells also have receptors inside the cells. Usually, water-soluble molecules adrift in the extracellular fluids that bathe the cells can lock only onto the receptors on the cell membrane. They cause an inner, or second, messenger (thought to be calcium in some cases) to take the message and trigger a cascade of events within the cell and even its DNA, causing the cell to do, or stop doing, its special activity, for example, protein synthesis.

▶ THERAPEUTIC DRUG LEVELS

Each pill, each teaspoon of fluid, each syringe of solution contains millions of molecules of shapes meant to fit the desired receptors on or in cells. To ensure a therapeutic blood level, the dose or volume of molecules must be large enough to lock into sufficient numbers of receptors to effect the desired result. Too few molecules of medication will have no effect. Too many molecules will cause toxicity. Intoxication may be a therapeutic goal as in anesthesia, where neurons are overwhelmed to render the patient unconscious for surgery or other procedures. The frequency of administration of the specific volume is also essential to attain and maintain a therapeutic level of the drug in the blood. Such dosage must take into account drug metabolism and excretion rates by the liver, second-pass rates as excreted drugs are reabsorbed from the gut, and the ability of the kidneys to excrete drug molecules.

▶ PHARMACOKINETICS: DRUG RECYCLING AND EXCRETION

The body has mechanisms to break down and recycle its own messenger molecules. It also breaks down and removes drug molecules. Drugs do not remain un-changed in the body, though often the synthetic drug molecule may remain unchanged longer than would a naturally occurring molecule. Through a process called metabolism the body changes drugs. The liver breaks down and detoxifies drugs. Preexisting liver impairment can interfere with the metabolism of many drugs including acetaminophen [Tylenol], chlorpromazine [Thorazine], methyldopa [Aldomet], the monoamine oxidase inhibitors (MAOIs), phenytoin [Dilantin], and tetracycline [Terramycin]. Jaundice may signal drug toxicity. In addition, the liver excretes unchanged drugs via the gallbladder. The gallbladder releases bile containing the excreted drug into the gut, where the drug may be reabsorbed and used in a second pass. The kidneys also excrete drugs. Renal failure decreases drug excretion and can lead to toxicity. Pharmacology makes use of kidney excretion of drugs to treat urinary tract infections; for example, penicillin is quickly excreted by the kidneys and thus can be used to fight an infection in the area. The lungs and skin can also excrete drugs, just as they can be a route of administration.

▶ AGONISTS, ANTAGONISTS, AND SYNERGISTS

Agonist drug molecules enhance a specific cell function. Antagonists are drugs with opposing actions that may compete for the same receptors, even bumping out a molecule already in the receptor. This antagonist action can be lifesaving in the case of opiate overdose when the antagonist naloxone displaces morphine in the opiate receptors (Fig. Intro–1). Sometimes drug molecules may work together, intentionally or not. This synergism may result in either a beneficial or a toxic effect on the target cells. Combining a tranquilizer with a drink of alcohol is an example of synergism that can prove toxic, whereas combining probenecid with penicillin exemplifies a beneficial synergism, because probenecid elevates and prolongs plasma concentrations of penicillins.

▶ ROUTES OF ADMINISTRATION

The route through which a drug is administered determines how rapidly it will act and where most of the therapeutic effect will take place. The routes include intravenous (IV), intramuscular (IM), subcutaneous (SC or subQ), oral (PO, from the Latin *per os* for "by mouth"), intradermal, buccal, nasal, inhalational, ocular (eyedrops [gtt]), aural (eardrops [gtt]), urethral, vaginal, rectal, and topical. Some drugs are also administered into the central nervous system fluid in the spinal canal (intrathecal) or directly into cavities and wounds.

Example: In an endorphin receptor...

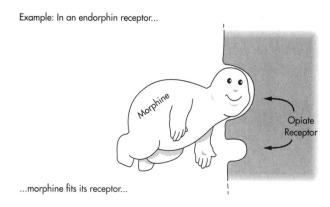

...morphine fits its receptor...

...but naloxone can displace opiates from their receptors

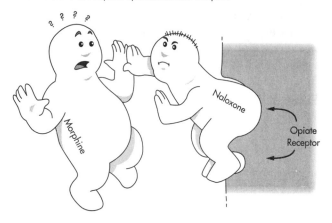

Figure Intro–1. Molecules and their receptor sites.

▶ HOW CELLS PROTECT THEMSELVES

For their own protection cells are selective about the water solubility of molecules vying for entry. Because the membranes of cells are "fat sandwiches," barriers made of two layers of lipids, they repel water and won't let water-soluble molecules enter. But they will readily let in oil-soluble molecules. For example, steroids like cortisone and testosterone are oil soluble. They slip right through the cell membrane and head for the cell nucleus, where they cause genetic changes (Fig. Intro–2).

▶ THE BLOOD–BRAIN BARRIER

The brain needs additional protection from potentially harmful molecules. The "feet" of astrocytes, star-shaped glial cells in the brain, lock together like the pieces of a jigsaw puzzle to form a second wall around the outside of the capillary walls in the brain. This extra wall, the blood–brain barrier (BBB), blocks or slows water-soluble substances, which can easily pass through capillary walls throughout the body (Fig. Intro–3). If, however, the brain needs those water-soluble molecules, a transport system is used to carry them across. Oil-soluble substances, on the other hand, can slip right through. For example, morphine and heroin are the same drug; however, heroin contains two acetyl wings that make it oil sol-

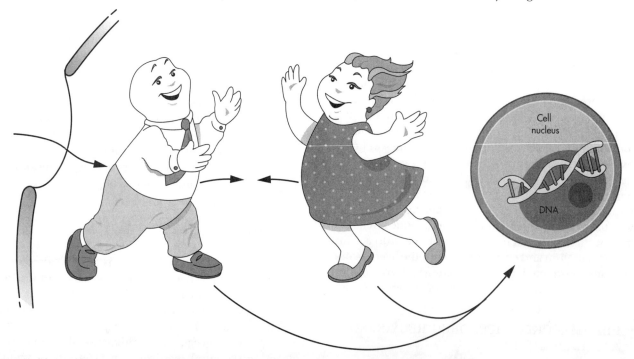

The oil-soluble hormone enters the cell, finds its receptor and together they move into the nucleus. There they trigger the transcription of specific genes and cause biochemical changes.

Figure Intro–2. How oil-soluble hormones affect cells.

uble and account for the "rush" heroin addicts describe as the drug passes through the BBB. Morphine, lacking heroin's oil solubility, takes longer to relieve pain. The size of the molecule also determines whether or not it will cross the BBB; smaller ones cross more easily. In addition, the BBB keeps essential molecules from escaping the central nervous system.

▶ THE FETUS, PLACENTA, AND DRUGS

During pregnancy the placenta forms a barrier too; however, the placenta does not block a very wide range of drugs, some of which can turn off, or on, genetic switches in the cells of developing fetal organs, as happened in the thalidomide tragedies of the 1970s, when babies were born with deformed or missing limbs to mothers who took thalidomide tranquilizers during the embryonic stage of limb development. Alcohol can also pass through the placenta, and excessive alcohol use during pregnancy can result in fetal alcohol syndrome, a form of mental retardation. Some drugs can addict the fetus, just as they do the mother.

▶ DRUGS, CHILDREN, AND THE ELDERLY

Metabolic and excretion rates differ in children and the elderly. Organs that break down and excrete drugs in children are immature. Body proportions and fluid balances are different. A child's body responds differently to drugs than a young or middle-aged adult's because of the immature structures. The elderly, too, may respond differently as their organs slow and become inefficient. The liver may not break down drugs as before. Kidneys may not excrete as well. A slowed, crippled heart won't circulate drug molecules effectively. Receptor sites decrease in number. What irony that the elderly may need the help of medications at the very time when their bodies may least be able to handle the drugs.

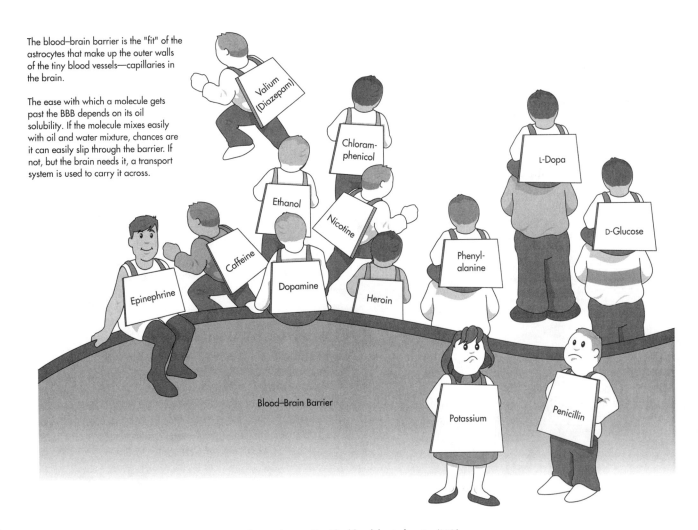

The blood–brain barrier is the "fit" of the astrocytes that make up the outer walls of the tiny blood vessels—capillaries in the brain.

The ease with which a molecule gets past the BBB depends on its oil solubility. If the molecule mixes easily with oil and water mixture, chances are it can easily slip through the barrier. If not, but the brain needs it, a transport system is used to carry it across.

Figure Intro-3. The blood–brain barrier (BBB).

▶ DRUG SIDE EFFECTS

The flip side of drug therapies is that drug molecules can also cause harm. No matter which of the physiologic systems a drug is aimed at, a drug may appear foreign to the immune system and trigger an allergic response. For example, angiotensin-converting enzyme inhibitors in the endocrine system, phenytoin in the nervous system, and penicillin in the immune system can induce an allergic response. Drugs can also cause potentially fatal blood dyscrasias, for example, bone marrow depression and aplastic anemia, when they alter the DNA in developing blood cells. Sometimes side effects can benefit, as is the case with aspirin's ability to make platelets less "sticky." Possibly the two most common side effects of drugs are nausea and vomiting. Drug side effects are commonly linked to dosage.

Plant Molecules and Pharmacology

Life on this planet consists of food chains, and each plant and creature is a link in the chain. A major feature of the linkage is that plants and animals share similar molecular features. Many of the plants we eat have molecules that can lock into receptors on our cells. For example, the parasympathetic system has receptors for molecules from mushrooms and also for nicotine molecules from plants. Pharmacology began as the study of the medicinal qualities of plants, known as *materia medica*, a branch of botany. Plant survival depends on producing molecules that affect our cells, either to entice us to eat them or to repel us. Humans discovered that some molecules, like those of the opium poppy, had pleasant effects that made us want to eat them, thus increasing the chance of depositing their seeds elsewhere. Opium derivatives have been used for thousands of years to relieve pain, coughing, and diarrhea. Other plants, for example, the castor plant, made us ill and its derivatives serve as cathartics. Indians of the Amazon tip their darts with curare from a plant of the genus *Strychnos* to paralyze the prey they shoot. Using variations, or analogs, of that same paralyzing plant molecule, the anesthesiologist paralyzes the patient in major surgery, to relax the abdominal muscles and ease the procedure, or in electroconvulsive therapy, to reduce the severity of the convulsion. Medicinal plants affect our cells' receptor sites because they produce molecules that fit those sites and simply mimic the languages "spoken" by cells in each of the three systems.

▶ SCIENTIFIC ADVANCEMENTS

The ancient Egyptians believed that the brain's function was to create mucus. They had no way of knowing otherwise. But over thousands of years we have acquired great stores of medical knowledge as health practitioners and scientists found better ways of unraveling the body's mysteries. Giants of medicine, from Hippocrates to Salk, have preceded us, and, as Isaac Newton wrote, "If I have seen further it is by standing on the shoulders of giants." In pharmacology we have classified drugs using the ancient methods based on the knowledge of where they act in the body or by botanical names or other assorted criteria. But we can see further and deeper now. We can see more than a heart, or a lung, or a kidney. We can see the receptors of the cells of the tissues that make up organs and organ systems. We can understand how cells communicate with other cells close by or at distant sites. These modern understandings need a new way of looking at drug classification.

▶ AN INVITATION

Cells talk and they speak the messages encoded in our DNA through the languages of the nervous system, the endocrine system, and the immune system for the ultimate survival of our DNA. The reader is invited to enjoy the wonder of cell language and how drugs imitate it in the Master Systems. We can see further now and we can hear cells talk.

I
section

The Nervous System and Drugs

▶ THE NERVOUS SYSTEM MASTER SYSTEM

The nervous system makes thought and movement possible. Our millions-of-years-old physiologic history is reflected in the way the nervous system is laid out, from the primitive, intrinsic, yet essential reflexive actions of the segmented spinal cord to the conscious, thinking activities of the higher cortical structures. All of these structures work together in highly organized networks and patterns to enhance survival.

The cells, or neurons, of the nervous system constitute the gray matter. White matter is made up of the fine and fragile filaments of axons and dendrites that branch out from the cells. **Axons** and **dendrites** are the wiring of the nervous system by which neurons send and receive messages. Axons carry the impulses or messages from the neurons, and dendrites receive incoming impulses. Dendrites branch and grow as we learn and practice new information or skills. **Neurons** produce chemical messenger molecules and secrete them from the ends of axons into the synapses, those spaces between neurons. Lightning fast, neurotransmitters are released into the synapses. The neurotransmitters lock into receptors on dendrites of neurons upstream or downstream.

Neuronal communication is based on the shapes of neurotransmitters and receptors. Like a key in a lock, neurotransmitters must fit the receptor sites. The insertion of a neurotransmitter sets off a chain reaction of ions. Sodium and chloride outside the neuron's membrane enter the cell through its respective channels (little trapdoors) and potassium exits the cell through its channels. This exchange results in an electrochemical wave of energy that sweeps over the cell from the dendrites to the axons. At the end of the energy sweep, calcium enters the axon and pushes the neurotransmitters out of their storage vesicles into yet other synapses. This ebb and flow of neuronal energy is as constant as the life of the individual, ceasing only at death.

▶ THE SPINAL CORD

Of all the structures of the nervous system, the spinal cord is the most primitive. Constructed in segments it carries messages back and forth the length of the body. Nerve fibers from anterior motor neurons in the cord innervate or stimulate skeletal muscle fibers. The simple action of swinging our arms and legs in walking is under the control of the spinal cord, but the brain signals purposeful action to start and stop the action. The spinal cord also contains reflex arcs that cause us to pull back from painful stimuli immediately without having to think first. The spinal cord is under the coordinating influence of higher brain structures that include the brain stem, the cerebellum, the basal ganglia, and, finally, the cerebral cortex. The crude stepping actions of a newborn's legs offer a good illustration of how the limbs work without coordination by the higher brain structures.

▶ THE BRAIN STEM

The brain stem tops off the spinal cord and sends down messages that provide for the most basic body functions of breathing, vasoconstriction, and cardiac action. Rising upward from the brain stem, the gossamer netting of the reticular system rouses us into consciousness. Ringing the brain stem, the limbic system acts as the gatekeeper of memory. With its appetites for food, sex, fight, and flight, it enables us to feel pain and passion.

In the twin and curving hippocampal structures, a discrete number of cells are responsible for encoding new memories. Damage to these cells leaves the individual without the ability to learn new skills or make new memories, doomed to live only in the past.

On each side of the limbic system, the thumbnail-sized, almond-shaped **amygdalae** react to threatening stimuli with fear. They may follow this with anger and rage to protect and defend. The amygdalae also have sexual functions and can produce copulating muscle activity.

The **thalamus,** in the center of the limbic system, also aids in memory and in the experience of pain. In humans the limbic system apparently stores memories for about 3 years, after which other cortical structures also store them.

Just below the thalamus in the limbic system, the **hypothalamus** monitors and controls hormonal activities. It is essential in the bonding of the mother with the newborn and responds to the infant's cry with milk let-down or protective actions. The hypothalamus oversees endocrine functions and monitors hormonal activities in glands throughout the body. It serves as a connection between mind and body. It is important to note that there is no organ called the mind. The mind is a function of limbic and cortical structures working together.

Topping off the nervous system, the convoluted **cortex** wraps around the limbic structures. Ancient parts of the temporal lobes of the cortex are considered to be part of the limbic system. The cortex, both new and old, is only about six layers thick. If it were to be spread out it would be about the size of a pie crust. The cortex rises up from the thalamus and is folded and wrinkled so that more surface area can be packed into the skull. Conscious control over movement, sensory interpretation, speech, and cognitive functions occurs here. The prefrontal lobes of the cortex set us apart from all other life on earth. They give us the ability to anticipate the future, make plans, and realize our mortality.

▶ THE CEREBELLUM

Tucked and folded under the cortex and snugged up against the brain stem lies the cerebellum, source of athletic grace. The **cerebellum** sends messages to the cord that smooth out the reflexive, crude actions of the limbs.

▶ THE PERIPHERAL SYSTEM

The brain cells and neuronal systems within systems maintain a barrage of communication. The **peripheral,** or **sensory, nervous system** sends constant information back to the brain about conditions inside and outside the body, for example, pressure, position, and temperature. The incoming stimuli may be visual, auditory, olfactory, or kinesthetic. Responding brain structures fire messages along nerve fibers that can extend as far as 3 ft, as do the long axons that make up the spinal cord, or short distances to neighboring cells or brain structures.

▶ THE MOTOR SYSTEM

SOMATIC SYSTEM

Using the neurotransmitter **acetylcholine,** the brain sends responses down through the motor system, which comprises two subsystems. One, the **somatic system,** has long, single axons going to specific skeletal muscles. The somatic system can override the second part of the motor system—the autonomic system.

THE AUTONOMIC SYSTEM

The **autonomic system** controls the essential, or vegetative, body functions of the stem at an unconscious level. It also divides into the parasympathetic nervous system and the sympathetic nervous system. The autonomic nervous system uses two neurons in its pathway. Preganglionic neurons originate in the brain and descend the cord to the ganglia. Postganglionic neurons then continue out from the ganglia. A ganglion is a synaptic switching station or junction.

Emerging from the ganglia, the parasympathetic system continues using acetylcholine, its only neurotransmitter, while the sympathetic system switches to using mostly the catecholamine neurotransmitter, norepinephrine. The sympathetic and the parasympathetic systems work as a team. When one is in control, the other is on stand-by.

The Parasympathetic Nervous System

The **parasympathetic nervous system,** using only the neurotransmitter acetylcholine, controls a vast range of behaviors from thoughts and feelings to visceral activities and muscle actions. The parasympathetic nervous system basically controls the body when we are engaged in day-to-day activities such as feeding, digestion, and elimination. It also has influence in higher cognitive functions of thoughts, dreams, and hallucinations. The parasympathetic nervous system has only one method of disposing of acetylcholine after its mission is completed. It uses the enzyme acetylcholinesterase to break down acetylcholine.

Many drugs, both ancient and modern, have been developed to mimic or block acetylcholine. Cholinergic and anticholinergic drugs are discussed later in this book.

The Sympathetic Nervous System

The **sympathetic nervous system** controls our responses to stressful events both joyful and terrifying: the flight-or-fight behaviors attributed to the limbic structures. Its neurons produce chemical messengers called the catecholamines: dopamine, epinephrine, norepinephrine. Dopamine plays a role in reward-motivated behaviors. Even though the sympathetic nervous system oversees emotionally charged responses, it uses acetylcholine to stimulate sweat glands; however, the apocrine glands in the axillae respond to threat with thick, smelly secretions in response to catecholamine stimulation. (Perhaps this is the smell of fear.)

The sympathetic nervous system can break down catecholamines using the enzyme monoamine oxidase, or it simply recycles the catecholamines whole through a reuptake process that returns the molecules back to the secreting neurons. In addition, though not termed an adrenergic, like dopamine, norepinephrine, and epinephrine, the neurotransmitter serotonin is also a monoamine. It is broken down by the enzyme monoamine oxidase, as are the other neurotransmitters. Serotonin plays a role in our affect or mood. It is also implicated in migraine headache and feeding behaviors. (A vast number of drugs mimic or oppose the neurotransmitters of the sympathetic nervous system. These drugs are discussed in Chapter 4.)

The Adrenal Medulla: Part of the Sympathetic Nervous System

The **adrenal medulla**, or middle of the adrenal glands, is part of the sympathetic nervous system, because it also makes catecholamines. Stress stimulates the chromaffin cells of the medulla with acetylcholine from the central nervous system to produce the adrenergic neurotransmitters dopamine, norepinephrine (noradrenalin), and epinephrine (adrenaline), which are released into the bloodstream to stimulate the heart, liver, and other target organs, such as fat cells, needed for emergencies (see Fig. I–1). At the same time, the chromaffin cells also release endorphins.

▶ THE PHARMACOLOGY OF THE NERVOUS SYSTEM

LEAD DRUGS

"LEAD" is a mnemonic, composed of the first letters of the four common drugs used in cardiovascular emergencies: lidocaine, epinephrine, atropine, and dopamine (see Fig. I–2). **Lidocaine** interferes with sodium channels to block potentially deadly electrical conduction abnormalities in heart muscle. **Epinephrine** speeds the heart, raises blood pressure, and stimulates the liver

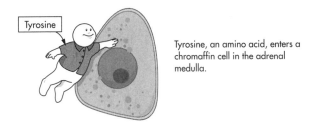

Tyrosine, an amino acid, enters a chromaffin cell in the adrenal medulla.

Inside...tyrosine hydroxylase turns tyrosine...

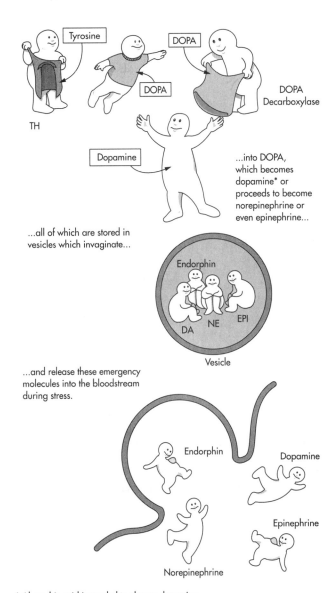

...into DOPA, which becomes dopamine* or proceeds to become norepinephrine or even epinephrine...

...all of which are stored in vesicles which invaginate...

...and release these emergency molecules into the bloodstream during stress.

* Abscorbic acid is needed to change dopamine into norepinephrine.

Figure I-1. How cells in the adrenal medulla make neurotransmitters used in stress.

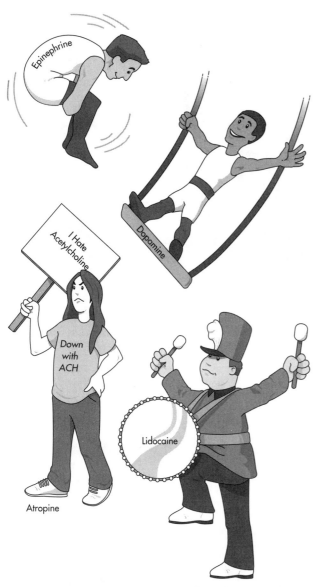

The catecholamines dopamine and epinephrine, along with atropine and lidocaine, are the four drugs noted in the mnemonic LEAD–the basic emergency drugs.

Figure I–2. LEAD—the basic emergency drugs.

to release stored energy. **Atropine** blocks acetylcholine and helps to speed a slowing heart. **Dopamine**, epinephrine's precursor, also has epinephrine's actions. These drugs are discussed more fully in the following chapters.

OTHER DRUGS FOR THE NERVOUS SYSTEM

Although LEAD drugs can save lives when used in cardiovascular emergencies, other drugs used in the nervous system can provide anesthesia or analgesia, treat psychiatric disturbances, and ease bowel and bladder disorders associated with neurotransmission. Drugs can interrupt life-threatening aberrant discharges in the brain or replace depleted neurotransmitters in such diseases as Alzheimer's, Parkinson's, or myasthenia gravis. Drugs for the nervous system are used to treat imbalances and depletions of neurotransmitters.

New discoveries produce new pharmaceutical strategies for treating nervous system disorders. At this time the major neurotransmitters have been identified and more than 60 lesser neurotransmitters have also been found. The science of pharmacology seeks an ever closer and specific fit of drug molecules to intended target receptors.

1

Sodium and Drugs That Affect the Action Potential

drug list

- adenosine [Adenocard]
- benzocaine [Americaine, Anbesol, Solarcaine, others]
- bupivacaine hydrochloride [Marcaine, Sensorcaine]
- chloroprocaine hydrochloride [Nesacaine, Nesacaine-CE]
- cocaine hydrochloride
- dibucaine hydrochloride [Nupercaine, Percaine, Cinchocaine]
- disopyramide phosphate [Norpace]
- etiodocaine hydrochloride [Duranest]
- flecainide [Tambocor]
- lidocaine hydrochloride [Xylocaine, others]
- mexiletine [Mexitil]
- phenytoin [Dilantin, others]
- pramoxine hydrochloride [Fleet Relief Anesthetic Hemorrhoidal, Prax, ProctoFoam, Tronolane, Tronothane]
- procainamide hydrochloride [Pronestyl, others]
- propafenone hydrochloride [Rhythmol]
- quinidine gluconate [Duraquin, others]
- quinidine polygalacturonate [Cardioquin]
- quinidine sulfate [Quinora, others]
- tetracaine hydrochloride [Amethocaine, Pontocaine]

Antiarrhythmic drugs and local anesthetics work on the principle of the action potential. Every individual is a walking sea of cells bathed in a solution of sodium and chloride ions called **electrolytes**. The cells contain potassium ions (Fig. 1–1). Cells also have trapdoors, or "channels," on their membranes that widen or narrow to allow or bar the exchange of ions specific to the channel. Chloride passes through its channels. Sodium has so-called fast channels. Potassium moves through its special channels. When a thought is generated or a muscle moves, intentionally or not, millions of cells are involved in a swap of ions through their cell membrane channels. This rapid-fire exchange of ions through their respective channels has a cascading domino effect called an "action potential," a sweep of electrochemical energy that washes over nerve cell membranes to the axons, where released neurotransmitters flood the synapses, or gaps, between nerve cells. The neurotransmitters lock into nerve endings across the space of the synapse, relaying the message and the action potential to downstream neurons.

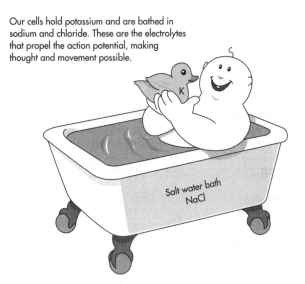

Our cells hold potassium and are bathed in sodium and chloride. These are the electrolytes that propel the action potential, making thought and movement possible.

Salt water bath NaCl

Figure 1-1. Nerve language and electrolytes.

▶ DEPOLARIZATION

Before the action potential makes its sweep, the involved cells have a positive charge on their surfaces and a negative charge on the inside. "Pluses" sit outside of the cell membrane and "minuses" sit inside. The ion swap through the little trapdoors of the cell membrane causes the "pluses" to move in and the "minuses" to move out. The event is called **depolarization**, a vulnerable moment for a cell, because it needs a fraction of time to recover before receiving a new stimulus. An aberrant discharge of energy from an ectopic source in cardiac conduction, especially in the ventricles, during depolarization can cause life-threatening medical emergencies. In the brain such a discharge can trigger a seizure. Ion exchange takes place in the **nodes of Ranvier**, junctions between the insulating Schwann cells. These nodes are permeated with channels through which potassium, sodium, and chloride make their exchange, propelling the action potential in normally rhythmic waves. Drugs that affect sodium and chloride concentrations can stabilize cells that emit ectopic electrical discharges (Fig. 1–2).

Because these drugs interfere with nerve conduction, it follows that side effects would include a potentially large array of impeded nervous system conduction responses such as flushing, dizziness, nausea, and respiratory difficulties. Additionally, because the parasympathetic system, using the neurotransmitter acetylcholine, is affected by the drugs' sodium channel interference, one would expect to see anticholinergic side effects.

▶ ANTIARRHYTHMIC DRUGS

Antiarrhythmic drugs interfere with the ionic influx of sodium to treat potentially lethal irregular heart rhythms.

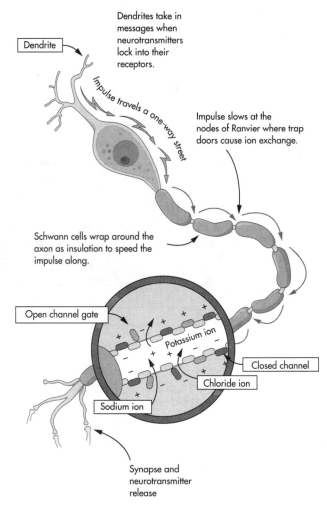

Dendrite

Dendrites take in messages when neurotransmitters lock into their receptors.

Impulse travels a one-way street

Impulse slows at the nodes of Ranvier where trap doors cause ion exchange.

Schwann cells wrap around the axon as insulation to speed the impulse along.

Open channel gate

Potassium ion

Closed channel

Chloride ion

Sodium ion

Synapse and neurotransmitter release

Ions have gates or channels specific to the ion.

Figure 1-2. The action potential: how nerves pass on their messages.

Adenosine [Adenocard] slows conduction through the atrioventricular (AV) and sinoatrial (SA) nodes, can interrupt the reentry pathways through the AV node, and is used for conversion to sinus rhythm of paroxysmal supraventricular tachycardia (PSVT). Depression of the left ventricular conduction is transient because of the short half-life of the drug.

Drug Interactions: Increased effect with dipyridamole. Effect blocked by theophylline. Increased risk of heart block with carbamazepine.

Side Effects

Nervous System: arrhythmias—prolonged asystole/atrial fibrillation/flutter/palpitations/ventricular tachycardia*/fibrillation, increased BP—transient, shortness

---

* Life-threatening side effect.

of breath/dyspnea, bronchospasm,* dizziness, headache, hypotension, lightheadedness, metallic taste, numbness, nausea, pain—chest/neck/back, psyche—apprehension, sensation of heaviness in arms, tingling in arms, vision—blurred.

Endocrine System: (Pregnancy Category C) facial flushing, sweating.

Immune System: none noted.

Dosage: 6-mg rapid IV bolus over 1–2 s. May repeat in 1–2 min with 12 mg IV push × 2 (total of 3 doses). Maximum recommended dose is 12 mg. Give in the vein or most proximal IV tubing port. Rapid flush with saline.

Disopyramide phosphate [Norpace] is used to treat premature ventricular contractions (PVCs) and ventricular tachycardia. It requires a pacemaker in second- and third-degree AV block, and can exacerbate ventricular dysfunction. Disopyramide has an anticholinergic effect, precluding use in patients with glaucoma. Atrial flutter and fibrillation must be treated before starting disopyramide.

Drug Interactions: Anticholinergic effects increased by other anticholinergic drugs such as antihistamines and tricyclic antidepressants. Increased toxicity with other antiarrhythmics. Possible increased metabolism of the drug with phenytoin; rifampin may decrease disopyramide levels. Increased hypoprothrombinemia with warfarin possible.

Side Effects

Nervous System: arrhythmias, cardiogenic shock,* CHF—worsened, convulsions,* bladder—frequency/hesitancy/retention/urgency, bowel—constipation, dizziness, dyspnea, fatigue, headache, heart block,* hypotension, laryngospasm,* muscle—aches/weakness, myasthenia gravis—precipitation, pain—abdominal/chest/epigastric, paresthesias, peripheral neuropathy, psyche—nervousness/psychosis, syncope, vision—blurred/precipitation of acute angle-closure glaucoma/>IOP/pupil enlargement.

Endocrine System: (Pregnancy Category C) drying of bronchioles/eyes/nose/throat, dry mouth, edema, renal insufficiency, uterine contractions—during pregnancy.

Immune System: agranulocytosis*—rare, photosensitivity, rash, thrombocytopenia.

Dosage: PO >50 kg: 100–200 mg q6h or 300 mg controlled-release cap q12h; <50 kg: 100 mg q6h or 200 mg controlled-release cap q12h.

Flecainide [Tambocor] suppresses PVCs as it decreases cardiac conduction throughout the heart, especially the His–Purkinje system. Not for use in chronic atrial fibrillation, second- or third-degree AV block, right bundle branch block associated with a left hemiblock (without a pacemaker). While effective in life-threatening ventricular arrhythmias, flecainide may have an excessive cardiac arrest rate. Dose-related side effects.

Drug Interactions: Levels may increase with cimetidine. May increase digoxin levels 15–25%. Possible additive negative inotropic effects with beta blockers.

Side Effects

Nervous System: arrhythmias*/cardiac arrest,* bladder—frequency/retention, bowel—constipation, CHF—worsened, cramps, dizziness, dyspnea, edema, fatigue, headache, lightheadedness, nausea, pain—chest, paresthesias, speech disorders, taste changes, vision—blurred/difficulty focusing.

Endocrine System: (Pregnancy Category C) edema, fever.

Immune System: leukopenia, thrombocytopenia.

Dosage: PO 100 mg q12h; may increase by 50 mg bid q4d to a max of 400 mg/d.

Lidocaine hydrochloride [Xylocaine, others] was originally a local anesthetic until its ability to control deadly arrhythmias was discovered. Lidocaine is given IV in acute myocardial infarction (MI) to control or prevent PVCs, ventricular tachycardia, and fibrillation. Normal potassium levels enhance its effectiveness. It must be used cautiously with sinus node dysfunction, second- and third-degree block, and bundle branch block. Toxicity is usually related to dose; the elderly are especially sensitive.

Drug Interactions: Decreased activity with barbiturates. Increased effect with beta blockers, cimetidine, quinidine. Increased cardiac depressant effects with phenytoin. Increased cardiac and neurologic effects with procainamide.

Incompatibilities

Solution/Additive: cefazolin, phenytoin.

Y-site: phenytoin.

Side Effects

Nervous System: arrhythmias, cardiac arrest,* cardiovascular collapse, convulsions,* dyspnea,* edema, heart block, nausea/vomiting, paresthesias, psyche—confusion/mood changes/psychosis, speaking difficulty, swallowing impaired, tremors, twitching, vision changes.

Endocrine System: (Pregnancy Category B) anorexia, edema, sweating.

Immune System: anaphylaxis,* edema, rash.

---

* Life-threatening side effect.

Dosage: IV 1–1.5 mg/kg bolus over 2–3 min; then a 0.5–0.75mg/kg bolus in 5–10 min to a total of 3 mg/kg; followed with a continuous IV at 1–4 mg/min (30 mL/h approximately) calibrated to prevent arrhythmias and toxicity. (Mix 2 g in 250 mL of D5W.) IM/SC 200–300 mg. May repeat once after 60–90 min. (Also see local anesthetics in this chapter.)

Mexiletine [Mexitil] shortens action potential duration and refractory period and improves resting potential; prolongs the His-to-ventricular interval if the patient has preexisting conduction disturbance. Used for acute and chronic ventricular arrhythmias, prevention of recurrent cardiac arrests, suppression of PVCs due to ventricular tachyarrhythmias. Unlabeled use for Wolff–Parkinson–White syndrome and supraventricular arrhythmias.

Drug Interactions: Levels may decrease with phenytoin, phenobarbital, and rifampin. Levels may increase with cimetidine.

Side Effects

Nervous System: arrhythmias—exacerbation, arthralgia, bladder—retention, bowel—constipation/diarrhea, dyspnea, dizziness, edema, headache, heartburn, hiccups, hypotension, impotence, incoordination, malaise, nausea/vomiting, numbness, pain—abdominal/chest, palpitations, paresthesias, psyche—nervousness, syncope, tremor, vision—blurred.

Endocrine System: (Pregnancy Category C) dry mouth, fever.

Immune System: rash.

Dosage: PO 200–300 mg q8h (max 1200 mg/d).

Phenytoin [Dilantin, others] is most easily recognized as an anticonvulsant, but is sometimes used for atrial and ventricular arrhythmias caused by digitalis toxicity or mitral valve collapse. The side effects are usually dose-related.

Drug Interactions: Decreased effect with alcohol. Increased or decreased levels with other anticonvulsants. Increased metabolism and decreased absorption of oral anticoagulants. Increased metabolism and decreased effectiveness of oral contraceptives. Increased levels with amiodarone, chloramphenicol, omeprazole. Decreased levels with antituberculosis agents. Decreased absorption possible of calcium, folic acid, vitamin D. Decreased absorption possible with enteral nutrition supplements.

Incompatibilities

Solution/Additive: amikacin, aminophylline, bretylium, cephapirin, codeine phosphate, 5% dextrose, dobutamine, insulin, levorphanol, lidocaine, lincomycin, meperidine, metaraminol, methadone, morphine, nitro-glycerin, norepinephrine, pentobarbital, procaine, secobarbital, streptomycin.

Y-site: amikacin, bretylium, dobutamine, heparin, lidocaine, potassium chloride, vitamin B complex with C.

Side Effects

Nervous System: arrhythmias—bradycardia/cardiovascular collapse*/ventricular fibrillation,* bowel—constipation, nausea/vomiting, psyche—confusion, seizures,* vision—blurred/diplopia/photophobia.

Endocrine System: (Pregnancy Category D) alkaline phosphatase elevations, fever, glycosuria, hyperglycemia, hypocalcemia, acute renal failure, TSH increase, weight—gain/loss.

Immune System: agranulocytosis,* aplastic anemia,* craniofacial abnormalities, gingival hyperplasia, toxic epidermal necrolysis, liver necrosis, lupus erythematosus,* pancytopenia, Peyronie's disease, pneumonitis, pulmonary fibrosis, rashes, Stevens–Johnson syndrome.

Dosage: IV in cardiac conditions 100 mg/5 min until the arrhythmia subsides or to a maximum of 1 g. Too rapid a rate of infusion can cause hypotension, bradycardia, arrest.

Procainamide hydrochloride [Pronestyl, others] is an analog of the local anesthetic procaine used when lidocaine fails; also used for atrial fibrillation and paroxysmal tachycardia. Not for use if the patient also has myasthenia gravis. An artificial pacemaker is needed when used in second- and third-degree block.

Drug Interactions: Increased therapeutic and toxic effects with other antiarrhythmics. Increased anticholinergic effects with other anticholinergic agents. Increased hypotensive effect with antihypertensive agents. Increased levels/toxicity with procainamide.

Incompatibilities

Solution/Additive: bretylium, ethacrynate.

Side Effects

Nervous System: arrhythmias—AV block/tachycardia/ventricular fibrillation,* bowel—diarrhea, dizziness, hypotension—severe, myalgia, nausea/vomiting, pain—joints/muscles/pleuritic, polyarthralgias, psyche—psychosis, taste—bitter.

Endocrine System: (Pregnancy Category C) anorexia, chills, fever, flushing.

---

* Life-threatening side effect.

Immune System: agranulocytosis*—with repeated use, angioedema,* rash, SLE-like syndrome—50% chance with large doses, thrombocytopenia.

Dosage: Ventricular tachycardia: IM (used only until PO is possible) 0.5–1 g q4–6h; PO 1 g followed by 250–500 mg q3h or 500 mg–1 g q6h sustained-release. PVCs: 50 mg/kg/d divided q3h, maintain on 50 mg/kg/d (SR) divided q6h. Atrial fibrillation and paroxysmal atrial tachycardia: start with 1.25 g; then in 1 h, if no ECG changes, give 0.75 g; then 0.5–1 g q2h until either the normal rhythm resumes or toxicity occurs; maintain on 0.5–1 g q4–6h. Arrhythmias of anesthesia or surgery: IV 100 mg q5min at 25–50 mg/min until either normal rhythm resumes, toxicity occurs, or the maximum dose of 1 g has been given; maintain on infusion of 2–6 mg/min based on body weight, circulation, and renal function.

Propafenone hydrochloride [Rhythmol] blocks sodium channels to stabilize myocardial membranes, reduces automaticity and the rate of single and multiple PVCs, and suppresses ventricular tachycardia.

Drug Interactions: Levels and toxicity increase with amiodarone and quinidine. May increase levels and toxicity of tricyclic antidepressants, cyclosporine, digoxin, beta blockers, theophylline, warfarin. May increase diltiazem levels. Phenobarbital decreases propafenone levels.

Side Effects

Nervous System: arrhythmias—various and heart block—AV/BBB/and complete sinus arrest/ventricular tachycardia,* bowel—constipation/abdominal discomfort, CHF, dizziness, fatigue, headache, hypotension, nausea/vomiting, paresthesias, somnolence, taste changes, vertigo, vision—blurred.

Endocrine System: (Pregnancy Category C) dry mouth.

Immune System: COPD worsening, granulocytopenia, hepatitis, leukopenia, rash.

Dosage: PO 150–300 mg q8h.

Quinidine gluconate [Duraquin, others], quinidine polygalacturonate [Cardioquin], quinidine sulfate [Quinora, others] all derive from quinine, the antimalarial drug from the bark of the cinchona tree. Dr. Karl Wenckebach, a Dutch cardiologist, discovered its usefulness in treating atrial fibrillation when a patient successfully self-medicated with the parent drug, quinine (Sneader, 1985). Quinidine, an isomer of quinine, is still used, almost 100 years later, for atrial fibrillation. It is also used to treat atrial flutter and paroxysmal tachycardia. It reduces ectopic beats and cre-

ates a longer refractory period in the Purkinje fibers. Quinidine suppresses the second pacemaker; therefore, it can cause ventricular standstill when there is AV block or a nodal or idioventricular pacemaker. Quinidine decreases the need for digoxin by half, increases warfarin action, and enhances beta blocker action.

Drug Interactions: Digoxin levels may double. Quinidine levels may increase with amiodarone, reserpine, and phenothiazines. Other antiarrhythmics increase cardiac depressant effects. Metabolism is increased by anticonvulsants, barbiturates, rifampin. Antacids decrease kidney elimination. Increased hypotension with verapamil. Increased clotting time with warfarin.

Side Effects

Nervous System: arrhythmias—atrial flutter/bradycardia/heart block*/QRS widening/ventricular arrhythmias,* bowel—diarrhea, CHF, hearing changes, hypotension, nausea/vomiting, psyche—apprehension/delirium, respiratory depression,* syncope with loss of consciousness, tremors, vascular collapse,* vertigo, vision changes.

Endocrine System: (Pregnancy Category C) fever, hypokalemia.

Immune System: agranulocytosis,* angioedema,* hemolytic anemia,* hypoprothrombinemia, leukopenia, liver dysfunction, rash, SLE, thrombocytopenia.

Dosage: Ectopic beats: quinidine sulfate PO 200–300 mg tid or qid. Ventricular arrhythmias: PO 400–600 mg q2–3h until arrhythmia ceases; then 200–300 mg tid or qid. Atrial flutter: PO 200 mg q2–3h × 5–8 doses until NSR restored or toxicity occurs to a max of 3–4 g; then 200–300 mg tid or qid. Quinidine gluconate: Tachycardia: PO 324 mg 1–2 tab q8–12h. IM 600 mg; then 400 mg q2h prn. IV 200–750 mg at 16 mg/min. Quinidine polygalacturonate [Cardioquin]: 275–825 mg q3–4h for 4 or more doses until arrhythmia terminates; then 137.5–275 mg bid or tid.

► ANESTHETICS THAT PREVENT SODIUM INFLUX: THE LOCAL ANESTHETICS

Earlier in this chapter, lidocaine was described for its antiarrhythmic qualities. Lidocaine is also a local anesthetic. Both amide and ester forms of local anesthetics elevate the threshold of electric excitation of the nerve by entering open, inactive sodium channels. The anesthetic closes the channel, blocking sodium influx, delaying the impulse, decreasing the action potential, and, finally, blocking conduction (Dripps, 1997). The membrane is stabilized at resting potential. Local anesthetics are often used as spinal anesthesia and are in-

* Life-threatening side effect.

jected into the subarachnoid space where they affect spinal nerve roots, the dorsal root ganglia, and the periphery of the spinal cord. Spinal anesthesia is used for operations of the lower abdomen. Spinal anesthesia provides hypotension, which decreases bleeding, relaxes muscle, and causes quiet respirations. Side effects include headache, which is not necessarily prevented by "keeping the patient supine in bed after lumbar puncture" (Dripps, 1997). For other side effects refer to the earlier reference to lidocaine in this chapter. Duration of action ranges from 60 to 150 minutes depending on the lipid solubility of the agent used. The amide compounds, in addition to lidocaine [Xylocaine], include the following.

Bupivacaine hydrochloride [Marcaine, Sensorcaine] creates slow-onset anesthesia of long duration. It is more cardiotoxic than lidocaine because it binds to the heart's sodium channels longer than lidocaine. But because it binds to open sodium channels longer, it is 16 times more potent than lidocaine in reducing cardiac contractility (Dripps, 1997).

Drug Interactions: Increased CNS depression with other CNS depressants. Risk of CVA if hypertension is treated with isoproterenol, ergonovine if used with epinephrine. Severe or prolonged hypotension or hypertension possible if used with epinephrine.

Side Effects

Nervous System: arrhythmias—bradycardia*/fatal bradycardia during delivery*/cardiac arrest*/myocardial depression/ventricular arrhythmias,* cardiac output—decreased, convulsions,* dizziness, drowsiness, hypotension, maternal hypotension, nausea/vomiting, psyche—unusual anxiety/excitement/nervousness, respiratory arrest,* sneezing, syncope, unconsciousness, vision—blurred/double/pupillary constriction. (Associated with epidural anesthesia: bladder—retention, bowel—incontinence, loss of perineal sensation/sexual function, paresthesia persistent analgesia.)

Endocrine System: (Pregnancy Category C) chills, crosses placenta, diaphoresis, hyperthermia, labor—slowed/increased incidence of forceps/cranial nerve palsies [with inadvertent intrathecal injection] sweating.

Immune System: anaphylactoid reactions,* anaphylaxis,* angioneurotic edema* (including laryngeal edema), cutaneous lesions, sneezing, tinnitus, urticaria. Injection site: inflammation, sepsis.

Dosage: IM, local, sympathetic: 0.25% solution. Lumbar epidural: 0.25, 0.5, 0.75% solutions. Caudal, peripheral

---

* Life-threatening side effect.

nerve block: 0.25% solution. Retrobulbar block: 0.75% solution.

Dibucaine hydrochloride [Nupercaine, Percaine, Cinchocaine] is used to relieve the pain and discomfort of anorectal disorder, minor insect bites, minor burns, cuts, and scratches. It is not to be used on the eyes.

Drug Interactions: None noted.

Side Effects

Nervous System: none noted.

Endocrine System: (Pregnancy Category C) none noted.

Immune System: contact dermatitis, irritation, rectal bleeding with suppository.

Dosage: Topical 0.5% cream or 1% ointment to a maximum of 1 oz/24 h. Rectal suppository 1% am and hs and after bowel movement.

Etidocaine hydrochloride [Duranest] is a newer drug, similar to lidocaine.

Drug Interactions: None noted.

Side Effects

Nervous System: arrhythmias, cardiac arrest,* backache, convulsions*—followed by drowsiness/unconsciousness/respiratory arrest,* edema, fetal bradycardia during delivery,* headache, maternal hypotension, myocardial depression,* nausea/vomiting, psyche—anxiety/excitement/nervousness, vision—blurred/pupillary constriction.

Endocrine System: (Pregnancy Category B) none noted.

Immune System: anaphylactoid reactions,* anaphylaxis,* skin rash, tinnitus. Injection site: inflammation and pain.

Dosage: Percutaneous: 0.5% solution. Caudal, peripheral nerve block: 0.5–1% solution. Central neural block: 0.5 or 1.5% solution. Maximum single dose: 300 mg. Maximum single dose with epinephrine: 400 mg.

► **ESTER COMPOUNDS**

The ester compounds are local anesthetics that include the original compound, cocaine, and procaine hydrochloride [Novocain], which is scarcely used today because of allergic responses and short duration of action.

Benzocaine [Americaine, Anbesol, Solarcaine, others] is an ethyl ester of *para*-aminobenzoic acid with a chemical structure similar to that of procaine and is used as a topical anesthetic. It is available as an aerosol, cream, gel, lotion, lozenge, ointment, and otic drops.

Drug Interactions: May antagonize action of sulfonamides.

Side Effects

Nervous System: none noted.

Endocrine System: (Pregnancy Category C) none noted.

Immune System: anaphylaxis,* local allergic reactions, methemoglobinemia in infants.

Dosage: topical in lowest effective dose for least length of time necessary.

Chloroprocaine hydrochloride [Nesacaine, Nesacaine-CE], though similar to procaine, is one of the safest compounds, and often is used in continuous epidural anesthesia, especially for labor.

Drug Interactions: None noted.

Side Effects

Nervous System: arrhythmias—various/bradycardia/cardiac arrest*/myocardial depression, convulsions*—followed by drowsiness, nausea/vomiting, paresthesia—circumoral, psyche—anxiety/nervousness, respiratory arrest,* vision—blurred or double, sedation, sneezing, tremors. With caudal/epidural: backache/headache, bladder—incontinence/retention, bowel—incontinence, labor slowed—increased incidence of forceps delivery.

Endocrine System: (Pregnancy Category C) edema.

Immune System: anaphylactoid reactions,* delayed onset of cutaneous lesions, sneezing, tinnitus. With caudal/epidural: status asthmaticus.

Dosage: Infiltration and nerve block: 1–2% solution. Maximum dose with epinephrine is 1 g; without epinephrine, 800 mg. Caudal and epidural [Nesacaine-CE]: 2–3% solution (maximum 800 mg without epinephrine and 1 g with epinephrine).

Cocaine hydrochloride, a Schedule II drug, is made from the leaves of *Erythroxylon coca*. Sigmund Freud suggested its use as a local anesthetic after he tried it and noted its numbing effect on the mucous membranes (Snyder, 1986). Systemic use causes euphoria and indifference to pain or hunger. It gives a sensation of great strength, endurance, and mental capacity. The indigenous people of the Andes Mountains have used it for generations to give them endurance to carry great loads up and down steep mountains. It is also used as a tea for altitude sickness in South America. In this country it is used legally as a topical anesthetic for ENT, vaginal, and rectal procedures.

It is sometimes an ingredient in Brompton's cocktail for the pain in terminal illness.

Drug Interactions: Risk of severe hypertension and arrhythmias with epinephrine. Increased effect with MAOIs.

Side Effects

Nervous System: angina pectoris, arrhythmias—tachycardia/ventricular fibrillation,* CNS depression*—respiratory/circulatory failure, CNS stimulation, nausea/vomiting.

Endocrine System: (Pregnancy Category C) anorexia.

Immune System: cornea—clouding/pitting/ulceration, formication ("cocaine bugs"), hypersensitivity reactions, lung damage with chronic cocaine smoking, nasal septum perforation, pneumonia.

Dosage: Topical: 1–10% solution. Maximum single dose: 1 mg/kg. Use with caution if over 4% solution.

Lidocaine hydrochloride as a local anesthetic. (See this chapter for lidocaine's antiarrhythmic uses and side effects.)

Dosage: Infiltration: 0.5–1% solution. Nerve block: 1–2% solution. Epidural: 1–2% solution. Caudal: 1–1.5% solution. Spinal: 5% with glucose. Saddle block: 1.5% with glucose. Topical: 2.5–5% jelly, ointment, cream, or solution.

Pramoxine hydrochloride [Fleet Relief Anesthetic Hemorrhoidal, Prax, ProctoFoam, Tronolane, Tronothane] is a topical and mucosal anesthetic that does not depress the gag reflex. Not for use in eyes or nasal membranes.

Drug Interactions: None noted.

Side Effects

Nervous System: topical burning/stinging.

Endocrine System: (Pregnancy Category C) none noted.

Immune System: rectal bleeding.

Dosage: Topical: 1% cream or lotion q3–4h. Rectal suppository analgesic effect may last up to 5 h.

Tetracaine hydrochloride [Amethocaine, Pontocaine] is a common spinal anesthetic with high lipid solubility (making it more potent and longer-acting). It is also used for local anesthesia for ocular, nose, and throat procedures as well as for pain, itching, and burning of the skin.

Drug Interactions: None noted.

* Life-threatening side effect.

Side Effects

Nervous System: arrhythmias—various/bradycardia, convulsions,* cough reflex—prolonged depression, faintness, headache, postspinal headache, hypotension, psyche—anxiety/nervousness, spinal nerve paralysis, syncope.

Endocrine System: (Pregnancy Category C) mucous membranes—dry.

Immune System: anaphylaxis,* corneal erosion/retardation or prevention of healing of corneal abrasion, transient pitting/sloughing of corneal surface.

Dosage: Spinal: 1% solution diluted in an equal volume of 10% dextrose. Ophthalmic: 0.5% solution 1–2 gtt; 0.5% ointment 1.25 to 2.5-cm line in lower conjunctival fornix prior to procedure.† Topical: 0.5% ointment or solution to nose or throat prior to procedure.

Chapter Highlights

- Sodium flows into the neuron through its "fast channels," helping to propel the sweep of the action potential over the neuron.

- In the split second when the positive charge on the cell has become negative, the cell has been depolarized and cannot take on a new stimulus.

- In cardiac conditions, ectopic beats occurring during depolarization can cause potentially fatal arrhythmias.

- By blocking sodium influx, the antiarrhythmic drugs stabilize the myocardium.

- The local anesthetics, some of which are also used to treat arrhythmias, also block sodium channels.

---

* Life-threatening side effect.
† Eye related.

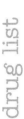

Drugs That Affect Calcium, Phosphorus, and the Completion of the Action Potential

- aminophylline (theophylline ethylenediamine) [Phyllocontin, Somophyllin, Somophyllin-DF, Truphylline]
- amlodipine [Norvasc]
- amrinone lactate [Inocor]
- dantrolene [Dantrium]
- digitoxin [Crystodigin, Purodigin]
- digoxin [Lanoxicaps, Lanoxin]
- digoxin immune-Fab [Digibind]
- diltiazem [Cardizem]
- dipyridamole [Persantine]
- erythrityl tetranitrate [Cardilate]
- ethaverine hydrochloride [Ethaquin, Ethatab, Ethavex-100, Isovex]
- felodipine [Plendil]
- hydralazine hydrochloride [Apresoline]
- isosorbide dinitrate [Isordil, Sorbitrate]
- isradipine [DynaCirc]
- milrinone lactate [Primacor]
- minoxidil [Loniten, Rogaine]
- nicardipine hydrochloride [Cardene, Cardene SR]
- nifedipine [Adalat, Adalat CC, Procardia, Procardia XL]
- nimodipine [Nimotop]
- nitroglycerin [Deponit, Minitran, Nitro-Bid, Nitro-Bid IV, Nitrocap, Nitrodisc, Nitro-Dur, Nitrogard, Nitrogard-SR, Nitroglyn, Nitrol, Nitrolingual, Nitrong, Nitrong SR, Nitrospan, Nitrostat, Nitrostat IV, Nitro-TD, Transderm-Nitro, Tridil]
- nitroprusside, sodium [Nipride, Nitropress]
- oxtriphylline [Choledyl, Choledyl-SA, Choline Theophyllinate]
- papaverine hydrochloride [Cerespan, Genabid, Pavabid, Pavased, Pavatym, Paverolan]
- pentaerythritol tetranitrate [Peritrate]
- quinine sulfate [Quinamm, Quiphile]
- sildenafil citrate [Viagra]

- theophylline [Bronkodyl, Elixophyllin, Lanophyllin, Quibron-T, Respbid, Slo-Bid, Slo-Phyllin, Somophyllin, Theo-24, Theo-Dur, Theolair, Theospan-SR, Uni-Dur, Uniphyl]
- theophylline sodium glycinate [Synophylate]
- verapamil hydrochloride [Isoptin, Calan]

No thought, feeling, or muscle movement can occur without calcium. The exchange of sodium, chloride, and potassium through their specific channels depolarizes the cell membrane and creates the action potential. As this electrochemical impulse sweeps over the neuron and reaches the end of the axons, calcium enters the neuron and pushes the neurotransmitter storage vesicles to the cell membrane, where they open up and their contents flood into the synapse or neuromuscular junction, helping to further propel the action potential to its final task (Fig. 2–1).

In muscle cells calcium is stored just under the cell membrane. Here, when the action potential stimulates the cell membrane, calcium channels open and calcium goes deeper into the cell. In the fibrils and sarcoplasm, rich in potassium, magnesium, phosphate, enzymes, and mitochondria, calcium binds with troponin, causing muscle contraction. In the heart muscle cells, calcium creates greater muscle contractility (inotropic) and enhanced current for chronotropic response. Drugs that enhance or interfere with calcium are used to treat disorders of cardiac muscle, vascular muscle, and skeletal muscles.

Phosphorus plays a role with calcium in muscle action. In smooth muscle, phosphorus decreases calcium's ability to bind with troponin in the cell. As a result the muscle cells relax. In heart muscle cells, however, phosphorus increases calcium binding with troponin and increases cell contractility.

▶ DRUGS USED TO TREAT ANGINA AND HYPERTENSION

Angina, a paroxysmal thoracic pain that most commonly comes on with exertion, the result of a decreased oxygen supply to cardiac muscle, may be relieved by drugs that dilate the coronary arteries. The Prinzmetal form occurs at rest and may be caused by coronary artery spasms without vessel blockage. The treatment goal for angina is to decrease the heart's workload, thus decreasing its need for oxygen. Blocking the action of calcium in arterial muscles decreases contractility, which both lowers blood pressure and reduces the work of the heart when it pumps against less resistance as blood is pooled elsewhere and less volume is pumped.

CALCIUM CHANNEL BLOCKERS

Calcium channel blockers block calcium's entry specifically into the muscles lining the artery walls. The search for calcium channel blockers was spurred by the need for a drug that did not metabolize as rapidly as the nitrates. The calcium channel blockers decrease blood pressure by relaxing vascular muscles. They relieve angina and are being used more often instead of digitalis for CHF. Calcium blockers can be used in combination with the nitrates and beta blockers to relieve angina; however, when combined they can cause CHF.

Amlodipine [Norvasc] is used to treat mild to moderate hypertension and angina.

Drug Interactions: Possible bradycardia with adenosine.

Side Effects

Nervous System: arrhythmias—bradycardia/tachycardia, arthralgia, bladder—frequency/nocturia, bowel—constipation/diarrhea, dyspepsia, dysphagia, dyspnea, fatigue, flatulence, headache, hypotension—postural, lightheadedness, myalgia, nausea/vomiting, pain—abdominal/chest, palpitations, sexual dysfunction, syncope.

Endocrine System: (Pregnancy Category C) anorexia, edema—facial/peripheral flushing.

Immune System: rash.

Dosage: PO 5–10 mg qd.

Diltiazem [Cardizem] is used to treat angina (especially Prinzmetal's) and hypertension. Both diltiazem and verapamil affect the SA and AV nodes and can slow conduction.

Drug Interactions: Possible intoxication if used with digitalis.

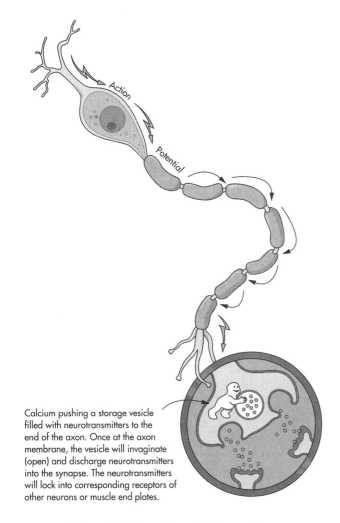

Calcium pushing a storage vesicle filled with neurotransmitters to the end of the axon. Once at the axon membrane, the vesicle will invaginate (open) and discharge neurotransmitters into the synapse. The neurotransmitters will lock into corresponding receptors of other neurons or muscle end plates.

Figure 2-1. The action potential: completion.

Side Effects

Nervous System: angina, arrhythmias—second-/third-degree AV block/bradycardia, asthenia, bowel—constipation/diarrhea, dizziness, drowsiness, fatigue, gait abnormalities, headache, hypotension, nausea/vomiting, palpitations, psyche—confusion/insomnia/nervousness, syncope, taste impairment, tremor.

Endocrine System: (Pregnancy Category C) anorexia, edema, flushing, weight increase.

Immune System: rash.

Dosage: Angina: PO 30 mg qid to a maximum of 360 mg/d. Hypertension: 60–120 mg SR bid. Atrial fibrillation: IV 0.25 mg/kg IV bolus over 2 min; if poor response, may repeat in 15 min with 0.35 mg/kg, followed by a continuous infusion of 5–10 mg/h to a maximum of 15 mg/h for 24 h.

Felodipine [Plendil], like the other calcium channel blockers, is selective for vascular muscle calcium channels.

By relaxing arterial muscle it relieves mild to moderate hypertension.

Off Label: Also used to treat angina, CHF, severe hypertension, pulmonary hypertension.

Drug Interactions: Carbamazepine, phenobarbital, phenytoin may lower bioavailability and serum concentrations. Cimetidine may increase bioavailability.

Side Effects

Nervous System: arrhythmias—bradycardia/tachycardia, bowel—diarrhea/flatulence, dizziness, dyspepsia, fatigue, headache, nausea, palpitations.

Endocrine System: (Pregnancy Category C) edema—peripheral, flushing.

Immune System: slight decrease—Hct/Hb/RBC count.

Dosage: PO 5–10 mg qd to a maximum of 20 mg/d.

Isradipine [DynaCirc] is used to treat mild to moderate hypertension.

Off Label: Angina, CHF.

Drug Interactions: It may prolong bradycardia with adenosine and increase cyclosporine levels and toxicity.

Side Effects

Nervous System: abdominal discomfort, arrhythmias—tachycardia, bowel—constipation, CHF, dizziness, dyspnea, fainting, fatigue, headache, hypotension, nausea/vomiting, pain—chest, palpitations, psyche—sleep disturbances, skin—decreased sensation, vertigo.

Endocrine System: (Pregnancy Category C) edema—ankle, flushing.

Immune System: increased liver enzymes, rash.

Dosage: Hypertension: PO 1.25–10 mg bid to a maximum of 20 mg/d. Angina: PO 2.5–7.5 mg tid to a maximum of 15 mg/d.

Nicardipine hydrochloride [Cardene, Cardene SR] is used to treat both angina (effort-associated, chronic, stable) and hypertension, and is more selective to cells in vascular smooth muscle than those of cardiac muscle. It is sometimes used in combination with nitroglycerine or beta blockers.

Drug Interactions: Plasma levels increased by cimetidine. Increases cyclosporine levels.

Side Effects

Nervous System: angina—increased, arrhythmias—tachycardia, arthralgia, bowel—constipation/diarrhea, dizziness, drowsiness, dyspepsia, fatigue, headache, hypotension, nausea/vomiting, palpitations, psyche—

anxiety/depression/insomnia/nervousness, paresthesias.

Endocrine System: (Pregnancy Category C) anorexia, dry mouth, edema—pedal, flushing.

Immune System: arthritis, pruritus, rash.

Dosage: Angina/hypertension: PO 20–40 mg tid. Begin with 20 mg tid. SR 30–60 mg bid. IV: In a drug-free patient start with 5 mg/h; increase by 2.5 mg/h q15 min or faster to a maximum of 15 mg/h. Severe hypertension: 4–7.5 mg/h. Postop hypertension: Start with 10–15 mg/h; then 1–3 mg/h (25 mg in 250 mL D5W or NS—0.1 mg/mL for continuous IV infusion).

Nifedipine [Adalat, Adalat CC, Procardia, Procardia XL] is especially effective with Prinzmetal's and severe or malignant hypertension and angina. In addition, it does not have the same SA and AV node effect as verapamil and diltiazem. It has a noticeable dilating effect on cerebral vessels.

Drug Interactions: Increased risk of CHF with beta blockers. Increased risk of phenytoin toxicity.

Side Effects

Nervous System: arrhythmias—tachycardia, balance difficulty, bowel—constipation/diarrhea/flatulence, cough, cramps, dizziness, drowsiness, dyspepsia, headache, hypotension, insomnia, lightheadedness, nausea/vomiting, palpitations, psyche—mood changes/nervousness, sexual difficulties, vision—blurred, weakness, wheezing.

Endocrine System: (Pregnancy Category C) edema—peripheral, fever, flushing, heat sensation, sweating.

Immune System: gingival hyperplasia, inflammation, MI,* nasal congestion, sore throat, urticaria, wheezing.

Dosage: PO. Angina: 10–20 mg tid to a maximum of 180 mg/d. Hypertension: 10–20 mg tid–qid to a maximum of 180 mg/d. SR 30–90 mg qd to a maximum of 180 mg/d. It can also be cut open and squirted sublingually for prompt action in acute hypertension. Hypertensive emergency: PO 10–20 mg q20–30 min if necessary.

Nimodipine [Nimotop] is oil soluble, making it useful for cerebral artery spasms.

Drug Interactions: Increased hypotension with other calcium channel blockers.

Side Effects

Nervous System: headache, hypotension.

Endocrine System: (Pregnancy Category C) none noted.

Immune System: hemorrhage—GI, liver function tests—slight transient rise.

Dosage: PO 60 mg q4h for 21 d. Start within 96 h of subarachnoid hemorrhage.

Verapamil hydrochloride [Isoptin, Calan], a papaverine derivative, does not affect blood calcium levels. It is used to treat angina, hypertension (especially malignant), and supraventricular arrhythmias. It is now the drug of choice for PAT, and is also used to treat atrial fibrillation and flutter.

Drug Interactions: arrhythmias—bradycardia, heart block, hypotension, and edema with concurrent use of beta blockers. Quinidine and digoxin levels can increase 50–70% if used with verapamil.

Side Effects

Nervous System: arrhythmias—AV block*/bradycardia/ventricular tachycardia,* CHF, constipation, discomfort, dizziness, edema—peripheral/pulmonary, fatigue, headache, hypotension, insomnia, nausea, psyche—depression/insomnia, syncope, vertigo.

Endocrine System: (Pregnancy Category C) edema, flushing, sweating.

Immune System: liver enzymes—elevated, pruritus.

Dosage: Angina: PO 80 mg q6–8h; may increase up to 320–480 mg/d in divided doses. Hypertension: PO 40–80 mg tid or 90–240 mg SR 1–2 times/d up to 480 mg/d. Supraventricular tachycardia, atrial fibrillation: PO 240–480 mg/d in divided doses. IV 5–10 mg push; repeat in 15–30 min if needed.

OTHER CARDIOVASCULAR DRUGS THAT BLOCK CALCIUM

Although the following drugs do have an effect on calcium in arterial walls, they are not specific to the calcium channels of only vascular muscle. Thus, some of them may be used for treatment of other muscular disorders.

Ethaverine hydrochloride [Ethaquin, Ethatab, Ethavex-100, Isovex], an opium derivative, is used to treat peripheral and cerebral vascular insufficiency associated with arterial spasm and spastic conditions of the GI and GU tracts.

Drug Interactions: May decrease effect of levodopa. Morphine is a possible antagonist.

Side Effects

Nervous System: abdominal distress, arrhythmias, drowsiness, fatigue, headache, hypotension, lassitude, malaise, nausea, respiratory depression,* vertigo.

---

* Life-threatening side effect.

Endocrine System: (Pregnancy Category C) anorexia, flushing, sweating, dry throat.

Immune System: anemia, anaphylaxis,* angioedema, leukopenia, rash, thrombocytopenia.

Dosage: PO 100–200 mg tid.

Hydralazine hydrochloride [Apresoline] dilates arteries by interfering with calcium's movement in vascular muscle so that the muscle cannot contract efficiently. Besides essential hypertension, it is used for CHF, preeclampsia, and eclampsia. Sometimes hydralazine is used in combination with nitrates in managing CHF.

Drug Interactions: Hypotension increased with beta blockers and other antihypertensive drugs.

Side Effects

Nervous System: angina, arrhythmias—tachycardia/various with overdose, arthralgia, bladder—dysuria, bowel—constipation/diarrhea/paralytic ileus, chills, cramps—muscle, dizziness, headache, lacrimation, nausea/vomiting, pain—abdominal, palpitations, paradoxical pressor response, shock with overdose,* tremors.

Endocrine System: (Pregnancy Category C) edema, fever, flushing.

Immune System: agranulocytosis,* anemia, eosinophilia, glomerulonephritis, Hct/Hb—decrease, hepatitis, jaundice, MI,* nasal congestion, rash, SLE-like syndrome.

Dosage: PO 10–50 mg qid to control BP. IM 10–50 mg q4–6h. IV 10–20 mg q4–6h.

Minoxidil [Loniten, Rogaine] is sometimes used for resistive hypertension, as well as for bilateral nephrectomy candidates. This drug impedes calcium's passage through the cell membrane and relaxes arterial muscles, but has an adrenergic action of speeding up the heart. It is used with both a beta blocker and a diuretic. Minoxidil's most famous use is for treating alopecia.

Drug Interactions: Excessive cardiac stimulation with epinephrine and norepinephrine. Orthostatic hypotension with guanethidine.

Side Effects

Nervous System: angina, arrhythmias—tachycardia, CHF, ECG changes, edema and pulmonary edema, fatigue, rebound hypertension,

Endocrine System: (Pregnancy Category C) edema—salt/water retention, flushing.

Immune System: rash, Stevens–Johnson syndrome; topical: dermatitis.

Dosage: PO start with 5 mg qd; if needed, increase q3d to 10, 20, and then 40 mg qd or divided doses to a maximum of 100 mg/d. Baldness: 2% solution 1 mL bid; therapeutic value is lost if the treatment is discontinued.

Nitroprusside, sodium [Nipride, Nitropress] interferes with both calcium's entry into the vascular smooth muscle cell and its usual activity within the cell, which would ordinarily result in muscle cell contraction. Nitroprusside is used for acute MI and CHF when diuretics and nitrates fail. It is the drug of choice in hypertensive crisis because of its brief immediate action as it dilates arteriolar and venous beds and relieves pre- and postload on the heart. This drug requires constant BP monitoring. Nitroprusside metabolizes to cyanide. Because it is chemically unstable, it must be shielded from light and discarded after 4 hours or if discolored.

Drug Interactions: none reported.

Side Effects

Nervous System: arrhythmias—bradycardia/tachycardia, dizziness, ECG changes, headache, nausea/retching, pain—abdominal, palpitations, psyche—apprehension/restlessness, pulse changes, retrosternal discomfort, twitching. Overdose or >48 h: disorientation, fatigue, heart sounds—faint, hypotension—profound, loss of consciousness,* muscle spasms, nausea/vomiting, psychosis, reflexes—absent, vision—blurred.

Endocrine System: (Pregnancy Category C) plasma cobalamins—rise/fall, serum creatinine—increase, sweating. Overdose or >48 h: metabolic acidosis.

Immune System: Overdose or >48 h: toxicity.

Dosage: Hypertensive crisis. IV: dilute 50 mg in 250–500 mL D5W and titrate to BP, 0.5–10 μg/kg/min (average 3 μg/kg/min).

Papaverine hydrochloride [Cerespan, Genabid, Pavabid, Pavased, Pavatym, Paverolan], an opium derivative with no narcotic action, acts on cerebral, coronary, peripheral, and pulmonary arteries. In the myocardium it slows conduction, decreases irritability, and prolongs refractory period. It also stimulates respiration and relaxes smooth muscles.

Drug Interactions: May decrease levodopa effectiveness and antagonize morphine.

Side Effects

Nervous System: arrhythmias—paroxysmal tachycardia/transient ventricular ectopic rhythms, BP—slight rise, bowel—constipation/diarrhea, dizziness, drowsiness, headache, nausea, respiration—increased depth. Rapid IV: apnea,* arrhythmias, AV block,* priapism, respiratory depression.* Overdose: coma,* diplopia,

---

* Life-threatening side effect.

drowsiness, respiratory depression,* vision—nystagmus, weakness.

Endocrine System: (Pregnancy Category C) anorexia, dry mouth/throat, flushing, sweating.

Immune System: eosinophilia, hepatotoxicity,* jaundice liver function tests—abnormal.

Dosage: PO for cerebral and peripheral ischemia 100–300 mg 3–5×/d; 150 mg SR q8–12h. IM/IV 30–120 mg q3h prn.

▶ DRUGS USED TO TREAT MUSCLE SPASMS BY INTERFERING WITH CALCIUM

The sweep of the action potential over a neuron ends with the influx of calcium ions through their channels at the axon. The calcium causes storage vesicles of acetylcholine to fuse with the cell membrane of the neuron and rupture, releasing acetylcholine into the synapse. The acetylcholine propels the action potential across the synapse to the target muscle. Calcium stored in the sarcoplasmic reticulum that wraps around bundles of myofibrils is then released into those muscle fibers, causing the muscle to contract. Drugs that prevent calcium's release from storage in the sarcoplasmic reticulum are used to prevent spasticity.

Dantrolene [Dantrium] blocks the passage of calcium from its storage place in the muscle cell's sarcoplasmic reticulum into the cell, where it can cause muscle contraction. Dantrolene is a risky drug of last resort for unyielding spasticity; it is also used for the muscle rigidity of malignant hyperthermia, the result of exposure to certain anesthetics. The drug is also used to treat the spasticity of multiple sclerosis. Dantrolene is potentially fatal in the presence of liver disease.

Drug Interactions: Increased risk of ventricular fibrillation and cardiovascular collapse with IV dantrolene. CNS depression increased with other CNS depressants. Increased risk of liver toxicity with estrogens.

Side Effects

Nervous System: arrhythmias—tachycardia, BP—erratic, bladder—burning/enuresis/frequency/nocturia/retention, bowel—constipation/diarrhea (severe), cramps—abdominal, dizziness, drowsiness, dysphagia, erection difficulties, extreme fatigue, headache, insomnia, lightheadedness, nausea/vomiting, psyche—confusion/depression/euphoria/nervousness, seizures, speech disturbances, taste changes, vision—blurred/diplopia/ photophobia, weakness.

---

* Life-threatening side effect.

Endocrine System: (Pregnancy Category C) anorexia, crystalluria.

Immune System: eosinophilic pleural effusion, GI bleeding, hepatic necrosis,* hepatitis, hepatomegaly, jaundice, pericarditis,* photosensitivity, rash.

Dosage: PO. Antispasmodic: 25 mg bid to qid; increase every 4–7 d to a maximum of 100 mg bid or qid. Malignant hyperthermia: IV 4–8 mg/kg tid or qid for 1–2 d prior to surgery; last dose 3–4 hours preop; continue PO 1–2 mg/kg qid after surgery for 1–3 d to prevent relapse; if a crisis occurs during surgery, discontinue anesthesia, and give IV 1 mg/kg rapidly to relieve the crisis or to the maximum dose of 10 mg/kg.

Quinine sulfate [Quinamm, Quiphile], the classic antimalarial drug, also blocks the passage of calcium. It has a curare-like action on motor end plates, making it useful in relieving night leg cramps.

Drug Interactions: Raises digoxin serum levels. Potentiates warfarin. Cholinergic agents may antagonize cardiac effects. Anticholinergics increase quinine's vagolytic actions. Anticonvulsants, barbiturates, rifampin increase metabolism of quinine. Quinine's antimalarial properties are discussed in Section III.

Side Effects

Nervous System: angina, bowel—diarrhea, dizziness, headache, hearing—decreased auditory acuity/tinnitus, psyche—apprehension/confusion/delirium/excitement, vertigo, vision—impairment. Toxicity: arrhythmias—tachycardia, cardiovascular collapse,* decrease in BP/respiration, coma,* convulsions.*

Endocrine System: (Pregnancy Category X) fever, flushing. Toxicity: hypothermia.

Immune System: agranulocytosis,* hemolytic anemia, hypoprothrombinemia, leukopenia, pruritus, thrombocytopenia. Toxicity: blackwater fever, ie, intravascular hemolysis with renal failure,* death.*

Dosage: PO for nocturnal leg cramps 1 tab hs or 1 tab ac and hs (supplied as 200, 260, 300, 360 mg per tablet).

▶ DRUGS THAT MAKE MORE CALCIUM AVAILABLE TO THE HEART: THE CARDIAC GLYCOSIDES

Although many drugs described in this chapter block calcium's action in the cardiovascular system, the cardiac glycosides make it more available to the heart. One of the oldest cardiac drugs, **digitalis**, a folk medicine, was brewed as a tea and given for a condition known as "dropsy," what we now call edema. Because of its inotropic quality, digitalis, or foxglove, relieves edema by making the heart muscle contract more powerfully as more calcium enters cardiac muscle cells. With improved circulation, blood is less likely to pool and leak its watery components into dependent parts of the body. Digitalis increases AV node conduction time and the refractory period, slowing the heart, a chronotropic quality. Although digitalis and its compounds are called cardiac glycosides, their action on the heart is indirect. The cardiac glycosides disperse throughout the body, binding to the potassium receptors of the potassium–sodium pumps in muscle cells. Most muscles have such pumps, but the heart has calcium–sodium pumps. Cardiac glycosides tie up sodium throughout the body and even more sodium is drawn away from its calcium–sodium pumps in the heart muscle, freeing up the calcium that would have been used in the calcium–sodium pumps to wander into cardiac muscle cells, where it causes stronger contractions (Fig. 2–2). The therapeutic value of cardiac glycosides has recently been called into question; however, they are still used for CHF and CHF with atrial fibrillation, though calcium channel blockers, which relax blood vessels and take the pumping load off of the heart, are often preferred treatment. Other uses for the cardiac glycosides include atrial flutter and fibrillation and paroxysmal tachycardia.

Drug Interactions: Digitalis levels are raised by spironolactone and quinidine. Low potassium levels increase potential for toxicity. Toxicity is treated by discontinuing the drug, giving digoxin antibody fragments if necessary, and using dilantin and lidocaine for the ectopic beats.

Note: Always obtain an apical pulse before administering cardiac glycosides to monitor against intoxication. Hold the drug and notify the physician if the patient's pulse is below 60. A good practice to cultivate is to advise the physician when the apical pulse is around 60.

Digitoxin [Crystodigin, Purodigin] is the more toxic of the two forms of cardiac glycoside, because it binds more tightly to proteins. (Think of "toxin" in its name.) It comes from the "purple foxglove," the plant used as medicinal tea so long ago. Digitoxin is metabolized by the liver and excreted in bile through the gut and reabsorbed. Eventually the inactive metabolites are excreted through the kidneys.

Drug Interactions: Treatment with quinine can cause vertigo, blurred vision, deafness, tinnitus, GI upset, and skin rash. For side effects, see *digoxin.*

Dosage: Rapid digitalization initial 0.6 mg; followed by 0.4 mg, then 0.2 mg q4–6h. Slow loading 0.2 mg bid × 4 days. PO, IM, IV: 0.1–0.15 mg qd in divided doses. Maintain on 0.05–0.3 mg qd.

Digoxin [Lanoxicaps, Lanoxin] comes from *Digitalis lanata* or "woolly foxglove," and is less toxic because it binds less

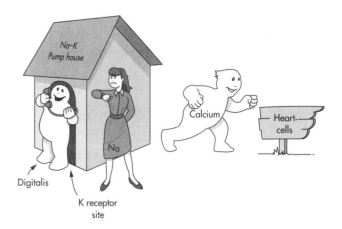

Throughout the body, digitalis ties up the sodium–potassium pumps, causing more sodium to be used in excessive numbers of pumps. Sodium is drawn away from the heart's sodium–calcium pumps, and the calcium wanders off into cardiac muscle cells.

Figure 2–2. Digitalis ties up the sodium–potassium pump.

tightly to proteins, freeing it to act faster and be excreted faster by the kidneys. Kidney function in the elderly may be impaired, and, in addition, their decreased muscle mass may put them at greater risk for toxicity.

Drug Interactions: Metabolism is speeded by anticonvulsants, antihistamines, barbiturates, oral hypoglycemics, and thyroid hormone, causing toxicity. Antacids and antidiarrheals can decrease its absorption.

Side Effects

Nervous System: arrhythmias—various/AV block,* bowel—diarrhea, dizziness, drowsiness, dysphagia, fatigue, headache, hypotension, malaise, nausea/vomiting, neuralgia—facial, paresthesias, psyche—agitation/confusion/depression/hallucinations, vision—disturbances, weakness.

Endocrine System: (Pregnancy Category A) anorexia, sweating.

Immune System: rare reactions.

Dosage: To start: PO 10–15 µg/kg in divided doses over 24–48 h. IV 10–15 µg/kg (1 mg) in divided doses. Maintain on PO/IV 0.1–0.375 mg/d. Only half the daily dose of digoxin is needed with quinidine or verapamil.

Digoxin Immune-Fab [Digibind] is the antidote for life-threatening digoxin (and sometimes digitoxin) intoxication. The drug is produced from sheep that are immunized with a digoxin–albumin conjugate. Named Fab because it consists of fragments of antidigoxin antibodies, the drug prevents digoxin or digitoxin from binding at receptor sites. It is later excreted by the

---

* Life-threatening side effect.

kidneys. The side effects include the effects of digitalis withdrawal on the heart, hypokalemia, and only rare allergy. This drug may be given in a bolus if necessary to prevent cardiac arrest.

Side Effects

Nervous System: arrhythmias, CHF, increased heart rate.

Endocrine System: (Pregnancy Category C) hypokalemia.

Immune System: rare allergic reactions (skin test with drug prior to administration).

Dosage: IV slowly over 30 min. Use 0.22-mm filter. Calibrate dosage based on serum digoxin level or amount ingested if possible, or 800 mg (20 vials).

▶ DRUGS THAT AFFECT PHOSPHORUS

Phosphorus increases calcium–troponin binding in heart muscle cells and strengthens contractions. In smooth muscle it decreases such bonding and relaxes contractility. Thus, phosphorus can both strengthen the heartbeat and relax vascular muscles.

Amrinone lactate [Inocor], an inotropic agent and a vasodilator, inhibits the enzyme phosphodiesterase, resulting in an increase in intracellular cAMP. It is used for short-term treatment of CHF when digitalis, diuretics, and vasodilators do not fully control the condition. The vasodilation it causes may result in hypotension.

Drug Interactions: Possible excessive hypotension with disopyramide.

Side Effects

Nervous System: arrhythmias, cramps—abdominal, dyspnea, hypotension, hypoxemia.

Endocrine System: (Pregnancy Category C) anorexia, hypokalemia, nephrogenic diabetes insipidus.

Immune System: ascites, jaundice, myositis, pericarditis, pleuritis, thrombocytopenia, vasculitis.

Dosage: IV 0.75 mg/kg IV bolus slowly over 2–3 min. May give a second bolus of the same dosage after 30 min. Maintain on infusion of 5–10 μg/kg/min to maximum of 10 mg/kg/d.

Dipyridamole [Persantine] is used to treat angina because it decreases coronary vascular resistance and increases blood supply and oxygen to cardiac muscle. This drug inhibits phosphodiesterase, causing it to increase platelet cAMP and making it an antiplatelet drug too. Its anticoagulant properties are discussed further in Section III because clotting is an immune system function.

Side Effects

Nervous System: abdominal distress, bowel—diarrhea, dizziness, faintness, headache, nausea/vomiting, peripheral vasodilation, syncope, weakness.

Endocrine System: (Pregnancy Category C) flushing.

Immune System: pruritus, rash.

Dosage: PO 75–400 mg/d tid or qid. IV 0.14 mg/kg/min × 4 min to a maximum of 60 mg.

Milrinone lactate [Primacor] is an inotropic/vasodilator agent used for short-term management of CHF. Like amrinone, it inhibits phosphodiesterase to increase cAMP in cardiac and smooth vascular muscle. Thus it increases myocardial contractility and vasodilation. Off label: Increases cardiac function prior to heart transplant.

Drug Interactions: Excessive hypotension with disopyramide.

Side Effects

Nervous System: angina—increased arrhythmias—increased ectopics/supraventricular arrhythmias/PVCs ventricular fibrillation*/ventricular tachycardia,* hypotension.

Endocrine System: (Pregnancy Category C) hypokalemia.

Immune System: none noted.

Dosage: IV loading dose: 50 μg/kg over 10 min; maintain on 0.375–0.75 μg/kg/min.

▶ PHOSPHORUS AND NITROGLYCERIN

Nitrates have been used for angina pectoris since the mid-1800s. They are also used in acute MI. As vasodilators they divert blood to the ischemic area after an MI. Nitrates also benefit CHF by dilating peripheral blood vessels, thus diverting or sidetracking blood. This decreases the load a heart in CHF must pump and the vessel resistance a weakened heart must pump blood out against. Dilation of blood vessels provides increased blood flow to the coronary arteries during the anginal spasms caused by oxygen deprivation. Although nitroglycerin decreases the heart's work as the blood volume drops in the dilated vessels, the heart beats faster to compensate for what seems to be a loss of blood. The increased heart rate is treated with beta blockers, and the ultimate goal of taking the load off the heart is achieved; the heart needs less oxygen. In the muscle cells of the blood vessels, nitroglycerin begins to work as sodium floods in through its channels. The nitrates activate guanylate cyclase. This increases synthesis of cGMP in smooth muscle. cGMP is similar to cAMP, another in-

---

* Life-threatening side effect.

tracellular mediator, and both may be found in the same cell, tending to different tasks.

Nitrates form reactive free radical nitric oxide, which interacts with and activates guanylate cyclase. A cGMP-dependent protein kinase is stimulated, altering phosphorylation of proteins in smooth muscle and interfering with muscle contractions. This occurs because a contraction requires the phosphorylation of specific proteins within the muscle cell. cGMP analogs can also relax vascular and bronchial smooth muscle. Nitrogen oxide-containing vasodilators and related drugs become nitric oxide and act as vasodilators.

Nitroglycerin [Deponit, Minitran, Nitro-Bid, Nitro-Bid IV, Nitrocap, Nitrodisc, Nitro-Dur, Nitrogard, Nitrogard-SR, Nitroglyn, Nitrol, Nitrolingual, Nitrong, Nitrong SR, Nitrospan, Nitrostat, Nitrostat IV, Nitro-TD, Transderm-Nitro, Tridil]

is used to treat angina by reducing preload and afterload, thereby decreasing oxygen need in the myocardium.

Sublingual tablets of nitroglycerin are used for relief of an attack in progress. The tablets are stored in air- and moisturetight, dark bottles to protect their potency. Lack of a tingle when the pill is under the tongue may signal loss of drug potency. Sublingual nitroglycerin is usually potent for about 6 months.

Although the sublingual tablets and sprays may relieve an attack in progress, topical nitrates prevent the onset of an attack. The patches are never cut in half. In some instances the patient is purposely instructed to not wear them at times to avoid building up tolerance.

Nitroglycerin is available in sublingual spray form for relief of an attack. This form does not lose potency as easily as the tablets. The spray container gives about 200 doses. The following are other sublingual tablet forms with durations of action of hours.

Angina attacks may also be prevented by giving long-acting oral nitrates; however, the long-acting forms often cause severe headaches that result in poor patient compliance. On the other hand, remembering to take the shorter-acting doses is not easy.

Note: The topical forms may cause skin allergy.

Drug Interactions: Hypotensive effects are compounded by alcohol and antihypertensive agents. IV nitroglycerin may antagonize heparin. All forms of nitroglycerin have similar side effects and are noted as follows.

Side Effects

Nervous System: angina, apprehension, arrhythmias—bradycardia/tachycardia, bladder—incontinence, bowel—incontinence, circulatory collapse,* dizziness, faintness, headache, hypotension—postural, nausea/vomiting, pain—abdominal, palpitations, psyche—

apprehension, twitching, vasodilation, vertigo, vision—blurred. (A sizzling sensation in the mouth as sublingual forms dissolve serves as an indicator that the drug has not lost potency.)

Endocrine System: (Pregnancy Category C) sweating.

Immune System: anaphylaxis,* angioedema,* methemoglobinemia, rash.

Dosage: SL 0.3–0.6 mg tablet q3–5 min prn to a maximum of 3 doses in 15 min. SL 1–2 sprays (0.4–0.8 mg). PO 1.3–9 mg q8–12h. IV start with 5 mcg/min and titrate q3–5 min until desired response attained. Transdermal apply qd for 24 h or DC for 10–12h for a nitrate-free period. Ointment apply 1.5–5 cm (½–2 in.) of ointment q4–6h.

Erythrityl tetranitrate [Cardilate] is used for prophylaxis and long-term treatment of angina. PO or sublingual 5–10 mg tid or qid to a maximum of 100 mg/d.

Isosorbide dinitrate [Isordil, Sorbitrate]

Dosage: Acute sublingual 2.5–10 mg q2–3h. Chewable 5–30 mg prn. Prophylaxis PO 2.5–30 mg qid ac and hs. SR PO 40 mg q6–12h.

Pentaerythritol tetranitrate [Peritrate]

Dosage: PO 10–40 mg q6h. Extended-release form: 30–80 mg q12h.

INTRAVENOUS NITRATES

The nitrates can also be given intravenously. This route requires monitoring the blood pressure and pulmonary capillary wedge pressure. The IV route after an MI can decrease the infarction. Intravenous nitrates not only dilate veins, but also dilate the coronary arteries, increasing flow of blood and oxygen to the heart's collateral circulation. Not only does the damaged area benefit, but the heart works against less resistance and requires less oxygen.

Dosage: IV. Start with 5 µg/min; then 5 µg/min increments q 3–5 min. If no response at 20 µg, increase increments to 10–20 µg. Reduce dosage once BP responds.

INHALANT NITROGLYCERIN

Nitroglycerin can also be inhaled as amyl nitrite.

Dosage: 0.18–0.3 mL prn.

► PHOSPHORUS AND BRONCHODILATORS

Bronchodilators are used to treat asthma, a condition of the immune system. **Asthma,** a COPD, results when mast

---

* Life-threatening side effect.

cells in the immune system explode in response to allergens and release SRSA. Muscles in the bronchial tree constrict and a thick, tenacious mucus is secreted. Bronchodilators are given to counter the bronchial muscle contraction.

Methylxanthines, like theophylline, dilate and relax the bronchi by preventing the breakdown of cAMP through inhibition of the enzyme phosphodiesterase. In addition, they relax pulmonary blood vessels, stimulate respiration, and have a diuretic effect. Blood levels must be measured for signs of methylxanthine toxicity: The most meaningful specimens are drawn 1–2 h after giving the immediate-acting drug form and 4 h after giving the SR form. The therapeutic range is 10–20 µg/mL. Toxicity can be caused by liver impairment, which increases blood levels, and by fever, a diet high in carbohydrate and low in protein, cimetidine, erythromycin, and flu vaccine.

Note: Lactating mothers should feed infants before taking the medication.

Aminophylline (theophylline ethylenediamine) [Phyllocontin, Somophyllin, Somophyllin-DF, Truphylline] is a salt of theophylline. It is used to prevent and relieve symptoms of acute bronchial asthma and to treat bronchospasm associated with chronic bronchitis and emphysema.

Off Label: Respiratory stimulant in Cheyne–Stokes respiration; for treatment of apnea and bradycardia in premature infants; as cardiac stimulant and diuretic for CHF.

Drug Interactions: Increased lithium excretion. Increased levels with cimetidine, high-dose allopurinol (600 mg/d), ciprofloxacin, erythromycin, troleandomycin possible.

Incompatibilities

Solution/Additive: amikacin, bleomycin, cephalosporins, chlorpromazine, ciprofloxacin, clindamycin, codeine phosphate, dimenhydrinate, dobutamine, dopamine, doxapram, doxorubicin, epinephrine, hydralazine, hydrazine, insulin, isoproterenol, levorphanol, meperidine, methadone, methylprednisolone, morphine, nafcillin, norepinephrine, oxytetracycline, papaverine, penicillin G, pentazocine, procaine, prochlorperazine, promazine, promethazine, tetracycline, verapamil, vitamin B complex with C.

Y-site: amiodarone, ciprofloxacin, clindamycin, codeine phosphate, dobutamine, dopamine, epinephrine, levorphanol, meperidine, methadone, morphine, norepinephrine, phenothiazines, verapamil.

---

* Life-threatening side effect.

Side Effects

Nervous System: angina, cardiac arrhythmias,* bowel—diarrhea, convulsions,* dizziness, muscle hyperactivity, nausea/vomiting, pain—epigastric, psyche—depression/irritability/insomnia. Rapid IV: cardiac arrest,* chest pain, hyperventilation hypotension—severe.

Endocrine System: (Pregnancy Category C) anorexia.

Immune System: hematemesis.

Dosage: By ideal body weight. Loading dose: IV 6 mg/kg over 30 min. Maintenance: Continuous infusion at a slow rate to prevent angina, BP drop, syncope; PO in divided doses q6h. Nonsmoker: PO/IV 0.5 mg/kg/h q6h. Smoker: IV 0.75 mg/kg/h PO 0.75 mg/kg divided q6h. With CHF or cirrhosis: PO/IV 0.25 mg/kg/h.

Oxtriphylline [Choledyl, Choledyl-SA, Choline Theophyllinate], a choline salt of theophylline, is used as a bronchodilator.

Drug Interactions: Increased lithium excretion. Increased levels with cimetidine, high-dose allopurinol (600 mg/d), ciprofloxacin, erythromycin, troleandomycin.

Side Effects

Nervous System: arrhythmias—tachycardia, bladder—transient frequency, bowel—diarrhea, convulsions,* dizziness, hypotension, muscle, nausea/vomiting, pain—epigastric, palpitations, restlessness, twitching.

Endocrine System: (Pregnancy Category C) anorexia, dehydration, fever, flushing.

Immune System: kidney irritation, peptic ulcer—activation, urticaria.

Dosage: By ideal body weight. PO 4.7 mg/kg (usual dose 200 mg) q8h (q6h for smoker).

Theophylline [Bronkodyl, Elixophyllin, Lanophyllin, Quibron-T, Respbid, Slo-Bid, Slo-Phyllin, Somophyllin, Theo-24, Theo-Dur, Theolair, Theospan-SR, Uni-Dur, Uniphyl], theophylline sodium glycinate [Synophylate], the xanthine prototype, relaxes smooth muscle in the respiratory and GI systems. It also stimulates cardiac muscle, making it useful in cardiac dyspnea and CHF edema.

Drug Interactions: Increased lithium excretion. Increased levels with cimetidine, high-dose allopurinol (600 mg/d), ciprofloxacin, erythromycin, troleandomycin possible.

Incompatibilities

Solution/Additive: amikacin, bleomycin, cephalosporins, chlorpromazine, ciprofloxacin, clindamycin, codeine phosphate, dimenhydrinate, dobutamine, dopamine, doxapram, doxorubicin, epinephrine, hydralazine, hydrazine, insulin, isoproterenol, levorphanol, meperidine, methadone, methylprednisolone, morphine, nafcillin, norepinephrine, oxytetracycline, papaverine, penicillin G, pentazocine, procaine, prochlorperazine, promazine, promethazine, tetracycline, verapamil, vitamin B complex with C.

Y-site: amiodarone, codeine phosphate, ciprofloxacin, clindamycin, phenothiazines, epinephrine, dobutamine, dopamine, levorphanol, morphine, meperidine, methadone, norepinephrine, verapamil.

Side Effects

Nervous System: angina, arrhythmias—extrasystoles/tachycardia, bladder—transient frequency, bowel—diarrhea, circulatory collapse,* dizziness, headache, hyperexcitability, marked hypotension, insomnia, irritability, nausea/vomiting, pain—epigastric or abdominal, respiratory arrest,* restlessness, drug-induced seizures.*

Endocrine System: (Pregnancy Category C) albuminuria, anorexia, dehydration, fever, possible urinary catecholamine excretion.

Immune System: kidney irritation, peptic ulcer—irritation and activation.

Dosage: By body weight. Loading dose: PO/IV 5 mg/kg. Maintenance: PO 0.4 mg/kg divided q6h or (SR q8–12h). IV 0.4 mg/kg/h continuous infusion. Maintenance for smoker: PO 0.6 mg/kg divided q6h (q8–12h SR). IV 0.6 mg/kg/h continuous infusion. CHF or cirrhosis: PO 0.2 mg/kg divided q6h (q8–12h SR) IV 0.2 mg/kg continuous infusion.

▶ A DRUG USED TO TREAT IMPOTENCE

Impotence, the inability to have an erection, can be a source of distress for men. The quest for aphrodisiacs spans centuries. Most products are of questionable value and include folk remedies. Most likely they have a placebo effect. The following drug does treat impotence. It is not an aphrodisiac and is effective only when the man is sexually aroused.

<u>Sildenafil citrate [Viagra]</u> is used to treat erectile dysfunction by enhancing the effect of nitric oxide by inhibiting phosphodiesterase, the enzyme that degrades cGMP in the corpus cavernosum. Erection occurs when sexual stimulation causes the release of nitric oxide in the corpus cavernosum. Nitric oxide activates the enzyme guanylate cyclase, and results in increased levels of cGMP. The result is smooth muscle relaxation and the inflow of blood. Sildenafil is ineffective in the absence of sexual arousal.

Drug Interactions: Increased levels with cimetidine, erythromycin, itraconazole, ketoconazole, mibefradil. Contraindicated with other organic nitrates.

Side Effects

Nervous System: angina, arrhythmias—arrest*/AV block/tachycardia, arthralgia, asthenia, ataxia, bowel—diarrhea, cough—increased, dizziness, dyspepsia, dysphagia, dyspnea, edema, headache, hearing—deafness/tinnitus, hypertonia, hyperesthesia, hypotension and postural hypotension, myalgia, myasthenia, neuralgia, palpitations, pain—abdominal/back/bone/chest/ear/eye, paresthesia, psyche—depression/abnormal dreams/insomnia/somnolence, reflexes decreased, tremor, vertigo, vision—mild and transient color tinge/mydriasis/photophobia, vomiting.

Endocrine System: (Pregnancy Category B) chills, unstable diabetes, edema and peripheral edema, flushing, gout, hyperglycemia, hypernatremia, hyperuricemia, dry mouth, sweating, thirst.

Immune System: accidental injury, allergic reaction, anemia, arthritis, asthma, bronchitis, cerebral thrombosis,* colitis, facial edema, esophagitis, gastritis, gastroenteritis, gingivitis, glossitis, herpes simplex, eye—cataract/conjunctivitis/dryness/hemorrhage, laryngitis, leukopenia, liver function tests—abnormal, myocardial ischemia,* pharyngitis, photosensitivity, sinusitis, rectal hemorrhage, skin—contact dermatitis/exfoliative dermatitis/pruritus/rash/ulcer/urticaria, sputum increase, stomatitis, tendon rupture, tenosynovitis.

Dosage: PO 50 mg as needed 1 h before sexual activity or 4–0.5 h before sexual activity. Dose may be increased to 100 mg or decreased to 25 mg based on individual need. Maximum recommended dosing frequency is once per day.

 Chapter Highlights

- Calcium is released from the synapse at the end of the passage of the action potential.

- Calcium makes muscle contraction possible.

- Calcium and phosphorus have an inverse relationship in muscle contraction.

- Drugs that affect muscle cells' use of these two elements have important uses in the treatment of cardiovascular muscle and in maintaining an airway in COPD.

---

* Life-threatening side effect.

Cholinergic and Anticholinergic Drugs

- atracurium besylate [Tracrium]
- atropine
- belladonna extract or tincture
- benztropine mesylate [Cogentin]
- bethanechol chloride [Urecholine]
- biperiden hydrochloride [Akineton]
- dexpanthenol (pantothenic acid) [Ilopan]
- diphenhydramine hydrochloride [Benadryl, others]
- donepezil [Aricept]
- echothiophate iodide [Phospholine Iodide]
- edrophonium chloride [Tensilon]
- hyoscyamine sulfate [Anaspaz]
- methscopolamine bromide [Pamine]
- meclizine hydrochloride [Bonine, Antivert, others]
- neostigmine bromide, neostigmine methylsulfate [Prostigmin]
- oxybutynin chloride [Ditropan]
- pancuronium bromide [Pavulon]
- physostigmine salicylate [Antilirium, Isopto Eserine]
- physostigmine sulfate [Eserine Sulfate]
- pilocarpine [Salagen]
- pilocarpine hydrochloride [Akarpine, Isoptocarpine]
- pilocarpine nitrate [PV Carpine Liquifilm]
- pilocarpine ocular therapeutic system [Ocusert Pilo-20 and -40]
- pralidoxime chloride [Protopam Chloride, PAM]
- procyclidine hydrochloride [Kenadrin]
- propantheline bromide [Pro-Banthine]
- pyridostigmine bromide [Mestinon, Regonol]
- scopolamine
- succinylcholine chloride [Anectine]
- tacrine [Cognex]
- trihexyphenidyl hydrochloride [Artane]
- tubocurarine chloride
- vecuronium [Norcuron]

Drugs that oppose or block acetylcholine are called anticholinergic. Drugs that increase or imitate acetylcholine are called cholinergic, cholinomimetic, or parasympathomimetic. In contrast to the sympathetic nervous system, which uses many neurotransmitters, the parasympathetic nervous system uses only one neurotransmitter, acetylcholine; however, acetylcholine singlehandedly makes possible a vast array of functions from dreaming to digestion (Fig. 3–1). The parasympathetic nervous system takes care of routine matters when all is quiet. It makes digestive juices flow (think of salivating in response to food), moves and empties the gastrointestinal tract, empties the bladder, constricts the pupils, and makes the heart beat slowly. Acetylcholine also cools the heated body with sweat, even when perspiration is the result of fight or flight, which are under the control of the sympathetic nervous system (Fig. 3–2).

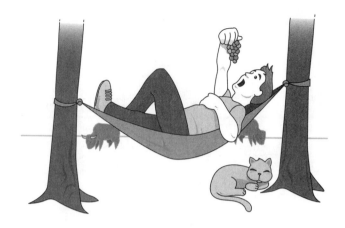

It's the caretaker system in charge when all is quiet. It makes the GI tract move, the bladder empty, the pupils constrict (the better to see our food), the digestive juices flow (think of saliva), and the heart beat slowly.

Figure 3–2. The parasympathetic nervous system is for grazing.

▶ ACETYLCHOLINE AND THE GANGLIA

A **ganglion** might be described as a neuronal switching station for nerves as they leave the spinal cord. Emerg-

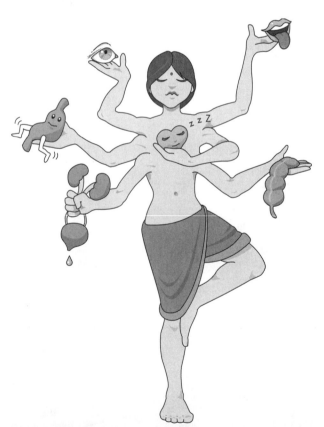

Acetylcholine is the neurotransmitter of the parasympathetic nervous system. It is referred to as cholinergic.

Figure 3–1. Acetylcholine has many functions.

ing from the cord, preganglionic neurons are cholinergic in both the parasympathetic and sympathetic nervous systems. Thus, cholinergic and anticholinergic drugs have the potential to activate or block both the sympathetic and parasympathetic systems. The result can be side effects far beyond the organ targeted for therapeutic intervention.

▶ ACETYLCHOLINESTERASE

Unlike the sympathetic nervous system, which can recycle its neurotransmitters through both enzyme activity and a reuptake process, the parasympathetic nervous system has no reuptake ability for recycling acetylcholine. Instead, using the enzyme acetylcholinesterase, it takes apart acetylcholine once its job is done in the synapse. Thus, there are no drugs to block the reuptake of acetylcholine.

▶ NICOTINIC AND MUSCARINIC RECEPTORS

Though the parasympathetic nervous system uses only the one neurotransmitter, acetylcholine, it has two types of receptors for acetylcholine, muscarinic and nicotinic, which have slightly different shapes. *Muscarinic* means "mushroom," and mushroom poisoning involves these receptors. **Muscarinic receptors** are found in all effector cells stimulated by postganglionic neurons of the parasympathetic system, including the receptors that control potassium channels in heart cells. The ancient drug atropine, other belladonna derivatives, and scopolamine block muscarinic receptors.

Nicotinic receptors, found in synapses between *both* the pre- and postganglionic neurons of *both* parasympathetic and sympathetic neuromuscular junctions, respond to nicotine. Nicotinic receptors can be blocked by curare derivatives, resulting in total paralysis. Hexamethonium blocks nicotinic receptors between the spinal cord and the ganglia. Drugs that paralyze muscles are used in abdominal surgeries where muscle relaxation speeds the procedures.

▶ CHOLINERGIC DRUGS

Two drug strategies make more acetylcholine available. One is inhibition of the enzyme acetylcholinesterase, which prevents the breakdown of acetylcholine. The other is simply replacement of acetylcholine. Only synthetic acetylcholine can be used. Because acetylcholinesterase cannot break down the synthetic acetylcholine drugs as easily as it does the body's natural acetylcholine, the synthetics remain longer everywhere in the body, except the brain. The ordinarily temporary conditions treated by increasing acetylcholine include urinary retention, paralytic ileus, and the chronic diseases of myasthenia gravis, glaucoma, and Alzheimer's disease. Myasthenia gravis results from damage to or destruction of acetylcholine receptors by viral infection or an autoimmune process. Glaucoma is a group of eye diseases caused by increased intraocular pressure resulting from blocked drainage of aqueous humor from the eye. Alzheimer's disease is a progressive destruction of neurons that first manifests as memory loss.

Because insects also have nervous systems that use acetylcholine, infestations of lice and scabies are treated with insecticides that contain cholinergic agents.

DRUGS THAT REPLENISH ACETYLCHOLINE DEFICIENCIES

The following drugs increase acetylcholine levels. Because they are synthetic, they are not broken down as readily as naturally occurring acetylcholine. When treating a patient with drugs that increase acetylcholine levels, it is prudent to have atropine readily available to block any acetylcholine toxicity.

<u>Bethanechol chloride [Urecholine]</u>, a synthetic acetylcholine, is used to treat unobstructed urinary retention and paralytic ileus.

Side Effects

Nervous System: arrhythmias—atrial fibrillation (hyperthyroid patient)/reflex tachycardia/transient complete heart block, belching, bladder—urgency, borborygmi, bowel—diarrhea/incontinence/urgency, cramps—abdominal, dizziness, dyspnea, headache, hypotension, malaise, nausea/vomiting, pain/pressure—substernal, vision—blurred/lacrimation/miosis.

Endocrine System: (Pregnancy Category C) flushing hypothermia.

Immune System: acute asthma.

Dosage: PO 10–50 mg bid–qid to a maximum of 120 mg/d. SC 2.5–5 mg tid or qid prn.

<u>Dexpanthenol (pantothenic acid) [Ilopan]</u>, the alcohol analog of pantothenic acid and a precursor of coenzyme A, a cofactor in making acetylcholine, is used postoperatively to prevent paralytic ileus.

Side Effects

Nervous System: bowel—diarrhea, BP—slight drop, dyspnea, nausea/vomiting.

Endocrine System: (Pregnancy Category C) none noted.

Immune System: dermatitis.

Dosage: IM 250–500 mg; repeat in 2 h; then q4–12h until danger has passed. IM 500 mg for adynamic ileus; repeat in 2 h, every 6 h prn. IV 500 mg diluted in glucose or lactated Ringer's; infuse slowly.

<u>Edrophonium chloride [Tensilon]</u>, a short-acting cholinergic agent, is used to diagnose myasthenia gravis and also to distinguish between cholinergic and myasthenia crisis, as these diseases have similar symptoms, ie, respiratory distress or failure, the first from too much acetylcholine, the latter from too little. In addition, edrophonium is an antidote for atropine, which blocks acetylcholine.

Drug Interactions: Decreased effects possible with procainamide, quinidine. Increased heart sensitivity to edrophonium with digitalis glycosides. Prolonged neuromuscular blockade possible with succinylcholine, decamethonium.

Side Effects

Nervous System: arrhythmias—bradycardia/irregular pulse, bladder—frequency/incontinence, bowel—constipation/diarrhea, bronchospasm*/laryngospasm,* convulsions,* cramps—abdominal/muscle, dysarthria, dysphagia, hypotension, nausea/vomiting, psyche—depression, vision—blurred/diplopia/lacrimation/miosis, respiratory arrest,* weakness.

Endocrine System: (Pregnancy Category C) excessive salivation, sweating.

Immune System: pulmonary edema.

Dosage: Diagnosis of myasthenia gravis: IV 2–4 mg; may repeat to a total of 10 mg if smaller dose has no effect; IM 10 mg in one dose. Evaluation of myasthenia treatment:

---

* Life-threatening side effect.

IV 1–2 mg 1 h after last PO dose of anticholinesterase medication. Curare antagonist: IV 10 mg over 30–45 s. Repeat q5–10min prn to maximum of 40 mg.

GLAUCOMA

Glaucoma has about seven different causes, any one of which results in the blocked drainage of aqueous humor from the eye. The resulting pressure on the optic nerve can cause blindness. **Parasympathomimetics** unblock drainage by constricting the pupil, opening the angle, and acting on the **ciliary body**; a muscle of visual accommodation, to release the trapped buildup of aqueous humor.

Pilocarpine hydrochloride [Akarpine, Isoptocarpine], pilocarpine nitrate [PV Carpine Liquifilm], pilocarpine ocular therapeutic system [Ocusert Pilo-20 and -40] are ophthalmic solutions applied as drops directly to the affected eye. The Ocusert unit is placed in the affected eye's cul-de-sac every week for slow release of pilocarpine.

Pilocarpine [Salagen] is the oral form used to treat dry mouth (xerostomia).

Drug Interactions: Increased effects of both pilocarpine (oral) and carbachol. Conduction disturbances possible with beta blockers. Decreased effects of anticholinergics. Decreased absorption with high-fat food.

Side Effects (with oral forms)

Nervous System: arrhythmias—tachycardia, bladder—frequency, bowel—diarrhea, bronchospasm,* cramps—abdominal, epigastric distress, nausea/vomiting, tremors, vision—blurred/ciliary spasm with browache/diminished in poor lighting/reduced acuity/lacrimation/miosis/pain when focus changes/eyelid twitching.

Endocrine System: (Pregnancy Category C) chills, salivation, sweating.

Immune System: cataract, conjunctival irritation, contact allergy, follicular conjunctivitis, retinal detachment.

Dosage: Ophthalmic.† Glaucoma: Use with a systemic carbonic anhydrase inhibitor and osmotic agent to decrease aqueous humor. [Not for use in conjunctivitis, keratitis, retinal detachment, or if intense miosis is needed.] Pilocarpine ophthalmic comes in 0.5%, 1%, 2%, 3%, 4%, and 6% strength drops. Apply to affected eye. 1 gtt of 1–2% solution q5–10min for 3–6 doses, then 1 gtt q1–3h until IOP is reduced. Chronic glaucoma: 1 gtt of 0.5–4% solution q4–12h or 1 ocular system q 7d. PO for xerostomia: 5 mg tid. May increase up to 10 mg tid.

ACETYLCHOLINESTERASE INHIBITORS

Acetylcholine is broken down by the enzyme acetylcholinesterase. Drugs that inhibit the enzyme increase available acetylcholine in conditions such as Alzheimer's disease, glaucoma, and myasthenia gravis.

Echothiophate iodide [Phospholine Iodide] is a long-acting cholinesterase inhibitor and organophosphate used in open-angle glaucoma to make more acetylcholine available to the ciliary muscle and iris sphincter muscle. It is available strengths of 0.03%, 0.06%, 0.125%, and 0.25%.

Drug Interactions: Increased systemic cholinergic effects with ambenonium, edrophonium, neostigmine, pyridostigmine. Prolonged apnea, cardiovascular collapse possible with succinylcholine.

Side Effects

Nervous System: arrhythmias—bradycardia and others, bladder—frequency/incontinence, bowel—diarrhea, cramps—abdominal, dyspnea, head/browache, nausea/vomiting, vision—blurring/dimness/lacrimation/lid twitching/spasms of accommodation/stinging.

Endocrine System: (Pregnancy Category C) salivation, sweating.

Immune System conjunctival redness/thickening, iris cysts, nasal congestion.

Dosage: Ophthalmic 1–2 gtt qd in conjunctival sac.†

Neostigmine bromide, neostigmine methylsulfate [Prostigmin] are used to treat myasthenia gravis and also to help relieve urinary retention by increasing the amount of acetylcholine available to the muscles of urination (Fig. 3–3). Overdose can be fatal.

Drug Interactions: Prolonged phase I block or reverse phase II block possible with succinylcholine decamethonium. Antagonized effects of atracurium, pancuronium, procainamide, quinidine, tubocurarine, vecuronium. Effects antagonized by atropine.

Side Effects

Nervous System: arrhythmias—bradycardia, belching, bladder—incontinence/difficulty, bowel—diarrhea, chest tightness, convulsions,* cough, cramps—muscle, dizziness, drowsiness, dyspepsia, dysphagia, dyspnea, fatigue, hyper-/hypotension, nausea/vomiting, pallor, paralysis,* psyche—agitation/fear, respiratory depression,* vision—blurred/lacrimation/miosis, twitching.

Endocrine System: (Pregnancy Category C) edema, salivation, sweating.

Immune System: secretions—bronchial.

Dosage: Diagnosis of myasthenia gravis: IM 0.022 mg/kg to maximum of 0.031 mg/kg if lower dose is inconclusive.

* Life-threatening side effect.
† Eye related.

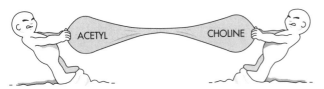

The enzyme acetylcholinesterase takes apart acetylcholine.

Drugs that inhibit this enzyme make more acetylcholine available. Physostigmine and neostigmine both inhibit the enzyme. They are used...

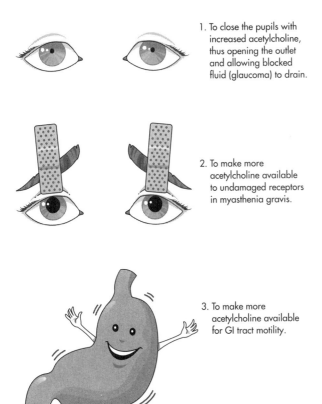

1. To close the pupils with increased acetylcholine, thus opening the outlet and allowing blocked fluid (glaucoma) to drain.

2. To make more acetylcholine available to undamaged receptors in myasthenia gravis.

3. To make more acetylcholine available for GI tract motility.

Figure 3-3. Cholinergic drugs make more acetylcholine available.

Treatment of myasthenia gravis: 15–375 mg/d in 3–6 divided doses; IM/IV 0.5–2.5 mg. Reversal of nondepolarizing neuromuscular blockade: IV 0.5–2.5 mg slowly. Urinary retention: IM 0.25 mg q4–6h for 2–3 d.

Physostigmine salicylate [Antilirium, Isopto Eserine], physostigmine sulfate [Eserine Sulfate] act as antidotes for anticholinergic overdose by inhibiting cholinesterase, thus increasing acetylcholine concentrations.

Drug Interactions: Antagonized effects of echothiophate, isoflurophate.

Side Effects

Nervous System: arrhythmias—bradycardia/irregular pulse, ataxia, bladder—incontinence, bowel—diarrhea/incontinence, bronchospasm,* cholinergic crisis,* collapse,* convulsions,* dizziness, drowsiness, dyspepsia, dysphagia, dyspnea, headache, hyper-/hypotension, nausea/vomiting, restlessness, pain—brow/epigastric/eye, psyche—hallucinations/depression/transient decrease in manic symptoms, vision—blurring/dimness/lacrimation/miosis, respiratory paralysis,* tremors, twitching, weakness.

Endocrine System: (Pregnancy Category C) salivation, sweating.

Immune System: chronic conjunctivitis, dermatitis, follicular cysts, iris—color changes, rhinorrhea.

Dosage: IM or slow IV 0.5–3 mg (1 mg/min IV). Ophthalmic ointment (physostigmine sulfate): 0.25–0.5% hs or salicylate solution 0.25% or 0.5% 1–2 gtt tid or qid.†

Pyridostigmine bromide [Mestinon, Regonol] has anticholinesterase activity to block the breakdown of acetylcholine in the treatment of myasthenia gravis.

Drug Interactions: Antagonized by atropine, nondepolarizing.

Side Effects

Nervous System: arrhythmias—bradycardia, bowel—diarrhea, bronchoconstriction,* fasciculation, hypotension, nausea/vomiting, vision—miosis, weakness.

Endocrine System: (Pregnancy Category C) salivation, sweating.

Immune System: bronchial secretions, rash, thrombophlebitis (after IV administration).

Dosage: PO 60 mg–1.5 g/d. May use SR tablets if patient needs hs dose. Maximum daily dosage: 1500 mg. IM or IV: 1/30 of PO dose.

ALZHEIMER'S DISEASE

Alzheimer's disease is manifested by a premature loss of mental abilities similar to those losses seen in extreme old age. In the brain large areas are filled with amyloid plaques. Areas affected include the cerebellum, cortex, basal ganglia, hippocampus, and thalamus. The hippocampus and thalamus are essential to memory, and one of the signs of Alzheimer's disease is profound memory loss. Though its cause is still unknown, Alzheimer's disease results in a lack of acetylcholine in the brain.

---

* Life-threatening side effect.
† Eye related.

Sometimes referred to as senile dementia, the disease eventually results in death as the neurons produce less and less acetylcholine. No cure exists, although medication can buy the patient some time in this progressive disease. In addition to a lack of acetylcholine in Alzheimer's, there is also a lack of acetylcholinesterase, the enzyme that takes acetylcholine apart, because the enzyme is stored in acetylcholine-producing nerves devastated by the disease. At this time very little can be done to treat the disease.

Donepezil [Aricept] inhibits acetylcholinesterase to make more acetylcholine available in the treatment of Alzheimer's disease. It does not appear to change the course of the disease.

Drug Interactions: Decreased levels possible with carbamazepine, dexamethasone, ketoconazole, phenobarbital, quinidine, rifampin.

Side Effects

Nervous System: arrhythmias—atrial fibrillation/bradycardia, bladder—frequency/incontinence/nocturia, bowel—bloating/diarrhea/incontinence, cramps—muscle, dyspnea, headache, hypertension, hypotension, pain—chest/epigastric/general/tooth, psyche—depression/abnormal dreams/somnolence, syncope, vision—blurred.

Endocrine System: (Pregnancy Category C) anorexia, dehydration, hot flashes, sweating, weight loss.

Immune System: arthritis, bleeding, bone fracture, bronchitis, ecchymosis, GI bleeding, influenza, pruritus, sore throat, urticaria, vision—cataract/irritation.

Dosage: PO. Start with 5 mg hs. Maximum 10 mg qh after 4–6 wk.

Tacrine [Cognex] inhibits acetylcholinesterase, slowing the breakdown of acetylcholine (ACh). As a cholinergic agent, it has systemic actions that result in a wide range of parasympathetic side effects. Toxic to the liver, it requires weekly liver function tests.

Drug Interactions: Increased levels with cimetidine. Increased levels of theophylline. Prolonged action of succinylcholine and possibly other neuromuscular blocking agents.

Side Effects

Nervous System: abdominal discomfort, ataxia, belching, bladder—frequency/incontinence with UTI, bowel—diarrhea, dizziness, drowsiness, nausea/vomiting, psyche—agitation/confusion/hallucinations/insomnia.

Endocrine System: (Pregnancy Category C) anorexia, sweating.

Immune System: hepatotoxicity, purpura, UTI.

Dosage: PO 10 mg qid between meals. Increase 40 mg/d over 6 wk to maximum of 160 mg/d.

A DRUG TO REVERSE ANTICHOLINESTERASE ACTIVITY

Pralidoxime chloride [Protopam Chloride, PAM] reactivates cholinesterase inhibited by organophosphorous insecticides, related compounds, and anticholinesterase drugs. It is effective against the nicotinic receptor symptoms of anticholinesterase compounds, that is, cramps, muscle twitching, weakness. For the muscarinic side effects of bronchoconstriction, diarrhea, and increased secretions, atropine is more effective.

Off Label: Reversal of toxicity of echothiophate ophthalmic solution.

Drug Interactions: None noted.

Side Effects

Nervous System: arrhythmias—tachycardia, dizziness, drowsiness, headache, hypertension, hyperventilation, nausea, vision—blurred/diplopia/impaired accommodation, weakness. With rapid IV: laryngospasm,* muscle rigidity, tachycardia.

Endocrine System: (Pregnancy Category C) none noted.

Immune System: none noted.

Dosage: Organophosphate poisoning: IV 1–2 g in 100 mL of saline over 15–30 min; or 1–2 g as 5% solution of sterile H_2O over not less than 5 min; repeat p̄1h; then q4–8h as poisoning persists. SC or IM in presence of pulmonary edema or when IV is not possible. Anticholinesterase overdose in myasthenia gravis: IV first dose as above, then 250 mg q5min prn. PO for mild organophosphate poisoning 1–3 g. Repeat as needed in 5 h.

Atropine, the prototype of all anticholinergic drugs, is given concurrently with pralidoxime chloride.

Dosage: IM, IV 1–2 mg q5–60min until muscarinic blockade is broken and symptoms abate.

▶ ANTICHOLINERGIC DRUGS

When acetylcholine is blocked, everyday functions are blocked. The body cannot sweat or spit. The heart speeds up. Digestion is blocked. Urinary retention and constipation set in. Anticholinergic drugs, or cholinergic blocking agents, take the parking places or receptor sites used by acetylcholine. In fatally large doses they first

---

* Life-threatening side effect.

stimulate the CNS, then depress it. Anticholinergic drugs speed the heartbeat, dilate the bronchi, and decrease respiratory tract secretions (Fig. 3–4). They decrease GI tract muscle activity, but do not affect gastric secretions. Anticholinergic drugs dilate pupils and are contraindicated in glaucoma. In addition, anticholiner-

gic drugs decrease sweat and saliva and relax the ureters, bladder, detrusor muscle, and smooth muscle in the gallbladder and bile duct. Anticholinergic drugs can prevent laryngospasm during surgery by blocking acetylcholine, the neurotransmitter responsible for the muscle spasms that constrict the airway.

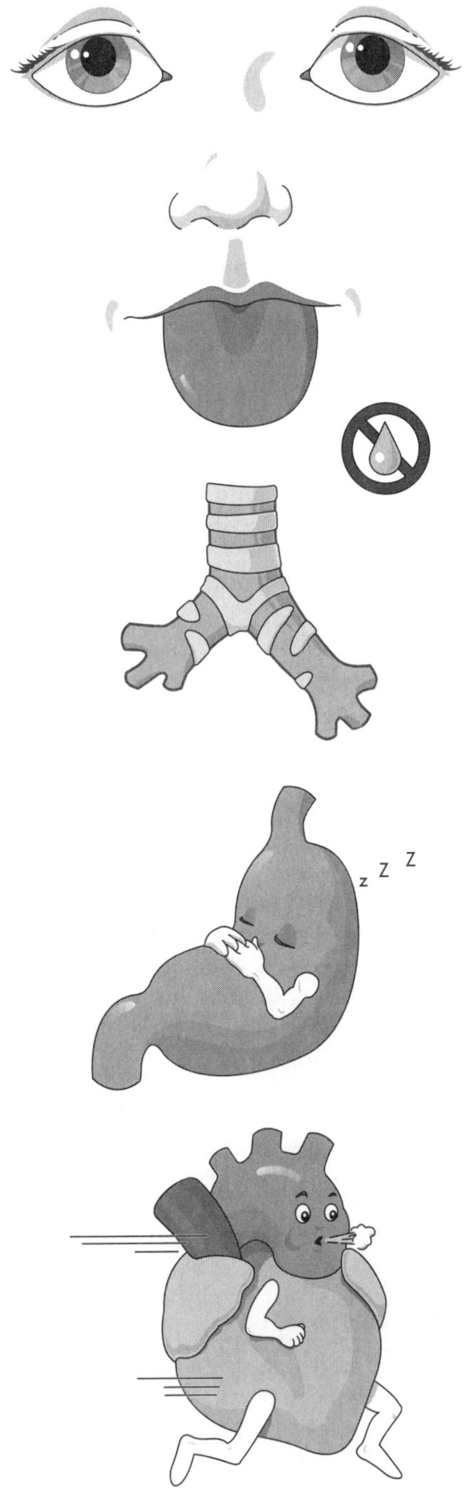

CONDITIONS TREATED WITH ANTICHOLINERGIC DRUGS

Anticholinergic drugs are used to treat GI tract spasms, bradycardia and heart block, Parkinson's and pseudo-Parkinson's (also called extrapyramidal symptoms) diseases, urinary tract spasms, and inadequate bladder capacity. They are used to dilate the pupil for eye examinations and eye surgery. Used preoperatively, anticholinergic drugs decrease secretions that might interfere with the airway and they relax the abdominal muscles. In ECT they decrease muscle contraction. Anticholinergic drugs are contraindicated in prostatic hypertrophy, glaucoma, tachyarrhythmias, MI, CHF (unless there is a bradycardia), and hiatal hernia, in which they will increase reflux.

Atropine is the classic anticholinergic drug. Atropine blocks acetylcholine receptors, most specifically the muscarinic receptors (Fig. 3–5). The oldest of the known anticholinergics, atropine serves many functions. Though water soluble, atropine crosses the BBB, where it acts as a CNS stimulant, but becomes a depressant in toxic doses. The kidneys rapidly excrete atropine. Atropine can be used to treat bradyarrhythmias, for example, sinus bradycardia and first-, second-, and third-degree heart block. Atropine tilts the balance to the sympathetic nervous system, which speeds the heartbeat, improving and increasing sinus node automaticity. It improves AV conduction. In an acute MI, atropine relieves the hypotension and PVCs. There is a danger that a speeded heartbeat may extend an infarction or ischemia. Atropine relieves bronchospasm in asthma by blocking acetylcholine as it stimulates the bronchial muscle cells to contract due to the allergic response of the immune system.

Drug Interactions: Increased anticholinergic effects with amantadine, antihistamines, disopyramide, procainamide, quinidine, tricyclic antidepressants. Decreases effects of levodopa. EPS possible with methotrimeprazine. Decreased absorption of phenothiazines increases psychotic behavior.

Side Effects

Nervous System: antral stasis, ataxia, arrhythmias—atrial fibrillation, AV dissociation/paradoxical bradycardia/ventricular fibrillation*/tachycardia, bladder—dysuria/hesitancy/retention, bowel—constipation/

1. Dilate pupils (Mydriasis)

2. Decrease secretions in eyes, mouth, nose, and airway

3. Slow the GI tract...

4. and speed up the heart.

Figure 3–4. Anticholinergic drugs.

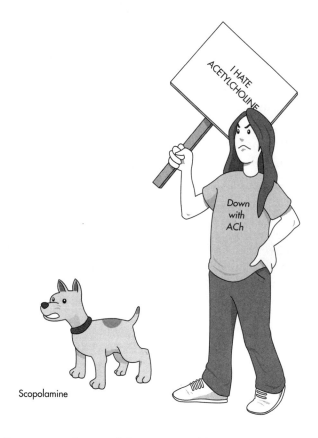

Scopolamine

This is Atropine. She is named after Atropos, one of the three Fates who spin the thread of life. Atropos was the one who cut the thread. The dog is Scopolamine. He acts much like Atropine.

Atropine blocks acetylcholine receptors. It is an anticholinergic, as is any drug that interferes with acetylcholine.

Figure 3–5. Atropine.

diarrhea/paralytic ileus, convulsions,* cramps, dizziness, drowsiness, dysphagia, fatigue, gastric emptying—slowed, headache, hyper-/hypotension, impotence, nausea/vomiting, palpitation, psyche—confusion/depression/disorientation/excitement/irritability, taste loss, vision—blurred/cycloplegia/increased intraocular pressure/mydriasis/photophobia.

Endocrine System: (Pregnancy Category C) anhidrosis, dryness—eyes/mouth/skin, flushing, thirst.

Immune System: allergic conjunctivitis, dermatitis, fixed drug eruption.

Dosage: PO/SC 0.3–1.2 mg q4–6h. Preop: IM/IV/SC 0.2–1 mg 30–60 min before anesthesia. Bronchoconstriction: 0.025 mg/kg in saline in a nebulizer tid or qid. Arrhythmias: IM/IV 0.5–1 mg; may repeat q1–2h prn to maximum of 2 mg.

Note: Maximum of no more than 2 mg cumulatively per day.)

Ophthalmic solution 0.5%, 2%, 3% strength.† Uveitis: 1–2 gtt or 0.3 cm qd–tid. Cycloplegia procedure: 1 gtt or small amount of ointment 1 h prior to procedure. Organophosphate antidote: IV/IM 1–2 mg q5–60min until muscarinic signs and symptoms subside (may need up to 50 mg). Usually given concomitantly with pralidoxime chloride, which is used to treat the nicotinic receptor symptoms.

<u>Belladonna extract or tincture</u> (a tincture contains alcohol) is used to treat spasms of the GI tract. Like atropine, belladonna is an old drug. Its name means "pretty lady"; long ago women used to put drops of belladonna into their eyes to make their pupils dilate, a sign of beauty.

Drug Interactions: Increased anticholinergic effects with amantadine, antihistamines, disopyramide, procainamide, quinidine, tricyclic antidepressants. Decreased effects of levodopa. EPS possible with methotrimeprazine. Decreased absorption of phenothiazines increases psychotic behavior.

Side Effects

Nervous System: arrhythmias—tachycardia/palpitations, bladder—retention/urgency, bowel—constipation, psyche—confusion/delirium/excitement—children/elderly, vision—blurred/mydriasis/photophobia.

Endocrine System: (Pregnancy Category C) none noted.

Immune System: none noted.

Dosage: PO extract 15–30 mg or tincture 0.6–1 mL tid–qid.

<u>Hyoscyamine sulfate [Anaspaz]</u> is a belladonna-like drug, also used for the relief of GI tract spasms.

Drug Interactions: Increased anticholinergic effects with amantadine, antihistamines, disopyramide, procainamide, quinidine, tricyclic antidepressants. Decreased effects of levodopa. EPS possible with methotrimeprazine. Decreased absorption of phenothiazines increases psychotic behavior.

Side Effects

Nervous System: arrhythmias—tachycardia, bladder—retention, bowel—constipation, drowsiness, excitement—elderly, headache, psyche—confusion, vision—blurred/cycloplegia/increased intraocular tension/mydriasis, weakness.

Endocrine System: (Pregnancy Category C) anhidrosis, lactation—suppressed.

Immune System: none reported.

Dosage: PO/SL 0.125–0.25 mg tid–qid prn. IM/SC/IV 0.25–0.5 mg q6h to control symptoms, then DC.

---

* Life-threatening side effect.

† Eye related.

Methscopolamine bromide [Pamine] is more specific for blocking vagal impulses than scopolamine or atropine; and less potent and longer-acting than atropine.

Drug Interactions: See *scopolamine*.

Side Effects

Nervous System: bladder—hesitancy/retention, bowel—constipation, dizziness, drowsiness, vision—blurred.

Endocrine: (Pregnancy Category C) dry mouth, flushing.

Immune System: allergy.

Dosage: PO 2.5–5 mg 30 min ac and hs.

Oxybutynin chloride [Ditropan], like atropine, inhibits acetylcholine on muscarinic receptors. Although it relaxes smooth muscle, it has only one-fifth the anticholinergic activity of atropine, but is up to 10 times more potent as an antispasmodic for the bladder.

Drug Interactions: None noted.

Side Effects

Nervous System: arrhythmias—tachycardia, bladder—hesitancy/retention, bloated feeling, bowel—constipation, dizziness, drowsiness, impotence, nausea/vomiting, palpitations, psyche—psychotic behavior/insomnia/restlessness, vision—blurred/cycloplegia/increased ocular tension.

Endocrine System: (Pregnancy Category C) dry mouth, fever, flushing, lactation—suppressed, sweating—decreased.

Immune System: allergy—severe, rash.

Dosage: PO 5 mg bid or tid to maximum of 20 mg/d.

Scopolamine is similar to atropine in action, but with some different central effects, eg, the sense of balance, which makes it useful as a patch for motion sickness. Given parenterally to affect the CNS, it causes drowsiness, euphoria, relaxation, amnesia, and sleep before therapeutic procedures.

Drug Interactions: Increased anticholinergic effects with amantadine, antihistamines, disopyramide, procainamide, quinidine, tricyclic antidepressants. Decreased effects of levodopa. EPS possible with methotrimeprazine. Decreased absorption of phenothiazines increases psychotic behavior.

Side Effects

Nervous System: arrhythmias—bradycardia, bladder—retention, bowel—constipation, dizziness, drowsiness, fatigue, psyche—disorientation/hallucinations/toxic psychosis, respirations—depressed,* restlessness, vision—blurred/dilated pupils/photophobia,

Endocrine System: (Pregnancy Category C) dryness—mouth/throat.

Immune System: allergy to adhesive, follicular conjunctivitis, local irritation, rash.

Dosage: Motion sickness: PO 0.25–0.6 mg 1 h before trip or 1 transdermal disk q72h starting 12 h before travel. Preop: PO 0.5–1 mg. IM/IV/SC 0.3–0.6 mg. Scopolamine ophthalmic dilates pupils (mydriasis). Dosage: 0.2–0.25% 1–2 gtt per affected eye prn up to qid.†

AN ANTICHOLINERGIC DRUG THAT DOES NOT CROSS THE BLOOD–BRAIN BARRIER

The inability of a drug to cross the BBB results in the patient being less likely to experience side effects such as confusion, convulsions, disorientation, and other CNS manifestations that can interfere with the patient's routines and safety.

Propantheline bromide [Pro-Banthine], used to treat irritable bowel and other spastic conditions of smooth muscle, has similar side effects to other anticholinergics drugs.

Drug Interactions: None noted.

Side Effects

Nervous System: bladder—dysuria, bowel—constipation, drowsiness, libido—decreased, vision—blurred/mydriasis/increased IOP.

Endocrine: (Pregnancy Category C) dry mouth.

Immune System: allergy.

Dosage: PO 15 mg tid ac and 30 mg hs to a maximum of 120 mg/d.

ANTICHOLINERGIC DRUGS THAT PARALYZE

Paralyzing drugs derived from curare, a compound the Amazon Indians discovered to paralyze prey, are used in major surgery on the abdomen to block acetylcholine and relax the abdominal muscles. When these drugs are used, the anesthesiologist must artificially "breathe" for the patient, because the respiratory muscles use acetylcholine and are also paralyzed. Skeletal neuromuscular junctions have acetylcholine receptors that are blocked by these agents, resulting in a flaccid paralysis, a condition considered desirable in abdominal surgery. These drugs help prevent bone fractures during ECT by decreasing the force of muscle contractions during the induced seizure. They are also used to make mechanical ventilation easier. Because they do block acetylcholine,

---

* Life-threatening side effect.
† Eye related.

special caution must be used with patients who have myasthenia gravis. In addition, these agents cause histamine release. They are initially administered just as the skin is incised or as the ECT treatment commences, and then only by anesthesiologists or anesthetists.

Atracurium besylate [Tracrium] causes neuromuscular blockade by competing with acetylcholine for receptors at neuromuscular junctions. It is given with general anesthesia after unconsciousness has been induced by other drugs. This timing is essential, as atracurium has no analgesic action and the paralyzed patient would be unable to signal that she or he was alert and feeling the procedure.

Drug Interactions: Increased duration and magnitude of neuromuscular blockade with general anesthetics. Increased neuromuscular blockade with aminoglycosides, bacitracin, clindamycin, lidocaine, parenteral magnesium, polymyxin B, quinidine, quinine, trimethaphan, verapamil. Increased or decreased blockade with diuretics. Prolonged blockade with lithium. Possible additive respiratory depression with narcotic analgesics. Increased onset and depth of blockade with succinylcholine. Resistance or reversal of blockade with phenytoin.

Side Effects

Nervous System: arrhythmias—bradycardia/tachycardia, respiratory depression.*

Endocrine System: (Pregnancy Category C) increased salivation.

Immune System: anaphylaxis.*

Dosage: IV bolus. Start with 0.4–0.5 mg/kg. Maintain with 0.08–0.1 mg/kg 20–45 min p̄ first if needed. Less is needed with isoflurane and enflurane (0.25–0.35 mg/kg) and halothane (0.3–0.4 mg/kg). Mechanical ventilation: IV 5–9 μg/kg/ min by continuous infusion.

Pancuronium bromide [Pavulon] is a synthetic curariform neuromuscular blocking agent that is up to five times as potent as tubocurarine. Because it produces little or no histamine release and no ganglionic blockade, it does not cause bronchospasm or hypotension. At high doses, it directly blocks acetylcholine receptors in the heart, and thus may increase heart rate, cardiac output, and arterial pressure. It is used to induce skeletal muscle relaxation during surgery and facilitate mechanical ventilation.

Drug Interactions: Increased neuromuscular blocking and duration of action with general anesthetics. Increased neuromuscular blockade with aminoglycosides, bacitracin, clindamycin, lidocaine, magnesium, polymyxin B, quinidine, quinine, trimethaphan, verapamil.

Increased/decreased neuromuscular blockade with diuretics. Prolonged duration of neuromuscular blockade with lithium. Increased respiratory depression possible with narcotic analgesics. Increased onset and depth of neuromuscular blockade with succinylcholine. Resistance or reversal of neuromuscular blockade possible with phenytoin.

Side Effects

Nervous System: arrhythmias—ventricular, extrasystoles, heart rate/BP increased, respiratory depression,* skeletal muscle weakness, vein—burning sensation.

Endocrine System (Pregnancy Category C) salivation.

Immune System: transient acneiform rash.

Dosage: IV 0.04–0.1 mg/kg initial dose. Additional doses of 0.01 mg/kg may be given at 30- to 60-min intervals.

Succinylcholine chloride [Anectine] is another paralyzing drug used during surgical procedures or ECT.

Drug Interactions: Prolonged neuromuscular blockade possible with aminoglycosides, colistin, cyclophosphamide, cyclopropane, echothiophate, halothane, iodide, lidocaine, magnesium salts, MAOIs, methotrimeprazine, narcotic analgesics, organophosphamide insecticides, phenothiazines, procaine, procainamide, propranolol, quinidine, quinine. Increased risk of arrhythmias with digitalis glycosides.

Incompatibilities

Solution/Additive: sodium bicarbonate, thiopental.

Side Effects

Nervous System: apnea,* arrhythmias—bradycardia/sinus arrest/tachycardia, bronchospasm,* GI—decreased tone/motility, hyper-/hypotension, hypoxia, muscle—fasciculations/pain/profound and prolonged relaxation, respiratory arrest,* vision—IOP.

Endocrine System: (Pregnancy Category C) hyperkalemia, malignant hyperthermia,* salivation—excessive.

Immune System: myoglobinemia, salivary glands—enlarged.

Dosage: Surgical procedures: IV 0.3–1.1 mg/kg over 10–30 s; maintain with 0.04–0.07 mg if needed. IM up to 2.5–4 mg/kg; maximum: 150 mg total. Prolonged muscle relaxation: IV 0.5–10 mg/min continuous infusion.

Tubocurarine chloride, by competing for cholinergic receptors on skeletal muscle end plates, blocks acetylcholine and causes relaxation/paralysis.

---

* Life-threatening side effect.

Side Effects

Nervous System: apnea,* arrhythmias—bradycardia/sinus arrest/tachycardia, bronchospasm,* circulatory collapse,* GI—decreased tone/motility, hypotension, hypoxia, muscle—fasciculations/pain/profound and prolonged relaxation, respiratory arrest,* vision—IOP.

Endocrine System: (Pregnancy Category C) hyperkalemia, malignant hyperthermia,* salivation—excessive.

Immune System: bronchial secretions—increased, hypersensitivity reactions.

Dosage: With anesthesia: IV 6–9 mg over 1–1.5 min; follow with 3–4.5 mg 3–5 min later, if needed. ECT: IV 0.165 mg/kg slowly. Diagnosis of myasthemia gravis: IV 0.004–0.033 mg/kg.

<u>Vecuronium [Norcuron]</u> binds to acetycholine at motor endplate receptors to relax skeletal muscle during surgery. Because it causes little histamine release, it has minimal cardiovascular action.

Drug Interactions: Increased neuromuscular blocking and duration of action with general anesthetics. Increased neuromuscular blockade with aminoglycosides, bacitracin, clindamycin, lidocaine, parenteral magnesium, polymyxin B, quinidine, quinine, trimethaphan, verapamil. Decreased neuromuscular blockade possible with diuretics. Prolonged neuromuscular blockade with lithium. Increased respiratory depression possible with narcotic analgesics. Increased onset and depth of neuromuscular blockade with succinylcholine. Resistance or reversal of neuromuscular blockade possible with phenytoin.

Side Effects

Nervous System: respiratory depression,* skeletal muscle weakness.

Endocrine System (Pregnancy Category C) malignant hyperthermia.*

Immune System: none noted.

Dosage: IV 0.04–0.1 mg/kg initially. After 25–40 min may give 0.01–0.15 mg/kg q12–15min or 0.001 mg/kg/min by continuous infusion.

ANTICHOLINERGIC ANTIEMETICS

Acetylcholine causes peristalsis, the rhythmic movements of the GI tract that keep moving nutrients through the intestinal tract; however, acetylcholine in the vomiting center reverses peristalsis or vomiting. Thus blocking acetylcholine in the center can have an antiemetic effect.

<u>Meclizine hydrochloride [Bonine, Antivert, others]</u> blocks acetylcholine in the vomiting center with its input from the chemoreceptor trigger zone, though peripheral anticholinergic effects may also help. It also has antihistamine activity.

Drug Interactions: none noted.

Side Effects

Nervous System: drowsiness, fatigue, vision—blurred.

Endocrine System: (Pregnancy Category B) dry mouth.

Immune: none noted.

Dosage: PO 25–50 mg 1 h before travel, then q24h throughout the trip. Vertigo: PO 25–100 mg daily in divided doses.

ANTICHOLINERGICS FOR PARKINSON'S DISEASE AND PSEUDO-PARKINSON'S DISEASE

Parkinson's disease is caused by a lack of dopamine, a sympathetic nervous system neurotransmitter or neurohormone in the CNS. Usually in Parkinson's the paired adrenal medullas continue production of dopamine, which is released into the bloodstream, but the dopamine molecules cannot pass the BBB. The treatment goal for Parkinson's is to increase dopamine levels in the CNS. Early in the disease anticholinergic drugs are used to block some acetylcholine and reestablish a balance, decreased though it is, between the sympathetic and parasympathetic systems.

By blocking the action of acetylcholine, these drugs slow gastric emptying. (If a patient is also on levodopa, the levodopa sits in the stomach longer, degrading and making less dopamine available.) Of course, anticholinergic drugs also cause dry mouth, blurred vision, dizziness, nausea, constipation, bladder retention, tachycardia, palpitations, nervousness, and pedal edema. In the extreme, dry mouth can cause parotitis. Other worst-case scenarios include paralytic ileus, confusion, hallucinations, agitation, and psychosis.

Pseudo-Parkinson's Disease in Schizophrenia

Treatment of schizophrenia consists of drugs that block excessive dopamine receptors. Antipsychotic drugs are not selective; therefore, they also block the motor pathways, thus causing a pseudo-Parkinson's disease, or EPS, as the balance tilts to acetylcholine, which in turn causes muscle spasms. Anticholinergic drugs are used to treat this pseudo-Parkinson's.

---

* Life-threatening side effect.

Cogwheeling

When in doubt if the person is showing early signs of EPS, the nurse may check for "cogwheeling" by placing fingers over the client's antecubital space. The nurse flexes the person's forearm and then slowly lowers it, feeling for tension in the tendons as they stiffly give way to release the arm, rather like cogwheels slowly turning in a machine.

The following drugs have CNS anticholinergic effects and are used in early Parkinson's and for EPS.

Benztropine mesylate [Cogentin] helps to reestablish the balance between the sympathetic and the parasympathetic systems by blocking acetycholine.

Drug Interactions: Increased effect with alcohol, CNS depressants. Increased anticholinergic effects and possible confusion, hallucinations, paralytic ileus with amantadine, MAOIs, phenothiazines, procainamide, quinidine, tricyclic antidepressants.

Nervous System: arrhythmias—palpitations/tachycardia, ataxia, bladder—dysuria, bowel—constipation/distension/paralytic ileus, dizziness, drowsiness, muscle—inability to move certain muscle groups/weakness, nausea/vomiting, paresthesias, psyche—agitation/irritability/confusion/delirium/hallucinations/insomnia/nervousness/restlessness/toxic psychosis, vision—blurred/mydriasis/photophobia.

Endocrine System: (Pregnancy Category C) none noted.

Immune System: none noted.

Dosage: Acute EPS: IM/IV 1–2 mg q6h. Less acute EPS: PO 0.5–1 mg with gradual increase to 6 mg/d. Parkinson's PO 0.5–1 mg/d to a maximum of 6 mg/d.

Biperiden hydrochloride [Akineton] is an antiparkinsonian drug that blocks acetylcholine in the extrapyramidal system in Parkinson's and pseudo-Parkinson's diseases.

Drug Interactions: Increased sedation with alcohol and other CNS depressants. Increased risk of anticholinergic side effects with haloperidol, opiates, phenothiazines, quinidine, tricyclic antidepressants.

Side Effects

Nervous System: arrhythmias—tachycardia, bowel—constipation, dizziness, drowsiness, lack of coordination, muscle weakness, nausea/vomiting, postural hypotension—mild transient (after IM), psyche—agitation/confusion/disorientation/euphoria, vision—blurred/photophobia.

Endocrine System: (Pregnancy Category C) dry mouth.

Immune System: none noted.

Dosage: PO 2 mg tid or qid. IM/IV 2 mg injected slowly. May repeat q30min up to 8 mg/24 h.

Diphenhydramine hydrochloride [Benadryl, others], primarily an antihistamine, also has anticholinergic activity.

Drug Interactions: Increased CNS depression with alcohol, other CNS depressants.

Side Effects

Nervous System: arrhythmias—tachycardia, bladder—dysuria/frequency/retention, cardiovascular collapse,* bowel—constipation/diarrhea, dizziness, drowsiness, epigastric distress, fatigue, headache, hyper-/hypotension—mild, insomnia, nausea/vomiting, psyche—confusion/euphoria/excitement/nervousness, restlessness, tight chest sensation, tinnitus, tingling/weakness/heaviness—hands, vertigo, vision—blurred/diplopia/dry eyes, wheezing.

Endocrine System: (Pregnancy Category C) anorexia, dry mouth/nose/throat, fever, sweating.

Immune System: anaphylaxis,* photosensitivity, bronchial secretions—thickened, rash, urticaria.

Dosage: Allergy/EPS/motion sickness/nighttime sedation/Parkinson's: PO 25–50 mg tid or qid to maximum of 300 mg/d. IM/IV 10–50 mg q4–6h to maximum of 400 mg/d. Nonproductive cough: PO 25 mg q4–6h to maximum of 100 mg/d.

Procyclidine hydrochloride [Kenadrin] is also used to relieve EPS and parkinsonian cholinergic effects.

Drug Interactions: None noted.

Side Effects

Nervous System: arrhythmias—palpitation/tachycardia, bladder—retention, bowel—constipation/paralytic ileus,* dizziness, epigastric distress, headache, hypotension, lightheadedness, muscle—feeling of weakness, nausea/vomiting, psyche—confusion/psychotic-like symptoms, vision—blurred, mydriasis/photophobia.

Endocrine System: (Pregnancy Category C) flushing, sweating—decreased.

Immune System: acute suppurative parotitis, skin eruptions.

Dosage: PO 2–5 mg tid pc to maximum of 45–60 mg/d.

Trihexyphenidyl hydrochloride [Artane] is used to treat EPS and early acetylcholine unbalance in Parkinson's disease.

---

* Life-threatening side effect.

Off Label: Huntington's chorea, spasmodic torticollis.

Drug Interactions: Decreased effects of chlorpromazine, haloperidol, phenothiazines. Increased levels of digoxin. Increased effect with MAOIs.

Side Effects

Nervous System: arrhythmias—palpitations/tachycardia, bladder—hesitancy/retention, bowel—constipation, dizziness, drowsiness/insomnia, glaucoma—closed-angle, hypotension and orthostatic hypotension, nausea, psyche—agitation/confusion/delirium/euphoria/psychotic manifestations (CNS stimulation in high doses), vision—blurred/mydriasis/photophobia.

Endocrine System: (Pregnancy Category C) dry mouth.

Immune System: hypersensitivity reactions.

Dosage: Parkinson's: PO 1 mg day 1, 2 mg day 2; then increase by 2 mg q3–5d up to 6–10 mg/d tid or qid with meals and hs maximum 15 mg/d. EPS: PO 5–15 mg/d in divided doses.

 Chapter Highlights

- The parasympathetic nervous system, with its single transmitter, acetylcholine, balances the sympathetic nervous system.

- The neurotransmitter acetylcholine and the parasympathetic system control vast areas of the body.

- The receptors are termed muscarinic and nicotinic.

- Cholinergic drugs replace missing acetylcholine.

- Parasympathomimetic drugs ease the pressure of glaucoma by constricting the pupil.

- Anticholinergic drugs are used to treat EPS caused by phenothiazines, early Parkinson's disease, bradycardia, heart block, GI tract spasms, and urinary tract muscle spasms.

- The parasympathetic system has only one mode of recycling, its lone neurotransmitter.

- The drugs of the parasympathetic system take care of basic, but vital, functions.

4 Drugs of the Sympathetic Nervous System

- amantadine hydrochloride [Symmetrel]
- amiodarone hydrochloride [Cordarone, Amio-Aqueous]
- amitriptyline hydrochloride [Elavil, others]
- amitriptyline hydrochloride & chlordiazepoxide [Limbitrol]
- amitriptyline hydrochloride & perphenazine [Triavil]
- amoxapine [Ascendin]
- amphetamine sulfate [Racemic Amphetamine Sulfate]
- apomorphine hydrochloride
- atenolol [Tenormin]
- bretylium tosylate [Bretylol]
- brimonidine tartrate [Alphagan]
- bromocriptine mesylate [Parlodel]
- bupropion hydrochloride [Wellbutrin]
- cabergoline [Dostinex]
- caffeine, caffeine & sodium benzoate, citrated caffeine [Caffedrine, No Doz]
- carbidopa [Lodosyn]
- carbidopa & levodopa [Sinemet]
- carvedilol [Coreg]
- chlorpromazine hydrochloride [Thorazine, others]
- chlorprothixene [Taractan]
- clomipramine hydrochloride [Anafranil]
- clonidine hydrochloride [Catapres]
- clozapine [Clozaril]
- cocaine
- cyclobenzaprine hydrochloride [Cycoflex, Flexeril]
- desipramine hydrochloride [Norpramin]
- dextroamphetamine sulfate [Dexedrine]
- dobutamine hydrochloride [Dubutrex]
- dolasetron mesylate [Anzemet]
- dopamine [Intropin]
- doxepin hydrochloride [Sinequan, others]
- dronabinol [Marinol]
- droperidol [Inapsine]

drug list

- epinephrine [Bronkaid Mist, Epi-E-Zpen, Epinephrine Pediatric, EpiPen Auto-Injector, Primatene Mist Suspension]
- epinephrine bitartrate [Asthma-Haler, Bronkaid Mist Suspension, Bronitin Mist Suspension, Epitrate, Medihaler-Epi, Primatene Mist Suspension]
- epinephrine hydrochloride [Adrenalin Chloride, Bronkaid Mistometer, Dysne-Inhal, Epifrin, Glaucon]
- epinephrine, racemic [AsthmaNefrin, Dey-Dose Epinephrine, micro-Nefrin]
- epinephryl borate [Epinal, Eppy/N]
- ergonovine [Ergotrate]
- ergotamine tartrate [Ergomar]
- fluoxetine hydrochloride [Prozac]
- fluphenazine [Prolixin]
- fluvoxamine [Luvox]
- guanabenz acetate [Wytensin]
- guanadrel sulfate [Hylorel]
- guanethidine sulfate [Ismelin]
- haloperidol [Haldol]
- imipramine hydrochloride [Tofranil]
- ipecac
- isocarboxazid [Marplan]
- isoproterenol hydrochloride [Isuprel]
- labetalol hydrochloride [Normodyne]
- levodopa (L-dopa) [Dopar, Larodopa]
- loxapine hydrochloride [Loxitane]
- maprotiline hydrochloride [Ludiomil]
- mesoridazine besylate [Serentil]
- methotrimeprazine hydrochloride [Levoprome]
- methoxamine hydrochloride [Vasoxyl]
- methyldopa [Aldomet]
- methylphenidate hydrochloride [Ritalin]
- methysergide [Sansert]
- metoclopramide hydrochloride [Reglan]
- metoprolol tartrate [Lopressor]
- midodrine [ProAmatine]
- mirtazapine [Remeron]
- molindone hydrochloride [Moban]
- nadolol [Corgard]
- nefazodone [Serzone]
- norepinephrine bitartrate [Levarterenol, Levophed, Noradrenalin]
- nortriptyline hydrochloride [Aventyl, Pamelor]
- olanzapine [Zyprexa]
- paroxetine [Paxil]
- pemoline [Cylert]

drug list

- pergolide [Permax]
- perphenazine [Phenazine, Trilafon]
- phenelzine sulfate [Nardil]
- phenmetrazine hydrochloride [Preludin]
- phenoxybenzamine hydrochloride [Dibenzyline]
- phentolamine mesylate [Regitine]
- phenylephrine hydrochloride [Neo-Synephrine]
- pindolol [Visken]
- pramipexole [Mirapex]
- prazosin hydrochloride [Minipress]
- prochlorperazine [Compazine]
- promazine hydrochloride [Proziner, Sparine]
- promethazine hydrochloride [Phergan, others]
- propranolol [Inderal]
- protriptyline hydrochloride [Vivactil]
- quetiapine fumarate [Seroquel]
- reserpine [Serpasil]
- risperidone [Risperdal]
- ropinirole [Requip]
- selegiline hydrochloride (L-deprenyl) [Eldepryl]
- sertraline hydrochloride [Zoloft]
- sibutramine hydrochloride [Meridia]
- sumatriptan [Imitrex]
- tamsulosin hydrochloride [Flomax]
- thioridazine hydrochloride [Mellaril]
- thiothixene hydrochloride [Navane]
- timolol maleate [Blocadren, Timoptic, others]
- tizanidine hydrochloride [Zanaflex]
- tranylcypromine sulfate [Parnate]
- trazodone [Desyrel, Desyrel Dividose]
- trifluoperazine HCl [Stelazine]
- trimipramine maleate [Surmontil]
- venlafaxine [Effexor]
- zolmitriptan [Zomig]

The sympathetic nervous system responds to stress, both painful and pleasant. Its neurotransmitters prepare the body for fight, flight, or fun as the heart races and blood pressure rises. The mundane tasks of the parasympathetic nervous system must wait until the excitement, danger, and tension have passed (Fig. 4–1). The sympathetic balances the parasympathetic with neurotransmitters called catecholamines. **Catecholamines** are derived from the amino acid tyrosine and contain the catechol moiety that gives them their name. The basic catecholamine is dopamine from which the more complex norepinephrine or noradrenaline evolves. The third and most complex is epinephrine, or adrenaline (Fig. 4–2).

The catecholamines are involved in appetite, reward, drinking, vomiting, Parkinson's disease, tachycardia,

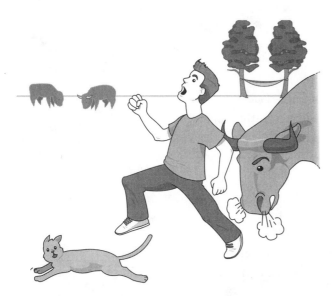

The sympathetic nervous system is activated by excitement, danger, or pleasure. The heart beats faster, the bronchi open up, the pupils dilate, blood vessels constrict, and breathing speeds up. The GI tract and bladder must now wait until the excitement is past.

The catecholamines—dopamine, norepinephrine, and epinephrine (the last two are derived from dopamine)—are neurotransmitters of the sympathetic nervous system. They are called adrenergic.

Figure 4–1. The sympathetic nervous system is for gallop.

schizophrenia, depression, and in the form of hypertension caused by the response of vascular muscle to catecholamines. In what may seem like a paradox, the alerting catecholamines are also involved in sleeping and, in certain neural pathways, decreased cardiovascular response. Catecholamines dilate the pupils, speed the heart, constrict vascular muscles to increase blood pressure, slow and even reverse peristalsis, fill the bladder, and make the liver change its stored glycogen into sugar. The ability to effect gluconeogenesis requires special consideration in the management of diabetes. The catecholamine dopamine is implicated in schizophrenia, and manifestations of psychosis can occur as side effects of drugs that increase its presence.

Traditionally, the drugs discussed in this chapter have been divided into drugs for cardiac conditions, Parkinson's disease, schizophrenia, depression, stimulants, and so on. But that is not the way the body functions. The reader is invited to see the connections, to see why, for example, drugs that are used to treat conditions influenced by decreased or increased dopamine can manifest psychotic side effects or why an antidepressant may cause cardiac arrhythmias.

▶ ALPHA AND BETA RECEPTORS AND BLOCKERS

The sympathetic nervous system has two major kinds of receptors: alpha and beta. Usually the alphas excite

and the betas inhibit. For example, alphas constrict blood vessels in the bronchi to decrease congestion and edema. The alpha receptors also cause contraction of intestinal sphincters, pilomotor muscles, and bladder sphincters. They also dilate the iris and cause the intestine to relax.

Betas relax bronchial muscles. Beta receptors are further classified as beta-1 (β_1) and beta-2 (β_2) shapes. Beta-1 receptors have an affinity for both norepinephrine and epinephrine. Beta-2 receptors have a greater affinity for epinephrine. Beta-1 receptors speed the heart, increase its contractility, and make it more efficient. Beta-2 receptors relax the bladder wall, the intestine, and the uterus. They cause vasodilation, bronchodilation, calorigenesis, and glycogenolysis.

▶ RECYCLING THE CATECHOLAMINES

The sympathetic nervous system recycles catecholamines by pumping them back into presynaptic neuronal storage vesicles from the synapse after use. Whatever leaks into or remains in the synapse after the action potential passes is taken apart by the enzyme monoamine oxidase. Drug therapies to increase available sympa-

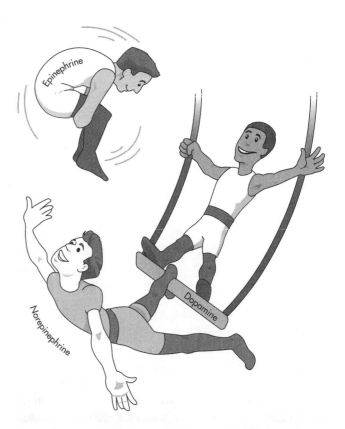

Derived from the amino acid tyrosine, all have the catechol moiety, thus the name catecholamine. Dopamine is the first of these, then the more complex norepinephrine and the most complex—epinephrine.

Figure 4–2. The exciting catecholamine family.

thetic neurotransmitters, besides supplementing the catecholamines in emergencies and blocking the reuptake process, include blocking the enzyme breakdown of the catecholamines.

▶ PARKINSON'S DISEASE AND DRUGS TO RESTORE AND REPLACE DOPAMINE

Parkinson's disease, a chronic, progressive disorder, results from a depletion in dopamine production by damaged or destroyed neurons in the substantia nigra that project to the basal ganglia, caudate nucleus, putamen, pallidum, and neostriatum. So abundant is the production of dopamine that the patient may not even be aware of the condition until production has been reduced by 80%. Even though the adrenal medullas continue adequate production of dopamine, the neurotransmitter cannot pass the BBB into the CNS.

Depletion of dopamine in these neural pathways results in motor control symptoms. The patient exhibits tremor with the classic "pill-rolling" of the thumb and fingers, muscle rigidity, and slowness of movement (bradykinesia). In treating the Parkinson's patient, the nurse must never hurry the patient, and must look and listen for other cues to his or her needs because facial expressions may be impaired and the voice may be weak. Difficulty in swallowing may cause drooling and choking. Decreased dopamine stimulation of receptors in the GI tract results in delayed gastric emptying, nausea, and constipation (Wilson, 1995). The patient's muscle rigidity can be painful and the patient may also suffer psychic manifestations of depression and sleep disorders. The ultimate paralysis after decades results in death.

This CNS depletion of dopamine tilts the normal sympathetic–parasympathetic balance to the parasympathetic. Disruption of homeostasis has implications for the early treatment of Parkinson's. Anticholinergic drugs are first-line drugs used in early Parkinson's to block acetylcholine and reestablish the balance that tilts to the parasympathetic due to decreased dopamine production; however, as dopamine levels continue to decline, treatment is aimed at increasing available dopamine. The treatment becomes less effective over years. Sometimes it helps to decrease the dose and increase the frequency. Some patients may experience "on–off" exacerbations of symptoms. Dopaminergic antiparkinsonian drugs can cause schizophrenic-like side effects, just as drugs used to treat schizophrenia by blocking dopamine can cause parkinsonian side effects. Increasing dopamine to motor areas of the brain to treat Parkinson's increases dopamine in the emotional centers of the brain as well. The neuroleptic drug clozapine is sometimes used to treat hallucinations and confusion, and it may even help the depression some patients experience.

Amantadine hydrochloride [Symmetrel], an antiviral drug, increases dopamine release in the brain as a side effect. Amantadine is less effective than levodopa.

Drug Interactions: Alcohol can enhance CNS effects. Amantadine can also potentiate anticholinergic effects.

Side Effects

Nervous System: ataxia, convulsions,* dizziness, dyspnea, peripheral edema, headache, orthostatic hypotension, insomnia, irritability, lightheadedness, nausea/vomiting, psyche—anxiety/concentration difficulties/confusion/hallucinations/mood and mental changes/nervousness/nightmares, vision—blurring/loss.

Endocrine System: (Pregnancy Category C) dry mouth, peripheral edema.

Immune System: leukopenia, rashes.

Dosage: EPS PO 100 mg qd or bid to a maximum of 400 mg/d. Parkinson's: 100 mg qd or bid. Start with 100 mg qd if patient is on other antiparkinsonian drugs.

Bromocriptine mesylate [Parlodel] stimulates dopamine receptors in the brain, making more dopamine receptors available and reducing the "on–off" phenomenon; however, its efficacy lasts only about 6 months. Bromocriptine is added to the regimen of levodopa/carbidopa in the later stages of Parkinson's. If taken with antihypertensive drugs, bromocriptine may increase hypotension. (Bromocriptine is also used for female infertility and to prevent lactation. This drug is discussed further in Section II.)

Side Effects

Nervous System: angina—exacerbation, arrhythmias—extrasystoles, ataxia, bowel—constipation/diarrhea, cramps—abdominal, dizziness, dyskinesia, dysphagia, fainting, fatigue, headache, hypertension—postpartum, hypotension—orthostatic, insomnia, nausea/vomiting, pain—epigastric, psyche—anxiety/depression/mania/nervousness/nightmares/Raynaud's phenomenon, sedation, shock,* taste—metallic, vertigo, vision—blepharospasm/blurred/diplopia.

Endocrine System: (Pregnancy Category C) anorexia, dry mouth.

Immune System: erythromelalgia, extremities—edematous/hot/red/tender, eyes—burning sensation, MI—acute,* nasal congestion, peptic ulcer, rash.

Dosage: PO. Parkinson's: Start with 1.25 mg bid with meals. Increase 2.5 mg q2wk to 100 mg/d maximum. Female infertility/amenorrhea/glactorrhea: PO 1.25–2.5 mg/d to a maximum of 2–5 mg tid. Postpartum lactation

---

* Life-threatening side effect.

suppression: PO 2.5 mg bid 4 h p̄ delivery × 14–21 days. Acromegaly: PO 1.25–2.5 mg/d × 3d; then increase 1.25–2.5 mg q3–7d until desired effect is achieved.

<u>Cabergoline [Dostinex]</u> is a dopamine receptor agonist that inhibits secretion of prolactin for the treatment of hyperprolactinemic disorders, either idiopathic or caused by pituitary adenomas.

Drug Interactions: Increased activity of D_2 antagonists, eg, butyrophenones, metoclopramide, phenothiazines, thioxanthenes.

Side Effects

Nervous System: arthralgia, asthenia, bowel—constipation/diarrhea/flatulence, dizziness, dyspepsia, fatigue, headache, hypotension, nausea/vomiting, pain—abdominal/breast/tooth, palpitation, paresthesia, psyche—anxiety/impaired concentration/depression/insomnia/nervousness/somnolence, syncope, vertigo, vision—abnormal.

Endocrine System: (Pregnancy Category B) anorexia, dependent edema, dry mouth, dysmenorrhea, hot flashes.

Immune System: acne, influenza-like symptoms, periorbital edema, pruritus, rhinitis, throat irritation.

Dosage: PO. Start with 0.25 mg 2×/wk. Increase by 0.25 mg twice weekly to a maximum of 1 mg 2×/wk based on serum prolactin level.

<u>Carbidopa [Lodosyn]</u> alone cannot be used to treat Parkinson's. It is given in combination with levodopa (see *Sinemet*) because it helps to keep levodopa intact so more of it can cross the BBB and the duration of levodopa activity is extended. Levodopa and carbidopa in combination usually have fewer side effects, and administering the combination is the preferred method. The drugs are given after meals to help avoid nausea. Carbidopa can be given in additional doses in tandem with levodopa when more is needed. Its side effects are attributed to the levodopa.

Side Effects

Nervous System: none noted.

Endocrine System: (Pregnancy Category C) none noted.

Immune System: none noted.

Dosage: For patients on levodopa: PO start as 20–25% of initial dose of levodopa.

<u>Carbidopa and levodopa [Sinemet]</u> are supplied in tablets of carbidopa 10 mg/levodopa 100 mg, carbidopa 25 mg/levodopa 100 mg, and carbidopa 25 mg/levodopa 250 mg.

Drug Interactions: MAOIs may precipitate hypertensive crisis. Tricyclic antidepressants potentiate postural hypotension. Phenothiazines, haloperidol may antagonize effects of levodopa. Anticholinergic agents may enhance levodopa effects, but can exacerbate involuntary movements. Methyldopa, guanethidine increase hypotensive and CNS effects. Phenytoin, papaverine may interfere with levodopa effects.

Side Effects

Nervous System: ataxia, arrhythmias—tachycardia, bladder—incontinence/retention, bowel—constipation/diarrhea, breathing irregularities, delirium, edema, fatigue, hand tremors—increased, headache, hypertension/hypotension—orthostatic, muscle—blepharospasm/bradykinetic episodes/bruxism/dilated pupils/opisthotonos/tremors/trismus/twitching, nausea/vomiting, numbness, priapism, palpitations, psyche—agitation/anxiety/confusion/depression/euphoria/hallucinations/hypomania/insomnia/nightmares/paranoia/suicidal ideation, vision—blepharospasm/blurred/diplopia/miosis/mydriasis/oculogyric crisis, seizures, taste changes, tongue—burning sensation.

Endocrine System: (Pregnancy Category C) anorexia, BUN, edema, hair loss, neuroleptic malignant syndrome,* sweat—dark.

Immune System: agranulocytosis,* anemia—hemolytic/nonhemolytic, hoarseness, liver function tests—abnormal, phlebitis, rash, thrombocytopenia.

Dosage: PO. Start with the 10 mg/100 mg or 25 mg/100 mg strength tablets tid with meals. Increase 1 tablet q2–3d. May be taken as often as q2–3h. To a maximum of 6 tabs/d if not on concurrent levodopa.

<u>Levodopa (L-dopa) [Dopar, Larodopa]</u>, the dopamine precursor, crosses the BBB, whereas oral dopamine cannot. Approximately 95% of the levodopa is broken down into dopamine and remains in the body. The remaining 5% enters the brain. The patient must not supplement the diet with vitamin B_6 because it breaks down levodopa into dopamine, which cannot cross the BBB.

Drug Interactions: Levodopa may possibly interact with antihypertensive agents to potentiate hypotension, but with MAOIs may cause a hypertensive crisis. In addition, haloperidol, methyldopa, papaverine, phenothiazines, phenytoin, and reserpine are dopamine antagonists. *Note:* Muscle twitching can be an early sign of overdose.

Side Effects

Nervous System: ataxia, arrhythmias—tachycardia, bladder—incontinence/retention, bowel—constipation/diarrhea/flatulence, dysphagia, edema, fatigue,

---

* Life-threatening side effect.

headache, hypertension/hypotension—orthostatic, muscle— blepharospasm/bradykinetic episodes/bruxism/opisthotonos/tremors/trismus/twitching, nausea/vomiting, priapism/increased sex drive, palpitations, psyche—agitation/anxiety/confusion/depression/euphoria/hallucinations/hypomania/insomnia/nightmares/paranoia/suicidal ideation, vision—blurred/diplopia/pupils dilated, taste changes, tongue—burning sensation.

Endocrine System: (Pregnancy Category C) growth hormone/PBI hypokalemia—elevated, anorexia, flushing, glucose tolerance—decreased, edema, hair loss, postmenopausal bleeding, sweating, weight—gain/loss.

Immune System: alkaline phosphatase/ALT/AST/bilirubin—increased, Hct/Hb/ WBC—decreased, GI bleeding, hepatotoxicity, rash, rhinorrhea.

Dosage: PO. Start with 500 mg–1 g bid or more. May increase 100–750 mg q3–7d to optimal response or maximum of 8 g/d. In combination with carbidopa, decrease levodopa dose by 75–80%.

Pergolide [Permax] is used as an adjunct to levodopa/carbidopa in treating Parkinson's. A dopamine agonist, it stimulates both D_1 and D_2 receptors.

Off Label: acromegaly, hyperprolactinemia.

Drug Interactions: Use with levodopa increases risk of dyskinesia.

Side Effects

Nervous System: arrhythmias—PVCs/other ventricular arrhythmias, bowel—constipation, edema, headache, hypotension—orthostatic, lightheadedness, nausea/vomiting, Parkinson's symptoms worsened, psyche—anxiety/confusion/hallucinations/nightmares/paranoia, somnolence—transient.

Endocrine System: (Pregnancy Category B) edema.

Immune System: rash, rhinitis.

Dosage: PO. Parkinson's: Start with 0.05 mg qd for 2 d; then increase by 0.1 or 0.15 mg/d q3d for the next 12 d; then may increase by 0.25 mg every third day until desired therapeutic response is achieved; give in divided doses tid to maximum of 5 mg/d. Acromegaly: 0.1–1.5 mg qd. Hyperprolactinemia: 0.025–0.6 mg qd.

Pramipexole [Mirapex] is a dopamine agonist used to treat Parkinson's disease. It probably works by stimulating dopamine receptors in the striatum.

Drug Interactions: Increased levels with cimetidine. Decreased effect possible with dopamine antagonists.

Side Effects

Nervous System: asthenia,[1,2] bladder—frequency[2]/incontinence[2], bowel—constipation,[1,2] dizziness,[1,2] dyspnea,[2] dysphagia,[1] edema,[1,2] hyperesthesia,[1] hypotension—orthostatic,[2] libido—decreased,[1]/impotence,[1] malaise,[1,2] muscle—EPS[2] akathisia[1,2]/dyskinesia[2]/dystonia[1,2]/hypertonia[2]/gait abnormalities[2]/myasthenia[2]/myoclonus[1]/twitching,[2] nausea,[1] pain—chest,[2] psyche—amnesia[1,2]/confusion[1,2]/delusions[2]/dream abnormalities[2]/hallucinations[1,2]/insomnia[1,2]/paranoia/somnolence[1,2]/thinking abnormalities,[1,2] vision—abnormalities[1,2]/accommodation abnormalities[1,2]/diplopia.[2]

Endocrine System: (Pregnancy Category C) anorexia,[1] creatine phosphokinase—increased,[2] dry mouth,[2] fever,[1] peripheral edema,[1,2] weight loss.[1]

Immune System: arthritis,[2] bursitis,[2] injury—accidental,[2] pneumonia,[2] rhinitis,[2] UTI.[2]

Dosage: PO. Start with 0.375 mg in three divided doses; not to be increased more frequently than q5–7d. Maintain on 1.5–4.5 mg/d with or without concomitant levodopa (approximately 800 mg/d). In combination with pramipexole, a reduction of levodopa should be considered.

Ropinirole [Requip] is a dopamine that agonist binds to dopamine receptors to treat Parkinson's disease.

Drug Interactions: Increased mean steady state of L-dopa. Increased levels with ciprofloxacin. Reduced oral clearance with estrogens. Decreased effectiveness possible with dopamine antagonists.

Side Effects

Nervous System: arrhythmias—atrial fibrillation[1]/extrasystoles[1]/tachycardia,[1] arthralgia,[2] asthenia,[1] bowel—constipation[2]/diarrhea[2]/flatulence,[1,2] dizziness,[1,2] dyskinesia,[2] dyspepsia,[1] dysphagia,[2] falls,[2] fatigue,[1] headache,[2] hyperesthesia,[1] hyperkinesia,[1] hypokinesia,[2] hypertension,[1] hypotension[1,2] and orthostatic hypotension,[1] impotence,[1] nausea[1,2]/vomiting[1,2], pain—abdominal[1,2]/chest,[1,2], palpitations,[1] paresis,[2] paresthesia,[2] psyche—amnesia[1,2]/anxiety[2]/impaired concentration[1]/confusion[1,2]/abnormal dreams[2]/hallucination[1,2]/nervousness[2]/somnolence,[1,2] syncope,[1,2] tremor,[1,2] vertigo,[1] vision—abnormalities,[1] yawning.[1]

Endocrine System: (Pregnancy Category C) alkaline phosphatase—increase,[1] anorexia,[1] drug level—increase,[2] dry mouth,[1,2] flushing,[1] edema—dependent/leg, saliva—increased,[2] sweating—increased,[1,2] vision—dry eyes,[1] weight increase.[2]

Immune System: anemia,[2] arthritis,[2] bronchitis,[1] ischemia—peripheral,[1] pharyngitis,[1] rhinitis,[1] sinusitis,[1] upper respiratory infection,[2] UTI,[1] viral infection.[1]

---

[1] Early Parkinson's.
[2] Advanced Parkinson's.

Dosage: Week 1: 0.25 mg tid. Week 2: 0.5 mg tid. Week 3: 0.74 mg tid. Week 4: 1.0 mg tid.

<u>Selegiline hydrochloride (L-deprenyl) [Eldepryl]</u> blocks the breakdown of dopamine by inhibiting MAO type B activity. It may also interfere with reuptake from the synapse. Severe CNS toxicity is possible with tricyclic antidepressants.

Drug Interactions: Fluoxetine, sertraline, paroxetine may cause CNS toxicity and muscle rigidity. Potentially severe reactions may occur with meperidine.

Side Effects

Nervous System: dyskinesia, hypotension, psyche—agitation/confusion/sleep disturbance.

Endocrine System: (Pregnancy Category C) anorexia.

Immune System: none noted.

Dosage: PO 5 mg bid with breakfast and lunch.

▶ DOPAMINE AND VOMITING

Vomiting is reverse peristalsis. In extreme cases vomiting can persist long enough to bring up fecal material. Dopamine transmits the vomit stimulus in the vomiting center of the medulla received from afferent parasympathetic and sympathetic nerves when they signal an irritated or overdistended stomach or duodenum (Fig. 4–3). In addition, vomiting can be caused by stimulation of the chemoreceptor trigger zone in the brain. Drugs such as digitalis, morphine, and apomorphine cause vomiting in this manner. The drug ipecac induces vomiting through GI tract irritation messages both to the vomiting center and to the chemoreceptor trigger zone.

<u>Droperidol [Inapsine],</u> related to the neuroleptic haloperidol, a major tranquilizer, opposes neurotransmitters of the sympathetic nervous system. Like haloperidol, droperidol can cause EPS. Some blocking of alpha-adrenergic receptors with resulting hypotension is possible. Its antiemetic action takes place in the CTZ. It can block the action of the emetic apomorphine. It is used to tranquilize and to reduce nausea and vomiting during surgical and diagnostic procedures. It is also used for induction and as a part of maintaining anesthesia, both general and regional, usually with fentanyl to reduce motor activity and to create indifference to pain and environmental stimuli.

Off Label: IV as an antiemetic during cancer chemotherapy.

Incompatibilities: Incompatible in solution and at Y-site with fluorouracil, furosemide, heparin, leucovorin,

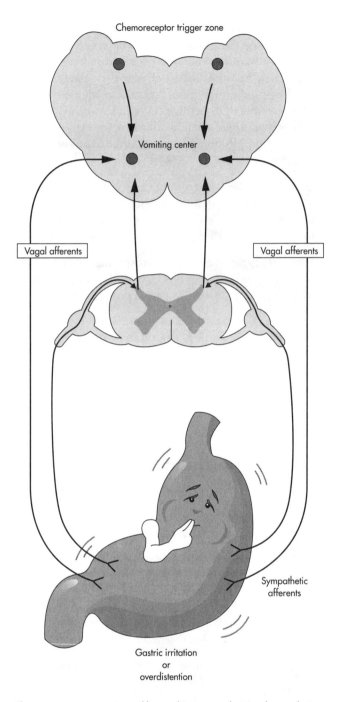

The message to vomit is triggered by vagal (parasympathetic) and sympathetic afferent signals from an irritated, or overdistended stomach or duodenum to the vomiting center of the medulla. In addition, the brain itself can induce vomiting by stimulating the chemoreceptor trigger zone. Certain drugs like digitalis, morphine, and apomorphine cause vomiting in this manner. The drug ipecac induces vomiting through both GI tract irritation messages to the vomiting center and by the chemoreceptor trigger zone.

Figure 4–3. Vomiting.

methotrexate, pentobarbital. Also incompatible at Y-site with nafcillin.

Side Effects

Nervous System: akathisia, arrhythmias—tachycardia, bronchospasm,* dizziness, drowsiness, dystonia, EPS, hypotension, laryngospasm,* psyche—anxiety/depression/hallucination/restlessness, vision—oculogyric crisis.

Endocrine System: (Pregnancy Category C) chills, shivering.

Immune System: none noted.

Dosage: IM 2.5–10 mg 30–60 min before procedure. Anesthesia induction: IM/IV 0.22–0.275 mg/kg and 1.25–2.5 mg to maintain as adjunct to anesthesia. For nausea/vomiting: IM/IV 2.5–5 mg q3–4h prn.

Metoclopramide hydrochloride [Reglan] tilts the balance back to the parasympathetic and its neurotransmitter, acetylcholine, by interfering with dopamine from the sympathetic and its effect on the CTZ. This tilt makes the gut empty faster, relieves nausea and vomiting, causes the pyloric sphincter to relax, and increases the speed and force of peristalsis in the duodenum and jejunum with no effect on the colon. Metoclopramide is used to treat the severe emesis of chemotherapy, to speed gastric emptying for x-ray procedures and surgery, for diabetic gastroparesis, and to decrease esophagitis and reflux.

Drug Interactions: Opiates and anticholinergics antagonize metoclopramide. In turn, metoclopramide increases the absorption of drugs like acetaminophen, alcohol, levodopa, and tetracycline from the small intestine. Metoclopramide decreases effects of drugs absorbed from the stomach, like digoxin and penicillin V. Use of diphenhydramine [Benadryl] helps prevent possible EPS. The incidence of EPS with metoclopramide increases if the patient is also on major tranquilizers. Insulin needs may change to reflect changes in digestion. Metoclopramide is never used in the presence of GI bleeding, perforation, or obstruction, epilepsy, EPS, possible breast cancer, or with medications like the thioxanthenes, butyrophenones, MAOIs, tricyclics, or adrenergics. Such drugs are discontinued 2 wk before treatment with metoclopramide.

Side Effects

Nervous System: bowel—constipation/diarrhea, fatigue, headache, hypertensive crisis,* impotence, muscle—acute EPS, nausea, psyche—agitation/disorientation/restlessness, sedation.

Endocrine System: (Pregnancy Category B) altered drug absorption, amenorrhea, galactorrhea, gynecomastia.

Immune System: edema—glossal/periorbital, methemoglobinemia, rash.

Dosage: Gastroparesis: PO 10 mg 30 min ac and hs for 2–8 wk. With chemotherapy: IV 2 mg/kg 30 min before treatment and IV 1–2 mg/kg 3 h after treatment to total of 5 doses. PO 2 mg/kg 1 h before antineoplastic administration. May repeat q2h for 3 more doses. X-ray procedures: IV 10 mg over 1–2 min.

PHENOTHIAZINES USED TO TREAT NAUSEA AND VOMITING

The phenothiazines used to block dopamine receptors in the treatment of schizophrenia can also block dopamine in the vomiting center to treat nausea and vomiting. The dosages are smaller than those needed in psychiatry.

Chlorpromazine Hydrochloride [Thorazine, others] is discussed later in this chapter under Phenothiazines.

Dosage: PO 10–25 mg q4–6h prn. IM/IV 25–50 mg q3–4h prn. Rectal: 50–100 mg q6–8h. Intractable hiccups: PO/IM/IV 25–50 mg tid–qid.

Prochlorperazine [Compazine] controls severe nausea and vomiting. It is sometimes used in the management of psychotic disorders, but it has more potential to cause EPS than chlorpromazine.

Drug Interactions: It increases CNS depression with other CNS depressants. It should be administered 2 h apart from antacids and antidiarrheals because they decrease its absorption. Phenobarbital increases its metabolism. With general anesthetics it increases excitation and hypotension. It antagonizes antihypertensive action of guanethidine. It may cause sudden death with phenylpropanolamine. Its hypotensive and anticholinergic effects increase with tricyclic antidepressants. It lowers seizure threshold, and anticonvulsant dosage may need to be increased.

Incompatibilities

Solution/Additive: aminophylline, amphotericin B, ampicillin, calcium gluceptate, calcium gluconate, cephalothin, chloramphenicol, chlorothiazide, dimenhydrinate, hydrocortisone, hydromorphone, methohexital, midazolam, penicillin G sodium, pentobarbital, phenobarbital, sodium bicarbonate, thiopental.

Side Effects

Nervous System: dizziness, drowsiness, EPS, hypotension, psyche—acute catatonia, tardive dyskinesia, vision—blurred.

---

* Life-threatening side effect.

Endocrine System: (Pregnancy Category C) amenorrhea, galactorrhea.

Immune System: agranulocytosis,* leukopenia, photosensitivity.

Dosage: PO 5–10 mg tid–qid; SR 10–15 mg q12h. IM 5–10 mg q3–4h to a maximum of 40 mg/d. IV 2.5–10 mg q6–8h to a maximum of 40 mg/d. Rectal: 25-mg suppository bid.

Promazine hydrochloride [Sparine] has weak antipsychotic and extrapyramidal activity.

Drug Interaction: Antacids inhibit absorption of oral form.

Side Effects

Nervous System: bowel—constipation, drowsiness, hypotension—orthostatic, seizures.*

Endocrine System: (Pregnancy Category C) none noted.

Immune System: agranulocytosis,* leukopenia, photosensitivity, risk of Reye's syndrome under age 12.

Dosage: PO, IM 25–50 mg q4–6h to maximum of 1000 mg/d.

Promethazine hydrochloride [Phenergan, others] is a long-acting phenothiazine derivative with infrequent EPS activity. Its antihistamine action gives it antiserotonin, anticholinergic, and anesthetic action. It acts in the CTZ to relieve nausea and vomiting. It is commonly used pre- and postoperatively and in obstetrics for its sedating quality and as an adjunct to analgesics for pain relief.

Drug Interactions: synergistic with other CNS depressants.

Incompatibilities

Solution/Additive: aminophylline, carbenicillin, cefotetan, chloramphenicol, chlorothiazide, diatrizoate, dimenhydrinate, heparin, hydrocortisone, methicillin, methohexital, iodipamide, iothalamate, nalbuphine, penicillin G sodium, pentobarbital, phenobarbital, thiopental.

Y-site: carbenicillin, cefotetan, heparin.

Side Effects

Nervous System: bladder—retention, bowel—constipation, coordination—disturbed, dizziness, drowsiness, hyper-/hypotension—transient, nausea/vomiting, psyche—confusion/restlessness, respirations—irregular, sedation, vision—blurred. Acute toxicity: cardiorespiratory symptoms,* CNS stimulation/abnormal movements, coma,* convulsions,* EPS, respiratory depression.*

Endocrine System: (Pregnancy Category C) anorexia, mouth/nose/throat— dry.

Immune System: agranulocytosis,* leukopenia, photosensitivity.

Dosage: PO, IM, rectal, IV 12.5–25 mg q4–6h prn. Motion sickness: PO/PR/IM/IV 25 mg bid. Preoperative and sedation: 25–50 mg. The IV solution should not exceed 25 mg/mL. Do not give faster than 25 mg/min.

CANNABINOIDS

These synthetic derivatives of tetrahydrocannabinol (THC) are used only for the nausea and vomiting associated with chemotherapy.

Dronabinol [Marinol], a Schedule II drug, is used to treat the nausea and vomiting of chemotherapy for cancer when other antiemetics are ineffective. It is also used to stimulate appetite in AIDS patients.

Off Label: glaucoma.

Side Effects

Nervous System: ataxia, arrhythmias—tachycardia, bowel—diarrhea/incontinence, dizziness, drowsiness, headache, hypertension, hypotension—orthostatic, insomnia, myalgia, paresthesias, psyche—anxiety/confusion/depersonalization/ depression/disorientation/ euphoria/irritability/memory lapse/nightmares/paranoia, sensory difficulty, speech difficulty, syncope.

Endocrine System: (Pregnancy Category B) flushing, sweating.

Immune System: allergy.

Dosage: PO 5 mg/m² 1–3 h before chemotherapy and q2–4h after for a total of 4–6 doses to maximum of 15 mg/m². Appetite stimulant (AIDS related): start with 2.5 mg before lunch and dinner. Titrate to maximum 20 mg/d.

▶ EMETICS

Sometimes vomiting can be lifesaving. **Emetics** are given to initiate vomiting of potentially harmful ingestion of intoxicating drugs or plants. The patient must be conscious and the substance not caustic, oily, or highly viscous and apt to cause further trauma or respiratory complications. Apomorphine or ipecac may be used to induce vomiting. Both of these drugs affect the CTZ, though ipecac has a local action on the gastric mucosa as well.

Apomorphine hydrochloride, a Schedule II drug, is a powerful and potentially dangerous emetic and may cause

---

* Life-threatening side effect.

violent emesis and severe CNS depression. It is not used in opiate or CNS depressant overdose or cardiac depression. Almost 100% reliable for emesis, apomorphine works in 2–15 min. The adult patient is given 200–300 mL of water just before administration of the drug to have a better emetic effect.

Drug Interactions: In large doses, it may potentiate heart block with digitalis or precipitate convulsions with convulsant drugs.

Side Effects

Nervous System: arrhythmias—tachycardia, drowsiness, hypotension—orthostatic, nausea, restlessness, syncope, tremors, vomiting—severe, weakness. Large doses: bradycardia, acute circulatory failure,* CNS depression,* coma,* depressed respirations,* retching, violent and persistent vomiting.

Endocrine System: (Pregnancy Category C) none noted.

Immune System: none noted.

Dosage: SC 2–10 mg one time only. (Average dose 5–6 mg.) Give patient 10 oz of water first.

Ipecac, though not quite as effective as apomorphine, is 90% reliable in 30 min, and does not have the severe CNS side effects if it is vomited back and not absorbed or overdosed. It is used to induce vomiting of unabsorbed ingested poisons.

Side Effects

Nervous System: arrhythmias—atrial fibrillation/tachycardia, coma,* convulsions,* cramps— abdominal, dyspnea, hypotension, muscles—achy/stiff, severe myopathy—cardiomyopathy*/cardiotoxicity,* pain—chest, sensory disturbances, tremors, vomiting—persistent.

Endocrine System: (Pregnancy Category C) none noted.

Immune System: bloody diarrhea, fatal myocarditis,* gastroenteritis.

Dosage: PO 5–30 mL, depending on patient's weight and size. Follow with 8–16 oz of water. May repeat once in 20 min if necessary.

▶ THE CATECHOLAMINES AND ADRENERGIC DRUGS AS VASOPRESSORS

Vasoconstriction is intended to save life, and more neural pathways are dedicated to vasoconstriction than to vasodilation. Drugs that mimic catecholamines are used in the emergencies of cardiogenic, septic, and

allergic shock, standstill, and allergic obstruction of airways. The catecholamines and adrenergics trigger gluconeogenesis and require cautious monitoring in diabetes. They also increase the need for oxygen.

Dobutamine hydrochloride [Dobutrex] is used for CHF, after cardiac surgery, and for acute heart failure. Similar to dopamine, dobutamine affects beta receptors. It is ino- and chronotropic. Dobutamine can be combined with nitroprusside for CHF and with dopamine for improved renal and cardiac function. Dobutamine can increase the ventricular rate in atrial fibrillation, tachycardia, and other arrhythmias. The MI patient may need more oxygen with dobutamine. Because catecholamines spur gluconeogenesis by the liver, dobutamine can also increase insulin need. Dobutamine instantly raises BP, so infusion requires careful, frequent monitoring of vital signs.

Drug Interactions: Serious arrhythmias may result when cyclopropane or halothane has sensitized the myocardium to adrenergics. Not for use with beta blockers. Pressor effects are increased with MAOIs and tricyclic antidepressants.

Incompatibilities

Solution/Additive: aminophylline, bretylium, bumetanide, calcium chloride, calcium gluconate, diazepam, doxapram, digoxin, epinephrine, furosemide, heparin, insulin, magnesium sulfate, phenytoin, potassium chloride, potassium phosphate, sodium bicarbonate.

Y-site: acyclovir, aminophylline, sodium bicarbonate.

Side Effects

Nervous System: angina, arrhythmias—PVCs,* BP—increased, cramps—legs, dyspnea, fatigue, headache, nausea/vomiting, pain—chest, palpitations, paresthesias, pulse—increased, psyche—nervousness, tremors.

Endocrine System: (Pregnancy Category C) blood sugar level increased.

Immune System: MI—extension.*

Dosage: IV 2.5–10 µg/kg/min per microdrip in D5W. (Maximum dose: 40 mcg/kg/min.)

Dopamine [Intropin], the "D" in the mnemonic LEAD, is the least complex molecule of the catecholamines dopamine, norepinephrine, and epinephrine. It is used to treat hemodynamic hypotension. Given by IV microdrip pump and titrated to the patient's BP, it must be monitored closely. MAOIs increase available catecholamines in the synapse, so patients on MAOIs receive only one-tenth the regular dosage. At the lowest effective dose dopamine dilates the renal vasculature. Heart rate and

---

* Life-threatening side effect.

contractility increase with a corresponding dose increase, until finally, there is vasoconstriction. Dopamine reverses peristalsis and can cause nausea, vomiting, angina, headache, and, paradoxically, hypotension.

Off Label: acute renal failure, barbiturate intoxication, cirrhosis, hepatorenal syndrome.

Drug Interactions: Increased alpha-adrenergic effects with MAOIs, ergot alkaloids, furazolidone. Guanethidine and phenytoin may decrease dopamine action. Alpha blockers antagonize peripheral vasoconstriction. Beta blockers block cardiac effects. Hypertension and ventricular arrhythmias risk with cyclopropane and halothane.

Incompatibilities

Solution/Additive: aminophylline, amphotericin B, ampicillin, cephalothin, penicillin G, sodium bicarbonate.

Y-site: acyclovir, aminophylline, amphotericin B, sodium bicarbonate.

Side Effects

Nervous System: angina, arrhythmias—aberrant conduction/bradycardia/ectopics/tachycardia/widened QRS, dyspnea, headache, hypertension/hypotension, nausea/vomiting, palpitations, vasoconstriction—elevated diastolic.

Endocrine System: (Pregnancy Category C) azotemia.

Immune System: gangrene.* With extravasation: necrosis/sloughing.

Dosage: Shock: IV 2–5 µg/kg/min in 250 mL of D5W. Increase gradually up to 20–50 µg/kg/min. Titrate to vital signs. Renal failure: IV 2–5 µg/kg/min.

Epinephrine [Bronkaid Mist, Epi-E-Zpen, Epinephrine Pediatric, EpiPen Auto-Injector, Primatene Mist Suspension], epinephrine bitartrate [Asthma-Haler, Bronkaid Mist Suspension, Bronitin Mist Suspension, Epitrate, Medihaler-Epi, Primatene Mist Suspension], epinephrine hydrochloride [Adrenalin Chloride, Bronkaid Mistometer, Dysne-Inhal, Epifrin, Glaucon], epinephrine, racemic [AsthmaNefrin, Dey-Dose Epinephrine, microNefrin], epinephryl borate [Epinal, Eppy/N]. Epinephrine, the "E" in the LEAD drugs, is used to treat ventricular fibrillation and standstill. Epinephrine, the most complex of the three catecholamines, increases the amplitude in atrial fibrillation, making the heart more responsive to cardioversion. It is used in CPR for alpha stimulation, to raise diastolic pressure in the aorta and increase myocardial perfusion. Characteristic of the catecholamines, epinephrine will increase the need for oxygen. It has ophthalmic uses. In addition, it may be added to local anesthetics to decrease local bleeding, eg, in dentistry. Epinephrine is also used

to override the immune response in asthma and anaphylactic shock. Epinephrine affects both alpha and beta receptors.

Drug Interactions: Possible increased hypotension in circulatory collapse or hypotension caused by phenothiazines. Alpha and beta blockers block its actions. Increased toxicity with other adrenergics. Cardiac irritability with general anesthetics.

Incompatibilities

Solution/Additive: aminophylline, cephapirin, hyaluronidase, mephentermine, sodium bicarbonate, warfarin.

Y-site: aminophylline, sodium bicarbonate.

Side Effects

Nervous System: arrhythmias—tachycardia/ventricular fibrillation,* bladder—retention, CVA,* dizziness, dyspnea, headache, hypertension, insomnia, nausea/vomiting, pallor, palpitations, pain—precordial, psyche—altered perceptions and thought/anxiety/fear/psychosis, syncope, tremors, weakness.

Endocrine System: (Pregnancy Category C) blood glucose—transient elevations, metabolic acidosis, serum lactic acid—elevated, sweating.

Immune System: edema—bronchial/pulmonary,* MI,* necrosis—with repeated injections

Dosage: Anaphylaxis: SC 0.1–0.5 mL of 1:1000 q10–15 min prn. IV 0.1–0.25 mL of 1:1000 q10–15min. Cardiac arrest: IV 0.5–1 mg q5min. Intracardiac: 0.1–1 mg. Asthma: SC 0.1–0.5 mL of 1:1000 q20min–4h. Inhalation: 1 inhalation q4h prn. Glaucoma: 1–2 gtt 0.25–2% solution qd or bid.† Ocular mydriasis, nasal hemostasis: 1–2 gtt 0.1% ophthalmic or 0.1% nasal solution.† Topical hemostasis: 1:50,000–1000 or 1:500,000–1:50,000 mixed with a local anesthetic.

Note: Epinephrine can also be administered through an endotracheal tube or injected into the heart muscle, though this last procedure can cause coronary artery laceration, pneumothorax, and even cardiac tamponade.

Isoproterenol hydrochloride [Isuprel] mimics the sympathetic nervous system, affecting beta-1 and beta-2 receptors. Beta-2 receptors dilate blood vessels in skeletal muscles and dilate the bronchi. Isoproterenol is the antidote to the calcium channel blocker verapamil. Because isoproterenol is not a vasopressor, it is not used in cardiac arrest; however, its bronchodilating property makes it useful in the treatment of asthma.

Drug Interactions: Isoproterenol can interact with the MAOIs or oxytocin to increase BP.

---

* Life-threatening side effect.

† Eye related.

Incompatibilities

Solution/Additive: aminophylline, sodium bicarbonate.

Side Effects

Nervous System: angina, arrhythmias—tachycardia/ventricular,* BP—unstable, headache, nausea, palpitations, psyche—anxiety/excitement/insomnia/nervousness, taste—bad, tremors.

Endocrine System: (Pregnancy Category C) flushing, sweating.

Immune System: bronchial edema/irritation, buccal irritation, parotid swelling.

Dosage: Sublingual 10–20 mg q3–4h. Not to exceed 60 mg/d. IV 0.02– 0.06 mg bolus, then 5 μg/min infusion. SC 0.15–0.2 mg prn. Bronchospasm: MDI 1–2 inhalations 4–6×/d, to maximum of 6 inhalations in any hour of a 24-h period. IPPB: 0.5 mL of 0.5% solution diluted to 2–2.5 mL with water or saline over 10–20 min up to 5×/d.

Methoxamine hydrochloride [Vasoxyl] acts mainly on alpha-adrenergic receptors to cause peripheral vasoconstriction and a corresponding rise in BP. It may also cause a reflex bradycardia and reduced renal blood flow. Vital signs must be closely monitored.

Drug Interactions: Atropine blocks reflex bradycardia and enhances vasopressor effects. Beta blockers may increase available methoxamine at receptor sites. Hypertensive crisis possible with MAOIs, vasopressin, and ergot alkaloids. Phenothiazines and phentolamine block vasopressor response.

Side Effects

Nervous System: arrhythmias—bradycardia, bladder—urgency, BP—high, headache—severe, paresthesias, restlessness, vomiting—projectile.

Endocrine System: (Pregnancy Category C) sense of coldness.

Immune System: none noted.

Dosage: Hypotension during anesthesia: IM 5–20 mg; IV 3–5 mg slowly. Paroxysmal supraventricular tachycardia: IM 10–20 mg; IV 5–15 mg over 3–5 min.

Midodrine [ProAmatine], an alpha agonist, raises standing, sitting, and supine systolic and diastolic blood pressure by activating alpha-adrenergic receptors in arteriolar and venous vasculature.

Drug Interactions: Increased pressor effects with alpha-adrenergics. Decreased effects with alpha-adrenergic

blocking agents. May enhance or precipitate bradycardia, AV block, or arrhythmia with cardiac glycosides. Supine hypertension possible with fludrocortisone acetate.

Side Effects

Nervous System: bladder—dysuria/frequency/impaired/retention/urgency, headache, hyperesthesia/paresthesia/scalp paresthesia, pain—abdominal/increased pain, piloerection, psyche—anxiety/confusion/nervousness, supine hypertension.

Endocrine System: (Pregnancy Category C) chills, dry mouth, flushing.

Immune System: pruritus/scalp pruritus, rash.

Dosage: PO 10 mg on rising in the morning, midday, and late afternoon, but not later than 6 PM.

Norepinephrine bitartrate [Levarterenol, Levophed, Noradrenalin], more complex than dopamine, is also used for refractory hypotension. It affects alpha receptors and stimulates the beta-1 receptors in the heart. Norepinephrine restores BP in blood transfusion and drug reactions, MI, pheochromocytomectomy, poliomyelitis, septicemia, shock, spinal anesthesia, and sympathectomy. It is used to treat cardiac arrest (as an adjunct drug) and requires constant vital sign monitoring: q2min until stabilized at the desired level, then q5min for the duration of administration. Norepinephrine's effect is rapid and reversible. It is inotropic and chronotropic. Like the other catecholamines, it increases the patient's need for oxygen.

Drug Interactions: Its actions are blocked by alpha and beta blockers. Pressor effects are potentiated by ergot alkaloids, furazolidone, guanethidine, methyldopa, and tricyclic antidepressants.

Incompatibilities

Solution/Additive: aminophylline, amobarbital, whole blood, cephapirin, chlorothiazide, chlorpheniramine, pentobarbital, phenobarbital, phenytoin, secobarbital, sodium bicarbonate, sodium iodide, streptomycin, thiopental.

Side Effects

Nervous System: arrhythmias—reflex bradycardia/fatal arrhythmias,* BP—elevated, dizziness, dyspnea, headache, pallor, palpitations, psyche—anxiety/insomnia/restlessness, tremors, weakness. Overdose/sensitivity: CVA,* convulsions,* headache—severe, hypertension—severe, pain—pharyngeal/retrosternal, vision—blurred/photophobia, vomiting.

Endocrine System: (Pregnancy Category D) Overdose/sensitivity: hyperglycemia, sweating—severe. Prolonged use: edema, plasma volume depletion.

---

* Life-threatening side effect.

Immune System: MI extension,* necrosis at extravasation site. Prolonged use: hemorrhage, necrosis—hepatic*/intestinal/renal.*

Dosage: IV 8–12 µg/min. Titrate to vital signs q2–5 min.

Phenylephrine hydrochloride [Neo-Synephrine], like epinephrine, stimulates both alpha- and beta-adrenergic receptors; however, the beta stimulation is weak. Systolic and diastolic blood pressure is raised as the drug constricts arterioles. This rise in BP can cause a reflex bradycardia. Vital signs must be closely monitored. Long use is precluded because of reduction of renal blood flow. It is used to maintain BP during anesthesia, to treat vascular failure in shock, and to overcome paroxysmal supraventricular tachycardia. Topical use treats rhinitis of the common cold and allergy and sinusitis. It may also be used to treat wide-angle glaucoma. It is a mydriatic in eye examination and surgery and to relieve uveitis.

Drug Interactions: Alpha and beta blockers block its actions. Arrhythmia risk increases with halothane and digoxin. Its pressor actions are increased with ergot alkaloids, guanethidine, reserpine, and tricyclic antidepressants. Oxytocin causes persistent hypertension.

Side Effects

Nervous System: arrhythmias—bradycardia/extrasystoles/tachycardia, BP—elevated, dizziness, dyspnea, headache, lightheadedness, pain—precordial, pallor, palpitation, psyche—anxiety/insomnia, tingling, tremors, severe visceral or peripheral vasoconstriction,* weakness. With eye use: browache, headache, lacrimation, vision—blurred.

Endocrine System: (Pregnancy Category C) sweating.

Immune System: Infiltrated IV site: necrosis. With eye use: allergy. Intranasal: rebound congestion.

Dosage: IM, SC 2–5 mg q10–15min prn. IV per infusion: start with 100–180 µg/min, then 40–60 µg/min; the infusion solution is prepared by diluting 10–20 mg of phenylephrine in 500 mL of IV fluid to create a concentration of 20–40 µg/mL. Ophthalmic: 2.5–10% solution (children 2.5%). Eye examination: 1 gtt prior to exam.† Chronic mydriasis: 1 gtt bid–tid. Vasoconstriction: 0.12–0.15% 2 gtt q3–4h prn.

OTHER USES FOR ADRENERGIC DRUGS

The eyes have adrenergic receptors that decrease aqueous humor production and increase the uveoscleral out-

flow. Adrenergic agonists also inhibit the release of prolactin. In addition, they can relieve muscle spasticity.

Brimonidine tartrate [Alphagan] is an alpha-adrenergic receptor agonist in an ophthalmic solution used to reduce aqueous humor production and increase uveoscleral outflow.

Drug Interactions: None noted.

Side Effects

Nervous System: drowsiness, fatigue, headache, vision—blurring/burning/foreign body sensation/stinging.

Endocrine System: (Pregnancy Category B) hyperemia.

Immune System: allergy, conjunctive follicles, pruritus.

Dosage: Ophthalmic: 1 gtt affected eye tid approximately 8 h apart.†

Cabergoline [Dostinex] is an antiparkinsonian agent described on page 50.

Tizanidine hydrochloride [Zanaflex] is an alpha-2-adrenergic receptor agonist. It reduces muscle spasticity by increasing presynaptic inhibition of motor neurons.

Drug Interactions: Effect of acetaminophen delayed. Increased effect with alcohol. Increased levels with oral contraceptives.

Side Effects

Nervous System: arrhythmias—bradycardia, asthenia, bladder—frequency, bowel—constipation/diarrhea/flatulence/impaction, dizziness, dyskinesia, dyspepsia, dysphagia, hypotension, migraine, pain—abdominal/back, psyche—nervousness/somnolence, speech disorder, syncope, vision—blurred, vomiting.

Endocrine System: (Pregnancy Category C) cholelithiasis, dry mouth, fever, flushing, sweating.

Immune System: flu syndrome, infection, pharyngitis, rash, rhinitis, SGPT/ALT—increased, UTI.

Dosage: PO. Start with 4 mg in a single dose to relieve spasticity. Increase gradually in 2- to 4-mg steps to optimum effect. (Maximum: 3 doses or 36 mg/24 hr.) Effect peaks at 1–2 h and dissipates between 3 and 6 h.

CATECHOLAMINES AND MIGRAINE

Migraine headaches appear to be the result of dilated blood vessels in the head. Though the cause is not clearly understood, in theory an ischemic event triggers the vasodilation and inflammation of cerebral vessels and resultant pain. Several neurotransmitters may be involved,

* Life-threatening side effect.
† Eye related.

including norepinephrine, epinephrine, prostaglandins, and serotonin. Platelets release serotonin into the bloodstream, and serotonin appears to be the main culprit in migraine headaches (Beckett, 1997). Although new drugs that counter serotonin's actions have become available, vasoconstricting drugs are frequently prescribed for migraines to counter the vasodilation.

Ergotamine tartrate [Ergomar], closely related to ergonovine [Ergotrate], an ergot derivative, is specific for the treatment and relief of migraine headache.

Drug Interactions: Possibility of additive vasoconstrictor effects with high doses of beta-adrenergic blockers. Erythromycin, troleandomycin may cause severe peripheral vasospasm.

Dosage: PO, SL 1–2 mg at onset of headache. Repeat q30–60min, then qh until headache is relieved; not to exceed 6 mg/24 h or 10 mg/wk. Spray form: 1 inhalation. If no relief in 5 min, repeat; maximum: 6 inhalations/24 h or 15/wk.

Side Effects

Nervous System: aftertaste—unpleasant, angina, arrhythmias—bradycardia/tachycardia, ataxia, bowel—diarrhea, claudication—intermittent, convulsions, dizziness, drowsiness, headache, hyper-/hypotension, nausea/vomiting, numbness, pain—abdominal/muscle/precordial, paresthesias, psyche—agitation/delirium/insomnia, pulse absence in extremities, Raynaud's phenomenon.

Endocrine System: (Pregnancy Category X) sweating.

Immune System: gangrene of digits/ears/nose/part of tongue.

Dosage: PO 1–2 mg followed by 1–2 mg q30min until headache ends or to a maximum of 6 mg/24 h or 10 mg/wk. Inhalation: 1 inhalation of 360 µg q5min to maximum of 6 in 24 h or 15/wk. Rectal: 2 mg qh to maximum of 4 mg/24 h or 10 mg/wk.

▶ DRUGS THAT BLOCK CATECHOLAMINE RELEASE, REUPTAKE, OR RECEPTORS

Hypertension may occur when blood volume is essentially normal, but the muscles that line the blood vessels contract, narrowing the vessel lumen, or the vessels have been narrowed by fatty deposits. A primary approach to lower blood pressure is to decrease blood volume by administering diuretics; however, most diuretics actually affect sodium balance. (Because the endocrine system monitors and regulates sodium levels, diuretics are discussed in section II.) Another approach to treating

hypertension is the use of ACE inhibitors; however, ACE is part of a feedback loop for blood volume control in the endocrine system. (This information is also discussed in Section II.) What remains are drugs that lower blood pressure by their effect on the sympathetic nervous system and the muscle cells lining the blood vessels. These drugs have many similar side effects.

Side Effects

Nervous System: arrhythmias—bradycardia/tachycardia, arthralgia, ataxia, bladder—frequency, bowel—constipation/diarrhea, dizziness, drowsiness, dyspepsia, dysphagia, dyspnea, edema, fatigue, headache, hypotension—orthostatic, myalgia, nausea/vomiting, pain—chest, psyche—agitation/depression/insomnia, vision—blurred, sexual dysfunction, taste changes.

Endocrine System: (Pregnancy: Category C) dry mouth, edema.

Immune System: possible allergy.

ALPHA-ADRENERGIC BLOCKERS

Under normal conditions the vasomotor center continuously maintains vascular tone throughout the body via the sympathetic nervous system. It is under the control of higher brain structures and responds immediately to excitatory or inhibitory impulses. In turn it increases or decreases heart rate and vascular tone. Norepinephrine is the neurotransmitter secreted at the endings of the vasoconstrictor nerves to constrict blood vessels, acting specifically on the alpha receptors of vascular smooth muscle. Any muscle activity is perceived as stress in the vasomotor center, whether it is caused by strenuous exercise or fight/flight responses. Interpretation of environmental stimuli is done by higher brain centers. The task of the vasomotor center is strictly stimulation of cardiovascular muscle to respond to normal and extraordinary requirements (Guyton, 1996). The alpha-adrenergic blocker drugs lower blood pressure by blocking alpha receptors, as their name implies.

Clonidine hydrochloride [Catapres], an alpha-adrenergic blocker, is used to treat hypertensive crisis, and in psychiatric setting it is used to treat the cardiovascular effects of drug detoxification. Clonidine initially constricts vessels by stimulating peripheral alpha-adrenergic receptors, but its action on the brain's vasocenter alpha-2 receptors ultimately decreases sympathetic stimulation of cardiovascular organs.

Drug Interactions: Other CNS depressants increase clonidine's depressant action, and tricyclic antidepressants may decrease its antihypertensive action.

Side Effects

Nervous System: arrhythmias—bradycardia/ECG changes/tachycardia, ataxia, bowel—constipation/diarrhea/flatulence/pseudoobstruction, dizziness, drowsiness, dyspnea, fatigue, headache, hypotension—postural (mild), impotence/loss of libido, nausea/vomiting, pain—abdominal, paresthesias, psyche—agitation/anxiety/behavior changes/depression/vivid dreams/hallucination/insomnia/nervousness/nightmares/restlessness, Raynaud's phenomenon, sedation, taste changes. Withdrawal: Rapid increase in BP with rapid withdrawal. Rebound hypertension may occur within 12–18 h of stopping the medication.

Endocrine System: (Pregnancy Category C) dry mouth, edema—peripheral, flushing, sodium retention/weight gain, sweating, vision—dry eyes.

Immune System: hair thinning, hyperbilirubinemia, pruritus, psoriasis exacerbation, rash.

Dosage: PO. Start with 0.1 mg bid or tid; increase by 0.1–0.2 mg/d as needed to control hypertension to maximum of 2.4 mg/d. Transdermal: 0.1-mg patch once q7d; may increase by 0.1 mg q1–2 wk.

Guanabenz acetate [Wytensin], an alpha-2-adrenergic agonist, interferes with sympathetic nervous system messages from the bulbar area to decrease peripheral resistance and thus relax vessels. Guanabenz is also used for opiate withdrawal.

Drug Interactions: CNS depression compounded by alcohol and other CNS depressants. Tricyclic antidepressants may reduce its antihypertensive actions.

Side Effects

Nervous System: abdominal discomfort, aches—muscles/extremities, ataxia, arrhythmias—various, bladder—frequency, bowel—constipation/diarrhea, dizziness, drowsiness, dyspnea, headache, impotence/loss of libido, nausea/vomiting, pain—chest/epigastric, palpitations, psyche—anxiety/depression/sleep disturbances, sedation, taste changes, vision—blurred, weakness. Overdosage: bradycardia, hypotension, irritability, lethargy, miosis, nervousness, somnolence, unusual fatigue/weakness.

Endocrine System: (Pregnancy Category C) dry mouth, edema.

Immune System: nasal congestion, pruritus, rash.

Dosage: PO 4–32 mg bid. Opiate withdrawal: 4 mg bid or qid.

Methyldopa [Aldomet] is metabolized to α-methyl norepinephrine. As a synthetic neurotransmitter, methyldopa stimulates the central alpha receptors that de-

crease sympathetic transmission from the CNS and is used to treat hypertension and preeclampsia.

Drug Interactions: It potentiates other antihypertensive drugs and tolbutamide. It makes lithium and haloperidol more toxic.

Incompatibilities

Solution/Additive: amphotericin B, methohexital, verapamil.

Y-site: fat emulsion.

Side Effects

Nervous System: abdominal distention, arrhythmias—bradycardia, bowel—constipation/diarrhea, dizziness, drowsiness, dyspnea, fatigue, headache, hypotension—postural, impotence/loss of libido, nausea/vomiting, parkinsonism, psyche—amnesia-like syndrome/concentration impairment/decreased mental acuity/depression/mild psychosis/nightmares/restlessness, sedation, sluggishness, syncope, vertigo, weakness. Paradoxic hypertensive reaction, especially with IV administration.

Endocrine System: (Pregnancy Category C) dry mouth, fever (with allergy) gynecomastia, hypothermia with large doses, lactation, malabsorption syndrome, sodium retention/weight gain.

Immune System: direct Coombs'—positive common (especially in African-Americans), eosinophilia, flu-like symptoms, granulocytopenia,* granulomatous skin lesions, hepatic necrosis,* hepatitis, jaundice, liver function tests—abnormal, lupus/rheumatoid factors—test positive, lymphadenopathy, nasal stuffiness, sialoadenitis, skin eruptions, tongue—sore or black, ulcerations—soles of feet.

Dosage: PO 250 mg bid or tid; may increase to maximum of 3 g/d in divided doses. IV 250–500 mg q6h over 30–60 min to maximum of 1 g q6h.

Phenoxybenzamine hydrochloride [Dibenzyline] has actions and side effects similar to those of phentolamine. It is used in the treatment of pheochromocytoma, but its therapeutic effects may not manifest for several weeks.

Off Label: Adjunctive treatment of shock, hypertensive crisis, to improve circulation in peripheral vasospastic conditions.

Side Effects

Nervous System: arrhythmias—tachycardia, dizziness, drowsiness, eyelids—droop, fainting, headache, hypotension—postural, lethargy, psyche—confusion, sedation, sexual dysfunction, shock,* tiredness, weakness. Large doses: CNS stimulation.

---

* Life-threatening side effect.

Endocrine System: (Pregnancy Category C) dry mouth.

Immune System: allergic contact dermatitis, nasal congestion.

Dosage: PO. Start with 5–10 mg bid. Increase by 10 mg every few days up to 60 mg (even higher for some patients). A pulse over 120 may also require a beta blocker.

Phentolamine mesylate [Regitine] IV and IM is used for the hypertensive crisis of MAOI interaction with the amino acid tyramine or for withdrawal from clonidine. It blocks alpha-2 receptors from an excess of catecholamines. In addition, it is used to treat the hypertensive crisis of pheochromocytoma (chromaffin cell tumors of the adrenal medulla that secrete norepinephrine and epinephrine) and counter vessel constriction caused by catecholamines. The onset is slow; the effect long-lasting.

Off Label: Prevention of dermal necrosis and sloughing following IV administration or extravasation of norepinephrine.

Side Effects

Nervous System: angina, arrhythmias—tachycardia and others, bowel—diarrhea, cerebrovascular spasm, dizziness, hypotension—orthostatic/also acute and prolonged, nausea/vomiting, pain—abdominal, shock-like state,* weakness.

Endocrine System: (Pregnancy Category C) flushing.

Immune System: conjunctival infection, MI,* nasal stuffiness, peptic ulcer exacerbation.

Dosage: IM/IV 2–5 mg q5min until BP is brought under control. To prevent necrosis when administering norepinephrine add 10 mg/L phentolamine to the fluid containing norepinephrine. Extravasation: 5–10 mg/10 mL 0.9% NaCl into affected area within 12 h of incident. Test for pheochromocytoma: IM/IV 5 mg.

Prazosin hydrochloride [Minipress] blocks postsynaptic alpha-1-adrenergic receptors and dilates arterial and venous systems. BP drops and cardiac output increases. To avoid orthostatic hypotension, the patient should take the first dose at bedtime.

Drug Interactions: Hypotensive effects are increased by other hypotensive agents.

Side Effects

Nervous System: abdominal discomfort/pain, angina, arrhythmias—tachycardia, arthralgia, bladder—frequency/incontinence, bowel—constipation/diarrhea, dizziness, drowsiness, dyspnea, edema, headache, hypotension—postural, nausea/vomiting, palpitations,

paresthesia, psyche—depression/insomnia/nervousness, sexual dysfunction—impotence/priapism (especially with sickle cell anemia), syncope, vertigo, vision—blurred.

Endocrine System: (Pregnancy Category C) BUN—increased, dry mouth, edema, serum uric acid—increased, sweating.

Immune System: alopecia, epistaxis, leukopenia—transient, lichen planus, nasal congestion, pruritus, sclerae-reddened, tinnitus.

Dosage: PO. Start with 1 mg hs, then 1 mg bid to a maximum 20 mg qid.

Tamsulosin hydrochloride [Flomax] causes smooth muscle relaxation in the prostate gland by alpha-1A-adrenoreceptor blockade. Benign prostatic hypertrophy has two components: static and dynamic. The static component is the proliferation of smooth muscle cells. The dynamic component is the increase in muscle tone of the smooth muscle cells of the prostate and bladder. Tamsulosin relaxes those muscle cells and improves urine flow.

Drug Interactions: Levels increased with cimetidine.

Side Effects

Nervous System: asthenia, bowel—diarrhea, cough increase, dizziness, nausea, pain—back, psyche—insomnia/somnolence, sexual function—ejaculation abnormal/libido decrease, vision—blurred.

Endocrine System: (Pregnancy Category B) none noted.

Immune System: infection, pharyngitis, rhinitis, sinusitis, tooth disorder.

Dosage: PO 0.4 mg qd 0.5 h after the same meal each day. May increase to 0.8 qd after 2–4 wk if needed.

BETA BLOCKERS

Just as atropine-like drugs block acetylcholine in the parasympathetic nervous system, there are drugs to block sympathetic nervous system receptor sites. Beta blockers stabilize cell membranes by blocking adrenergic receptors and preventing passage of the action potential. These beta-adrenergic blockers or, more simply, beta blockers, are used to treat essential hypertension and other conditions caused by the catecholamines of the sympathetic nervous system, eg, open-angle glaucoma, stage fright, anxiety, migraine headaches, cardiac responses to thyrotoxicosis, hypertrophic subaortic stenosis, supraventricular arrhythmias, anginas (except Prinzmetal's), and tachyarrhythmias of digitoxin. The beta blockers have value in decreasing the mortality rate after myocardial infarction. Beta blockers can also be used for stable chronic ventricular ectopic beats and arrhythmias

* Life-threatening side effect.

during anesthesia. Though beta blockers are fairly safe, pulse and blood pressure should be monitored to maintain the normal range. They must be avoided in COPD, bronchospasm, bradycardia, CHF, cardiogenic shock, and second- and third-degree block. In addition, beta blockers mask the symptoms of hypoglycemia.

Drug Interactions: Beta blockers must not be used with verapamil or nifedipine. They are not for use with MAOIs and can potentiate the bradycardia of digitalis.

Side Effects

Nervous System: arrhythmias—bradycardia/dysrhythmias, bronchospasm,* CHF, depression, diarrhea, dizziness, drowsiness, dyspnea, fatigue, headache, hypotension, insomnia, myalgia, nausea/vomiting, pain—legs, sexual ability—decrease.

Endocrine System: (Pregnancy Category C) may mask signs of hypoglycemia.

Immune System: pulmonary edema.

Atenolol [Tenormin] is long-acting and cardioselective. It may be used alone or with a diuretic to treat hypertension. It is also used in the treatment of angina and MI.

Off Label: Arrhythmias, mitral valve prolapse, pheochromocytoma, thyrotoxicosis, as prophylactic for vascular headaches. Atenolol is used with caution in patients with CHF, COPD, diabetes mellitus, impaired renal function, hyperthyroidism.

Drug Interactions: Anticholinergics cause increased absorption from the GI tract. NSAIDs may decrease hypotensive effects. Atenolol may mask hypoglycemia of insulin and sulfonylureas. It may increase lidocaine levels and toxicity and increase therapeutic/toxic effects of verapamil. Prazosin, terazocine may increase first-dose hypotension.

Side Effects

Nervous System: arrhythmias—bradycardia/dysrhythmias, bronchospasm,* bowel—diarrhea, CHF, dizziness, drowsiness, dyspnea, fatigue, headache, hypotension, lethargy, lightheadedness, nausea/vomiting, pain—legs, psyche—depression/insomnia/mental changes, sexual function—decrease, syncope, vertigo, weakness.

Endocrine System: (Pregnancy Category C) cold extremities may mask signs of hypoglycemia.

Immune System: pulmonary edema.

Dosage: Hypertension and angina: PO 25–50 mg qd to maximum of 100 mg/d. MI: IV 5 mg q5min for 2 doses; start first PO dose 10 min after second IV dose and continue PO as for hypertension schedule.

Metoprolol tartrate [Lopressor] is used in the treatment of mild to severe hypertension, either alone or combined with a thiazide or vasodilator or both. And being cardioselective, it is also used in the treatment of angina. Although it does reduce the mortality risk after MI, it has some life-threatening side effects.

Drug Interactions: Possible decrease in effects with barbiturates and rifampin and increase with cimetidine, methimazole, propylthiouracil, and oral contraceptives. Increased bradycardia with digoxin.

Side Effects

Nervous System: angina, arrhythmias—bradycardia/worsened AV block/AV dissociation/complete heart block,* bowel—constipation/diarrhea/flatulence, bronchospasm—high doses,* cardiac arrest,* CHF, dizziness, dyspepsia, dyspnea, fatigue, headache, intermittent claudication, laryngospasm,* myalgia, pain—gastric/throat, palpitations, psyche—depression/dreaming increase/insomnia, Raynaud's phenomenon.

Endocrine System: (Pregnancy Category C) cold extremities, dry skin, fever, hypoglycemia.

Immune System: agranulocytosis,* eosinophilia, pruritus, rash, thrombocytopenia.

Dosage: Hypertension: PO 100–450 mg qd in divided doses. Angina: PO 50–100 mg qd. MI: IV 5 mg q2min for 3 doses; then PO 50 mg q6h for 48 h, then 100 mg bid.

Nadolol [Corgard] is a nonselective beta-adrenergic blocking agent used to treat hypertension and angina pectoris. It has the convenience of once-a-day dosing. Nadolol has many of metoprolol's side effects, especially life-threatening laryngospasm. Abrupt withdrawal may precipitate MI or thyroid storm.

Drug Interactions: NSAIDs may decrease hypotensive effects. Sulfonylureas, prazosin, terazosin may increase severe hypotensive response to first dose.

Side Effects

Nervous System: arrhythmias—bradycardia/conduction or rhythm disturbances, bronchospasm,* dizziness, fatigue, headache, hypotension—postural, impotence, laryngospasm,* palpitations, paresthesias, psyche—behavior changes, Raynaud's phenomenon, vision—blurred/dry eyes.

Endocrine System: (Pregnancy Category C) dry mouth, dry skin, masks signs of hypoglycemia.

Immune System: rash, pruritus.

Dosage: Angina and hypertension: PO 40 mg qd to maximum of 320 mg/d in divided doses.

---

* Life-threatening side effect.

Pindolol [Visken] is a partial beta agonist–antagonist and has many of the beta blocker side effects, plus life-threatening bronchospasm and agranulocytosis.

Drug Interactions: Hypotensive effect is increased with diuretics and other hypotensive agents. NSAIDs blunt pindolol's effect. Pindolol decreases glyburide's hypoglycemic effect.

Side Effects

Nervous System: arrhythmias—bradycardia, bowel—constipation/diarrhea/flatulence, bronchospasm,* CHF, dizziness, drowsiness, dyspnea, fainting, fatigue, headache, hypotension, impotence/decreased libido, nausea, pain—back/joint, psyche—confusion/insomnia.

Endocrine System: (Pregnancy Category B) masks signs of hypoglycemia.

Immune System: agranulocytosis,* antinuclear antibodies, pulmonary edema.

Dosage: Hypertension: PO 5 mg bid; may increase 10 mg/d q2–3 wk to maximum of 60 mg/d in divided doses. Angina: PO 15–40 mg/d tid or qid.

Propranolol [Inderal], the beta blocker prototype, has uses ranging from cardiovascular to psychiatric. Propranolol is used in the treatment of arrhythmias, MI, angina pectoris, hereditary essential tremor, hypertension (alone or with other agents), pheochromocytoma, tachyarrhythmias associated with digitalis intoxication, anesthesia, and thyrotoxicosis.

Drug Interactions: Decreased clearance and increased effects with cimetidine. Bradycardia with atropine or tricyclic antidepressants. Increased hypotension with phenothiazines. Decreased effects with beta-adrenergic agonists.

Side Effects

Nervous System: angina, arrhythmias—AV heart-block/bradycardia/tachycardia, bowel—constipation/diarrhea/flatulence, bronchospasm,* cardiac stand-still,* CHF—acute,* cramps—abdominal, dizziness, drowsiness, dyspepsia, dyspnea, fatigue—legs, headache, hearing loss/tinnitus, hypotension, insomnia, laryngospasm,* myalgia, nausea/vomiting, paresthesia—hands, psyche—agitation/delusions/depression/hallucinations (visual)/decreased libido/organic brain syndrome (reversible)/psychosis/sleep disturbances/ vivid dreams, Raynaud-like syndrome, syncope, vertigo, vision—disturbances, weakness.

Endocrine System: (Pregnancy Category C) edema, fever, flushing, hyper/hypoglycemia, hypocalcemia in hyperthyroidism, masks signs of hypoglycemia, weight gain.

Immune System: agranulocytosis,* alopecia (reversible), cheilostomatitis, colitis—ischemic, hyperkeratoses, lupus-like reaction, pancreatitis, thrombosis—mesenteric arterial.

Dosage: Angina: PO 10–20 mg bid or tid to maximum of 320 mg/d in divided doses. Arrhythmias: PO 10–30 mg tid or qid. IV 1–3 mg not to exceed 1 mg/min for acute conditions. (A second dose may be given after 2 min and subsequent doses q4h.) Migraine prophylaxis: PO 80 mg/d in divided doses. Hypertension: PO 160–480 mg qd divided doses.

Timolol maleate [Blocadren, Timoptic, others] is a long-acting antihypertensive, antianginal, and antiarrhythmic that blocks beta-1 and beta-2 receptors. It shares many of the beta blocker side effects, but not the most serious, except for bronchospasm. It is also used as an ophthalmic drug to reduce aqueous humor formation in the treatment of aphakic glaucoma, open-angle glaucoma, secondary glaucoma, and ocular hypertension.

Drug Interactions: Effects potentiated by other antihypertensive drugs and hypotensive effects may be antagonized by NSAIDs.

Side Effects

Nervous System: arrhythmias—AV heart block/bradycardia, bronchospasm,* CHF,* dizziness, drowsiness, dyspepsia, dyspnea, fatigue, headache, hypotension, lethargy, nausea, palpitations, peripheral vascular insufficiency—aggravated, psyche—anxiety/confusion/depression/dissociation, syncope, weakness.

Endocrine System: (Pregnancy Category C) anorexia, edema, fever, hypoglycemia, hypokalemia.

Immune System: rash, urticaria. Ophthalmic: irritation—conjunctivitis/blepharitis/keratitis/superficial punctate keratopathy.

Dosage: Hypertension: PO 10–60 mg qd in divided doses. Angina: PO 15–45 mg in 3 divided doses. Ophthalmic: 1 gtt 0.25 or 0.5% solution bid. Apply gel qd.†

Propranolol and timolol, being water soluble, do not cross the BBB readily, resulting in fewer CNS problems.

INHIBITION OF ALPHA AND BETA RECEPTORS

Amiodarone hydrochloride [Cordarone, Amio-Aqueous], a fairly safe drug, inhibits both alpha- and beta-adrenergic stimulation. It is used to treat ventricular tachyrhythmia by dilating coronary arteries and prolonging the action

---

* Life-threatening side effect.

† Eye related.

potential and, thus, the refractory period of both the atrial and ventricular muscles.

Drug Interactions: Increases digoxin levels. Increases effects, therapeutic and toxic, of disopyramide, flecainide, lidocaine, procainamide, quinidine. Oral anticoagulant effect is enhanced. Amiodarone may potentiate AV block, sinus bradycardia, or sinus arrest. Amiodarone may increase cyclosporine levels and toxicity. Levels may be increased by cimetidine.

Incompatibilities

Solution/Additive: sodium bicarbonate.

Y-site: aminophylline, cefamandole, cefazolin, heparin, mezlocillin, sodium bicarbonate.

Side Effects

Nervous System: arrhythmias—AV block/bradycardia/left ventricular dysfunction/sinus arrest*/worsened ventricular arrhythmias,* cardiogenic shock,* CHF, bowel—constipation, dizziness, dry cough, dyskinesia and abnormal gait, dyspnea, fatigue, headache, hypotension (with IV), muscle—numbness/tingling, nausea/ vomiting, paresthesias, vision—blurred.

Endocrine System: (Pregnancy Category D) fever, fetal hyper-/hypothyroidism, hyper-/hypothyroidism, increased liver enzymes.

Immune System: alveolitis, corneal microdeposits, fibrosis—pulmonary, photosensitivity, pigment—slate blue, pneumonitis rash.

Dosage: PO: load with 800–1600 mg/d in 1–2 doses for 1–3 wk, then 400–600 mg qd or bid. IV: load with 150 mg over 10 min; follow with 360 mg over next 6 h. To convert from IV to PO: PO after less than 1 wk, 800–1600 mg. If 1–3 wk give 600–800 mg PO. If > 3 wk, give 400 mg PO.

Carvedilol [Coreg] has both alpha- and beta-blocking activity and is used to treat CHF. It decreases cardiac output, reduces exercise- or isoproterenol-induced tachycardia, reduces reflex orthostatic hypotension, causes vasodilation, and reduces peripheral vascular resistance.

Drug Interactions: Decreased levels with rifampin. Increased levels with cimetidine. Increased levels of digoxin.

Side Effects

Nervous System: arrhythmia, bowel—diarrhea, bradycardia, dizziness, dyspnea, fatigue, hypotension—postural, pain—abdominal/back, psyche—insomia/somnolence.

Endocrine System: (Pregnancy Category C), edema, hypertriglyceridemia.

Immune System: bladder infection, pharyngitis, rhinitis, thrombocytopenia, viral infection.

Dosage: PO. Start with 6.25 mg bid if patient tolerates with a standing systolic pressure about 1 hr after dosing; maintain dosage for 7–14 d. Increase to 12.5 mg bid if needed based on trough blood pressure. May increase after 1–2 wk to 25 mg bid if tolerated and needed. Not to exceed 50 mg/d. Reduce dosage if P is less than 55.

Labetalol hydrochloride [Normodyne] relieves hypertension by selectively blocking alpha-1 receptors and nonselectively blocking beta receptors.

Drug Interactions: Its bioavailability is increased with cimetidine. It also blunts nitroglycerin's reflex tachycardia.

Side Effects

Nervous System: angina, arrhythmias—bradycardia/others after IV, bladder—difficult voiding/retention, bowel—constipation/diarrhea, bronchospasm,* cholestasis, cramps—muscle, dizziness, dyspepsia, dyspnea, fatigue, headache, hypotension—postural, hypertension—paradoxical (pheochromocytoma), impotence/ejaculation/failure/Peyronie's, loss of libido, malaise, myalgia, nausea/vomiting, numbness—after IV, pain—IV site, palpitations, paresthesias, psyche—depression/drowsiness/nightmares/sleep disturbances, vision disturbances, syncope, taste changes.

Endocrine System: (Pregnancy Category C) dry eyes/mouth, edema—pedal/peripheral, extremities—cold, flushing, serum transaminase—increase, sweating.

Immune System: antimitochondrial antibodies, positive antinuclear antibodies, nasal stuffiness, pruritus, rash, rhinorrhea, SLE syndrome, toxic myopathy.

Dosage: PO 100 mg bid and increase by 100 mg bid over 2 or 3 d depending on standing BP; maintain on 200–400 mg bid. IV 20 mg slowly over 2 min; may be followed in 10-min intervals with 40- to 80-mg injections q10min to a total of 300 mg. May be diluted in 160 mL IV fluid and administered at 2 mL/min (2 mg/min) as a slow continuous infusion up to 300 mg total dose.

CARDIOVASCULAR DRUGS THAT BLOCK CATECHOLAMINE RELEASE OR REUPTAKE

Catecholamines, as neurotransmitters of the sympathetic nervous system, speed the heart, constrict vascular muscle, and raise blood pressure. Although their actions are intended to be life-enhancing, they can cause life-threatening cardiovascular conditions. Such conditions are often treated with drugs that block the action of catecholamines. Drugs that block catecholamines are com-

---

* Life-threatening side effect.

monly called adrenergic antagonists, blocking agents, or sympatholytics to name a few terms.

Bretylium tosylate [Bretylol] is used to treat ventricular tachycardia and fibrillation when other treatments, such as lidocaine and cardioversion, fail. Bretylium blocks norepinephrine release and reuptake, raises the fibrillation threshold, and decreases the difference in the refractory period between healthy and ischemic heart tissue. This action probably prevents takeover by ectopic ischemic tissue beats. Bretylium cannot be given PO because its absorption from the GI tract is unreliable. Its slow onset of action precludes use as a first-line antiarrhythmic drug.

Drug Interactions: Its antiarrhythmic action may be antagonized by lidocaine, procainamide, propranolol, and quinidine. These same drugs may increase hypotension. Digitalis toxicity may worsen arrhythmias.

Incompatibilities

Solution/Additive: dobutamine, nitroglycerin, phenytoin.

Y-site: phenytoin.

Side Effects

Nervous System: arrhythmias—bradycardia/increased PVCs*/digitalis-induced arrhythmias exacerbated, dizziness, faintness, hypertension—transitory, hypotension, lightheadedness, nausea/vomiting, respiratory depression,* syncope.

Endocrine System: (Pregnancy Category C) none noted.

Immune System: none noted.

Dosage: IV: First bolus 5 mg/kg; then 10 mg/kg; maximum of 30 mg over 15- to 30-min intervals; may repeat in 6 h. Also by continuous infusion at 1–2 mg/min. IM 5–10 mg/kg; repeat in 1–2 h if arrhythmia persists; maintain on 5–10 mg/kg q6–8h.

Guanadrel sulfate [Hylorel] depletes norepinephrine (NE) by blocking its release from the adrenal medulla and adrenergic nerve endings. Guanadrel has most of the side effects of norepinephrine-depleting drugs. Most of its side effects are dose related.

Drug Interactions: Alcohol increases orthostatic hypotension and sedation. Reserpine may intensify orthostatic hypotension and bradycardia. Guanadrel may enhance the actions of epinephrine, norepinephrine, methoxamine. Its hypotensive action may be antagonized by ephedrine, MAOIs, phenothiazines, tricyclic antidepressants.

Side Effects

Nervous System: bladder—frequency/nocturia/retention/urgency, bowel—constipation/diarrhea/increased stools, drowsiness, fatigue, headache, hypotension—orthostatic (morning and day), indigestion, musculoskeletal—aches/pains, nausea/vomiting, pain—abdominal (and distress)/chest, palpitations, paresthesias, psyche—confusion/depression/ other psychological problems/sleep disorders, sexual dysfunction, shortness of breath—with exercise or rest, tremors, vision—disturbances, weakness.

Endocrine System: (Pregnancy Category B) anorexia, dry mouth, thirst weight gain/loss—excessive.

Immune System: glossitis, hematuria, musculoskeletal inflammation, nasal stuffiness.

Dosage: PO 5 mg bid. May increase to maximum of 75 mg/d in 2–4 divided doses.

Guanethidine sulfate [Ismelin] blocks norepinephrine reuptake so it cannot be recycled and depletes its stores. Decreased norepinephrine in the synapse decreases the postganglionic neuron action potentials. The sympathetic responses of vasoconstriction, increased heart rate, and cardiac output are blocked; however, the endocrine system interprets the decreased cardiac output and resulting drop in blood volume being filtered by the kidneys as a real loss of blood. In response, the endocrine system causes renal retention of sodium and thus, water, to compensate for the drop. A diuretic is needed to remove the extra sodium and decrease the load the heart must pump.

Drug Interactions: Tricyclic antidepressants and amphetamines compete with guanethidine for entry into the neuron; however, guanethidine does not easily cross the BBB. Hypotensive action is intensified by alcohol, diuretics, other hypotensive agents, levodopa. MAOIs may antagonize hypotensive effects. Norepinephrine, pseudoephedrine, other decongestants, phenothiazines block hypotensive activity.

Side Effects

Nervous System: arrhythmias—bradycardia/complete heart block/sick sinus syndrome, bladder—incontinence/nocturia/urinary retention, bowel—severe diarrhea, CHF, edema, fatigue, hypotension—orthostatic/exertion, impotence/ejaculation impeded, myalgia, nausea/vomiting, paresthesias—chest, psyche—depression, vision—blurred/ptosis.

Endocrine System: (Pregnancy Category C) BUN—increase, edema/weight gain.

Immune System: asthma, congestion—nasal, polyarteritis nodosa.

---

* Life-threatening side effect.

Dosage: PO 10 mg qd to start. Maximum: 300 mg/d.

Reserpine [Serpasil] depletes catecholamines throughout the sympathetic nervous system. Such global actions lead to decreased cardiac output and vasodilation, but also to depression, which can be so severe as to lead to suicide. It can also cause EPS, nausea, and diarrhea.

Drug Interactions: Reserpine is not used with digoxin, guanethidine, hydralazine, MAOIs, quinidine, thiazides.

Side Effects

Nervous System: angina, appetite increase, arrhythmias—AV conduction increase/bradycardia, bladder—dysuria, bowel—diarrhea, colic—biliary, CHF, cramps—abdominal, dizziness, drowsiness, dyspepsia, edema, EPS, headache, hypotension—orthostatic, muscle ache, myalgia, nausea/vomiting, psyche—anxiety/depression—suicidal ideation/increased dreaming/nightmares, respiratory depression,* sexual dysfunction, vision—blurred/ lacrimation/miosis/ptosis.

Endocrine System: (Pregnancy Category D) appetite increase, breast engorgement, edema, feminization, galactorrhea, gynecomastia, hypothermia, menstrual irregularities, salivation/dry mouth.

Immune System: anemia, bleeding time prolonged, congestion—conjunctival/nasal, epistaxis, peptic ulcer reactivation, rash, thrombocytopenic purpura.

Dosage: PO. Start with 0.5 mg qd. Decrease to 0.1–0.25 mg/d.

▶ CATECHOLAMINES IN THE LIMBIC SYSTEM

FIGHTING, FLEEING, FEEDING, AND SEX: THE LIMBIC SYSTEM AND WILL

People take action or do nothing for only two reasons: the relief of pain and the quest for pleasure and reward, even enduring some pain if the reward is great enough. Emotions and pain are clearly connected and painful stimuli go no farther into the brain than the thalamus at the top of the limbic system, though higher cortical centers do process pain in a cognitive manner. The limbic system, deeply involved in the sensing and relief of pain and the quest for pleasure and reward, with connections to all of the brain, including sensory neurons, places an emotional tag on all sensory input that must pass through it. The limbic system contains reward centers and punishment centers. It is of interest that in animal studies stimulation of punishment centers in the limbic system for 24 h or longer causes the animal to sicken or even die (Guyton, 1996). Without commentary on the treatment of the animal subjects, this information can be

extrapolated to the human experience of prolonged suffering, sickness, and death and the importance of compassionate nursing care.

No response or action can ever be entirely "objective" because the limbic system has the final say on responses as they leave the brain. This mammalian brain contains the structures that cause us to fight, flee, feed, reproduce, and feed and nurture our offspring. The limbic system is the gateway to the mind.

THE LIMBIC SYSTEM AND MEMORY

The hippocampus in the limbic system serves as the gatekeeper of memory and without it we cannot store new memories. Though sometimes painful memories are repressed to protect the psyche, we remember best those events that caused us great pain or pleasure. Preverbal memories from early childhood are encoded in feelings, not words. We are our memories; to lose them causes distress and destroys who we are. ECT, meant to clear up the pain of depression, causes amnesia by affecting the mediotemporal area of the hippocampus. In fact, in the 1980s, L. Squire and S. Zola-Morgan studied patients receiving ECT as part of their research on memory. Perhaps their seminal work was the research that led to their discovery of the specific cells in the hippocampus that make laying down new memories possible. This discovery came from working with an amnesic patient who had suffered decreased cerebral blood perfusion after a coronary artery procedure. (Author's note: As a visitor, working in Zola-Morgan's research laboratory at UCSD, I was privileged to observe the brain of the subject R.B. R.B. had suffered a postoperative bleed following cardiac surgery. At no time was he without oxygen, but the decreased blood flow to his brain destroyed specific cells in the hippocampus, resulting in permanent retrograde amnesia as measured by L. Squire. Zola-Morgan, Squire, and D. Amaral were able to pinpoint the very cells on which we depend to encode memory.)

THE LIMBIC SYSTEM, PAIN, AND EMOTIONS

The twin almond-shaped amygdalae create our fear, rage, and anger, as well as aspects of sexual function in feedback loops with the rest of the limbic system and the rest of the brain. The limbic system nestles over the hypothalamus, which connects to the master gland, the pituitary (Fig. 4–4). It is at this juncture that mind and glandular body meet. Drugs used to treat the emotions, ie, psychiatric conditions, act in the limbic system.

NEUROTRANSMITTERS OF THE LIMBIC SYSTEM

The limbic system uses the same neurotransmitters as the rest of the CNS, and drugs that affect the limbic sys-

---

* Life-threatening side effect.

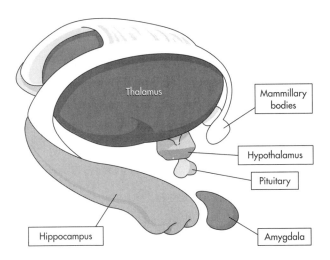

Figure 4–4. The limbic system.

tem can also affect other parts of the CNS or body. For example, treating psychotic conditions by blocking the influence of dopamine on the emotion centers of the brain may tilt the CNS's neurochemistry balance over to the parasympathetic system. Anticholinergics are then used to reestablish a balance. In addition to the catecholamines, the neurochemistry of our emotions includes the monoamine neurotransmitter serotonin (5-hydroxytryptamine [5-HT]), derived from tryptophan. Serotonin-enhancing antidepressants have become useful in treating, not only depression, but other psychiatric conditions as well. The immune system also uses serotonin, storing it in red blood cells for release if they are damaged, to cause vasoconstriction. Serotonin is used by the nervous system to stimulate the viscera to help contract smooth muscle.

▶ DOPAMINE AND PSYCHOSIS

The catecholamine dopamine, an alerting neurotransmitter, serves an important function in the way we experience the world. It helps us to feel adequate and capable. Drugs used to treat thought disorders interfere with dopamine transmission. The thought disorder schizophrenia, with its four characteristic A's—autism, associations, ambivalence, and affect—most defines psychosis with its bizarre thoughts, perseveration of thoughts, flight of ideas, unusual, often unrealistic linking of ideas, and autistic behaviors. The nature of schizophrenia has been debated ever since Eugen Bleuler (1857–1939) established its characteristics. Some argue that the condition is genetic. Seymour Kety, a neuroscientist, was one of the first to posit that schizophrenia has a biologic basis and studied a national population for years. He stated that both nature and nurture play roles in schizophrenia. "You can't have one without the other. They are

both important" (Kety, UCSD, personal communication). Still other experts argue that schizophrenia is not a disease at all, but a response to stress; that the twin studies are flawed; and that the drugs used to treat schizophrenia cause the neurologic changes seen in brain studies. Probably the one thing that can be agreed on is that the debate will continue.

Schizophrenia is considered a psychosis, but not all psychotic conditions are labeled schizophrenia. People can also be psychotically depressed or extremely manic and psychotically euphoric. This tilt toward the extremes of human thought and behavior is what medicine treats with the neuroleptics or antipsychotics. The neuroleptics do not cure schizophrenia; they simply block dopamine receptors found in overabundance in the illness. In the case of the psychotic affective (mood) disturbance, the neuroleptics are used only in the acute state, if at all; the antidepressants or lithium are specific for affective disorders.

Note: *Patients with schizophrenia sometimes feel alarmed when told they are receiving antipsychotic drugs. The nurse might best refer to the drug in question as a "tranquilizer," as tranquilizers are fairly commonplace today, and, after all, the drug is a tranquilizer of sorts.*

▶ TARDIVE DYSKINESIA

Long-term use of the older neuroleptics, in almost all instances, causes an irreversible condition wherein the body fights the drugs' actions by growing new dopamine receptors in unusual sites on the neurons; this condition is called tardive dyskinesia and results in restlessness, unusual gait, and involuntary movements. Because of their side effects, the major tranquilizers are not used for personality disorders, alcoholism, drug abuse, anxiety, or nonpsychotic assaultive behavior. Tardive dyskinesia must not be confused with the early and reversible side effect resulting from a blockade of the motor system pathways' dopamine receptors that resembles Parkinson's disease. Referred to as pseudo-Parkinson's or extrapyramidal symptoms (EPS), this condition is treated with anticholinergics. Some of the newer neuroleptics are less apt to cause tardive dyskinesia.

▶ THE DISCOVERY OF NEUROLEPTICS

In the late 1940s a French Navy surgeon, Henri Laborit, stationed in Tunisia, experimented with antihistamines, looking for drugs to prevent postsurgical shock, caused when the immune system creates fluid shifts in response to trauma. Antihistamines had the anticholinergic action he wanted. Intrigued by the calmness of patients facing major surgery after being medicated with the antihistamine chlorpromazine [Thorazine], a chlorinated form of promazine [Sparine], he suggested it to psychiatrists in Paris (Sneader, 1985). Chlorpromazine calmed thousands of agitated psychotic patients, ending the wild atmosphere of psychiatric hospitals.

Most of the major tranquilizers, or neuroleptics, are variations on a chemical theme that began with the antihistamines. Although antihistamines block histamine receptors, small changes in their molecular structure cause them to affect dopamine and norepinephrine receptors too. Chlorination of the phenothiazine antihistamine promazine [Sparine] led to the antipsychotic drug chlorpromazine. Continued modification, changing the nitrogen atom in chlorpromazine's middle ring, created the thioxanthenes chlorprothixene [Taractan] and thiothixene [Navane]. Psychiatrists have a long list of antipsychotic drugs to choose from, but because of the infinite variety of human responses to drugs, the challenge is to fit the right drug and dosage to the individual's needs.

▶ NEUROLEPTIC SIDE EFFECTS

Given the wide area of influence, the dopaminergic and histamine actions, the neuroleptics have a wide range of potential side effects, which include many of the following.

Nervous System: ataxia, arrhythmias—ECG changes/tachycardia, bladder—frequency/retention, bowel—adynamic ileus*/constipation, cholestatic jaundice, convulsions,* cough reflex—depressed, dizziness, drowsiness, edema—cerebral/idiopathic, EEG changes, EPS, headache, hypotension—orthostatic, insomnia, laryngospasm,* palpitations, psyche—agitation/restlessness, sedation/sleep—bizarre dreams/reduced REM, sexual function—inhibition of ejaculation/decreased libido/priapism, syncope, sudden unexplained death,* tardive dyskinesia, vision—blurred/mydriasis/photophobia, weakness.

Endocrine System: (Pregnancy Category C) anovulation, appetite—increased, dry mouth, edema, galactorrhea, glycosuria, gynecomastia, hirsutism, hypothermia,* hyper-/hypoglycemia, inability to sweat, infertility, menstrual irregularity, neuroleptic malignant syndrome,* pseudopregnancy, weight gain.

Immune System: agranulocytosis,* anaphylaxis,* dermatitis, eczema, fixed drug eruption, muscle necrosis—after IM, pancytopenia*—rare, parotid gland enlargement, peptic ulcer—aggravation, photosensitivity, rash, SLE-like syndrome, thrombocytopenic purpura.

Note: Because people with schizophrenia often dislike the effect that the antipsychotic drugs have on them, they may pretend to take the pills, but hide them in their mouths ("cheek the pills"), only to spit them out later.

*Life-threatening side effect.

The nurse must make a habit of checking the patient's mouth after administering the drug and also checking the paper medicine cups sometimes used to administer drugs, as some people may palm the pills or quickly wad them up in the paper medicine cup. Many of the major tranquilizers come in liquid form to foil patients who refuse to swallow the pills. Their taste is easier to tolerate if mixed with juice. Although they may form a precipitate with some juices, they usually mix well with orange juice.

▶ NEUROLEPTIC DRUG CLASSIFICATION

The neuroleptics are classified in groups according to their chemical structures as follows.

BENZISOXAZOLES

Risperidone [Risperdal] blocks dopamine from locking into D_2 receptors in the limbic system and it also blocks 5-HT$_2$ receptors and alpha-adrenergic receptors in the occipital cortex. It is used to treat the psychotic symptoms of schizophrenia.

Drug Interactions: Carbamazepine may decrease and clozapine may increase risperidone levels. Risperidone may increase the effects of some antihypertensive agents and antagonize the effects of levodopa and dopamine agonists.

Side Effects

Nervous System: arrhythmias—tachycardia, bladder—retention, bowel—constipation, dizziness, drowsiness/sedation, fatigue, headache, psyche—agitation/catatonia/disinhibition/insomnia, vision—transient blurring, weakness.

Endocrine System: (Pregnancy Category C) dry mouth, sweating.

Immune System: elevated liver function tests—AST, ALT.

Dosage: PO 1–6 mg bid. Start with 1 mg bid. With elderly and renal insufficiency: begin with 0.5 mg bid to a maximum of 1.5 mg bid.

BUTYROPHENONES

Haloperidol [Haldol], the most powerful of the neuroleptics when compared with the benchmark drug, chlorpromazine, is especially useful for the emergency treatment and management of agitated psychosis. On the other hand, it is sometimes misused for staff convenience in the "behavior management" of the elderly in some skilled nursing facilities. Haloperidol has the same actions as the other antipsychotic medications, but it is chemically quite different. In addition to the typical side effects, it may also cause life-threatening respiratory depression.

Drug Interactions: CNS depression is increased with other CNS depressants, eg, alcohol and opiates. It may antagonize oral anticoagulant action and increase intraocular pressure with anticholinergics. Methyldopa may precipitate dementia.

Side Effects

Nervous System: arrhythmias—ECG changes/tachycardia, bladder—retention, bowel—constipation/diarrhea, bronchospasm,* extrapyramidal reactions—akathisia/ataxia/dystonia/parkinsonian symptoms/tardive dyskinesia (after long-term use)/tremor, drowsiness, fatigue, headache, hypotension, laryngospasm,* nausea/vomiting, psyche—agitation/anxiety/confusion/depression/euphoria/exacerbation of psychotic symptoms/insomnia/restlessness, respiration—depression*/increased depth, seizures—grand mal,* weakness. With overdosage: hypertension.

Endocrine System: (Pregnancy Category C) anorexia, dry mouth/hypersalivation, galactorrhea, gynecomastia, hyper-/hypoglycemia, hyponatremia, hyperthermia, lactation, menstrual irregularities, neuroleptic malignant syndrome,* sweating.

Immune System: agranulocytosis*—rare, bronchopneumonia, leukopenia—mild/transient, photosensitivity, rash—acneiform/maculopapular.

Dosage: PO 0.2–5 mg bid or tid. Severe psychosis: 3–5 mg bid–tid to maximum of 100 mg/d. IM lactate 2–5 mg; May repeat qh prn until agitation abates, then q4–8h prn. IM decanoate for the unreliable chronic patient: 50–100 mg q4wk. Elderly: PO 0.5–1.5 mg to start, then 2–4 mg daily.

DIBENZOXAZEPINES

Clozapine [Clozaril], developed in Switzerland more than 20 years ago, may help some people with schizophrenia who have not responded to other antipsychotic drugs. A pregnancy category B drug, it also has a high incidence of risk for agranulocytosis and seizures. Patients must have weekly CBCs while on the drug and for 4 wk after it is discontinued. Of benefit is its decreased risk of EPS, which is probably due to its acting more in the limbic system than in striatal dopamine receptors. Specifically, it binds with D_1 and D_2 receptors. The decreased risk of EPS may foretell a decrease in incidence of tardive dyskinesia, a delayed side effect.

Drug Interactions: Anticholinergics increase clozapine's anticholinergic actions. Antihypertensives may potentiate hypotension. CNS depressants increase depressant activity.

Side Effects

Nervous System: arrhythmias—ECG changes/tachycardia, bladder—retention, bowel—constipation, hypotension—orthostatic, nausea, sedation, seizures.*

Endocrine System: (Pregnancy Category B) dry mouth/hypersalivation, fever—transient.

Immune System: agranulocytosis.*

Dosage: Start with 25 mg qd or bid, increasing by 25–50 mg/d. Maintain on 350–450 mg/d to maximum of 900 mg in three divided doses.

Loxapine hydrochloride [Loxitane] works in the limbic system to affect emotional manifestations of schizophrenia. Compared with chlorpromazine it is less sedating, but has similar anticholinergic activity. Patients with a history of seizures may benefit. It has antiemetic activity.

Drug Interactions: Increased effects with alcohol and other CNS depressants. Decreased effects of epinephrine.

Side Effects

Nervous System: akathisia, arrhythmias—tachycardia, bladder—retention, bowel—constipation, dizziness, drowsiness, EEG changes, EPS, hypertension, hypotension—orthostatic, muscle—weakness/staggering gait, paresthesias, sedation, syncope, tardive dyskinesia, vision—blurred/ptosis.

Endocrine System: (Pregnancy Category C) dry mouth, hyperpyrexia, malignant neuroleptic syndrome,* menstrual irregularities, polydipsia, weight gain/loss.

Immune System: dermatitis, facial edema, leukopenia—transient, nasal congestion, photosensitivity, pruritus, tinnitus.

Dosage: PO 10–50 mg divided to maximum of 250 mg/d. IM 12.5–50 mg q4–6h.

DIHYDROINDOLONES

Molindone hydrochloride [Moban] may work in the ascending reticular system. It appears to lower the seizure threshold.

Drug Interactions: None noted.

Side Effects

Nervous System: arrhythmias—tachycardia, bladder—retention, bowel—constipation, drowsiness—transient, EPS—dose related, psyche—euphoria/insomnia, sexual function—premature ejaculation/increased libido, vision—blurred.

---

* Life-threatening side effect.

Endocrine System: (Pregnancy Category C) amenorrhea, dry mouth, galactorrhea, gynecomastia, menses—heavy, neuroleptic malignant syndrome,* weight changes.

Immune System: hepatotoxicity,* nasal congestion, photosensitivity—mild, SLE-like syndrome, xerostomia.

Dosage: PO 50–75 mg/d in 3 or 4 divided doses to maximum of 225 mg/d.

PHENOTHIAZINES

Chlorpromazine [Thorazine, others], the original antihistamine neuroleptic recommended by the French naval surgeon, serves as the benchmark by which all neuroleptics are measured.

Drug Interactions: Absorption of antacids/antidiarrheals is decreased; give 2 h before or after chlorpromazine. CNS depression is increased with depressants. Metabolism is increased with phenobarbital. Increases excitation/hypotension with general anesthetics. With guanethidine/ phenylpropanolamine, antagonizes antihypertensive action and poses possibility of sudden death. With anticonvulsants, may decrease seizure threshold.

Incompatibilities

Solution/Additive: aminophylline, amphotericin B, ampicillin, chloramphenicol, chlorothiazide, cimetidine, dimenhydrinate, heparin, methicillin, methohexital, penicillin G, pentobarbital, phenobarbital, ranitidine, thiopental.

Y-site: aminophylline, amphotericin B, ampicillin, chloramphenicol, chlorothiazide, methicillin, methohexital, penicillin G, phenobarbital, thiopental.

Side Effects

Nervous System: ataxia, arrhythmias—ECG changes/tachycardia, bladder—frequency/retention, bowel—adynamic ileus*/constipation, convulsions, cough reflex—depressed, dizziness, drowsiness, edema—cerebral/idiopathic, EEG changes, EPS, headache, hypotension—orthostatic, insomnia, laryngospasm,* palpitations, psyche—agitation/restlessness/sedation/sleep—bizarre dreams/reduced REM, sexual function—inhibition of ejaculation/decreased libido/priapism, sudden unexplained death,* syncope, tardive dyskinesia, vision—blurred/mydriasis/photophobia, weakness.

Endocrine System: (Pregnancy Category C) anovulation, appetite—increased, dry mouth, edema, galactorrhea, glycosuria, gynecomastia, hirsutism, hypothermia,*

hyper-/hypoglycemia, inability to sweat, infertility, menstrual irregularity, neuroleptic malignant syndrome,* pseudopregnancy, weight gain.

Immune System: agranulocytosis,* anaphylaxis,* dermatitis, eczema, fixed drug eruption, cholestatic jaundice, muscle necrosis—after IM, pancytopenia*—rare, parotid gland enlargement, peptic ulcer—aggravation, photosensitivity, rash, SLE-like syndrome, thrombocytopenic purpura.

Dosage: PO 25–1000 mg/d divided. IM/IV 25–50 mg q4–6h to maximum of 600 mg.

Promazine hydrochloride [Prozine, Sparine], compared with its chlorinated form, is a weak antipsychotic drug, but may be used to reduce the psychotic effects of alcohol withdrawal.

Side Effects

Nervous System: bowel—constipation, drowsiness, hypotension—orthostatic, seizures in susceptible patients, vision—blurred.

Endocrine System: (Pregnancy Category C) none noted.

Immune System: agranulocytosis*—rare, leukopenia, photosensitivity.

Dosage: PO/IM 10–200 mg q4–6h up to 1000 mg/d.

A PHENOTHIAZINE FOR ANALGESIA

As a group the phenothiazines have no analgesic effect. Their value, other than as antipsychotics, is their ataractic, or calming, effect and their anticholinergic actions before and after surgery. One that does have an analgesic action is methotrimeprazine hydrochloride.

Methotrimeprazine hydrochloride [Levoprome] raises the pain threshold as it depresses the CNS and suppresses sensory input. Like chlorpromazine, it sedates and tranquilizes and has antihistamine and anticholinergic actions. It is used for preoperative sedation to relieve anxiety, and in obstetric analgesia because it does not depress respirations.

Drug Interactions: Methotrimeprazine's CNS depressant action is enhanced by other CNS depressants and its anticholinergic actions are intensified with other anticholinergics. Antihypertensives increase its antihypertensive actions and muscle relaxants extend the duration of its muscle relaxant action. Its pressor effects are antagonized by epinephrine.

Incompatibilities

Solution/Additive: ranitidine.

Y-site: heparin.

---

* Life-threatening side effect.

Side Effects

Nervous System: abdominal discomfort, arrhythmias—bradycardia/tachycardia, bladder—dysuria, drowsiness, dizziness, EPS, headache, hypotension—orthostatic with faintness, nausea/vomiting, palpitations, psyche—amnesia/delirium/disorientation/euphoria, respiratory depression,* sedation, speech—slurred, vision—blurred.

Endocrine System: (Pregnancy Category C) fever, chills, dry mouth. Prolonged high dosage: weight gain.

Immune System: bladder—hematuria. Prolonged high dosage: jaundice, severe blood dyscrasias.*

Dosage: IM only, and for no longer than 30 days. Analgesia: 10–20 mg q4–6h prn. Obstetric analgesia: 15–20 mg based on patient's needs. Preoperative: 2–20 mg 45 min to 3 h prior to surgery; if atropine is used, the dose, of course, would be less. Postoperative: 2.5–7.5 mg immediately postop. Then q4–6h prn.

PIPERAZINES

Most psychiatric patients wish that they did not have to take drugs. Long-acting, injectable neuroleptics were developed for people unable or unwilling to take the medications routinely by mouth.

Fluphenazine [Prolixin], in the decanoate or enanthate form, is a long-acting drug that does away with having to remember to take daily medication, especially on an outpatient basis. It is less sedating and hypotensive than similar drugs, but more apt to cause EPS.

Drug Interactions: Like the other antipsychotic drugs, fluphenazine can be potentiated by other CNS depressants, including alcohol.

Side Effects

Nervous System: arrhythmias—tachycardia, bladder—retention/frequency, bowel—constipation/fecal impaction, dizziness, drowsiness, EPS, headache, hyper-/hypotension, nausea, pain—epigastric, psyche—catatonic-like state/depression, sedation, seizures—grand mal,* sexual function—ejaculation inhibition, tardive dyskinesia, vision—blurred.

Endocrine System: (Pregnancy Category C) dry mouth, edema—peripheral, hyperprolactinemia, impaired temperature regulation,* vision—increased IOP.

Immune System: agranulocytosis,* contact dermatitis, cholecystic jaundice, leukopenia—transient, nasal congestion, photosensitivity.

Dosage: Decanoate: SC and IM 12.5–25 mg q1–4wk. Enanthate: SC/IM 25 mg q2wk. Short-acting tabs, elixir, parenteral forms: PO 0.5–10 mg/d divided to maximum of 20 mg/d; HCl: IM 2.5–10 mg/d q6h prn as tolerated to maximum of 10 mg/d.

Perphenazine [Phenazine, Trilafon] exerts antipsychotic action by blocking dopamine receptors. It also acts in the hypothalamus. Perphenazine blocks dopamine in the CTZ to relieve vomiting. Compared with chlorpromazine, it has fewer anticholinergic side effects, less hypotension, but more antiemetic action.

Drug Interactions: Other CNS depressants enhance its CNS depressant action and anticholinergics its anticholinergic action. Barbiturates and anesthetics increase hypotension and excitation.

Incompatibilities

Solution/Additive: midazolam, pentobarbital, thiethylperazine.

Y-site: cefoperazone, midazolam, pentobarbital.

Side Effects

Nervous System: akathisia, arrhythmias—bradycardia/ECG changes/tachycardia, bladder—retention, bowel—adynamic ileus*/constipation, convulsions,* EPS, hypotension—orthostatic, insomnia, laryngospasm,* pain—injection site, sedation, sexual function—inhibition of ejaculation, tardive dyskinesia, vision—blurred/mydriasis.

Endocrine System: (Pregnancy Category C) appetite—increased, dry mouth, galactorrhea, gynecomastia, hyperprolactinemia, menstrual irregularity, sweating—decreased, weight gain.

Immune System: agranulocytosis,* anaphylaxis,* angioneurotic edema, aplastic anemia* or hemolytic anemia, cholestatic jaundice, erythema, itching, liver function tests—abnormal, nasal congestion, thrombocytopenic purpura, urticaria, vision—corneal/lenticular deposits. Injection site: sterile abscess.

Dosage: PO 4–16 mg/d divided to maximum of 64 mg/d. SR 8–32 mg bid to maximum 64 mg/d. IM 5 mg q6h prn to maximum of 30 mg/d. IV 0.5 mg/mL in NS at no more than 1 mg q1–2min or 5 mg slow infusion. Nausea: PO 8–16 mg bid–qid. IM 5 mg q6h to maximum of 15 mg/d.

Trifluoperazine hydrochloride [Stelazine] is used to treat psychotic disorders and some manifestations of anxiety and tension seen in somatic or neurotic conditions.

Drug Interactions: Other CNS depressants increase its CNS depressant actions.

---

* Life-threatening side effect.

Side Effects

Nervous System: arrhythmias—tachycardia, bowel—constipation, cough reflex—depressed, dizziness, drowsiness, EPS, hypotension, psyche—agitation/insomnia, vision—blurred.

Endocrine System: (Pregnancy Category C) dry mouth, galactorrhea, gynecomastia, neuroleptic malignant syndrome,* sweating.

Immune System: agranulocytosis,* photosensitivity, rash, vision—pigmentary retinopathy.

Dosage: PO 1–20 mg/d divided. IM 1–2 mg q4–6h to maximum of 10 mg/d.

PIPERIDINE PHENOTHIAZINES

The goal of medicating schizophrenia is to tailor the drug molecule to the shape of the patient's dopamine receptors, to decrease side effects and increase efficacy. The piperidine derivatives of the phenothiazines offer more sedation than chlorpromazine.

Mesoridazine besylate [Serentil] is used to treat psychosis, but has more antiemetic action and has less frequency of EPS than the parent drug, chlorpromazine.

Drug Interactions: None noted.

Side Effects

Nervous System: arrhythmias—tachycardia, bladder—retention, bowel—constipation, dizziness, EPS, fainting, hypotension—orthostatic, sedation, vision—blurred.

Endocrine System: (Pregnancy Category C) dry mouth.

Immune System: contact dermatitis, nasal congestion.

Dosage: PO 10–50 mg/d divided to maximum of 400 mg/d. IM 25–175 mg/d divided. Hyperactivity: PO 25 mg tid to maximum of 75–300 mg/d. Alcohol dependence: PO 25 mg bid up to 50–200 mg/d. Anxiety and tension: PO 10 mg bid to maximum of 150 mg/d.

Thioridazine hydrochloride [Mellaril] is less specific for dopamine receptors than chlorpromazine.

Drug Interactions: CNS depressants increase its CNS depressant action.

Side Effects

Nervous System: arrhythmias—ventricular dysrhythmias, bladder—retention, bowel—constipation/paralytic ileus,* dizziness, drowsiness, EPS—infrequent, hypotension, psyche—nocturnal confusion/hyperactivity, sedation, vision—blurred.

Endocrine System: (Pregnancy Category C) amenorrhea, breast engorgement, dry mouth, galactorrhea, gynecomastia.

Immune System: nasal congestion, pigmentary retinopathy.

Dosage: PO 50–100 mg tid to maximum of 800 mg/d. Elderly: PO 10 mg tid to maximum of 200 mg/d. Marked depression: PO 25 mg tid to maximum of 200 mg/d.

THIOXANTHENES

The drugs in this group are similar in structure and action to the phenothiazines in blocking dopamine receptors.

Chlorprothixene [Taractan] produces a strong antiemetic effect as it inhibits the CTZ in the medulla. It treats psychosis by blocking dopamine receptors in the limbic system.

Drug Interactions: CNS depressants increase its CNS depressant action.

Side Effects

Nervous System: arrhythmias—Q and T wave distortions/tachycardia, ataxia, bladder—dysuria/retention, bowel—constipation, convulsions,* dizziness, drowsiness, EPS, lethargy, sedation, sexual function—impotence/increased libido, tardive dyskinesia, vision—blurring/disturbances.

Endocrine System: (Pregnancy Category C) amenorrhea, appetite—increased, galactorrhea, gynecomastia, thirst, uricosuria, impaired sweating, weight gain.

Immune System: agranulocytosis,* contact dermatitis, jaundice, leukopenia—transient, nasal stuffiness, photosensitivity, thrombocytopenic purpura, urticaria.

Dosage: PO 25–600 mg/d divided. IM 25–50 mg/d divided.

Thiothixene hydrochloride [Navane] is similar in structure to chlorprothixene.

Off-Label: antidepressant.

Drug Interactions: CNS depressants increase its CNS depressant action.

Side Effects

Nervous System: arrhythmias—tachycardia, bowel—constipation, cerebral edema, convulsions,* cough reflex—depressed, dizziness, drowsiness, EPS (dose related), hypotension—orthostatic (especially with IM), impotence, psyche—insomnia/paradoxical exaggeration of psychotic symptoms, sudden death.*

---

* Life-threatening side effect.

Endocrine System: (Pregnancy Category C) dry mouth, gynecomastia, thirst, uricosuria, impaired sweating, weight gain, neuroleptic malignant syndrome.*

Immune System: agranulocytosis,* contact dermatitis, jaundice, leukopenia—transient, nasal stuffiness, photosensitivity, thrombocytopenic purpura, urticaria.

Dosage: PO 5–60 mg/d divided. IM 4 mg bid–qid. Not to exceed 30 mg/d.

▶ DRUGS THAT BLOCK DOPAMINE AND SEROTONIN RECEPTORS TO TREAT PSYCHOSIS

Medical science keeps searching for more effective antipsychotic drugs that will be more effective and have fewer unpleasant side effects, ie, tardive dyskinesia. Some recent neuroleptics intentionally block serotonin, as well as dopamine.

Olanzapine [Zyprexa] is used to treat schizophrenia. This drug is antagonistic in dopamine D_1 to D_4 and $5\text{-}HT_{2A/2C}$ receptors. But it also binds to muscarinic, histamine, and beta-adrenergic receptors.

Drug Interactions: Increased effect of antihypertensive agents. Increased clearance and metabolism with carbamazepine. Increased CNS depression with other CNS depressants. Decreased effect of levodopa and dopamine agonists.

Side Effects

Nervous System: akathisia, arrhythmias—tachycardia, bowel—constipation, cough, dizziness, EPS, headache, hypotension—postural, hypertonia, pain—abdominal/back/chest/extremity/joint, psyche—agitation/amnesia/anxiety/euphoria/hostility/insomnia/nervousness/personality disorder, stuttering, tardive dyskinesia, tremor, twitching, vision—blurred.

Endocrine System: (Pregnancy Category C) appetite—increased, dry mouth, edema—peripheral, fever, neuroleptic malignant syndrome,* premenstrual syndrome, weight gain.

Immune System: ALT—elevations, blepharitis, corneal lesion, pharyngitis, rash, rhinitis.

Dosage: PO. Start with 5–10 mg qd. Target dose: 10 mg qd within 5–7 days. Maximum dose 20 mg/d.

Quetiapine fumarate [Seroquel] is an antipsychotic that blocks D_1 and D_2 receptors. In addition, it also blocks

$5\text{-}HT_{1A}$, $5\text{-}HT_2$, alpha-1, alpha-2, and H_1 receptors. Its antipsychotic action seems to be due to dopamine and serotonin blockage.

Drug Interactions: Increased action of alcohol and other centrally acting agents. Increased hypotension with antihypertensive agents. Decreased levels possible with carbamazepine, phenobarbital, rifampin or isoniazid, thioridazine. Increased effects with erythromycin, fluconazole, itraconazole, ketoconazole.

Side Effects

Nervous System: dizziness, dyspepsia, postural hypotension, palpitation, psyche—agitation/insomnia/somnolence, sedation.

Endocrine System: (Pregnancy Category C) anorexia, dry mouth, increased cholesterol/triglycerides, edema—peripheral, sweating, weight gain.

Immune System: dysarthria, flu syndrome, SGPT—elevated.

Dosage: PO. Start with 25 mg bid. Increase 25–50 mg two or three times a day to maximum of 400 mg/d.

▶ THE CATECHOLAMINES AND STIMULANTS

Mental stimulants mimic dopamine's action as seen in the paranoia of cocaine or methamphetamine abuse. The knowledge about the neurochemistry of psychosis came in large part from studying the effects of the abuse of cocaine and the amphetamines so tragically manifested in our society.

The rapid increase in catecholamines in the synapse caused by stimulants like cocaine and the amphetamines results in the increased alertness, strength, energy, and sense of well-being the individual experiences, in addition to paranoia. Cocaine interferes with the reuptake pumps for catecholamines, whereas the amphetamines displace or "shove" neurotransmitters out of their storage vesicles into the synapse.

The amphetamines were discovered in the search for an oral epinephrine to treat asthma as scientists looked for a synthetic form of ephedrine, a chemical similar to epinephrine, found in the rare ephedra plant (ma huang) of China. The chemist Gordon Alles created amphetamine to be inhaled by the patient during an asthma attack. The drug was called Benzedrine, and it was sold over the counter. It quickly caught on with the general public, especially with students cramming for exams (Sneader, 1985). Cocaine and amphetamines are Schedule II drugs.

Drug Abuse

As Freud noted, cocaine does temporarily relieve depression. The stimulants make people "feel good" as the

* Life-threatening side effect.

neurotransmitters dopamine and norepinephrine flood the synapse and plug into large numbers of receptors; however, the neurotransmitters are eventually depleted and the user "crashes" into despair and depression. Many people self-medicate for their emotional pain. The alcoholic calms his or her anxiety with GABA. The narcotic addict seeks blissful respite from pain and fear with opiates. The stimulant user seeks to feel stronger and smarter and more powerful to relieve his or her despair and sense of inadequacy. Many drug users are polydrug abusers, using drugs to affect not only the catecholamines, but GABA and the opiate receptors too. Drug use is a temporary solution for a deeper plague of despair and pain and hopelessness. Pain and fear drive the addiction.

▶ STIMULANTS AND CHILDREN

As legally controlled drugs, the stimulants are used to treat narcolepsy. Children are sometimes given stimulants for a condition labeled attention deficit hyperactivity disorder (ADHD). Stimulants do not calm the hyperactive child. They simply make him or her more alert and less distracted. They inhibit catecholamine reuptake from the synapse and by other means make more alerting neurotransmitters available in the synapse (Theeseu, 1997). Debate has long been waged over the wisdom of giving children psychoactive drugs and whether, in the long run, family therapy might be more useful. In many cases, abstention from the drug for short periods ("vacations") is part of the treatment. Though sometimes still used for obesity, stimulants cannot be used for more than a couple of weeks before losing effectiveness. Stimulant side effects involve the nervous system (BP elevation, euphoria/dysphoria, headache, hyperactive reflexes, impotence, insomnia, irritability, libido changes, palpitations, psychosis, restlessness, tachycardia) and endocrine system (anorexia, weight loss).

▶ STIMULANTS

Amphetamine sulfate [Racemic Amphetamine Sulfate], a Schedule II drug, is used for narcolepsy, obesity, and ADHD.

Drug Interactions: Decreased elimination with acetazolamide, sodium bicarbonate. Increased elimination with ammonium chloride, ascorbic acid. Barbiturate and amphetamine effects antagonized with concomitant use. Increased BP possible with and after gurazolidone. Decreased antihypertensive effect of guanethidine, guanadrel. Do not administer within 14 d of MAOIs, selegiline. Tricyclics increase effects. Increased adverse effects with beta agonists.

Side Effects

Nervous System: arrhythmias—tachycardia, BP—elevated, bowel—constipation/diarrhea, drowsiness, hyper-active reflexes, nausea/vomiting, psyche—dysphoria/euphoria/irritability/psychosis/restlessness, sexual function— impotence/libido changes

Endocrine System: (Pregnancy Category C) anorexia, dry mouth, weight loss.

Immune System: vasculitis, urticaria.

Dosage: Narcolepsy: PO 5–60 mg/d divided q4–6h. Obesity: PO 5–10 mg l h ac. ADHD (≥ 6 y): 5 mg bid increase to maximum of 40 mg/d.

Caffeine, caffeine and sodium benzoate, citrated caffeine [Caffedrine, No Doz] are socially accepted stimulants made from tea leaves. These are OTC drugs. Caffeine is also combined with some OTC analgesics, eg, acetylsalicylic acid, and with a non-OTC ergot; it is used for treatment of migraine headaches.

Drug Interactions: Increased effects of cimetidine possible. Increased cardiovascular stimulation of beta-adrenergic agonists. Increased theophylline toxicity possible.

Side Effects

Nervous System: arrhythmias—bradycardia/tachycardia/ventricular ectopic beats, bladder—increased urination, bowel—diarrhea, convulsions,* facial tingling, muscle—tremors/twitching, nausea/vomiting, psyche—agitation/confusion/delirium/insomnia/irritability/nervousness/restlessness, tachypnea, tinnitus, vision—scintillating scotomas.

Endocrine System: (Pregnancy Category C) diuresis, flushing.

Immune System: gastric irritation, hematemesis.

Dosage: PO 100–200 mg q3–4h prn. IM as circulatory stimulant 200–500 mg prn. IV for spinal puncture headache: 500 mg over 1 h; may repeat × 1 dose.

Cocaine, a Schedule II drug, is not used PO for medicinal purposes in the United States.

Drug Interactions: Risk of severe hypertension and arrhythmias with epinephrine. Its CNS stimulant effects are increased with MAOIs.

Side Effects

Nervous System: angina, arrhythmias—tachycardia/ventricular fibrillation,* CNS stimulation and depression (respiratory and circulatory failure),* nausea/vomiting, pain—abdominal.

Endocrine System: (Pregnancy Category C) anorexia.

---

* Life-threatening side effect.

Immune System: cornea—clouding/pitting, formication, hypersensitivity reactions, lung damage from chronic smoking, MI,* pneumonia, runny nose

Dosage: Ophthalmic 1–4% 1–2 gtt for ocular anesthesia.† Topical 1–10% solution. Use more than 4% solution with caution.

Dextroamphetamine sulfate [Dexedrine] is a Schedule II drug.

Off Label: In combination with other drugs to treat resistant depression.

Drug Interactions: Hypertensive crisis with MAOIs/selegiline. Tricyclic antidepressants increase CNS stimulation. Beta agonists increase cardiovascular adverse effects. Barbiturates antagonize dextroamphetamine CNS stimulation. Elimination increased with ammonium chloride, ascorbic and decreased with acetazolamide, sodium bicarbonate. Furazolidone may increase BP effects. Guanadrel, guanethidine antagonize antihypertensive actions.

Side Effects

Nervous System: arrhythmias—tachycardia, bowel—constipation/diarrhea, BP—elevated, drowsiness, headache, nausea/vomiting, palpitation, psyche—dysphoria/euphoria/insomnia/irritability/nervousness/psychosis/restlessness, reflexes—hyperactive, sexual function—impotence/libido changes, trembling, weakness.

Endocrine System: (Pregnancy Category C) anorexia, dry mouth, weight loss.

Immune System: urticaria.

Dosage: Narcolepsy: PO 5–20 mg bid. ADHD (≥ 6y): maximum of 40 mg daily in divided doses. Obesity: PO 5–10 mg qd or tid or SR 10–15 mg qd 30–60 min oc.

Methylphenidate hydrochloride [Ritalin], a Schedule II drug, is used to treat ADHD, mild depression, narcolepsy, and apathy/withdrawn senile behavior.

Drug Interactions: Antagonizes hypotensive effects of bretylium/guanethidine and may cause hypertensive crisis with MAOIs.

Side Effects

Nervous System: angina, arrhythmias—varied, BP/pulse changes, dizziness, drowsiness, nausea, psyche—insomnia/nervousness, vision—accommodation difficulties/blurred.

Endocrine System: (Pregnancy Category C) anorexia, dry throat, fever, growth suppression.

Immune System: arthralgia, erythema multiforme, exfoliative dermatitis,* hepatotoxicity,* rash, urticaria.

Dosage: Narcolepsy: PO 10–40 mg bid–tid 30–45 min pc. ADHD (≥ 6 y): PO 5–10 mg before breakfast and lunch; increase 5–10 mg/wk if needed to maximum of 60 mg daily in divided doses.

Pemoline [Cylert], a Schedule IV drug, has actions similar to those of amphetamine, but weak sympathomimetic ability. It is used in minimal brain dysfunction in children.

Off Label: Stimulant for geriatric patients.

Side Effects

Nervous System: bowel—diarrhea, convulsions,* discomfort—abdominal, dizziness, drowsiness, dyskinesia—eyes/body, fatigue, headache, malaise, nausea, psyche—mild depression/insomnia. Overdose: arrhythmias—tachycardia, psyche—agitation/excitement/hallucinations/restlessness.

Endocrine System: (Pregnancy Category B) anorexia. Overdose: elevated alkaline phosphatase level.

Immune System: jaundice, rash. Overdose: elevated ALT/AST levels.

Dosage: ADHD (≥ 6 y): PO 37.5–112.5 mg/d.

Phenmetrazine hydrochloride [Preludin], a Schedule II drug, is a CNS agent, a respiratory and cerebral stimulant. Structurally related to the amphetamines, phenmetrazine is used as an anorexiant.

Drug Interactions: Elimination is increased by ammonium chloride, ascorbic acid and decreased by acetazolamide, sodium bicarbonate; may antagonize barbiturates. Furazolidone may increase BP effects of amphetamines; interaction may last several weeks after discontinuation of furazolidone. Phenmetrazine antagonizes antihypertensive guanethidine, guanadrel effects. Hypertensive crisis with MAOIs, selegiline; amphetamines are contraindicated for 14 d before and after these drugs. Phenothiazines may block mood elevation. Tricyclic antidepressants increase amphetamine effects. Beta agonists increase adverse cardiovascular effects.

Side Effects

Nervous System: arrhythmias—tachycardia, bladder—frequency, BP—elevated, bowel—constipation, dizziness, headache, nausea, palpitations, psyche—nervousness, sexual function—impotence/libido changes, vision—blurred.

Endocrine System: (Pregnancy Category C) dry mouth, sweating.

Immune System: urticaria.

Dosage: PO 75 mg qd midmorning.

---

* Life-threatening side effect.
† Eye related.

▶ DEPRESSION: DOPAMINE, NOREPINEPHRINE, SEROTONIN, AND THE PUMP BLOCKER ANTIDEPRESSANTS

Dopamine, norepinephrine, and serotonin are "uppers," the "feel good" neurotransmitters. A lack of norepinephrine, or serotonin, whatever the cause, can result in depression. Some researchers have found that depressed people lacking serotonin are more seriously suicidal than those lacking norepinephrine. The earliest antidepressants evolved from the neuroleptic antihistamine, chlorpromazine. Removing the sulfur and chlorine atoms from the chlorpromazine molecule led to the tricyclic antidepressant imipramine [Tofranil]. Though the antidepressants begin to work immediately, there is a characteristic lag of to 2–4 wk before they begin to help alleviate depression.

Note: *A seriously suicidal patient may pretend to swallow his pills only to save them up for an overdose. The nurse must make sure each dose is swallowed.*

▶ CLASSIFICATION OF ANTIDEPRESSANTS

Antidepressants are classified according to their understood mechanisms of action. The tricyclics (TCA) have mixed serotonin and norepinephrine reuptake inhibition ability. The selective serotonin reuptake inhibitors block only serotonin. The mixed serotonin–catecholamine reuptake blockers drugs are less selective. And the monoamine oxidase inhibitors prevent catecholamine breakdown for recycling.

MIXED SEROTONIN–NOREPINEPHRINE REUPTAKE INHIBITORS

This group of antidepressants includes the tricyclics, which consist of the tertiary amines and secondary amines, aminoketones, the bicyclic venlafaxine, dibenzoxazepines, and tetracyclics.

Bicyclic Antidepressants

Venlafaxine [Effexor], a second-generation antidepressant chemically unlike the other antidepressants, selectively inhibits reuptake of serotonin, norepinephrine, and dopamine in descending order of potency.

Drug Interactions: Not to be combined with MAOIs. Cimetidine decreases clearance of venlafaxine.

Side Effects

Nervous System: arrhythmias—tachycardia, asthenia, BP—increased, bowel—constipation, dizziness, fatigue, headache, nausea/vomiting, palpitations, psyche—

anxiety/insomnia/somnolence, seizures, sexual dysfunction, tremors, vision—blurred.

Endocrine System: (Pregnancy Category C) dry mouth, serum cholesterol increase, sweating, weight loss.

Immune System: none noted.

Dosage: PO 25–125 tid. Start with a lower dose in the elderly.

Dibenzoxazepines

Amoxapine [Ascendin] is a mixed 5-HT/NE reuptake inhibitor used to treat agitated depression.

Drug Interactions: CNS depressants potentiate its CNS depression. Amoxapine may decrease response to antihypertensives, may increase hypoprothrombinemic effect of oral anticoagulants, and may increase sympathetic activity with sympathomimetics, including hypertension/hyperpyrexia. Possible severe reactions with MAOIs. Cimetidine, methylphenidate increase plasma TCA levels. Possibility of arrhythmias with thyroid drugs.

Side Effects

Nervous System: arrhythmias, bowel—constipation/diarrhea/flatulence, convulsions—overdose,* dizziness, drowsiness, dyspepsia, EPS, fatigue, headache, hypotension—orthostatic, nausea, psyche—panic attack, tardive dyskinesia, vision—blurred, taste—odd.

Endocrine System: (Pregnancy Category C) dryness—eyes/mouth, flushing.

Immune System: nephrotoxicity—overdose.

Dosage: PO 50 mg bid or tid; on day 3, may increase to 100 mg tid. Maintenance: Dose may be given hs.

Tetracyclic Antidepressants

This classification contains only one drug, maprotiline, which is similar to the tricyclic antidepressants.

Maprotiline hydrochloride [Ludiomil] is used to treat dysthymic disorder and manic–depressive illness, depressed type.

Drug Interactions: CNS depressant drugs may potentiate maprotiline CNS depression. May decrease some response to antihypertensives. Transient delirium with ethchlorvynol. Sympathomimetics, levodopa may cause sympathetic hyperactivity with hypertension and hyperpyrexia. With MAOIs may cause severe reactions, cardiovascular instability, toxic psychosis. Increased TCA plasma levels with methylphenidate or cimetidine. Possible arrhythmias with thyroid drugs. Possible hypoprothrombinemic effect increase with maprotiline.

---

* Life-threatening side effect.

Side Effects

Nervous System: arrhythmias—tachycardia, bladder—frequency/retention, bowel—constipation, convulsions,* dizziness, drowsiness, dyspepsia, hypertension, hypotension—orthostatic, nausea/vomiting, psyche—confusion/exacerbation of psychosis/excitement/hallucinations, tremors, vision—accommodation disturbances/blurred/mydriasis.

Endocrine System: (Pregnancy Category B) none noted.

Immune System: photosensitivity, rash, urticaria.

Dosage: Mild/moderate depression: PO 75 mg/d; gradually increase q2wk to maximum of 150 mg/d in single or divided doses. Severe depression: PO 100–150 mg/d; gradually increase to 300 mg/d in single or divided doses if needed.

Tricyclic Antidepressants

These three-ringed antidepressants block reuptake of norepinephrine for recycling after its release into the synapse, making more of the neurotransmitter available to the postsynaptic receptors and causing a lift in mood or affect. The first of these, imipramine, has a side chain exactly like the one on the antipsychotic drug chlorpromazine, which blocks dopamine receptors on the opposite side of the synapse. To some extent, tricyclics also block serotonin reuptake. Furthermore, the tricyclics block alpha-adrenergic, muscarinic–cholinergic, and H_1 and H_2 receptors, causing side effects associated with those receptors. Tricyclics can interfere with the action of beta blockers.

Amitriptyline hydrochloride [Elavil, others] is used to treat endogenous depression.

Off Label: Prophylaxis for cluster, migraine, chronic tension headaches; intractable pain; pathologic weeping and laughing secondary to forebrain disease; eating disorders associated with depression; sedation for nondepressed patient; increased muscle strength in myotonic dystrophy.

Side Effects

Nervous System: arrhythmias—ECG changes/tachycardia, bladder—retention, bowel—constipation, convulsions,* dizziness, drowsiness, EPS, fatigue, headache, hypotension—orthostatic, nausea/vomiting, psyche—insomnia/nervousness/restlessness, sedation, taste—metallic, vision—blurred/mydriasis.

Endocrine System: (Pregnancy Category C) appetite—increased/sweets preference, dryness—eyes/mouth, weight gain.

---

* Life-threatening side effect.

Immune System: bone marrow depression*—rare.

Dosage: PO 75–300 mg/d. IM 20–30 mg qid until able to take PO. In combination with perphenazine [Trilafon] and amitriptyline HCl are Triavil: 2–25 mg or 4–25 mg bid–qid or 4–50 bid (2–10 and 4–10 tablets give dosage flexibility). The combination of amitriptyline HCl with the GABA-like chlordiazepoxide is Limbitrol: PO amitriptyline HCl 12.5 mg with chlordiazepoxide 5 mg or DS 25 mg and 10 mg in divided doses with the largest hs.

Clomipramine hydrochloride [Anafranil] is used for obsessive–compulsive behavior.

Drug Interactions: See *amitriptyline.*

Side Effects

Nervous System: arrhythmias—tachycardia, bowel—constipation especially with abrupt withdrawal, convulsions,* dizziness, hypotension, psyche—mania, sexual function—anorgasmic/delayed ejaculation, tremor.

Endocrine System: (Pregnancy Category C) amenorrhea, galactorrhea, hyperprolactinemia, hyperthermia, neuroleptic malignant syndrome,* sweating, weight gain.

Immune System: anemia, thrombocytopenia.

Dosage: PO 75–300 mg/d in divided doses. Depression: PO 50–150 mg/d in single or divided doses.

Doxepin hydrochloride [Sinequan, others] is used to treat anxiety and depression and anxiety and depression associated with alcoholism, organic brain syndrome, psychotic depression, and, as a topical, pruritus.

Off Label: Neuralgia.

Drug Interactions: Same as for the other TCAs.

Side Effects

Nervous System: arrhythmias—tachycardia/ECG changes, bladder—delay/frequency/retention, bowel—constipation, dizziness, drowsiness, epigastric distress, fatigue, headache, hypertension, hypotension—orthostatic, palpitations, paresthesias, psyche—confusion/hypomania, vision—blurred/mydriasis/photophobia, sedation, tinnitus, weakness.

Endocrine System: (Pregnancy Category C) dry mouth, edema, sweating, weight gain.

Immune System: agranulocytosis,* photosensitivity, rash. Topical: burning/stinging at site.

Dosage: PO 30–300 mg/d hs or in divided doses. For pruritis: Topical qid, 3–4h between applications.

Imipramine hydrochloride [Tofranil] is used to treat depression by blocking norepinephrine and serotonin reuptake and also as an adjuvant treatment for enuresis in children >6 y.

Off Label: Depression with alcohol; cocaine withdrawal; in attention deficit disorder with or without hyperactivity; narcolepsy with amphetamines or methylphenidate; and panic disorders.

Drug Interactions: Similar to other TCAs.

Side Effects

Nervous System: abdominal cramps, ataxia, arrhythmias—ECG changes/heart block/tachycardia, bladder—delayed/frequency/nocturia, bowel—constipation/diarrhea/flatulence/paralytic ileus, CHF, convulsions*/EEG changes, dizziness, drowsiness, dyspnea, EPS, fatigue, upper GI—dyspepsia/gastric emptying slowed/nausea/reflux/vomiting, headache, hypotension—orthostatic, hypertension/hypotension, insomnia, paresthesias, psyche—agitation/anxiety/decreased concentration/confusion/delirium/vivid dreams/hallucinations/hypomania/mania/nervousness/exacerbation of psychoses/restlessness, salivation, sedation, sexual function—ejaculatory/erectile disturbances/libido changes/orgasm changes, tardive dyskinesia, taste changes, tremors, vasospasm—peripheral, vision—accommodation disturbances/blurred/mydriasis/nystagmus.

Endocrine System: (Pregnancy Category C) anorexia, appetite—excessive, dry mouth, flushing, blood glucose—depression/elevation, galactorrhea, gynecomastia, hair loss, porphyria—precipitation, SIADH secretion, sweating, temperature toleration changes.

Immune System: agranulocytosis,* angioedema,* black tongue, bone marrow depression,* drug fever, jaundice, photosensitivity, rash, thrombocytopenia.

Dosage: PO 75–300 mg/d in divided doses. IM 50–100 mg/d in divided doses.

Trimipramine maleate [Surmontil] is used to treat endogenous depression.

Drug Interactions: those typical of TCAs.

Side Effects

Nervous System: arrhythmias—tachycardia, bladder—retention, bowel—constipation/paralytic ileus, hypertension, hypotension—orthostatic, psyche—confusion, sedation, seizures,* tremors, vision—blurred.

Endocrine System: (Pregnancy Category C) dry mouth, sweating.

Immune System: photosensitivity.

---

* Life-threatening side effect.

Dosage: PO 75–300 mg/d in divided doses. Maintenance: 50–150 mg/d in divided doses.

Secondary Amines

This group of antidepressants affects norepinephrine levels and, to some degree, 5-HT levels also.

Desipramine hydrochloride [Norpramin], an active metabolite of imipramine, has many of the TCA side effects.

Drug Interactions: Those typical of TCAs.

Side Effects

Nervous System: arrhythmias—tachycardia/ECG changes/heart block, ataxia, bladder—delay/frequency/nocturia/retention, bowel—constipation/diarrhea, dizziness, drowsiness, fatigue, headache, hypotension and hypotension—postural, nausea, palpitations, psyche—confusion/depressive reaction/insomnia, sexual dysfunction, taste—bad, tinnitus, vision—accommodation disturbances/blurred/increased IOP/mydriasis.

Endocrine System: (Pregnancy Category C) craving for sweets, dry mouth, flushing, galactorrhea, hyperpyrexia, SIADH secretion, sweating, weight gain/loss.

Immune System: agranulocytosis,* bone marrow depression,* parotid swelling, photosensitivity, rash, urticaria.

Dosage: PO 75–300 mg/d in divided doses.

Nortriptyline hydrochloride [Aventyl, Pamelor] is thought to relieve depression by blocking the reuptake of norepinephrine.

Drug Interactions: CNS depression increased with other CNS depressants. May increase hypoprothrombinemic effect of oral anticoagulants. Transient delirium with ethchlorvynol. Possible increase in sympathetic activity with sympathomimetics.

Side Effects

Nervous System: bladder—retention, bowel—paralytic ileus, drowsiness, hypotension—orthostatic, psyche—confusion (especially in the elderly at high doses), tremors, vision—blurred.

Endocrine System: (Pregnancy Category D) dry mouth, sweating.

Immune System: agranulocytosis (rare),* photosensitivity.

Dosage: PO 25 mg tid or qid; gradually increase to 100–150 mg/d in divided doses.

Protriptyline hydrochloride [Vivactil] is used to treat depression, especially that with psychomotor retardation, apathy, and fatigue.

Drug Interactions: Those of the other TCAs.

Side Effects

Nervous System: arrhythmias—tachycardia, bladder—retention, bowel—constipation/paralytic ileus, headache, hypotension—orthostatic, psyche—confusion, vision—blurred.

Endocrine System: (Pregnancy Category C) change in heat or cold tolerance, dry mouth.

Immune System: angioedema, photosensitivity.

Dosage: PO 15–60 mg/d in divided doses.

AMINOKETONES

The aminoketone bupropion weakly raises synaptic levels of norepinephrine, serotonin, and dopamine. However, it also lowers the seizure threshold.

Bupropion hydrochloride [Wellbutrin] weakly blocks reuptake of norepinephrine and serotonin and, to some degree, dopamine. Bupropion, under the trade name Zyban, in combination with nicotine patches, helps long-time smokers to stop.

Side Effects

Nervous System: arrhythmias—tachycardia, bowel—constipation, convulsions* (especially in patients suffering anorexia nervosa, bulimia, or prior seizure), dizziness, headache, insomnia, nausea/vomiting, psyche—agitation/anxiety/confusion/delusions/hallucination/paranoia/psychotic episodes, vision—blurred, tremor.

Endocrine System: (Pregnancy Category B) dry mouth, weight—gain/loss.

Immune System: rash.

Dosage: PO 300 mg divided tid. Seizure risk with doses over 450 mg/d.

Mirtazapine [Remeron] is an antidepressant that enhances noradrenergic and serotonergic activity. It is also a potent antagonist of $5-HT_2$, $5-HT_3$, and H_1 receptors. The action on histamine receptors may account for its sedative effect.

Drug Interactions: Additive effect with alcohol, diazepam, and other drugs that enhance GABA effects.

Side Effects

Nervous System: asthenia, bladder—frequency, bowel—constipation, dizziness, dyspnea, edema, myalgia, pain—back, psyche—confusion/abnormal dreams/abnormal thinking/somnolence, tremor.

Endocrine System: (Pregnancy Category C) appetite—increased, dry mouth, edema—peripheral, weight gain.

Immune System: flu syndrome.

Dosage: PO 15 mg qd to maximum of 45 mg/d.

Monoamine Oxidase Inhibitors

In a different strategy for treating depression, the MAOIs interfere with monoamine oxidase, the enzyme that breaks off the amine group from the molecules of norepinephrine and serotonin that leak from their storage vesicles and protects our minds from the chaos of excess neurotransmitters. Inhibiting the enzyme makes more norepinephrine available in the synapse and helps relieve depression. In the 1950s MAOIs were derived from iproniazid, an antituberculosis drug derived from isoniazid. Iproniazid had a side effect of stimulating the CNS and lifting the mood of TB patients, sometimes to the point of euphoria. Because iproniazid sometimes caused jaundice, it was eventually supplanted by less toxic drugs (Sneader, 1985).

Tyramine, formed from the amino acid tyrosine in rotting food, is an analog of epinephrine. Eating tyramine while under MAOI therapy can cause a hypertensive crisis. After discontinuing use of MAOIs, the individual must refrain for 2 wk from eating tyramine-rich foods, including aged foods, broad bean pods, aged cheese, red wine, pickled herring, sausage, avocados, liver, yeast, chocolate, and yogurt. He or she must also avoid sympathomimetic drugs, eg, ephedrine, L-dopa, methyldopa, amphetamine, in addition to the drug reserpine, which depletes catecholamines. MAOIs are not to be given concurrently with the beta blockers, as beta blockers might defeat the purpose of treatment. MAOIs increase synaptic levels of norepinephrine and serotonin and constrict blood vessels. This action makes them useful in treating migraines.

Isocarboxazid [Marplan] is used to treat depression because it inhibits the enzymes that break down catecholamines, thereby leaving more norepinephrine in the synapse.

Drug Interactions: Headache, hypertensive crisis, hyperexcitability possible with tyramine-containing foods, TCAs, amphetamines, dopa, dopamine, ephedrine, fluoxetine, guanethidine, levodopa, phenylpropanolamine, reserpine, tryptophan. CNS depressants increase its CNS depressant activity. Fatal cardiovascular collapse possible with meperidine. Anesthetics increase CNS depression. Increased risk of seizures with metrizamide. Hypotensive effect increases with diuretics and antihypertensive agents.

---

* Life-threatening side effect.

Side Effects

Nervous System: arrhythmias—tachycardia/other arrhythmias, bladder—dysuria/incontinence/retention, bowel—constipation/diarrhea, dizziness, drowsiness, headache, hyperreflexia, hypertension—paradoxical,* hypotension—orthostatic, lightheadedness, muscle twitching, palpitations, psyche—confusion/hypomania/insomnia/mania/memory impairment/over activity, tiredness, tremors, vision—blurred/glaucoma/nystagmus.

Endocrine System: (Pregnancy Category C) anorexia, appetite—increased, chills, edema—peripheral, sweating, weight gain.

Immune System: black tongue, hepatitis, jaundice.

Dosage: PO 10–30 mg/d in divided doses.

<u>Phenelzine sulfate [Nardil]</u> is the MAOI antidepressant also used to treat migraines.

Drug Interactions: Possible hyperpyrexia or seizures with TCAs. Hypertensive crisis possible with sympathomimetics and foods containing tyramine. Fluoxetine, paroxetine, sertraline may cause delirium, diaphoresis, hyperthermia, tremors. Hypertensive crisis and circulatory collapse possible with meperidine. May cause hypertension with buspirone. Prolonged hypotensive and CNS depression with general anesthetics. Increased risk of seizures with dopamine, levodopa, methyldopa, metrizamide, tryptophan.

Side Effects

Nervous System: akathisia, ataxia, bowel—constipation, convulsions,* dizziness, drowsiness, fatigue, headache, hyperflexia, hypertensive crisis,* hypotension—orthostatic, nausea/vomiting, peripheral neuropathy, psyche—acute anxiety/confusion/delirium/euphoria/hallucinations/hypomania/insomnia/mania/memory impairment/toxic precipitation of schizophrenia, tremors, twitching, vertigo, vision—blurred, weakness. Overdose: circulatory collapse*/coma*/respiratory depression*/seizures,* opisthotonos.

Endocrine System: (Pregnancy Category C) anorexia, dry mouth, edema, sweating, weight gain.

Immune System: anemia, leukopenia, photosensitivity, rash.

Dosage: PO 15–90 mg/d.

<u>Tranylcypromine sulfate [Parnate]</u> inhibits the enzyme that breaks down catecholamines, making more norepinephrine available in the synapse.

---

* Life-threatening side effect.

Drug Interactions: Same as for other MAOIs.

Side Effects

Nervous System: abdominal discomfort, arrhythmias—varied, bowel—constipation/diarrhea, dizziness, headache, hypertensive crisis,* hypotension—orthostatic, impotence, tremors, twitching, vertigo, vision—blurred.

Endocrine System: (Pregnancy Category C) anorexia, edema—peripheral, sweating.

Immune System: rash.

Dosage: PO 30 mg/d divided into 20 mg AM and 10 mg PM to maximim 60/d.

SEROTONIN AND DEPRESSION

Serotonin, or 5-hydroxytryptamine (5-HT), a low-molecular-weight amine derived from tryptophan, has four types of receptors (5-HT$_1$, 5-HT$_2$, 5-HT$_3$, 5-HT$_4$), and each of those has many subtypes. In the nervous system the 5-HT$_1$ subtypes 1$_A$, 1$_C$, 1$_D$, and 1$_{like}$ have special significance. As with the catecholamine norepinephrine, decreased synaptic levels of serotonin contribute to some states of emotional depression.

Serotonin-enhancing antidepressants have become useful in treating, not only depression, but other psychiatric conditions such as obsessive–compulsive behaviors. Serotonin, like the monoamine norepinephrine, is broken down by MAO. Serotonin is also used by the nervous system to stimulate the viscera to help contract smooth muscle.

Selective Serotonin Reuptake Inhibitors in the Treatment of Depression

Some evidence links decreased serotonin levels in depression with an increased risk for suicide, and many of the recent antidepressants specifically inhibit serotonin reuptake. Antidepressants act immediately, but the body, to maintain homeostasis, blocks the action while neurons receptor sites adapt. Thus, the depressed patient experiences a 1- to 4-week lag before feeling the therapeutic effect.

<u>Fluoxetine hydrochloride [Prozac]</u> alleviates depression probably by blocking the reuptake of serotonin into presynaptic neurons. It is also used to treat obsessive–compulsive disorders.

Off Label: Obesity, bulimia nervosa.

Drug Interactions: May cause agitation/restlessness/GI distress with tryptophan. With selegiline, may increase risk of severe hypertensive reaction and death.

Side Effects

Nervous System: arthralgia, diarrhea, dizziness, drowsiness, dyspepsia, fatigue, headache, hypotension, myalgia, nausea, palpitations, pain—chest, psyche—anxiety/insomnia/nervousness, vision—blurred, sexual dysfunction.

Endocrine System: (Pregnancy Category B) appetite—increased, dry mouth, flushing, hyponatremia, menstrual irregularities, sweating.

Immune System: allergy, flu-like syndrome, pruritus, rash.

Dosage: PO 20 mg qam to maximum of 80 mg/d.

Fluvoxamine [Luvox] has actions similar to those of fluoxetine.

Drug Interactions: Increases TCA plasma levels, antagonizes beta-blocker antihypertensive actions. Increases prothrombin time with warfarin. Possible toxicity of carbamazepine. Possible neurotoxicity with lithium. Serotonin syndrome—mania/somnolence.

Side Effects

Nervous System: arrhythmias—bradycardia, bowel—constipation, convulsions,* dizziness, drowsiness, headache, hypotension—orthostatic, insomnia, nausea/vomiting, psyche—agitation, sexual dysfunction.

Endocrine System: (Pregnancy Category B) anorexia, dry mouth.

Immune System: toxic epidermal necrolysis,* Stevens–Johnson syndrome.*

Dosage: PO 50 mg qd. May slowly increase to 300 mg/d qhs or divided bid.

Paroxetine [Paxil] has most of the lesser side effects of the selective serotonin reuptake inhibitors plus elevated liver enzymes (rare). It is a highly selective inhibitor of serotonin reuptake into presynaptic CNS neurons. It is used to treat depression and obsessive–compulsive disorders.

Off Label: Diabetic neuropathy, myoclonus.

Drug Interactions: Reduced absorption with activated charcoal. Cimetidine increases paroxetine levels. Hypertensive crisis or death possible with MAOIs. Phenytoin may cause hepatic enzyme induction and result in lower paroxetine levels and shorter half-life. Increased risk of bleeding with warfarin.

_____

* Life-threatening side effect.

Side Effects

Nervous System: bladder—frequency/hesitancy, bowel—constipation/diarrhea/flatulence, dizziness, dyspepsia, headache, hypotension—postural, nausea/vomiting, paresthesias, psyche—agitation/anxiety/insomnia/nervousness, sedation, taste aversion tremors, vision—blurred.

Endocrine System: (Pregnancy Category B) appetite—increased, dry mouth sweating.

Immune System: elevated liver enzymes, pruritus, rash.

Dosage: PO 10–50 mg/d to maximum of 80 mg/d. Start with lower doses for elderly patients and those with renal or hepatic insufficiency.

Sertraline hydrochloride [Zoloft] is used to treat depression and obsessive–compulsive disorder.

Drug Interactions: Toxicity with MAOIs. Diazepam and tolbutamide clearance may be inhibited. Sertraline may displace tightly bound drug molecules like warfarin and digitoxin.

Side Effects

Nervous System: ataxia, arrhythmias—bradycardia, arthralgia, bowel—constipation/diarrhea/flatulence, bronchospasm,* cough, dizziness, drowsiness, dyspepsia, dyspnea, headache, hyper-/hypotension, nausea/vomiting, pain—abdominal/chest, palpitations, psyche—agitation/aggression/delusions/depersonalization/insomnia/abnormal dreams/emotional lability/hallucinations/paranoia/suicidal ideation, sexual dysfunction—male, syncope, vertigo, vision—blurred/diplopia/dryness/exophthalmos/mydriasis/photophobia/tearing.

Endocrine System: (Pregnancy Category B) anorexia, edema, gynecomastia.

Immune System: acne, alopecia, pharyngitis, rash, rhinitis, urticaria.

Dosage: Dosage: PO 50–200 mg qd.

Mixed Serotonin Effects: The Triazolopyridines
These drugs affect different types of serotonin receptors simultaneously, causing different effects.

Nefazodone [Serzone] is used to treat depression. It both inhibits reuptake of 5-HT and antagonizes 5-HT$_2$ receptors. Nefazodone is associated with a smaller incidence of anticholinergic side effects than other antidepressants.

Drug Interactions: none noted.

Side Effects

Nervous System: bowel—constipation, dizziness, drowsiness, headache, nausea, psyche—agitation/anxiety/asthenia/insomnia.

Endocrine System: (Pregnancy Category C) dry mouth.

Immune System: none noted.

Dosage: PO 50–100 mg bid to maximum of 600 mg/d in divided doses.

Trazodone [Desyrel, Desyrel Dividose] relieves depression by blocking serotonin reuptake.

Drug Interactions: CNS depressants increase CNS depressant action. Hypotension may be potentiated by antihypertensive agents and hypertensive crisis may occur with MAOIs. Trazodone may increase digoxin or phenytoin levels.

Side Effects

Nervous System: abdominal distress, ataxia, arrhythmias—bradycardia/tachycardia/PVCs*/ventricular tachycardia,* bladder—frequency/delayed flow, bowel—constipation/diarrhea/flatulence, dizziness, drowsiness, dyspnea, fatigue, headache, hyper-/hypotension (including orthostatic hypotension), lightheadedness, muscle twitches, nausea/vomiting, pain/aches—skeletal/chest, palpitations, psyche—agitation/disorientation/insomnia/decreases REM sleep/memory impaired, sedation, sexual function—priapism/inhibition of ejaculation, vision—blurred, speech—impaired, syncope, tinnitus.

Endocrine System: (Pregnancy Category C) dry mouth, menstrual cycle changes, sweating/clamminess, weight changes.

Immune System: acne, congestion—nasal/sinus, eye irritation, hematuria, photosensitivity, pruritus.

Dosage: PO 150 mg/d in divided doses may increase to maximum of 600 mg/d.

Serotonin and Migraine Headaches

Serotonin plays a role in the immune system, where it is stored in platelets and mast cells just as histamine is. Its release from platelets is a factor in migraines, and serotonin release from damaged platelets causes platelet aggregation as well. Serotonin appears to be the main culprit in migraine headaches (Beckett, 1997). Although new drugs that counter serotonin's actions have become available, vasoconstricting drugs are frequently prescribed for migraines to counter the vasodilation. Migraine headaches present as unilateral, excruciating, nonthrobbing pain that causes the victim to seek quiet darkness and sleep. Depression, personality, stress, epilepsy, hormonal changes, the environment, and diet all have been implicated as factors in various individuals.

Treatment modalities include addressing the prostaglandin release and platelet aggregation with NSAIDs. Calcium channel blockers may help in the initial vasoconstriction phase of an attack. (See Calcium Channel Blockers in Chapter 2.) The antiepilepsy drugs may be effective in migraine headaches associated with epilepsy (see Chapter 6.) The following drugs are specific to serotonin for the treatment of migraine headache.

Methysergide [Sansert] is an ergot derivative with weak oxytocic actions. In addition to being essential for good mental health, serotonin plays a role in vasoconstriction. During a migraine, serotonin levels drop. Initially, the cranial arteries involved constrict, but then dilate for the duration of the headache. Methysergide mimics the vasoconstricting action of serotonin and fits into serotonin receptors in cranial arteries. It is used prophylactically for migraines.

Off Label: GI symptoms of carcinoid disease, ie, diarrhea, malabsorption; postgastrectomy dumping syndrome.

Drug Interactions: None noted.

Side Effects

Nervous System: angina with effort, arrhythmias—ECG changes/tachycardia, arthralgia, ataxia, bowel—constipation/diarrhea, circulation impairment/claudication, drowsiness, dyspepsia, dyspnea, hyperesthesia, hypotension—postural, insomnia, myalgia, nausea/vomiting, pain—abdominal, paresthesias, psyche—anxiety/body image distortions/confusion/depersonalization/depression/euphoria/excitement/hallucinations/nightmares, telangiectasia, vertigo, weakness, vision—scotomas.

Endocrine System: (Pregnancy Category C) edema—peripheral, facial flushing, hyperchlorhydria, sweating, weight gain.

Immune System: Coombs test positive, eosinophilia, fibrosis of lungs/heart/peritoneum, hair loss, nasal stuffiness, neutropenia, rash, thrombophlebitis.

Dosage: PO 4–8 mg qd in divided doses with meals. A drug-free interval of 3–4 wk is necessary q6mo.

Sumatriptan [Imitrex] relieves migraine headache by vasoconstriction of cranial carotid arteries.

Off Label: Cluster headache.

---

* Life-threatening side effect.

Drug Interactions: Not concurrently with or 2 wk after MAOIs. MAOIs increase sumatriptan levels and toxicity (especially the oral form). Dihydroergotamine may cause a slight elevation in blood pressure.

Side Effects

Nervous System: BP—mild increase after IV doses of 8 μg or more, chest—pressure/tightness, dizziness, drowsiness, headache, pain on injection, sedation, seizure,* tingling, weakness.

Endocrine System: (Pregnancy Category C) warming sensation.

Immune System: none noted.

Dosage: PO 25 mg × 1 dose (maximum of 100 mg). SC 6 mg any time after onset of migraine; if no relief, may repeat with 6 mg SC at least 1 h after first injection (maximum: 12 mg/24 h).

Zolmitriptan [Zomig] relieves migraine by binding with 5-HT$_{1B/1D}$ receptor agonist and constricting cranial vessels, thus blocking release of proinflammatory neuropeptides.

Drug Interactions: Not for use with MAOIs and ergot-containing drugs.

Side Effects

Nervous System: dizziness, dyspnea, pain/tightness—jaw/neck/throat, paresthesias, somnolence, weakness.

Endocrine System: (Pregnancy Category C) sensations of warm/cold.

Immune System: angioedema, rash, wheezing.

Dosage: PO. Start with 2.5 mg or lower. May repeat in 2 h if headache returns. Not to exceed 10 mg in 24 h.

Serotonin and the Treatment of Nausea
The nausea and vomiting due to the toxicity of some cancer-fighting drugs pose a challenge. The following new drug is used to treat postoperative or chemotherapy-induced nausea and vomiting.

Dolasetron mesylate [Anzemet] is an antiemetic/antinausea agent and serotonin subtype 3 receptor antagonist. It is used for the prevention and treatment of nausea and vomiting after surgery or chemotherapy.

Drug Interactions: Possible QT prolongation with diuretics.

Side Effects

Nervous System: arrhythmia—ECG changes/tachycardia, bladder—retention, bowel—diarrhea, dyspepsia, fatigue, headache, hypotension, pain.

Endocrine System: (Pregnancy Category C) chills, shivering.

Immune System: none noted.

Dosage: IV to prevent chemotherapy-induced nausea/vomiting: 1.8 mg/kg up to maximum of 100 mg or a fixed dose of 100 mg. Give as a single dose approximately 30 min before chemotherapy over 30 s. Prevention and treatment of postoperative nausea and vomiting: 12.5 mg as a single dose approximately 15 min before cessation of anesthesia or administered as soon as nausea and vomiting present. PO to prevent postoperative nausea and vomiting: 100 mg within 2 h prior to surgery.

CONDITIONS OTHER THAN DEPRESSION AND HEADACHE

Muscle spasm may respond to drugs that block norepinephrine reuptake. In addition, a fairly new drug, sibutramine hydrochloride, blocks the reuptake of serotonin and dopamine and seems to help the obese patient lose weight.

Tricyclic Antidepressant Muscle Relaxants
In the sympathetic nervous system muscle spasm may be relieved by blocking norepinephrine reuptake. Structurally similar to the tricyclic antidepressants, this class of drugs acts in the CNS at the brain stem level, to relieve skeletal muscle spasm.

Cyclobenzaprine hydrochloride [Cycoflex, Flexeril] relieves muscle spasms at the cord or brain stem level.

Drug Interactions: CNS depressant action is increased with other CNS depressants. Cyclobenzaprine potentiates anticholinergic effects of phenothiazine and other anticholinergics. Hypertensive crisis possible with MAOIs.

Side Effects

Nervous System: arrhythmia—tachycardia (severe arrhythmias with high doses), asthenia, ataxia, bowel—diarrhea/paralytic ileus, convulsions,* dizziness, dyspepsia, dyspnea, fatigue, hypotension—orthostatic, insomnia, myalgia, pain—abdominal/chest, palpitations, paresthesias, psyche—disorientation/euphoria/mania, sexual function—impotence/libido changes, taste—unpleasant, tremors, twitching, weakness.

Endocrine System: (Pregnancy Category B) anorexia, sweating.

Immune System: alopecia, angioedema,* hepatitis, rash, tongue—coated/discolored.

* Life-threatening side effect.

Dosage: PO 20–40 mg/d in divided doses not to exceed 60 mg/d.

Sibutramine hydrochloride [Meridia] blocks serotonin and dopamine reuptake in the management of obesity in conjunction with reduced calorie intake for weight loss. It is a Schedule IV controlled drug.

Drug Interactions: Serotonin syndrome* with other serotonergic agents. A 2-wk period is required between the use of any other serotonin agent and sibutramine. Not to be used concomitantly with other serotonin agents. Decreased levels with ketoconazole, erythromycin. Increased effect of alcohol.

Side Effects

Nervous System: arrhytmias—tachycardia, arthralgia, asthenia, bowel—constipation, CNS stimulation, cough increase, dizziness, dyspepsia, ear—disorder/pain, headache, migraine, myalgia, nausea/vomiting, palpitations, pain—abdominal/back/chest/neck, paresthesia, psyche—anxiety/depression/emotional lability/insomnia/nervousness/somnolence, taste changes.

Endocrine System: (Pregnancy Category C) anorexia, appetite—increased, dry mouth, dysmenorrhea/menorrhagia, edema, flushing, sweating, thirst.

Immune System: acne, allergy, flu syndrome, gastritis, herpes simplex, injury accident, joint disorder, laryngitis, pharyngitis, rash, rectal disorder, rhinitis, sinusitis, tenosynovitis, UTI, vaginal monilia.

Dosage: PO 10 mg qd with or without food. After 4 wk may increase to 15 mg qd.

 Chapter Highlights

- The catecholamines dopamine, norepinephrine, and epinephrine of the sympathetic nervous system constitute a balance to the parasympathetic nervous system.

- The catecholamines, also called adrenergics or sympathomimetics, can be considered "uppers," making flight, fight, and fun possible.

- Cathecholamines are used as drugs in cardiovascular emergencies to raise blood pressure, constrict arteries, increase heart rate, and decrease bleeding by vasoconstriction.

- During emergency conditions, the sympathetic nervous system stimulates the adrenal medulla to secrete epinephrine, which, in turn, triggers gluconeogenesis in the liver and skeletal muscle and the lipolysis of stored fat into energy.

- Drugs that counter adrenergic vasoconstricting activity are used to treat hypertension.

- Dopamine plays an important role in the emotions of the limbic system.

- Dopamine is also implicated in schizophrenia, and drugs blocking its action are used to treat, but do not cure, the thought disorder of schizophrenia.

- Stimulant drugs make more catecholamines available in the synapse and are used in the treatment of attention deficit hyperactivity disorder and narcolepsy, and also as anorexic drugs in the short-term treatment of obesity.

- Like dopamine, norepinephrine, and epinephrine, serotonin is a monoamine and is broken down by MAOIs.

- Decreased levels of serotonin contribute to severe depression, and drugs that block the reuptake of serotonin into presynaptic neurons have proven to be effective antidepressants.

- Serotonin release from platelets causes an eventual decrease in available serotonin and results in migraine headaches.

- The cause of migraines varies from one individual to another and ranges from allergy to hormones, diet, and emotional factors.

- The neurotransmitters dopamine, norepinephrine, epinephrine, and serotonin are essential to life.

- The drugs that mimic or block these neurotransmitters are important adjuncts to saving and protecting life and making it worth living.

---

* Life-threatening side effect.

5

Histamine, Antihistamines, and H₂ Blockers

drug list

- astemizole [Hismanal]
- brompheniramine maleate [Dimetane]
- buclizine hydrochloride [Bucladin-S Softabs]
- cetirizine hydrochloride [Zyrtec]
- chlorpheniramine maleate [Chlor-Trimeton (CTM)]
- cimetidine [Tagamet]
- cyclizine hydrochloride [Marezine]
- cyproheptadine hydrochloride [Periactin]
- dimenhydrinate [Dramamine, others]
- diphenhydramine hydrochloride [Benadryl]
- famotidine [Pepcid]
- fexofenadine hydrochloride [Allegra]
- hydroxyzine hydrochloride [Atarax, Vistaril]
- loratadine [Claritin]
- olopatadine hydrochloride [Patanol]
- promethazine hydrochloride [Phenergan]
- ranitidine hydrochloride [Zantac]
- trimethobenzamide hydrochloride [Tigan]

The neurotransmitter histamine, formed from the essential amino acid histidine, is an alerting neurotransmitter in the brain with influences on nausea, vomiting, and blood pressure as well as alertness; however, it cannot be used therapeutically owing to the wide range of possible side effects. Its release from storage nerve cells requires calcium's help. In the nervous system, histamine molecules have shapes that imply relationships to the parasympathetic and the sympathetic nervous systems. Many antihistamines, drugs that block histamine receptors, also have anticholinergic activity, and one of the earliest antihistamines, promazine, became the molecular parent of the first-generation neuroleptics, which block dopamine receptors in the sympathetic

nervous system. In turn, the neuroleptic chlorpromazine became the molecular parent of the tricyclic antidepressants, which block reuptake of norepinephrine. Thus, these molecules can antagonize histamine, acetylcholine, and dopamine. Does this point to minute differences in the receptor sites as well as the neurotransmitters of the CNS?

Mast cells and basophils in the immune system contain histamine and release it in explosive responses to trauma or foreign invasion. Histamine in the immune system causes capillaries to become more permeable and release the watery constituents of the blood, even to the point of hypovolemic shock. The misery of allergies like hayfever is caused by the release of histamine. In the GI tract histamine, affecting H₂ receptors, mediates the

85

release of hydrochloric acid, once thought to be the sole cause of peptic ulcers (Fig. 5–1).

▶ ANTIHISTAMINES

Antihistamines for allergies block histamine-1 receptors. Because histamine is an alerting neurotransmitter in the brain, it stands to reason that antihistamines that cross the BBB may cause drowsiness. Antihistamines have at least four areas of influence: the decrease of alertness; the decrease of the release of fluids from the capillaries during the immune response; the decrease of the release

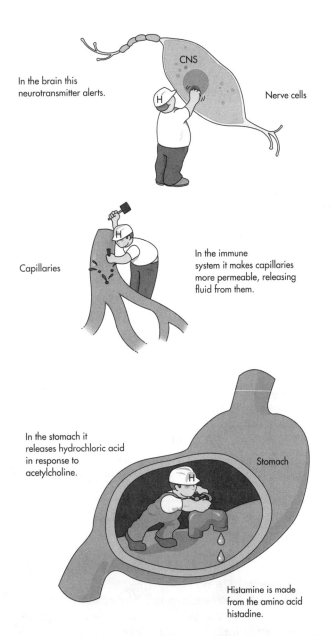

In the brain this neurotransmitter alerts.

CNS

Nerve cells

Capillaries

In the immune system it makes capillaries more permeable, releasing fluid from them.

In the stomach it releases hydrochloric acid in response to acetylcholine.

Stomach

Histamine is made from the amino acid histadine.

Figure 5-1. Histamine is hardworking.

of gastric acid secretions; and the relief of nausea and vomiting.

▶ PHENOTHIAZINE ANTIHISTAMINES

As described in Chapter 4, the phenothiazines, which were first recognized for their antihistamine and preoperative calming effects, also have antiemetic and antipsychotic actions. (See Chapter 4 for dosage and side effects of phenothiazines).

▶ ANTIHISTAMINES AS ANTIEMETICS

<u>Buclizine hydrochloride [Bucladin-S Softabs]</u> is used to treat motion sickness and vertigo.

Drug Interactions: Increased CNS depression with other CNS depressants and alcohol.

Side Effects

Nervous System: drowsiness, headache, nervousness, nausea.

Endocrine System: (Pregnancy Category C) dry mouth.

Immune System: none noted.

Dosage: PO 50 mg 30 min before a trip. Repeat q4–6h prn. Vertigo: PO 50 mg 1–3 ×/d.

<u>Cyclizine hydrochloride [Marezine]</u> is used to treat motion sickness and postoperative vomiting.

Drug Interactions: Increased CNS depression with other CNS depressants.

Side Effects:

Nervous System: arrhythmias—tachycardia, bowel—constipation/diarrhea, convulsions,* drowsiness, hypotension, nausea/vomiting, pain—IM site, psyche—euphoria/excitement/hallucinations (auditory, visual)/hyperexcitability, respiratory paralysis,* tinnitus, vision—blurred/diplopia.

Endocrine System: (Pregnancy Category B) anorexia, dryness—nose/mouth/throat, jaundice.

Immune System: rash, urticaria.

Dosage: PO 50 mg 30 min before a trip. Then q4–6h prn to maximum of 200 mg/d. IM 50 mg. Postop vomiting. IM preop, or 20–30 min before the end of surgery, or q4–6h prn.

---

* Life-threatening side effect.

Dimenhydrinate [Dramamine, others] is used to treat motion sickness, vertigo, nausea/vomiting of anesthesia, labyrinthitis, medications, Ménière's syndrome, radiation sickness, and stapedectomy.

Drug Interactions: Increased CNS depression with other CNS depressants.

Incompatibilities

Solution/Additive: aminophylline, amobarbital, butorphanol, chlorpromazine, glycopyrrolate, hydroxyzine, midazolam, pentobarbital, prochlorperazine, promazine, promethazine, thiopental.

Side Effects

Nervous System: bladder—dysuria/frequency, bowel—constipation/diarrhea, dizziness, drowsiness, headache, hypotension, incoordination, insomnia, nausea/ vomiting, nervousness, palpitations, restlessness, vision—blurred.

Endocrine System: (Pregnancy Category B) anorexia, dryness—nose/mouth/throat.

Immune System: rare responses.

Dosage: PO 50–100 mg q4–6h to maximum of 400 mg/ 24 h. IM 50 mg prn.

Diphenhydramine hydrochloride [Benadryl] is also used for its anticholinergic effects in Parkinson's. (See Chapter 3 for side effects.)

Dosage: Sedation: PO 25–50 mg hs. Motion sickness: PO 25–50 mg 30 min before a trip and ac. IM, IV 10–50 mg q4–6h to maximum 400 mg/d.

Hydroxyzine hydrochloride [Atarax, Vistaril] is a frequently used preop medication, valued for its ataractic effect as well as its antihistamine actions.

Drug Interactions: Increased CNS depression with other CNS depressants. Increased anticholinergic effects with other anticholinergics. May decrease pressor effects of epinephrine.

Incompatibilities

Solution/Additive: aminophylline, amobarbital, chloramphenicol, dimenhydrinate, penicillin G, pentobarbital, phenobarbital.

Side Effects

Nervous System: dizziness, drowsiness, dyspnea, EPS, headache, hypotension, sedation, wheezing.

Endocrine System: (Pregnancy Category C) dry mouth.

Immune System: erythema, IV (inadvertent) site reactions, rash.

Dosage: Anxiety: PO 25–100 mg tid–qid. IM 25–100 mg q4–6h. Pruritus: PO 25 mg tid or qid. IM 25 mg q4–6h. Nausea: IM 25–100 mg q4–6h.

Promethazine hydrochloride [Phenergan] is a phenothiazine commonly used for treating allergies, motion sickness, nausea, and for providing sedation.

Drug Interactions: Increased CNS depression with other CNS depressants. Anticholinergics increase anticholinergic action.

Incompatibilities

Solution/Additive: aminophylline, carbenicillin, cefotetan, chloramphenicol, chlorothiazide, diatrizoate, dimenhydrinate, heparin, hydrocortisone, iodipamide, iothalamate, methicillin, methohexital, nalbuphine, penicillin G sodium, pentobarbital, phenobarbital, thiopental.

Y-site: carbenicillin, cefotetan, heparin.

Side Effects

Nervous System: bladder—retention, bowel—constipation, CNS stimulation, coma,* convulsions,* coordination disturbances, dizziness, drowsiness, dyspnea/ respiratory depression,* EPS, hyper-/hypotension (mild), nausea/vomiting, psyche—confusion/restlessness, sedation/deep sleep, tremors, vision—blurred.

Endocrine System: (Pregnancy Category C) dryness—mouth/nose/throat.

Immune System: agranulocytosis,* photosensitivity.

Dosage: Allergies: PO/rectal/IM/IV 12.5 mg qid or 25 mg hs. Motion sickness: PO/rectal/IM/IV 25 mg bid. Nausea: PO/rectal/IM/IV 12.5–25 mg q4–6h prn. Sedation: PO/rectal/IM/IV 25–50 mg preop or hs.

Trimethobenzamide hydrochloride [Tigan] has only weak antihistamine action. Treats vomiting by acting in the CTZ of the medulla.

Drug Interactions: Increased CNS depression with other CNS depressants. Increased anticholinergic effects with belladonna alkaloids. EPS possible with phenothiazines.

Side Effects

Nervous System: bowel—diarrhea, cramps—muscle, EPS, hypotension, nausea—worsened.

Endocrine System: (Pregnancy Category C) none noted.

Immune System: acute hepatitis, jaundice, rash, Reye's syndrome.

---

* Life-threatening side effect.

Dosage: PO 250 mg tid–qid. IM, rectal 200 mg tid–qid.

▶ ANTIHISTAMINES FOR ALLERGY

<u>Brompheniramine maleate [Dimetane]</u> blocks histamine receptors.

Drug Interactions: Increased CNS depression with other CNS depressants.

Incompatibilities

Solution/Additive: Radiocontrast media.

Side Effects

Nervous System: bowel—constipation, coordination—disturbed, dizziness, drowsiness, dyspepsia, headache, hypotension, sedation.

Endocrine System: (Pregnancy Category C) dryness—mouth/nose/throat, sweating

Immune System: agranulocytosis,* hypersensitivity, photosensitivity, rash, urticaria.

Dosage: PO 4–8 mg tid or qid to maximum of 24 mg/24 h. SR: 8–12 mg bid or tid. IM/IV 5–20 mg q6–12h to maximum of 40 mg/24 h.

<u>Chlorpheniramine maleate [Chlor-Trimeton (CTM)]</u> is used to treat allergic responses.

Drug Interactions: Increased CNS depression with other CNS depressants.

Side Effects

Nervous System: arrhythmias—tachycardia, bladder—dysuria/frequency/retention, bowel—constipation/diarrhea, sensation of chest tightness, coordination impaired, dizziness, drowsiness, dyspepsia, fatigue, headache, mild hyper-/hypotension, insomnia, nausea/vomiting, palpitations, psyche—euphoria/nervousness, tremors, vertigo, vision—blurred/diplopia.

Endocrine System: (Pregnancy Category B) anorexia, dryness—mouth/nose/throat.

Immune System: bronchial secretions—thickened, acute labyrinthitis.

Dosage: PO tabs/syrup 2–4 mg tid or qid; 8–12 mg bid or tid to maximum of 24 mg/d. Allergic reactions to blood: SC/IM/IV 10–20 mg to maximum of 40 mg/d.

<u>Cyproheptadine hydrochloride [Periactin]</u> is used to increase appetite and to treat allergic reactions.

* Life-threatening side effect.

Drug Interactions: None noted.

Side Effects

Nervous System: bladder—dysuria/frequency/retention, dizziness, drowsiness, faintness, fatigue, headache, hypotension, nausea/vomiting, tremulousness.

Endocrine System: (Pregnancy Category B) appetite increase, dryness—nose/throat, transient decreases in FBS, serum amylase level increase, weight gain.

Immune System: rash, thickened bronchial secretions.

Dosage: PO 4 mg tid–qid. Maximum 0.5 mg/kg/d.

▶ THE BLOOD–BRAIN BARRIER AND ANTIHISTAMINES

Antihistamines that don't easily cross the BBB help allergy sufferers who must stay alert.

<u>Astemizole [Hismanal]</u> does not cross the BBB. Because food can decrease its absorption by 60%, the patient must take it 2 h pc and not eat for 1 h after medicating.

Drug Interactions: Increased risk of arrhythmias with erythromycin, itraconazole, ketoconazole.

Side Effects

Nervous System: arrhythmias, bowel—diarrhea, bronchospasm,* dizziness, headache, nausea, pain—abdominal, palpitations, psyche—depression/nervousness.

Endocrine System: (Pregnancy Category C) edema hunger, weight gain.

Immune System: angioedema,* conjunctivitis, epistaxis, pharyngitis, photosensitivity, pruritus, rash.

Dosage: PO 10 mg qd.

<u>Cetirizine hydrochloride [Zyrtec]</u> is used to treat seasonal and perennial allergic rhinitis and chronic idiopathic urticaria.

Drug Interactions: None noted.

Side Effects

Nervous System: bowel—constipation/diarrhea, drowsiness, headache, psyche—depression, sedation.

Endocrine System: (Pregnancy Category B) dry mouth.

Immune System: none noted.

Dosage: PO 5–10 mg qd. Chronic urticaria: PO 10 mg qd or bid.

<u>Fexofenadine hydrochloride [Allegra]</u> is an active metabolite of terfenadine and is used to treat seasonal allergic rhinitis.

Drug Interactions: None noted.

Side Effects

Nervous System: drowsiness, dyspepsia, fatigue, nausea.

Endocrine System: (Pregnancy Category C) dysmenorrhea.

Immune System: sinusitis, throat irritation, viral infection.

Dosage: PO 60 mg bid. Elderly or impaired renal function 60 mg qd.

Loratadine [Claritin] is an H_1 blocker for allergic rhinitis and idiopathic urticaria.

Drug Interactions: Increased levels with cimetidine, erythromycin, ketoconazole. Decreased levels of erythromycin.

Side Effects

Nervous System: arrhythmias—supraventricular tachyarrhythmias*/tachycardia, arthralgia, asthenia, bladder—incontinence/retention/changes, bowel—constipation/diarrhea/flatulence, bronchospasm,* coughing, cramps—leg, dizziness, dyspepsia, dysphonia, dyspnea, hiccup, hypotension/hypertension, hypertonia, malaise, migraine, myalgia, nausea/vomiting, pain—back/breast/chest/ear/eye/tooth, palpitations, paresthesia, psyche—agitation/anxiety/impaired concentration/confusion/depression/insomnia/irritability/paranoia, rigors, sexual function—impotence/decreased libido, sneezing, syncope, taste—altered, tinnitus, tremor, vertigo, vision—blepharospasm/blurred/altered lacrimation.

Endocrine System: (Pregnancy Category B) anorexia, appetite—increased, dysmenorrhea, fever, flushing, dry hair, menorrhagia, salivation—altered, dry skin, sweating, thirst, urinary discoloration, weight gain.

Immune System: bronchitis, dermatitis, angioneurotic edema, epistaxis, gastritis, hemoptysis, laryngitis, nasal dryness, pharyngitis, photosensitivity, pruritus, purpura, rash, sinusitis, stomatitis, urticaria, vaginitis, viral infection.

Dosage: PO 10 mg qd on empty stomach. Liver impairment: 60 mg qod.

Olopatadine hydrochloride [Patanol] is an H_1 antagonist that inhibits the release of histamine from mast cells during ophthalmic inflammation caused by allergens.

Drug Interactions: None noted.

Side Effects

Nervous System: burning/stinging, foreign body sensation, headache.

Endocrine System: (Pregnancy Category C) dry eyes.

Immune System: hyperemia, keratitis, lid edema, puritus.

Dosage: Ophthalmic solution 1–2 gtt to affected eye twice daily with a 6- to 8-h interval.†

▶ HISTAMINE-2 BLOCKERS

The original antihistamines blocked histamine-1 receptors in certain allergic conditions. The H_2 blockers block the histamine-2 receptors on gastric parietal cells, which are responsible for the release of gastric acid. The vagus nerve, under the influence of acetylcholine, triggers the release of histamine, which in turn triggers the release of hydrochloric acid (HCl). Too much HCl erodes the mucous lining of the stomach. H_2 blockers stop the histamine-mediated release of HCl in the stomach; they are given to prevent stress ulcers that occur in burns and other traumas and major illnesses and for GERD. A bacterial infection with *Helicobacter* seems to be the primary cause of ulcers and signals a new approach to the treatment of ulcers.

Cimetidine [Tagamet] blocks H_2 receptors on parietal cells to suppress gastric acid secretion.

Off Label: Prophylaxis of stress-induced ulcers, upper GI bleeding, aspiration pneumonitis; acetaminophen toxicity, GERD, chronic urticaria.

Drug Interactions: Decreased metabolism and increased toxicity of diazepam, lidocaine, phenobarbital, phenytoin, propranolol, warfarin. Decreased absorption possible with antacids.

Side Effects

Nervous System: arrhythmias and arrest after rapid IV bolus,* bowel—abdominal discomfort/constipation/diarrhea, dizziness/lightheadedness, drowsiness, headache, pain—IM site, psyche—confusion/depression/paranoia, sexual function—impotence.

Endocrine System: (Pregnancy Category B) fever, galactorrhea, gynecomastia, hypospermia, slight increase—BUN/creatinine/serum uric acid.

Immune System: alopecia, aplastic anemia,* arthritis exacerbation, neutropenia, PT—increase, Stevens–Johnson syndrome*, thrombocytopenia.

---

* Life-threatening side effect.

† Eye related.

Dosage: PO 300 mg qid with meals and hs, or 800 mg hs or 400 mg bid × 8 wk maximum. IV 300 mg in 20 mL D5W or saline over 2 min q6h or in 100 mL of dextrose in saline over 15–20 min q6h. IM 300 mg q6h. If there is renal impairment, give q8–12h. Maintenance: PO 400 mg hs.

Famotidine [Pepcid] is a thiazole derivative more potent than cimetidine or ranitidine. Give with food.

Drug Interactions: None noted.

Side Effects

Nervous System: bowel—constipation/diarrhea, dizziness, headache, hypotension, insomnia/somnolence, paresthesias, psyche—anxiety/confusion/depression, sexual function—libido decrease.

Endocrine System: (Pregnancy Category B) increased BUN/serum creatinine, flushing, dry skin.

Immune System: acne, pruritus, rash, thrombocytopenia.

Dosage: PO 40 mg hs or 20 mg bid. Maintenance: 20 mg hs. IV 20 mg q12h. Decrease to 20 mg hs (or 40 mg hs q3–4d) depending on response when kidneys are impaired (creatinine clearance less than 10 mL/min). Pain relief may not occur for several days into treatment. GERD, gastritis: PO 10 mg bid.

Ranitidine hydrochloride [Zantac] treats duodenal ulcer and GERD.

Drug Interactions: None noted.

Incompatibilities

Solution/Additive: amphotericin B, clindamycin, chlorpromazine, diazepam, hydroxyzine, methotrimeprazine, midazolam, nalbuphine, opium alkaloids.

Y-site: methotrimeprazine, midazolam, opium alkaloids, phenobarbital.

Side Effects

Nervous System: arrhythmias—bradycardia/tachycardia (with rapid IV push), bowel—constipation/diarrhea, dizziness, drowsiness, headache, insomnia, malaise, nausea, pain—abdominal, psyche—agitation/confusion/depression/hallucinations (elderly), vertigo.

Endocrine System: (Pregnancy Category B) none noted.

Immune System: anaphylaxis,* thrombocytopenia, WBC—reversible decrease.

Dosage: PO 150 mg bid or 300 mg hs. Maintenance: 150 mg hs. IV 50 mg in 20 mL D5W or 0.9% NaCl over 5 min q6–8h or 150–300 mg/24 h by continuous infusion. Give less often with renal impairment. Heartburn: PO 75 mg bid.

 ## Chapter Highlights

- Histamine is versatile, as a part of the immune system it causes vasodilation and capillary permeability.

- Antihistamines were originally used to counter the immune response to the tissue damage and fluid shifts that occur with the trauma of surgery.

- Histamine also acts as an alerting neurotransmitter in the nervous system where antihistamines have great value for their ataractic effects before and after surgery.

- Newer antihistamines have been developed that do not easily cross the BBB and are thus less sedating.

- Histamine plays a role in the release of gastric acid essential to digestion.

- Antihistamines that block H_2 receptors have value in treating ulcers and reflux (GERD).

---

* Life-threatening side effect.

6

Drugs That Affect GABA: Anxiolytics, Anticonvulsants, Hypnotics, and Muscle Relaxants

- acetazolamide [Diamox, others]
- alprazolam [Xanax]
- amobarbital [Amytal]
- amobarbital sodium [Amytal Sodium]
- baclofen [Lioresal]
- buspirone hydrochloride [BuSpar]
- butalbital + aspirin + caffeine [Fiorinal]
- carbamazepine [Tegretol]
- carisoprodol [Rela, Soma]
- chloral hydrate [Noctec]
- chlordiazepoxide hydrochloride [Librium]
- chlordiazepoxide + amytriptyline [Limbitrol]
- clonazepam [Klonopin]
- clorazepate dipotassium [Tranxene, Tranxene-SD]
- clorazepate dipotassium [Tranxene]
- diazepam [Valium]
- diazepam emulsified [Dizac]
- disulfiram [Antabuse]
- divalproex [Depakote]
- ethchlorvynol [Placidyl]
- ethosuximide [Zarontin]
- felbamate [Felbatol]
- flumazenil [Romazicon]
- flurazepam hydrochloride [Dalmane]
- gabapentin [Neurontin]
- glutethimde [Doriden, Doriglute]
- halazepam [Paxipam]
- lorazepam [Ativan]
- mephenytoin [Mesantoin]
- mephobarbital [Mebaral]
- methocarbamol [Robaxin, Marbaxin, Delaxin]
- methohexital sodium [Brevital]
- methsuximide [Celontin]

- methyprylon [Noludar]
- midazolam hydrochloride [Versed]
- oxazepam [Serax]
- pentobarbital [Nembutal]
- pentobarbital sodium [Nembutal Sodium]
- phenobarbital [Barbita, Luminal]
- phenobarbital sodium [Barbita, Luminal]
- phenobarbital sodium [Luminal Sodium]
- phensuximide [Milontin]
- phenytoin [Dilantin]
- primidone [Mysoline]
- quazepam [Doral]
- secobarbital [Seconal]
- secobarbital sodium [Seconal Sodium]
- temazepam [Restoril]
- thiamylal NA [Surital]
- thiopental sodium [Pentothal]
- topiramate [Topamax]
- triazolam [Halcion]
- valproic acid [Depakene]

Whereas acetylcholine and the catecholamines excite neurons, gamma-aminobutyric acid (GABA) created from the amino acid glutamate, applies the brakes. We make our own GABA as we engage in activities that bring us peace and tranquility, but some conditions require drugs to slow down cell firing (Fig. 6–1). The drugs that increase GABA's affinity for its receptors include sedatives, hypnotics, some anesthetics, and the anxiolytics. The oldest of the GABA drugs is alcohol, dating back to the earliest production of beer and wine. The barbiturates were first synthesized in 1864 by Adolph von Baeyer. Both alcohol and the barbiturates provide sedation and have excellent hypnotic qualities; however, these are drawbacks to allowing the patient to experience decreased anxiety yet remain awake and functional. The discovery of the first benzodiazepine, chlordiazepoxide [Librium] in 1960 and those that followed have improved the treatment of insomnia, anxiety, and epilepsy.

The brain achieves peace and tranquility in steps. First, a sedating molecule slides into the sedative-convulsant receptor. Next, the benzodiazapine receptor is engaged. The engagement of the first-step receptors increase GABA's affinity for its own receptor, and it then fits into its receptor, causing chloride channels to widen. As the chloride molecules enter the cell and reach equi-

librium on each side of the cell membrane, cell firing slows. For the cell to fire again more sodium is needed to depolarize the cell and overcome the inertia. If convulsants were to lock into the sedative convulsant receptor, chloride channels would narrow and seizures could result. For example, the insecticide lindane increases cell firing to the point of seizures and is treated with anticonvulsants that increase the affinity of GABA for its receptors (Fig. 6–2).

GABA receptors are postsynaptic, and GABA inhibits or tamps cell firing by blocking the spread of the action potential through cell networks that pass on and interpret stimuli from our surroundings. But when GABA is blocked in excitatory neurons, one can be inundated with stimuli beyond the normal ability to process and become alert, anxious, overwhelmed. In fact, the drug carboline fits the benzodiazepine receptor and causes unnaturally severe anxiety, even panic. If a drug exists that can cause panic, it stands to reason that we can endogenously produce alerting molecules that engage the GABA receptors to reduce GABA's affinity for its receptors and cause anxiety and panic. Such molecules would be necessary to alert us to danger.

GABA receptors abound on the dendrites of dopamine neurons in the limbic system, and GABA slows the firing rate of those ascending dopamine pathways.

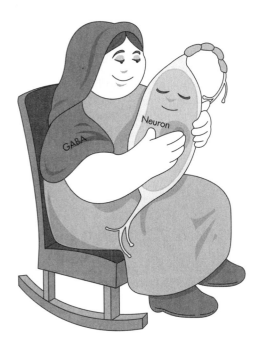

Figure 6–1. GABA quiets cell firing.

Dopamine plays a role in the paranoia of schizophrenia, and the anxiolytic drugs, because they increase GABA's affinity for its receptors, are contraindicated in the treatment of schizophrenia. Such drugs could decrease any inhibition the patient might have on acting out his or her destructive paranoid delusions and increase the possibility of the patient's being a danger to self or others.

GABA also inhibits the norepinephrine, serotonin, and acetylcholine pathways. The medulla in the brain stem, the amygdalae in the limbic system, and the cerebellum are rich in GABA receptors. The medulla is a major focus of seizures. In addition, the amygdalae, which cause fear, rage, and some pleasure and sexual responses, as well as other limbic structures play some role in memory. The benzodiazepines commonly cause posterograde amnesia by blocking the process of consolidating memories of new events. For example, patients typically have no recall of endoscopic examinations when given a benzodiazepine drug. GABA also influences the release of pituitary hormones like luteinizing hormone and prolactin—an example of the intertwining of the nervous and the endocrine systems.

▶ SEDATIVES AND HYPNOTICS

Sedation helps the patient tolerate the stress of diagnostic, therapeutic, and surgical procedures. Sleep is essential to health and healing. Sedatives and hypnotics increase GABA's affinity for its own receptors, resulting in

slowed cell firing so that the patient can relax or fall asleep. Sometimes the only difference between a sedative and a hypnotic is the dosage. Sometimes patients suffer insomnia or need sedation before or during a procedure. Hypnotics may be used to treat insomnia, but they cannot cure the condition, and should be used only for a short time to prevent habituation and tolerance. Meanwhile, the cause of the insomnia should be found and dealt with.

▶ ALCOHOL

The oldest drug to allay anxiety or sedate is alcohol. It fits into the sedative-convulsant receptor, causing GABA to drift into its receptor. One of the best examples of the effect of alcohol on human behavior is at a party. The chit-chat is stilted as it begins; then the alcohol gets served. One can imagine GABA drifting into its receptors as guests relax and the noise gets louder and louder. Anxiety, alcohol, and GABA go together in the alcoholic syndrome.

ALCOHOL-TYPE SEDATIVE/HYPNOTICS

The following drugs contain formulations of alcohol and engage the sedative-convulsant receptor, increasing

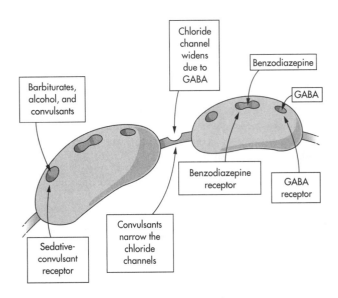

Until attracted to their receptors by the insertion of sedating, antianxiety, or anticonvulsant molecules, GABA molecules remain outside the GABA receptors. GABA receptor molecules are embedded in cell membranes. When GABA is attracted to its receptors, chloride channels widen. More chlorides enter the cell until equilibrium is reached on both sides of the cell membrane. The state of equilibrium requires more sodium to make the cell fire again.

Figure 6–2. GABA receptor molecules.

the affinity of GABA for its receptor. Because these medications are subject to abuse, they are Schedule IV drugs.

<u>Chloral hydrate [Noctec]</u>, a Schedule IV drug, has been used for over a hundred years. The chloral part of the molecule metabolizes in the liver to trichloroethanol, a form of alcohol that induces sleep. The infamous "Mickey Finn" is a mixture of chloral hydrate and alcohol.

Drug Interactions: Choral hydrate's CNS depressant action is compounded by other CNS depressants. It increases anticoagulant effect of oral anticoagulants. IV furosemide may cause BP changes, flushing, and sweating.

Side Effects

Nervous System: arrhythmias/cardiac arrest,* bowel—diarrhea, dizziness, headache, hypotension, incoordination, nausea/vomiting.

Endocrine System: (Pregnancy Category C) ketonuria.

Immune System: angioedema,* eczema, erythema, purpura, rash, urticaria. Chronic use: allergy, gastritis, kidney/liver damage, sudden death.*

Dosage: Sedation: PO/rectal 250 mg tid–pc. Hypnotic: PO/rectal: 500 mg–1 g hs or 30 min before surgery.

<u>Ethchlorvynol [Placidyl]</u>, a Schedule IV drug, is a short-acting tertiary acetylenic alcohol hypnotic; it decreases anxiety. It has anticonvulsant and muscle relaxant activity as well.

Drug Interactions: Ethchlorvynol's CNS depressant action is increased by other CNS depressants. It decreases anticoagulation with oral anticoagulants.

Side Effects

Nervous System: aftertaste, coma,* dizziness, facial numbness, hangover, headache, muscle—tremors/weakness, nausea/vomiting, nightmares, respiratory failure,* vision—blurred.

Endocrine System: (Pregnancy Category C) none noted.

Immune System: urticaria.

Dosage: PO. Sedative: 200 mg bid or tid. Hypnotic: 500 mg–1 g hs. Give 200 mg more if patient cannot sleep through the early AM.

▶ WHEN ALCOHOL IS THE PROBLEM

Alcohol, the oldest sedative, is sometimes misused and abused by those self-medicating psychic pain. Unfortu-

nately, using alcohol as a solution to life's problems leads to more problems. Therapy involves several modalities, including psychotherapy and GABA-like drugs to ease detoxification. The recovering alcoholic faces a daunting task to overcome alcohol addiction. Some recovering alcoholics, as additional motivation and only after careful consultation and education, agree to use the following drug, which can cause a toxic reaction if they ingest alcohol after taking it.

<u>Disulfiram [Antabuse]</u> intentionally poisons the patient who takes it and then uses alcohol. By inhibiting the enzyme acetaldehyde dehydrogenase, disulfiram prevents the metabolism of alcohol and causes a toxic reaction if the recovering alcoholic drinks. The individual must be motivated to stop drinking and consent to using disulfiram. It is never given to trick or punish. The patient must avoid use of any product containing alcohol, even colognes and aftershaves.

Drug Interactions: Toxic with any form of alcohol, also with IV cotrimoxazole and IV nitroglycerin. CNS symptoms with isoniazid. May increase blood levels and toxicity of barbiturates, paraldehyde, phenytoin, warfarin.

Side Effects

Nervous System: arrhythmias*—tachycardia, acute congestive heart failure,* convulsions,* death—sudden,* drowsiness, fatigue, gait—abnormal, GI disturbances—mild, headache, hyperventilation, hypotension, nausea/violent vomiting, pain—chest, palpitations, psyche—bizarre behavior/confusion/disorientation/personality changes/psychosis/restlessness/uneasiness, respiratory depression,* shock,* speech—slurred, taste—metallic or garlic, tremor, unconsciousness,* vertigo, vision—blurred, weakness.

Endocrine System: (Pregnancy Category X) flushing, sweating, thirst.

Immune System: allergic or acneiform dermatitis, fixed-drug eruption, hepatotoxicity,* hypersensitivity, optic neuritis, peripheral neuropathy, polyneuritis, urticaria.

Dosage: PO 250 mg qd for 1–2 weeks. Maintenance: 125–500 mg qd.

▶ BARBITURATES

Barbiturates, derived from barbituric acid and named after the feminine name Barbara, were once the most common sedatives and hypnotics; however, barbituates interfere with rapid eye movement (REM) sleep, patients quickly build tolerance, and the drugs have a long half-life of up to 42 hours resulting in daytime sleepiness or hang-

---

* Life-threatening side effect.

over. Most important, they are lethal in overdose. They are still used, some as short-acting anesthetics, but have given way to the benzodiazepines, which appear not to interfere with REM sleep. Barbiturates are Schedule II or IV drugs with the potential for dependence and abuse. (Note that the generic ending for barbiturates is "tal.")

<u>Amobarbital [Amytal], amobarbital sodium [Amytal Sodium]</u> are Schedule II drugs. Amobarbital is an anticonvulsant and sedative-hypnotic.

Drug Interactions: CNS depressants increase amobarbital's CNS depressant action. Possibility of nephrotoxicity with methoxyflurane. Antagonizes effects of phenmetrazine.

Incompatibilities

Solution/Additive: cimetidine, codeine phosphate, dimenhydrinate, hydrocortisone, hydroxyzine, insulin, levorphanol, meperidine, morphine, norepinephrine, pancuronium, penicillin G, pentazocine, phenothiazines, phenytoin, procaine, streptomycin, tetracycline, vancomycin.

Side Effects

Nervous System: dizziness, drowsiness, paradoxical excitement, hangover, hypotension, lethargy, respiratory depression.*

Endocrine System: (Pregnancy Category D) none noted.

Immune System: agranulocytosis,* angioedema,* rash, Stevens–Johnson syndrome, thrombocytopenia.

Dosage: Anticonvulsant: IV 65–500 mg to maximum of 1 g. Hypnotic: PO/IM 65–200 mg to maximum of 500 mg. Sedation: PO 30–50 mg bid or tid. Labor: PO 200–400 mg repeated at 1- to 3-h intervals to maximum of 1 g. Preop: PO/IM 200 mg 1 h before surgery.

<u>Pentobarbital [Nembutal], pentobarbital sodium [Nembutal Sodium],</u> Schedule II drugs, are short-acting barbiturates.

Drug Interactions: CNS depressant action is increased by other CNS depressants, antagonized by phenmetrazine. Risk of nephrotoxicity with methoxyflurane.

Incompatibilities

Solution/Additive: benzquinamide, cimetidine, many antihistamines and H_2 blockers, most opiates and synthetics, many phenothiazines, penicillin G, tetracyclines, vancomycin; some anxiolytics, hydrocortisone, insulin, phenytoin, succinylcholine.

Y-site: butorphanol, glycopyrrolate, midazolam, nalbuphine, perphenazine, ranitidine.

Side Effects

Nervous System: too rapid IV: apnea,* bronchospasm,* hypotension, laryngospasm,* respiratory depression.*

Endocrine System: (Pregnancy Category D) none noted.

Immune System: None noted.

Dosage: PO 100–200 mg hs. Sedative: PO 20–30 mg bid to qid. Preop sedation: PO 150–200 mg in 2 divided doses. IM 150–200 mg in 2 divided doses. IV 100 mg; may increase to 500 mg if necessary.

<u>Phenobarbital [Barbita, Luminal], phenobarbital sodium [Luminal Sodium]</u> are Schedule IV drugs. Phenobarbital, a sedative-hypnotic has many uses: sedation in anxiety or tension states, pre- and postoperative pediatric sedation, and pylorospasm in infants.

Off Label: Benzodiazepine withdrawal and management of chronic cholestasis. Its most frequent use is the management of seizure disorders. (See the anticonvulsants section of this chapter.)

Drug Interactions: CNS depression increased with other CNS depressants; phenobarbital may decrease absorption and increase metabolism of oral anticoagulants; increases metabolism of corticosteroids, oral contraceptives, anticonvulsants, digitoxin, possibly decreasing their effects; antidepressants potentiate adverse effects of phenobarbital; griseofulvin decreases absorption of phenobarbital.

Incompatibilities

Solution/Additive: benzquinamide, cephalothin, chlorpromazine, codeine phosphate, ephedrine, hydralazine, hydrocortisone, sodium succinate, hydroxyzine, insulin, levorphanol, meperidine, methadone, morphine, norepinephrine, procaine, prochlorperazine, promazine, promethazine, ranitidine, streptomycin, tetracyclines, vancomycin.

Side Effects

Nervous System: apnea,* arrhythmias—bradycardia, ataxia, bowel—constipation/diarrhea, bronchospasm,* circulatory collapse,* dizziness, hangover, headache, hypotension, hypoventilation, laryngospasm,* myalgia, nausea/vomiting, pain—epigastric, pain—at extravasation site, paresthesias, psyche—anxiety/confusion/depression/excitement/insomnia/irritability/nightmares, somnolence, vision—nystagmus. IV: coughing, hiccuping, laryngospasm.* Overdose: CNS depression,* coma,* death,* respiratory depression.*

Endocrine System: (Pregnancy Category D) deficiency—folic acid/vitamin D, fever, hypocalcemia, osteomalacia, rickets, sweating.

---

* Life-threatening side effect.

Immune System: megaloblastic anemia, agranulocytosis,* angioedema,* dermatitis, liver damage, rash, serum sickness, Stevens–Johnson syndrome,* thrombocytopenia. Extravasation: gangrene, redness, thrombosis.

Dosage: Sedation: PO/IM 30–120 mg bid–tid. IV/IM 100–200 mg/d. Hypnotic: PO 100–320 mg. Anticonvulsant: PO 100–300 mg/d. IM/IV 200–600 mg to maximum of 20 mg/kg.

Note: Use only large muscles for IM administration. Give IV only when prompt action is needed, and then administer slowly to prevent overdose. For example: start with 100 mg and evaluate.

<u>Secobarbital [Seconal], secobarbital sodium [Seconal Sodium]</u>, Schedule II, short-acting barbiturate sedative/hypnotic drugs, also have anticonvulsant uses.

Drug Interactions: CNS depressants increase CNS depression. Phenmetrazine antagonizes effects of secobarbital. Methoxyflurane increases risk of nephrotoxicity.

Incompatibilities

Solution/Additive: benzquinamide, codeine, cimetidine, ephedrine, erythromycin, glycopyrrolate, hydrocortisone, insulin, levorphanol, methadone, norepinephrine, pentazocine, phenytoin, procaine, sodium bicarbonate, streptomycin, tetracycline, vancomycin.

Y-site: cimetidine, glycopyrrolate.

Side Effects

Nervous System: drowsiness, paradoxical excitement—elderly, hangover. With rapid IV: hypotension/laryngospasm*/respiratory depression.*

Endocrine System: (Pregnancy Category D) none noted.

Immune System: none noted.

Dosage: Hypnotic: PO/IM 100–200 mg hs. Preop sedation: PO 100–300 mg 1-2 h before surgery. Sedation: PO 100–300 mg/d in 3 divided doses. Adjunct to spinal anesthesia: IV 50–100 mg to maximum of 250 mg/dose; slow infusion.

▶ NONBARBITURATE SEDATIVES
  AND HYPNOTICS

The nonbarbiturate formulations are also subject to abuse. They do not cure the cause of insomnia and should only be used for a short time.

<u>Glutethimide [Doriden, Doriglute]</u>, a Schedule III drug, is structurally related to methyprylon. Both of these drugs are piperidine derivatives with actions like those of the barbiturates. They depress REM sleep, and drug withdrawal can cause REM rebound with increased dreaming, nightmares, even insomnia. As with the other sedative-hypnotics, only short-term use is recommended. Because they stimulate hepatic microsomal enzymes, they can alter the metabolism of other drugs that are detoxified by this system. They have an anticholinergic effect too. The elderly can be quite sensitive to these drugs and become confused. These drugs can be deadly in overdose, and the patient should be evaluated for suicidal ideation beforehand.

Drug Interactions: Anticholinergic effects increased by tricyclic antidepressants. CNS depressants increase glutethimide's CNS depressant action. Decreases oral anticoagulants' effects.

Side Effects

Nervous System: apnea—sudden,* ataxia, arrhythmias—tachycardia, bowel—constipation/decrease motility/paralysis, coma,* convulsions,* cyanosis, dyspepsia, dyspnea, edema—cerebral/pulmonary, hangover, headache, hiccups, hypotension, muscle—flaccid/hyperreflexia/paralysis/spasticity/tremors/facial twitching, nausea/vomiting, psyche—agitation/excitement/hallucinations, respiratory depression,* vertigo, vision—blurred/diplopia/mydriasis. Fetal: CNS depression. Chronic or toxic: concentration/memory/speech—impairment, nystagmus.

Endocrine System: (Pregnancy Category C) fever, hypothermia, dry mouth.

Immune System: aplastic blood dyscrasias,* exfoliative dermatitis,* edema—pulmonary/cerebral, infections—severe, renal tube necrosis.

Dosage: PO 250–500 mg hs. May repeat once if 4 h remain until rising. The elderly: Do not exceed 500 mg hs. Preop sedation: PO 500 mg hs before surgery, then 500–1000 mg 1 h prior to anesthesia.

<u>Methyprylon [Noludar]</u>, a Schedule III drug, suppresses REM sleep as hypnotics do.

Drug Interactions: CNS depressants increase methyprylon's CNS depressant action.

Side Effects

Nervous System: bowel—diarrhea, convulsions,* dizziness, drowsiness—AM, dyspepsia, headache, nausea/vomiting, psyche—confusion/delirium/excitation/hallucinations. Toxicity: confusion, dyspnea, edema—pulmonary, respiratory depression,* shock,* somnolence, vision—pupil constriction.

Endocrine System: (Pregnancy Category B) exacerbation of intermittent porphyria. Toxicity: fever, hypothermia.

---

* Life-threatening side effect.

Immune System: rash.

Dosage: Insomnia: PO 200–400 mg hs. Not to exceed 400 mg/d.

▶ BENZODIAZEPINE HYPNOTICS

Some of the benzodiazepine hypnotics may also cause a daytime hangover; however, they appear not to interfere with REM sleep. Most benzodiazepines may cause the following side effect: mild hangover (in the first few days of treatment), aggression, anterograde amnesia, ataxia, impaired coordination, confusion, disorientation, excitement, irritation, and vertigo. No hypnotic heals the underlying cause of insomnia; the benzodiazepines are no exception. Long-term use may lead to tolerance. Because they have the potential for abuse and dependency, they are Schedule IV drugs.

Note: The generic names of most benzodiazepines end in "lam" or "pam".

Flurazepam hydrochloride [Dalmane] is a Schedule IV sedative-hypnotic, CNS agent, and anxiolytic.

Drug Interactions: Its CNS depressant action is increased with other CNS depressants. Levels may increase with cimetidine or disulfiram.

Side Effects

Nervous System: bowel—diarrhea, dizziness, drowsiness, headache, heartburn, hypotension, lightheadedness, nausea/vomiting, pain—abdominal, psyche—apprehension/depression/excitement/euphoria/hallucinations/hyperactivity/nervousness/nightmares/talkativeness, vision—blurred. Overdose: coma.*

Endocrine System: (Pregnancy Category X) none noted.

Immune System: allergy, burning eyes, granulocytopenia, jaundice.

Dosage: PO 15–30 mg hs.

Quazepam [Doral], Schedule IV, is an anxiolytic, sedative, and hypnotic. REM sleep is not changed and there are no observable withdrawal symptoms with quazepam.

Drug Interactions: CNS depressants, anticonvulsants increase CNS depression. Cimetidine increases quazepam plasma levels and increases toxicity. May decrease antiparkinsonian effects of levodopa. May increase phenytoin levels. Smoking decreases sedative action of quazepam.

Side Effects

Nervous System: dizziness, drowsiness, dyspepsia, fatigue, headache.

Endocrine System: (Pregnancy Category X) dry mouth.

Immune System: none noted.

Dosage: PO. Start with 15 mg; lower to 7.5 mg if needed.

Temazepam [Restoril], Schedule IV, has many of the benzodiazepine side effects.

Drug Interactions: CNS depressants increase temazepam CNS depressant actions. Cimetidine increases temazepam plasma levels and toxicity. May decrease antiparkinsonian effects of levodopa. May increase phenytoin levels. Smoking decreases sedative effects.

Side Effects

Nervous System: bowel—diarrhea, dizziness, drowsiness, palpitations, psyche—euphoria, weakness.

Endocrine System: (Pregnancy Category X) none noted.

Immune System: none noted.

Dosage: PO 15–30 mg hs.

Triazolam [Halcion], Schedule IV, has the typical benzodiazepine side effects.

Drug Interactions: CNS depressants increase CNS depression of triazolam. Cimetidine increases triazolam plasma levels, and thus its toxicity. May decrease antiparkinsonian effects of levodopa.

Side Effects

Nervous System: bowel—constipation, dizziness, drowsiness, EEG—minor changes, headache, lightheadedness, nausea/vomiting, psyche—nervousness/hyperactivity/talkativeness, vision disturbances.

Endocrine System: (Pregnancy Category X) none noted.

Immune System: none noted.

Dosage: PO 0.125–0.5 mg hs.

▶ BARBITURATES FOR ANESTHESIA

The barbiturates used for anesthesia produce unconsciousness rapidly, either as an induction agent used with general anesthesia or alone for brief procedures.

Methohexital sodium [Brevital], Schedule IV, is a short-acting anesthetic commonly used for cardioversion or ECT. It has similar side effects to thiopental.

Drug Interactions: Increased CNS depression with other CNS depressants.

Incompatibilities

Solution/Additive: atropine, chlorpromazine, glycopyrrolate, hydralazine, kanamycin, lidocaine, methi-

---

* Life-threatening side effect.

cillin, methyldopa, prochlorperazine, promazine, promethazine, streptomycin, tetracyclines.

Side Effects

Nervous System: apnea,* bowel—cramping/diarrhea, coughing, headache, hiccups, hypotension, laryngospasm,* muscle—involuntary movement/rigidity/tremor/twitching, nausea/vomiting, radial nerve palsy, respiratory depression,* seizures,* vascular collapse—peripheral.*

Endocrine System: (Pregnancy Category C) none noted.

Immune System: hemolytic anemia, rectal bleeding, thrombophlebitis.

Dosage: Induction: IV 5–12 mL of 1% solution (50–120 mg). Maintenance: 2–4 mL (20–40 mg) for 5–7 min.

Thiamylal NA [Surital] is a rapid and ultra-short-acting Schedule III barbiturate used to induce anesthesia and maintain it with intermittent IV injection for short procedures. It may be used, but with caution, in hypotension, shock, coronary artery disease, status asthmaticus, pain, or with impaired liver and/or kidneys.

Drug Interactions: As with other barbiturates.

Side Effects

Nervous System: retrograde amnesia, bronchospasm,* delirium during recovery, headache, hiccups, laryngospasm,* myocardial depression,* nausea/vomiting, respiratory depression,* salivation.

Endocrine System: (Pregnancy Category C) hypothermia.

Immune System: anaphylaxis,* thrombophlebitis. Injection site: pain, sloughing, swelling.

Dosage: After test dose of 2 mL of 2.5% for sensitivity: Induction: IV (intermittent) 1 mL q5s. Use newly prepared 2.5% solution, reconstituted with isotonic NaCl. Maintenance: 0.3% per intermittent injection or drip.

Thiopental sodium [Pentothal] is the classic short-acting Schedule III anesthetic, in use for over 50 years.

Drug Interactions: CNS depressants increase thiopental CNS depression. Phenothiazines increase risk of hypotension. Probenecid may prolong anesthesia.

Incompatibilities

Solution/Additive: amikacin, benzquinamide, cephapirin, chlorpromazine, codeine phosphate, dextrose Ringer's combination, 10% dextrose, dimenhydrinate,

diphenhydramine, doxapram, ephedrine, fibrinolysin, glycopyrrolate, hydromorphone, insulin, levorphanol, meperidine, metaraminol, methadone, morphine, norepinephrine, penicillin G, prochlorperazine, promazine, promethazine, sodium bicarbonate, succinylcholine, tetracycline.

Side Effects

Nervous System: arrhythmias, bowel—cramping/diarrhea, bronchospasm,* circulatory depression,* cough, emergence delirium, headache, hiccups, laryngospasm,* muscle—hyperactivity, myocardial depression,* nausea/vomiting, psyche—retrograde amnesia, respiratory depression*/apnea.

Endocrine System: (Pregnancy Category C) hypothermia, shivering.

Immune System: anaphylaxis,* bleeding—rectal, hypersensitivity reactions. Extravasation: sloughing/thrombosis.

Dosage: Test dose: IV 25–75 mg; then 3–4 mg/kg or 50–75 mg q 30–40 s until desired anesthetic response results.

▶ BENZODIAZEPINES FOR ANESTHESIA

The benzodiazepines are only infrequently used to induce anesthesia, but rather serve as premedication or adjuncts to regional or general anesthesia. They may be preferred over the barbiturates because they cause less cardiovascular and respiratory depression, but they require larger doses and act longer than the barbiturates (Dripps, 1997). Midazolam is the most commonly used benzodiazepine anesthetic, but diazepam and lorazepam may also be used. When used as anesthetics, only the anesthetist may administer them.

Midazolam hydrochloride [Versed], Schedule IV, is used for preoperative sedation and perioperative amnesia. (It is given by the nurse anesthetist for anesthesia induction or maintenance.)

Drug Interactions: CNS depressants increase midazolam's CNS depressant action. Cimetidine increases midazolam plasma levels, increasing its toxicity. May decrease antiparkinsonian effects of levodopa. May increase phenytoin levels. Smoking decreases sedative and antianxiety effects.

Incompatibilities

Solution/Additive: dimenhydrinate, pentobarbital, perphenazine, prochlorperazine, ranitidine.

Y-site: dimenhydrinate, pentobarbital, perphenazine, prochlorperazine, ranitidine. Midazolam has many of the typical benzodiazepine side effects plus the following.

---

* Life-threatening side effect.

Side Effects

Nervous System: cough, drowsiness, headache, hiccups, hypotension, laryngospasm,* nausea/vomiting, psyche—euphoria, respiratory arrest*, sedation—excessive, tachypnea, vision—blurred/diplopia/nystagmus/pinpoint pupils.

Endocrine System: (Pregnancy Category D) chills.

Immune System: hives. Injection site: burning/induration/swelling/pain.

Dosage: Preop: IM 0.07–0.08 mg/kg 1h before surgery. IV 1–1.5 mg; may repeat in 2 min. Intubated patient: 0.05–0.2 mg/kg/h continuous infusion. Induction for general anesthesia: Premedicated: IV 0.15–0.25 mg/kg over 20–30 s; allow 2 min to see effect. No premedication: IV 0.3–0.35 mg/kg over 20–30 s; allow 2 min to see effect.

▶ A BENZODIAZEPINE ANTAGONIST

The benzodiazepine antagonist reverses the action of benzodiazepines involved in recall, psychomotor impairment, and sedation. As would be expected, it has no effect on opiate overdose.

Flumazenil [Romazicon] reverses benzodiazepine anesthetic action and is used in overdose.

Off Label: For alcohol intoxication, hepatic encephalopathy, seizure disorders, and to facilitate weaning off mechanical ventilation.

Drug Interactions: Increased CNS depression with other CNS depressants.

Incompatibilities: None noted.

Side Effects

Nervous System: arrhythmias—bradycardia/tachycardia/PVCs, BP changes, dizziness, dyspnea, headache, hiccups, malaise, nausea/vomiting, pain—at injection site, psyche—agitation/anxiety/emotional lability, resedation, seizure,* tremor, vision—blurred, weakness.

Endocrine System: (Pregnancy Category C) dry mouth, hot flashes, shivering, sweating.

Immune System: none noted.

Dosage: Reversal of sedation: IV 0.2 mg over 15 s; may repeat 0.2 mg q60s for 4 additional doses or a cumulative dose of 1 mg. Benzodiazepine overdose: IV 0.2 mg over 30 s; if no response after 30 s, then 0.3 mg over 30 s; may repeat with 0.5 mg q60s for a maximum cumulative dose of 3 mg.

---

* Life-threatening side effect.

▶ GABA: BENZODIAZEPINES AND ANXIOLYTICS

Fear heightens our awareness of our surroundings and helps us survive, but sometimes fear, in the form of anxiety, can cripple us, leaving us unable to do anything but worry. Drugs that increase GABA's affinity for its receptors decrease neuronal cell firing, thus decreasing alertness and anxiety.

Benzodiazepines, also called minor tranquilizers or anxiolytics, help relieve anxiety, make withdrawal from alcohol and sedatives safer, and are used in anticonvulsant therapy. They also produce amnesia and ease discomfort in endoscopy and cardioversion. In addition, they help to relieve night terrors in children.

Though the benzodiazepines are fairly safe drugs and are quickly excreted by the kidneys, they are synergistic with other sedatives, like alcohol, and can be lethal in combination.

Alprazolam [Xanax], Schedule IV, is an anxiolytic and sedative-hypnotic.

Drug Interactions: CNS depressants increase alprazolam CNS depression. Cimetidine, disulfiram increase alprazolam effects by decreasing metabolism. Oral contraceptives may increase or decrease alprazolam effects.

Side Effects

Nervous System: arrhythmias—ECG changes/tachycardia, clumsiness, dizziness, drowsiness, dyspnea, fatigue, headache, hypotension, lightheadedness, psyche—depression/excitement/hallucinations/insomnia/nervousness/restlessness, rigidity, sedation, tremor, unsteadiness, vision—blurred.

Endocrine System: (Pregnancy Category D) none noted.

Immune System: none noted.

Dosage: PO 0.25–0.5 tid to a max of 4 mg/d. Panic attacks: PO 1–2 mg tid to maximum of 8 mg/d.

Chlordiazepoxide hydrochloride [Librium], Schedule IV, the earliest of the benzodiazepine anxiolytics, also has anticonvulsant, sedative, and skeletal muscle relaxant effects.

Off Label: essential, familial, and senile action tremors.

Drug Interactions: CNS depressants increase chlordiazepoxide CNS depression. Cimetidine increases chlordiazepoxide plasma levels, thus increasing toxicity. May decrease antiparkinsonian effects of levodopa. May increase phenytoin levels. Smoking decreases sedative and antianxiety effects.

Side Effects

Nervous System: arrhythmias—ECG changes/tachycardia, ataxia, bladder—frequency, bowel—constipation, dizziness, drowsiness, EEG changes, headache, hiccups, hypotension, lethargy, nausea/vomiting, psyche—confusion/delirium/depression/hallucinations/nightmares/vivid dreams/rage, respiratory depression,* syncope, tinnitus, vertigo.

Endocrine System: (Pregnancy Category D) appetite increase, dry mouth.

Immune System: jaundice, photosensitivity, rash. Injection site: edema, pain.

Dosage: Anxiety: PO 15–100 mg/d divided. Preop: IM/IV 50–100 mg 1 h before surgery. Alcohol detoxification: PO 50–100 mg prn to maximum of 300 mg/d. IM/IV 50–100 mg; may repeat in 2–3 h if necessary. Severe anxiety: 20–25 mg tid–qid. IM/IV 50–100 mg; then 25–50 mg tid or qid.

Chlordiazepoxide in combination with amitriptyline is [Limbitrol]. Chlordiazepoxide 5 mg (DS 10 mg) and amitriptyline 12.5 mg or (DS 25 mg).

Clorazepate dipotassium [Tranxene, Tranxene-SD], Schedule IV, is used to treat partial seizures and alcohol withdrawal, as well as anxiety.

Drug Interactions: CNS depressant action is increased with other CNS depressants. Clorazepate increases effects of cimetidine, disulfiram.

Side Effects

Nervous System: ataxia, dizziness, drowsiness, GI disturbances, headache, hypotension, psyche—confusion/excitement/insomnia, vision—blurred/diplopia.

Endocrine System: (Pregnancy Category C) none noted.

Immune System: allergic reactions, blood dyscrasias, decreased Hct, abnormal liver function tests, xerostomia.

Dosage: Anxiety: PO 15 mg/d hs to a maximum 60 mg/d divided doses. Acute alcohol withdrawal: PO 30 mg. Then 30–60 mg divided doses to maximum of 90 mg/d. Taper 15 mg/d over 4 d to 7.5–15 mg/d until stable. Partial seizures: PO 7.5 mg tid.

Diazepam [Valium], diazepam emulsified [Dizac] is still the drug of choice to treat status epilepticus.

Drug Interactions: CNS depressants increase diazepam CNS depressant action. Cimetidine increases diazepam plasma levels increases toxicity. May decrease antiparkinsonian effects of levodopa. May increase phenytoin levels. Smoking decreases sedative and antianxiety effects.

Incompatibilities

Solution/Additive: bleomycin, benzquinamide, dobutamine, doxapram, doxorubicin, fluorouracil, glycopyrrolate, heparin, nalbuphine.

Y-site: furosemide, heparin, potassium chloride, vitamin B complex with C. Emulsion also incompatible with morphine. Do not administer emulsion with any other drugs. Do not administer through polyvinyl chloride (PVC) infusion sets.

Side Effects

Nervous System: arrhythmias—tachycardia, ataxia, bladder—incontinence/retention, bowel—constipation, cardiovascular collapse,* cough, dizziness, drowsiness, EEG changes, fatigue, headache, hiccups, hypotension, laryngospasm,* pain—chest/throat, psyche—amnesia/rage/vivid dreams, slurred speech, tardive dyskinesia, tremors, vertigo, vision changes.

Endocrine System: (Pregnancy Category D) edema, menstrual irregularities, ovulation failure.

Immune System: hepatic dysfunction. Injection site: phlebitis, thrombosis.

Dosage: Anxiety, muscle spasm, convulsions: PO 4–40 mg/d divided. SR 15–30 mg/d. IM/IV 2–10 mg; repeat prn in 3–4 h.

Halazepam [Paxipam], Schedule IV, s an anxiolytic, sedative-hypnotic.

Drug Interactions: CNS depressants increase diazepam CNS depressant action. Cimetidine, disulfiram, oral contraceptives may increase effects of halazepam.

Side Effects

Nervous System: arrhythmias—bradycardia/tachycardia, bladder—distress, bowel—constipation, drowsiness, dyspnea, headache, hypotension, motion sickness, nausea/vomiting, paresthesia, psyche—confusion, respiratory disturbances, sedation, vision disturbances.

Endocrine System: (Pregnancy Category D) dry mouth, salivation increase.

Immune System: abnormal liver values.

Dosage: PO 20–40 mg tid or qid.

Lorazepam [Ativan], Schedule IV, is useful in anxiety, medical/surgical procedures.

Off Label: In status epilepticus and chemotherapy-induced nausea and vomiting.

Drug Interactions: CNS depressants increase lorazepam's CNS depressant action. Cimetidine increases lorazepam plasma levels increases toxicity. May decrease antiparkinsonian effects of levodopa. May increase phenytoin levels. Smoking decreases sedative and antianxiety effects. Lorazepam's side effects usually disappear with continued use or lowered dosage.

---

* Life-threatening side effect.

Incompatibilities

Y-site: ondansetron.

Side Effects

Nervous System: abdominal discomfort, dizziness, drowsiness, dyspnea, hearing disturbances, hypertension/ hypotension, nausea/vomiting, psyche—confusion/ depression/disorientation/hallucinations/restlessness, vision—blurred/diplopia

Endocrine System: (Pregnancy Category D) anorexia.

Immune System: None noted.

Dosage: PO 2–6 mg/d divided to maximum of 10 mg/d. Insomnia: PO 2–4 mg hs. Preop: IM 2–4 mg (0.05 mg/kg) at least 2 h before surgery. IV 0.044 mg/kg up to 2 mg 15–20 min before surgery.

Oxazepam [Serax], Schedule IV, is up to four times more potent than diazepam and treats anxiety and acute withdrawal symptoms of alcoholism.

Drug Interactions: CNS depressants increase oxazepam CNS depressant action. Cimetidine increases oxazepam plasma levels increases toxicity. May decrease antiparkinsonian effects of levodopa. May increase phenytoin levels. Smoking decreases sedative and antianxiety effects.

Side Effects

Nervous System: dizziness, drowsiness, edema, headache, hypotension, lethargy, nausea, psyche—confusion/depression/euphoria/excitement, slurred speech, sexual function—libido changes, syncope, tremor, vertigo.

Endocrine System: (Pregnancy Category C) edema, xerostomia.

Immune System: jaundice, leukopenia.

Dosage: PO 10–30 mg tid or qid. Alcohol withdrawal 15–30 mg tid or qid. Hypnotic 15–30 mg hs.

▶ A DIFFERENT ANXIOLYTIC

An emerging class of anxiolytics, aziperones, may have only minimal potential for abuse and little or no interaction with other CNS depressants. Unlike the benzodiazepines, this class has agonist effects on presynaptic dopamine receptors and a high affinity for serotonin receptors. Serotonin is an inhibitory neurotransmitter.

Buspirone hydrochloride [BuSpar], though not a benzodiazepine, may ultimately and indirectly bind to the GABA/chloride protein complex. Buspirone is used to treat generalized anxiety, but not panic disorders. Unlike the benzodiazepine anxiolytics, buspirone has no anticonvulsant, muscle relaxant, or sedative activity. Its being different from the benzodiazepine anxiolytics probably accounts for its minimal synergism with CNS depressants. It is not a controlled drug.

Drug Interactions: MAOIs—hypertension. Trazodone may increase liver transaminases. Increased haloperidol serum levels.

Side Effects

Nervous System: arrhythmias—tachycardia, arthralgia, bladder—frequency/hesitancy, bowel—abdominal and gastric distress/constipation/diarrhea, dizziness, drowsiness, dyspnea, edema, fatigue, headache, hyperventilation, lightheadedness, nausea/vomiting, nervousness, numbness, palpitations, paresthesias, psyche—concentration difficulties/confusion/depression/dream disturbances/excitement/mood changes, tremors, weakness, vision—blurred

Endocrine System: (Pregnancy Category B) edema, flushing, dry mouth, dry skin.

Immune System: bruising, hair loss, pruritus.

Dosage: PO. Start with 10–15 mg tid. Increase 5 mg/d q2–3d until the optimal therapeutic response is achieved. Maximum dose: 60 mg/d.

▶ TENSION HEADACHES AND GABA

Tension headaches, sometimes referred to as cluster headaches or muscle contraction headaches, are fairly common. Aspirin or acetaminophen alone is usually effective, but combining aspirin with the stimulant caffeine and the GABA-attracting butalbital may be beneficial. The caffeine helps constrict the dilated blood vessels that appear to play a role in the headache. The sedative-hypnotic helps decrease some of the patient's tension, which may be a factor.

Butalbital in combination with aspirin and caffeine [Fiorinal], a Schedule III drug, utilizes the GABA-like properties of the barbiturates to ease tension headaches. Each tablet or capsule contains butalbital 50 mg, ASA 325 mg, and caffeine 40 mg.

Dosage: PO 1–2 tabs or caps q4h to maximum of 6/d.

▶ ANTICONVULSANTS OR ANTIEPILEPTIC DRUGS (AEDs)

Epilepsy can result from brain trauma caused by blows, fever, or increasing intracranial pressure. Sometimes the cause is unknown. A seizure begins with an unstable neuronal membrane or a cluster of such destabilized cells. The site of electrical discharge may remain localized or the action potential may sweep over large areas of neurons. Seizure control is essential because the anoxia caused during a seizure can result in ischemia and "seizures can beget seizures," leading to further brain damage and different forms of seizures (Garnett, 1996).

Antiepileptic drugs or AEDs raise the seizure threshold. Most anticonvulsants fit into the sedative or benzodiazepine receptors that increase the affinity of GABA to its receptors or increase the amount of available GABA to slow or stop the wild firing of neurons. Careful observations help pinpoint the origin of a seizure and map the spread of cell involvement through the brain. GABA-like drugs are synergistic and anticonvulsants are often given in combination to control the seizures.

BARBITURATES AS ANTIEPILEPTIC DRUGS

The barbiturates are a mainstay of the management of seizure disorders. The ability of barbiturates to treat epilepsy was discovered in 1911 when a Dr. Hauptmann could not fall asleep in a room over a ward for epileptic patients due to the constant ruckus and commotion of patients' seizures downstairs. In desperation, he ordered phenobarbital for all the patients and went back to bed. The next day the nurses noted a decrease in seizure activity (Sneader, 1985). The barbiturates treat tonic–clonic and partial seizures (grand mal), partial seizures, eclampsia, febrile seizures in young children, and status epilepticus.

Mephobarbital [Mebaral] is a Schedule IV drug used to treat petit mal and grand mal epilepsy, alone or synergistically with other anticonvulsants. It is also used to manage delirium tremens and acute agitation and anxiety states.

Drug Interactions: Refer to phenobarbital.

Side Effects

Nervous System: constipation, dizziness, drowsiness, dyspnea/respiratory depression,* excitement, headache, nausea/vomiting, unsteadiness.

Endocrine System: (Pregnancy Category D) none noted.

Immune System: hypersensitivity reactions.

Dosage: PO 400–600 mg/d in divided doses. Delirium tremens: PO 200 mg tid–qid.

Phenobarbital sodium [Barbita, Luminal], the prototype barbiturate, is a Schedule IV drug.

Drug Interactions: It is intentionally synergistic with valproic acid. It is also synergistic with MAOIs, CNS depressants, and chloramphenicol, but decreases the plasma levels of oral anticoagulants, quinidine, digoxin, phenytoin, tricyclics, steroids, birth control pills, doxycycline, and griseofulvin.

Incompatibilities

Solution/Additive: benzquinamide, cephalothin, chlorpromazine, codeine phosphate, ephedrine, hydralazine, hydrocortisone hydroxyzine, insulin, levorphanol, meperidine, methadone, morphine, norepinephrine, procaine, prochlorperazine, promazine, promethazine, ranitidine, sodium succinate, streptomycin, tetracyclines, vancomycin.

Side Effects: See the section on barbiturate hypnotics.

Dosage: PO 100–300 mg/d. IM/IV 200–600 mg to maximum of 20 mg/kg. IV slow push 200–300 mg q6h prn for status epilepticus.

Primidone [Mysoline] metabolizes into phenobarbital and phenylethyl malonamide, both of which are anticonvulsants used for treating tonic–clonic and partial seizures. It is not a controlled drug.

Drug Interactions: Refer to phenobarbital.

Side Effects

Nervous System: ataxia, drowsiness, edema, extreme fatigue, headache, nausea/vomiting, psyche—confusion/emotional disturbances/excitement (children)/hyperirritability/acute psychoses with psychomotor epilepsy, sedation, sexual function—impotence, vision—diplopia/nystagmus.

Endocrine System: (Pregnancy Category D) edema, decreased serum folate levels, osteomalacia.

Immune System: anemia—megaloblastic, eosinophilia, leukopenia, LE-like syndrome, lymphadenopathy, rash, thrombocytopenia.

Dosage: PO 250 mg–2 g/d divided.

Secobarbital [Seconal], secobarbital sodium [Seconal Sodium] are Schedule II, short-acting anticonvulsants.

Drug Interactions: Phenmetrazine antagonizes effects of secobarbital. CNS depressants increase secobarbital CNS depression. MAOIs cause excessive CNS depression. Methoxyflurane increases risk of nephrotoxicity.

Incompatibilities

Solution/Additive: benzquinamide, codeine, cimetidine, ephedrine, erythromycin, glycopyrrolate, hydrocortisone, insulin, levorphanol, methadone, norepinephrine, pentazocine, phenytoin, procaine, sodium bicarbonate, streptomycin, tetracycline, vancomycin.

---

* Life-threatening side effect.

Y-site: cimetidine, glycopyrrolate.

Side Effects: See the barbiturate hypnotics in this chapter.

Dosage: Anticonvulsive, acute episode: IM 5.5 mg/kg; repeat q3–4h prn. IV 5.5 mg/kg at rate under 50 mg/15 s.

Thiopental sodium [Pentothal] is a Schedule III, ultra-short-acting drug. It causes rapid loss of consciousness and is used as a brief general anesthetic for 15-min operative procedures. It is also a supplement to other anesthetic agents and is used as an anticonvulsant, sedative-hypnotic, and for narcoanalysis and narcosynthesis in psychiatric disorders.

Drug Interactions: Refer to barbiturate anesthetics.

Incompatibilities: Refer to barbiturate anesthetics.

Side Effects: See barbiturate anesthetic section in this chapter.

Dosage: For convulsions: IV 75–125 mg. Narcoanalysis: 100 mg/min until confusion occurs.

HYDANTOINS

One of the drawbacks of the management of epilepsy is that the barbiturates, as sedative-hypnotics, are often too sedating for the patient and interfere with the routines of daily living. The hydantoins were derived from phenobarbital in a search for less sedating anticonvulsants.

Mephenytoin [Mesantoin] is used, usually with other anticonvulsants, in the management of focal, grand mal, Jacksonian, and psychomotor seizures in patients refractory to less toxic anticonvulsants. It is not a first-line anticonvulsant owing to serious side effects.

Drug Interactions: Toxic synergism with paramethadione, trimethadione. For others see phenytoin.

Side Effects

Nervous System: dizziness, drowsiness.

Endocrine System: (Pregnancy Category D) none noted.

Immune System: agranulocytosis,* aplastic anemia,* blood dyscrasias,* toxic epidermal necrolysis, erythema multiforme, exfoliative dermatitis,* hepatic damage, leukopenia,* neutropenia,* periarteritis nodosa, rash, SLE syndrome, thrombocytopenia.

Dosage: PO. Start with 50–100 mg/d for 1 wk; increase weekly to 200–600 mg/d in divided doses.

Phenytoin [Dilantin] was created from the phenyl group of the phenobarbital molecule over 60 years ago in the search for less sedating anticonvulsants. It fits into the

sedative receptor to slow cell firing in tonic–clonic, nonepileptic, and psychomotor seizures, and to prevent or treat seizures during or after neurosurgery.

Off Label: Used as an antiarrhythmic agent (see Chapter 2) and in the treatment of trigeminal neuralgia. It has been well studied and, therefore, has many well-known side effects. Despite the side effects, it is a fairly safe drug. Because it does not dissolve or mix well, it does not absorb evenly from the GI tract, causing fluctuations in dosage.

Drug Interactions: Phenytoin serum levels are raised by drugs that fit on the GABA molecule receptors: chlordiazepoxide, diazepam, disulfiram, ethosuximide, phenobarbital, primidone. The following drugs also raise serum levels: chloramphenicol, chlorpromazine, dicumarol, isoniazid, methylphenidate, phenylbutazone, propoxyphene, prochlorperazine, sulfamethoxazole.

Incompatibilities

Solution/Additive: amikacin, aminophylline, bretylium, cephapirin, codeine phosphate, 5% dextrose, dobutamine, insulin, levorphanol, lidocaine, lincomycin, meperidine, metaraminol, methadone, morphine, nitroglycerin, norepinephrine, pentobarbital, procaine, secobarbital, streptomycin.

Y-site: amikacin, bretylium, dobutamine, lidocaine, heparin, potassium chloride, vitamin B complex with C.

Side Effects

Nervous System: arrhythmias—bradycardia/cardiovascular collapse*/ventricular fibrillation,* bowel—constipation, nausea/vomiting, psyche—confusion, seizures,* vision—blurred/diplopia/photophobia.

Endocrine System: (Pregnancy Category D) alkaline phosphatase elevations, fever, glycosuria, hyperglycemia, hypocalcemia, acute renal failure, TSH increase, weight—gain/loss.

Immune System: agranulocytosis,* aplastic anemia,* craniofacial abnormalities, gingival hyperplasia, toxic epidermal necrolysis, liver necrosis, LE,* pancytopenia, Peyronie's disease, pneumonitis, pulmonary fibrosis, rashes, Stevens–Johnson syndrome.*

Dosage: PO. Load with 1 g or 15–18 mg/kg. Then 300 mg/d 1–3 divided doses. Status epilepticus: IV load with 17 mg/kg at 30–50 mg/min until seizures are controlled. IM 300–400 mg/d.

▶ BENZODIAZEPINES

The benzodiazepines (BZ) slow cell firing by locking into the BZ receptors and increasing the affinity of GABA

* Life-threatening side effect.

molecules for their respective receptors. As a result, chloride ions reach equilibrium on either side of the cell membrane, making the cell less responsive to the spread of the action potential. The benzodiazepines are potentiated by other CNS depressants. Breakthrough seizures may occur with tolerance. Diazepam and lorazepam are of special use for the treatment of status epilepticus. The benzodiazepines are Schedule IV drugs.

Clorazepate dipotassium [Tranxene], a Schedule IV drug, is used to treat partial seizures and alcohol withdrawal.

Drug Interactions: CNS depressant action is increased with other CNS depressants. Clorazepate increases effects of cimetidine, disulfiram.

Side Effects

Nervous System: ataxia, dizziness, drowsiness, GI disturbances, headache, hypotension, psyche—confusion/excitement/insomnia, vision—blurred/diplopia.

Endocrine System: (Pregnancy Category C) xerostomia.

Immune System: allergic reactions, blood dyscrasias, decreased Hct, abnormal liver function tests.

Dosage: For partial seizures PO 7.5 mg tid to a maximum of 90 mg/d in divided doses. Acute alcohol withdrawal: PO 30 mg followed by 30–60 mg/d in divided doses to a maximum of 90 mg/d. Taper by 15 mg/d over 4 d to 7.5–15 mg/d until stable.

Clonazepam [Klonopin] is a Schedule IV drug used with other AEDs for the treatment of atypical absence seizures, atonic seizures, infantile spasms, and myoclonic seizures and is of possible value for neonatal seizures and partial seizures. It is sometimes used for panic attacks.

Drug Interactions: CNS depressants increase clonazepam CNS depression. May increase phenytoin levels.

Side Effects

Nervous System: aphonia, ataxia, bladder—dysuria/enuresis/nocturia/retention, bowel—constipation/diarrhea, choreiform movements, coma,* drowsiness, dysarthria, dyspnea, edema, glassy-eyed appearance, headache, hemiparesis, hypotonia, insomnia, nausea, palpitation, psyche—aggression/confusion/depression/hallucinations/hysteria/suicidal ideation, respiratory depression,* sedation, sexual function—libido increase, slurred speech, tremor, vertigo, vision—abnormal eye movements/diplopia/nystagmus.

Endocrine System: (Pregnancy Category C) appetite increase, edema—ankle/face hirsutism, dry mouth, salivation.

---

* Life-threatening side effect.

Immune System: anemia, chest congestion, edema—ankle/facial, eosinophilia, hair loss, hypersecretion—upper respiratory tract, leukopenia, rash, rhinorrhea, thrombocytopenia, tongue—coated.

Dosage: PO 1.5 mg/d in 3 divided doses. Increase 0.5–1 mg q3d until seizures are controlled or side effects intolerable to maximum of 20 mg/d.

Diazepam [Valium], a Schedule IV drug, is still the drug of choice for status epilepticus.

Side Effects: Refer to anxiolytic section in this chapter.

Dosage: Status epilepticus: IM 5–10 mg q10–15min to 30 mg maximum. Repeat prn q2–4h. Emulsion: IV at 5 mg/min. Convulsions, alcohol withdrawal: PO 2–10 mg bid–qid or SR 15–30 mg. IM/IV 2–10 mg. Repeat 3–4 h prn.

SUCCINIMIDES

This group is used for absence, myoclonic, and akinetic seizures. Due to serious side effects, succinimides are not the first choice group.

Ethosuximide [Zarontin] is the most effective of the group.

Drug Interactions: Carbamazepine decreases ethosuximide levels. Isoniazid increases ethosuximide levels. Levels of both phenobarbital and ethosuximide may be altered with increased seizure frequency.

Side Effects

Nervous System: ataxia, bowel—constipation/diarrhea, dizziness, drowsiness, epigastric distress, fatigue, headache, hiccups, hyperactivity/restlessness, lethargy, muscle weakness, nausea/vomiting, pain—abdominal, psyche—aggression/anxiety/concentration difficulty/confusion/euphoria/hypochondriasis/irritability/night terrors/psychosis, exacerbation of seizures,* sleep disturbances, vision—myopia.

Endocrine System: (Pregnancy Category C) anorexia, hirsutism, weight loss.

Immune System: agranulocytosis,* aplastic anemia,* bleeding—vaginal, eosinophilia, gingival hyperplasia, leukopenia, pancytopenia,* rash, thrombocytopenia. Monthly CBCs are needed.

Dosage: PO 20–40 mg/kg/d or 500 mg–1.5 g/d divided.

Methsuximide [Celontin] is used to treat absence seizures refractory to other AEDs and in combination with other AEDs for mixed types of epilepsy.

Drugs Interactions: Carbamazepine decreases methsuximide levels. Isoniazid increases methsuximide levels. Both phenobarbital and methsuximide levels may be altered with increased seizure frequency.

Side Effects

Nervous System: ataxia, bowel—constipation/diarrhea, dizziness, drowsiness, headache, nausea/vomiting, pain—epigastric/abdominal, psyche—behavioral changes/insomnia/severe mental depression, vision—diplopia/photophobia. Hypersensitivity: hiccups.

Endocrine System: (Pregnancy Category C) anorexia, weight loss. Hypersensitivity: fever.

Immune System: Hypersensitivity: blood dyscrasia including aplastic anemia,* hyperemia, periorbital edema, skin eruptions.

Dosage: PO 300 mg–1.2 g/d divided doses.

Phensuximide [Milontin] is used to treat petit mal (absence seizures). Adjunct to other AEDs for petit mal when seen with other forms of epilepsy.

Drug Interactions: Carbamazepine decreases phensuximide levels. Isoniazid significantly increases phensuximide levels. Levels of phenobarbital and phensuximide may be altered with increased seizure frequency.

Side Effects

Nervous System: ataxia, dizziness, drowsiness, nausea/vomiting, weakness.

Endocrine System: (Pregnancy Category D) anorexia, flushing.

Immune System: alopecia, granulocytopenia,* nephropathy, periorbital edema, pruritus, rash.

Dosage: PO 0.5–1 g bid or tid.

MISCELLANEOUS ANTICONVULSANTS

Some AEDs do not fit into drug categories as easily as do the barbituates and diazepines.

Acetazolamide [Diamox, others] is used intermittently as an AED for petit mal, tonic–clonic, and focal seizures owing to rapid tolerance. A carbonic anhydrase inhibitor may act through induction of systemic metabolic acidosis.

Drug Interactions: Renal excretion of amphetamines, ephedrine, flecainide, quinidine, procainamide, tricyclic

antidepressants may be decreased, thereby enhancing or prolonging their effects. Renal excretion of lithium is increased. Excretion of phenobarbital may be increased. Amphotericin B and corticosteroids may accelerate potassium loss. Digitalis glycosides may predispose persons with hypokalemia to digitalis toxicity. Puts patients on high doses of salicylates at great risk for salicylate toxicity.

Side Effects

Nervous System: bladder—dysuria/frequency/polyuria, bowel—diarrhea, fatigue, malaise, nausea/vomiting, flaccid paralysis,* paresthesias, psyche—depression/disorientation, sedation, muscle weakness.

Endocrine System: (Pregnancy Category C) anorexia, crystalluria, increased excretion of calcium/potassium/magnesium/sodium, glycosuria, gout exacerbation, hyperylycemia, hyperuricemia, dry mouth, weight loss.

Immune System: agranulocytosis,* aplastic anemia,* hemolytic anemia, hepatic dysfunction, leukopenia, pancytopenia.

Dosage: PO 8–30 mg qd–qid.

Carbamazepine [Tegretol] is related to the tricyclic antidepressants, but it has an action similar to hydantoin. It is used to treat tonic–clonic, mixed, and psychomotor seizures. It also helps tic douloureux (trigeminal neuralgia).

Drug Interactions: Serum concentrations of other anticonvulsants may decrease because of increased metabolism. Verapamil, erythromycin may increase carbamazepine levels. Decreases hypoprothrombinemic effects of oral anticoagulants. Increases metabolism of estrogens, thus decreasing effectiveness of oral contraceptives.

Side Effects

Nervous System: akathisia, ataxia, arrhythmias/heart block, arthralgia, bladder—frequency/oliguria/retention, bowel—constipation/diarrhea, cholestatic jaundice, convulsions—minor motor, coordination disturbances, cramps—leg, dizziness, drowsiness, dyspepsia, dysphagia, dyspnea, edema, fatigue, headache, hearing—abnormal acuity, hyperreflexia, insomnia, myalgia, nausea/vomiting, pain—abdominal, paresthesias, psyche—aggression/agitation/confusion/visual hallucinations/activation of latent psychosis, respiratory depression,* sexual function—impotence, speech difficulty, syncope, tremors, vertigo, vision—blurred/diplopia/nystagmus/oculomotor disturbances/oscillopsia/scotoma.

Endocrine System: (Pregnancy Category C) anorexia, edema, hypothyroidism, increased SIADH excretion.

* Life-threatening side effect.

Immune System: agranulocytosis,* alopecia, aplastic anemia,* conjunctivitis, exfoliative dermatitis,* eosinophilia, hepatitis, jaundice, leukocytosis, leukopenia, abnormal liver function tests, multiforme—extreme, pancreatitis, photosensitivity, pigmentation changes, rash, SLE, Stevens–Johnson syndrome,* thrombocytopenia.

Dosage: PO 200 mg bid. Increase slowly to 800–1200 mg/d in 3–4 divided doses. Trigeminal neuralgia: PO 100 mg bid to maximum of 800 mg/d in 3–4 divided doses.

Felbamate [Felbatol] blocks repetitive neuronal firing, raises the seizure threshold, and prevents seizure spread. It acts as a glycine antagonist in treating Lennox–Gastaut syndrome and partial seizures.

Off Label: Alone or in combination with other AEDs for generalized tonic–clonic seizures.

Drug Interactions: Felbamate reduces serum carbamazepine levels by a mean of 25%, but increases levels of its active metabolite. Increases serum phenytoin levels approximately 20%. Increases valproic acid levels.

Side Effects

Nervous System: ataxia, bowel—constipation, dizziness, fatigue, headache, hiccups, indigestion, nausea/vomiting, psyche—aggression/agitation/emotional disturbances/hallucinations, taste disturbances, tremors—mild, vision—blurred/diplopia.

Endocrine System: (Pregnancy Category C) anorexia, appetite increase, serum cholesterol—slight increase, hypokalemia, hyponatremia, weight—gain/loss.

Immune System: aplastic anemia,* acute liver failure.*

Dosage: Partial seizures: PO. Start with 1200 mg/d in 3–4 divided doses. May increase by 600 mg/d q2wk to maximum of 3600 mg/d. If converting to monotherapy, reduce the dose of concomitant AED by ⅓ when initiating felbamate. Continue to decrease other AEDs by ⅓ with each increase in felbamate q2wk. If using as adjunctive therapy, decrease other AEDs by 20% when initiating felbamate. Further reductions in other AEDs may be needed to minimize side effects and drug interactions.

Gabapentin [Neurontin] The "gaba" in the generic name is a clue to the researchers' reasoning that gabapentin would be a GABA agonist. Instead, the drug binds with an amino acid carrier protein to act at a unique receptor in adjunctive therapy for partial seizures with or without secondary generalization in adults.

Off Label: As add-on therapy for generalized seizures.

Drug Interactions: May cause increase in phenytoin levels at higher doses (300–600 mg/d gabapentin). Does not

appear to affect serum levels of other anticonvulsants. Antacids reduce absorption of gabapentin about 20%.

Side Effects

Nervous System: concentration impaired, dizziness, drowsiness, fatigue, GI upset, headache, nausea/vomiting, partial seizure—increased frequency, speech slurred, tremor, vision—blurred/nystagmus.

Endocrine System: (Pregnancy Category C) weight gain.

Immune System: eczema, rash.

Dosage: As adjunctive therapy for seizures: PO. Start with 300 mg on day 1, 300 mg bid on day 2, and 300 mg tid on day 3. Continue to increase over 1 wk to an initial total dose of 400 mg tid (1200 mg/d). May increase to 1800–2400 mg/d depending on response. (Usual dose: 600–1800 mg/d in 3 divided doses.)

Topiramate [Topamax] is an anticonvulsant that blocks voltage-sensitive sodium channels, enhances the activity of GABA, and blocks the action of glutamate. Although it also inhibits carbonic anhydrase, this may not contribute to anticonvulsant activity, but may contribute to kidney stone formation.

Drug Interactions: Decreased digoxin levels. Decreased effect of oral contraceptives possible. Risk of kidney stone with other carbonic anhydrase inhibitors, eg, acetazolamide, dichlorphenamide.

Side Effects

Nervous System: asthenia, ataxia, bowel—constipation, coordination—abnormal, dizziness, dyspnea, dyspepsia, edema, hearing—decrease, hypoesthesia, myalgia, nausea, odor, pain—abdominal/back/breast (women)/chest/eye/leg paresthesias, psyche—aggression/agitation/apathy/confusion/depersonalization/depression/difficulties with attention, concentration, memory/lability/mood changes/nervousness/psychomotor slowing/somnolence, vision—abnormalities/blurred/nystagmus, rigors, speech problems, tremors.

Endocrine System: (Pregnancy Category C) anorexia, edema, flushing, menstrual disorders/dysmenorrhea, dry mouth, sweating, weight loss.

Immune System: epistaxis, gingivitis, hematuria, leukopenia, pruritus, rash, pharyngitis, sinusitis, URI.

Dosage: PO. Start with 50 mg hs for 1 wk. Increase to 50 mg AM and hs. Increase by 50 mg/wk over 8 wk to maximum of 200 mg AM and hs.

Valproic acid [Depakene], divalproex [Depakote] are used to treat absence, akinetic, atonic, myoclonic, tonic-clonic, and photosensitive seizures. Rather than fit the GABA molecule receptors, valproic acid makes more GABA available. Synergistic with clonazepam for absence seizures.

---

* Life-threatening side effect.

Drug Interactions: Valproic acid can raise blood levels of phenytoin and primidone and is synergistic with phenobarbital, hydantoin, and primidone. Chewing the tablets destroys tooth enamel.

Side Effects

Nervous System: alertness—increase, bowel—constipation/diarrhea, cramps—abdominal, diarrhea, dizziness, drowsiness, edema, indigestion, nausea/vomiting, psyche—aggression/agitation/emotional upset/hallucinations, seizures—breakthrough.

Endocrine System: (Pregnancy Category D) anorexia/weight loss, appetite increase/weight gain, edema, hyperammonemia, menses changes.

Immune System: anemia, bleeding time—prolonged, bone marrow depression,* death,* hair loss/curliness/waviness, hepatic failure,* hypofibrinogenemia, leukopenia, lymphocytosis, pulmonary edema, rash, thrombocytopenia.

Dosage: PO 15 mg/kg/d in divided doses. May increase after 250 mg to maximum of 60 mg/kg/d based on seizure control or developing side effects.

▶ MUSCLE RELAXANTS

<u>Baclofen [Lioresal]</u>, though not a benzodiazepine, decreases the transmission of monosynaptic extensor and polysynaptic flexor reflexes in the cord following upper motor lesions. It can relax the external sphincter in a hyperreflexive urinary bladder. It seems to have an anticholinergic action on involuntary bladder contractions. Take with food to decrease GI distress.

Drug Interactions: CNS depressants, MAOIs, antihistamines compound CNS depression. Insulin or sulfonylureas dosage may need to be increased.

Side Effects

Nervous System: ataxia, bladder—frequency, bowel—constipation, dizziness, drowsiness, fatigue, headache, hypotension, nausea/vomiting, psyche—confusion/insomnia, seizure control loss in epileptic patients, tinnitus, vertigo, vision—blurred/diplopia/miosis/mydriasis/nystagmus/strabismus. CNS depression is possible at high dosage.

Endocrine System: (Pregnancy Category C) may raise glucose levels.

Immune System: alkaline phosphatase and AST (SGOT)—increase, jaundice.

Dosage: PO 5 mg tid. May increase by 5 mg/dose q3d prn to maximum of 80 mg/d. Intrathecal: Initial bolus

of 50 μg/mL in not less than 1 min. Observe for 4–8 h. If muscle spasm response is less than desired, administer second bolus of 75 mcg/1.5 mL and observe 4–8 h. May repeat in 24 h with 100 mcg/2 mL bolus if necessary.

<u>Carisoprodol [Rela, Soma]</u> is used to relieve skeletal muscle spasm stiffness and pain in a variety of musculoskeletal disorders and to relieve spasticity and rigidity in cerebral palsy. The mechanism of action is not understood, but may be due to a sedative action.

Drug Interactions: CNS depressants potentiate carisoprodol CNS depression.

Side Effects

Nervous System: ataxia, arrhythmias—tachycardia, dizziness, drowsiness, hiccups, hypotension—postural, nausea/vomiting, psyche—depression/insomnia/irritability, syncope, vertigo.

Endocrine System: (Pregnancy Category C) fever, flushing.

Immune System: anaphylactic shock,* asthma, eosinophilia, erythema multiforme, pruritus, rash.

Dosage: PO 350 mg tid with last dose at hs.

<u>Methocarbamol [Robaxin, Marbaxin, Delaxin]</u> and carisoprodol are both propanediol-derivative monocarbamates, but methocarbamol reaches higher, faster, longer plasma levels. It works on neural pathways in the cord. For use also in tetanus.

Drug Interactions: CNS depressants increase methocarbamol CNS depression.

Side Effects

Nervous System: PO only: dizziness, drowsiness, headache, lightheadedness, nausea. Parenteral/PO: headache, vision—blurred. Parenteral only: bradycardia, convulsions,* hypotension, pain with extravasation, syncope, taste—metallic.

Endocrine System: (Pregnancy Category C) flushing. Parenteral/PO: fever.

Immune System: Parenteral/PO: anaphylaxis,* conjunctivitis, nasal congestion, pruritus, rash, urticaria. Parenteral: slight decrease in WBCs with extended use. Extravasation: sloughing, thrombophlebitis.

Dosage: PO. Start with 1.5 g qid for 2–3 d. Maintenance: 4–4.5 g divided into 3–6 doses. IM 0.5–1 g q8h. IV 1 g in not more than 250 mL of either sodium chloride or 5% dextrose for injection; not to exceed 3 g/d. Do not give for more than 3 consecutive days. Tetanus: 1–2 g (up to 3 g) into IV tubing at maximum rate of 300 mg/min; repeat q6h until it can be given per NG tube. Then give crushed tablets mixed in water to maximum of 24 g/d.

---

* Life-threatening side effect.

Chapter Highlights

- When gamma-amino butyric acid is attracted to its receptor site, chloride ions come to equilibrium on each side of the neuron's membrane, and cell firing slows.

- Drugs that fit into the sedative receptor, such as alcohol and barbiturates, or into the benzodiazepine receptor increase GABA's affinity for its own receptor site and slow cell firing.

- Drugs that increase GABA's affinity for its receptor include sedatives, hypnotics, some anesthetics, anxiolytics, and anticonvulsants.

Opiates and Opiate Blockers

- alfentanil hydrochloride [Alfenta]
- benzonatate [Tessalon]
- buprenorphine hydrochloride [Buprenex]
- butorphanol tartrate [Stadol]
- codeine
- codeine phospate
- codeine sulfate
- dextromethorphan hydrobromide [Romilar, others]
- diphenoxylate hydrochloride + atropine sulfate [Lomotil, others]
- fentanyl citrate [Duragesic]
- fentanyl citrate [Sublimaze]
- hydrocodone [Dicodid]
- hydrocodone bitartrate [Hycodan]
- hydrocodone bitartrate + acetaminophen [Vicodin]
- hydromorphone hydrochloride [Dilaudid]
- levorphanol tartrate [Levo-Dromoran]
- loperimide [Imodium, Imodium AD]
- meperidine hydrocholoride [Demerol]
- methadone [Dolophine]
- morphine sulfate
- nalbuphine hydrochloride [Nubain]
- naloxone hydrochloride [Narcan]
- naltrexone hydrochloride [Trexan]
- opium tincture [Laudanum]
- oxycodone
- oxycodone 5 mg + acetaminophen 325 mg [Percocet-5]
- oxycodone hydrochloride 4.5 mg + oxycodone terephthalate 0.38 mg
  + ASA 325 mg [Percodan]
- paregoric [Camphorated Opium Tincture]
- pentazocine hydrochloride [Talwin]
- propoxyphene hydrochloride [Darvon, others]
- propoxyphene napsylate [Darvon-N]
- remifentanil [Ultiva]
- sufentanil citrate [Sufenta]
- tramadol hydrochloride [Ultran, Zydol]

Long ago, from a lovely species of poppy, *Papaver somniferum,* in the Middle East came some of the most important medicines still in use. No one knows who first tasted the contents of the unripe opium poppy seed pod and discovered that it gave a sense of well-being, even euphoria; that it relieved coughs and diarrhea; and, above all, that it relieved pain. Knowledge of this miracle plant must have been passed on by word of mouth until the Sumerians in 2200 BC, writing on clay tablets, made note of the poppy's "joy juice." Thousands of years later, nothing has surpassed the analgesic effect of opium.

This wonder drug does have serious drawbacks. Opiates and their derivatives can cause physical addiction, and they can cause fatal respiratory depression. However, if administered carefully, their role in healing is invaluable.

▶ THE NATURE OF PAIN

Pain has value. It signals the victim to pay attention to injury and illness. Pain is often the only reason some patients will seek medical attention. On the other hand, fear of the pain resulting from treatment may make other patients reluctant to seek help. The nervous system experiences pain signals and responds to them, as do the immune and the endocrine systems. The endocrine system provides sugars for energy and proteins for healing. The immune system signals the nervous system with chemical messengers such as bradykinin, potassium, prostaglandins, serotonin, histamine, and proteolytic enzymes. Bradykinin plays a role in initiating the pain signal and prostaglandins enhance the nerve endings' sensitivity to pain. Dendrites in the trunk and limbs of the peripheral nervous system pick up the pain signals, felt as two different sensations, first a fast-sharp pain (phasic) and then a slow-burning pain (tonic). The signals exit the peripheral nervous system through primary sensory neuronal axons and enter the central nervous system via the spinothalamic nerve, which branches to become the paleospinothalamic and the neospinothalamic nerves.

Pain signals travel up this ancient mammalian neural tract more slowly, ending in the thalamus. Felt there as diffuse, gnawing, burning, and hard to pinpoint, this pain is also called chronic pain, and can become worse. As the slow-burning, or tonic, pain signal moves up the paleospinothalamic branch, it alerts the brain stem structures before reaching the limbic system, where structures in the limbic system respond emotionally in this pathway. The tonic pain signal continues to affect the emotional centers of the limbic system. Its diffuse quality makes the sufferer be still and "favor" the injured area. Over an extended time, pain causes the endocrine system to tilt away from protein production. The stress of pain causes cortisol levels to rise. Cortisol tilts the body toward making sugar for the energy to deal with the stress of chronic pain and away from wound healing.

NEOSPINOTHALAMIC TRACT—FAST PAIN

The fast, sharp, phasic pain is the emergency pain signal. It shoots up the neospinothalamic branch directly to the thalamus, where pain is felt as brief, immediate, or phasic pain such as suffered in stabbing and gunshot wounds, crush injuries, and fractures. Excruciating, acute, and overwhelming, this time-limited pain responds well to opiate analgesics. As the phasic pain stimulus ascends the neospinothalamic nerve branch, another branch continues up to the cerebral cortex, where pain is interpreted and evaluated in a cognitive, conscious manner.

REFERRED PAIN

Some body cells, organs, and structures cannot directly signal the central nervous system when injured or diseased. Abdominal or chest pain can be difficult to pinpoint because the organs have to send out or "refer" the pain signal from the actual location to body surface nerves that relay the message to the brain. Referred pain sends its message through visceral pathways from the affected organ based on the body segment in which the organ developed in the embryo. For example, the patient suffering a heart attack may complain of pain in the arm or jaw because the embryonic heart developed in the neck and upper thorax. In addition, the specifically affected area of the heart, for example, posterior, anterior, lateral, can be indicated by the location of the referred pain.

▶ OPIATE RECEPTORS

Not only is the limbic system the seat of emotions, the gatekeeper of memory, and an interpreter of pain, but structures within it, that is, the amygdala and the hypothalamus, are richly supplied with opiate receptors for the relief of pain and experience of pleasure and reward—the two motivators of behavior. Analgesic drugs relieve both physical and emotional pain by acting in this area. Downstream from the limbic system, the locus ceruleus in the brain stem also has great numbers of opiate receptors and plays a role in pain relief as well as reward-motivated behavior. The spinal cord also has opiate receptors.

Opiate receptors have differing shapes that influence the fit of corresponding opiate/opioid molecules. The receptors designated as mu (μ) produce the analgesia, euphoria, and respiratory depression associated with morphine and heroin. More specifically, mu-1 receptors produce analgesia, and mu-2 receptors produce constipation, euphoria, physical dependence, and respiratory depression. The delta (δ) receptors also produce analgesia. The sigma (σ) receptors stimulate respiratory and vasomotor activity as well as hallucinations and dysphoria. The kappa (κ) receptors influence spinal analgesia, sedation, and pupil constriction. Finally, the epsilon (ε) receptors produce analgesia.

Morphine and the opiate derivatives have an affinity for the mu and kappa receptors. The agonist–antagonist drugs, developed in the search for less addictive analgesia, can be agonistic or antagonistic at varying receptors.

▶ ENDOGENOUS OPIATES

The body manufactures opiates; we make our own analgesia. These endogenous opiates are neurotransmitters called endorphins, a word created out of two words: endogenous and morphine, to describe morphine produced by the body. They are sometimes referred to as enkephalins, a reference to the head, and are released by specific areas in the pituitary gland, the basal ganglia, the brain stem, and the spinal cord to relieve an emergency pain signal—the stabbing, crushing, burning, or throbbing pain of a fresh wound. The body rapidly takes apart endorphins with enzymes, making their actions shorter-lived than the botanical, synthetic, and semisynthetic opiates.

Note: The intestinal tract also is lined with opiate receptors.

▶ CONTROL DRUGS

Drugs that relieve physical or emotional pain attract abuse. Such drugs are listed on a controlled substances schedule created by Congress in the Controlled Substances Act of 1970.

Controlled Substances

Schedule I drugs, including heroin and LSD, are not used medicinally in the United States. (Heroin and morphine are the same drug. Heroin has two acetyl wings that make it oil soluble and able to enter the brain faster.)

Schedule II drugs, narcotics and cocaine, are used medicinally in this country.

Schedule III drugs include combinations of a narcotic plus a nonsteroidal antiinflammatory drug.

Schedule IV drugs enhance GABA's affinity for its receptors and result in decreased anxiety or in sedation.

Schedule V drugs usually have small amounts of narcotics used in antidiarrheal and antitussive preparations.

▶ DRUG DEPENDENCE AND TOLERANCE

Drug dependence occurs when a person develops a need for the drug and experiences withdrawal without it. Some evidence indicates that people who take narcotics for physical pain do not become addicted. In fact, opiates used for pain in fresh injuries or wounds speed healing by helping the patient to tolerate early, frequent movement, and by preventing the release of cortisols, which inhibit healing. But people who take opiates for emotional pain are more vulnerable to addiction. Also, with extended use of some drugs, not necessarily only opiates, cells may get accustomed to the amount of a drug the individual can "tolerate," and the person may require larger doses to get the original effect; thus the term, "tolerance."

▶ OPIATE ANALGESIA

Opiates, also called narcotics, fit the receptor sites that endorphins and enkephalins lock into. They affect the nervous system in important ways besides potent analgesia. Respiratory depression is their greatest immediate danger as they decrease brain stem sensitivity to CO_2. Opiates also suppress the cough reflex. They cause constipation by slowing peristalsis. Acting on the brain stem's chemoreceptor trigger zone, opiates can cause nausea and vomiting. Though they are well known to give a pleasant, even euphoric feeling, the opposite is possible too. They constrict the pupils and can cause spasms in some abdominal structures. In the immune system opiates also trigger histamine release, which can result in hypotension and allergic reactions.

Opiates relieve fast, sharp, acute, or phasic pain. They can be effective with slow, burning, or chronic pain, but a person with such pain may need other interventions. They are given to patients before, during, and after many surgical procedures in the smallest effective therapeutic dose. Parenteral forms have the most rapid onset and are most effective. Sometimes oral forms are combined with nonsteroidal antiinflammatory analgesics, which block prostaglandin release and decrease nerve endings' sensitivity to pain. Opiates raise the spinal cord's pain threshold and dull the limbic system's subjective response to pain, requiring a greater pain stimulus to surmount the threshold. Opiates also have a tranquilizing effect. The patient may be consciously aware of the pain through neocortical assessment, but the emotional response is blunted in the limbic system. This split response is the result of the way the pain message is split in two, with one message going to the thalamus and cortex via the neospinothalamic branch and the other taking the paleospinothalamic or old branch, stopping in the thalamus of the limbic system. Acting subcortically, opiates relieve pain and suffering, but leave the patient aware of pain in a cognitive way.

Side Effects of Opiates

Using the prototype and opiate gold standard, morphine, here are the potential side effects, usually dose-related, in each Master System.

NERVOUS SYSTEM: arrhythmias—bradycardia, bladder—dysuria/oliguria/retention/urgency, bowel—constipation/flatulence, cardiac arrest,* colic—biliary, coma,* convulsions*—infants/children, cough—decreased reflex, dizziness, drowsiness, dyspnea, edema, headache, hypotension (also orthostatic), insomnia, muscle—flaccidity, nausea/vomiting, palpitations, psyche—delirium/disorientation/dysphoria/euphoria, respiratory depression*/arrest,* sexual function—reduced libido/potency (prolonged use), sleep—deep, syncope, vision—disturbances/ miosis.

ENDOCRINE SYSTEM: (Pregnancy Category B) anorexia, edema, flushing—thorax and above, hypothermia (cold, clammy skin), precipitation of porphyria, prolonged labor, sweating, transaminase levels—elevated.

IMMUNE SYSTEM: anaphylaxis,* edema—pulmonary, pruritus, rash, urticaria/hemorrhagic urticaria.

THE OPIATES

Nothing more potent than opiates for the relief of pain, short of inducing unconsciousness, has been discovered. They all have similar side effects as noted above, the most life-threatening of which are anaphylactoid reaction, circulatory collapse, and respiratory depression.

Codeine phosphate, Schedule II, has the same uses, drug interactions, and side effects as the sulfate form.

Dosage: PO, SC, IM 15–60 mg q4h prn, to a max of 360 mg/d.

Codeine sulfate, a Schedule II drug, is an opium derivative used for decreasingly severe phasic pain and often in combination with ASA or acetaminophen.

Drug Interactions: Alcohol and other CNS depressants augment CNS depressant effects. Coma is possible when combined with chlordiazepoxide.

*Life-threatening side effect.

Side Effects

Nervous System: arrhythmias—bradycardia/tachycardia, bladder—retention, bowel—constipation, circulatory collapse,* convulsions,* dizziness, drowsiness, hypotension (also orthostatic), lethargy, lightheadedness, narcosis, nausea/vomiting, palpitations, psyche—agitation/euphoria/exhilaration/restlessness, respiratory depression,* sedation, shortness of breath, vision—miosis.

Endocrine System: (Pregnancy Category C) facial flushing, excessive perspiration.

Immune System: anaphylactoid reaction,* diffuse erythema, fixed—drug eruption, pruritus, rash urticaria.

Dosage: PO 15–60 mg q4h prn.

Hydrocodone bitartrate [Hycodan], a Schedule III drug, is a morphine derivative similar to codeine, though more addicting and with slightly more antitussive action. In the United States it is available only in formulation with other drugs.

Drug Interactions: Alcohol and other CNS depressants compound sedation and CNS depression.

Side Effects

Nervous System: bowel—constipation, dizziness, drowsiness, lightheadedness, nausea/vomiting, psyche—dysphoria/euphoria, respiratory depression,* sedation.

Endocrine System: (Pregnancy Category C) dry mouth.

Immune System: pruritus, rash.

Dosage: PO 5–10 mg q4–6h prn for pain.

Hydrocodone bitartrate combined with acetaminophen [Vicodin], a Schedule III drug, contains 5 mg of the narcotic and 500 mg of acetaminophen.

Side Effects

Nervous System: bowel—constipation, dizziness, drowsiness, lightheadedness, nausea/vomiting, psyche—dysphoria/euphoria, respiratory depression,* sedation.

Endocrine System (Pregnancy Category C) dry mouth.

Immune System: pruritus, rash.

Dosage: PO 5–10 mg q6h prn pain.

Methadone [Dolophine], a Schedule II drug, is a synthetic opiate derivative with actions similar to those of morphine.

Drug Interactions: CNS depressants increase CNS depression. Cimetidine adds to sedation. Amphetamines may potentiate CNS stimulation. Selegiline, furazolidone cause excessive and prolonged CNS depression/ convulsions/cardiovascular collapse with MAOIs. May cause withdrawal in TB patients on rifampin as rifampin lowers blood levels of methadone.

Side Effects

Nervous System: bowel—constipation, BP—transient fall, dizziness, drowsiness, lightheadedness, nausea/ vomiting, pain—bone/muscle, psyche—hallucinations, respiratory depression,* sexual function—impotence.

Endocrine System: (Pregnancy Category B; D with high doses at term) dry mouth.

Immune System: none noted.

Dosage: PO, SC, IM 2.5–10 mg q3–4h. Detoxification: PO 15–40 mg/d for 2–3 d. Decrease over 21 d. Maintenance: PO 20–120 mg q22–48h. Chronic pain: PO, SC, IM 5–20 mg q6–8h.

<u>Morphine sulfate,</u> Schedule II, the original "joy juice," has been refined, chemically defined, and synthetically imitated, but the active analgesic ingredient of the poppy, morphine, remains the gold standard by which all opioids are judged. Morphine has a twin, heroin, so named because its inventor, Heinrich Dresser, considered it a "heroic" drug (Snyder, 1986). Contrary to public belief, heroin is not stronger than morphine, just faster, accounting for the "rush" heroin addicts describe. Morphine and heroin differ only in that heroin contains two acetyl moieties, which make it oil soluble and able to penetrate the BBB more rapidly than morphine. However, heroin is not used legally in the United States.

Isolation of morphine in the 19th century coupled with the invention of the hypodermic syringe made opiates more potent and reliable than ever. Morphine is the drug of choice for myocardial infarction pain and pulmonary edema because it decreases anxiety, decreases dyspnea caused by left ventricular failure and pulmonary edema, and causes peripheral vasodilation, which decreases the pre- and postload on the heart.

Drug Interactions:
Morphine's CNS depressant action is increased with other CNS depressants. Hypertensive crisis possible with MAOIs. Phenothiazines may antagonize analgesia.

Incompatibilities

Solution/Additive: aminophylline, barbiturates, chlorothiazide, heparin, methicillin, phenytoin, sodium bicarbonate.

Y-site: minocycline, tetracycline.

*Life-threatening side effect.

Side Effects

Nervous System: arrhythmias—bradycardia, bladder—dysuria/oliguria/retention/urgency, bowel—constipation, colic—biliary, convulsions* (infants/children), cough—depressed reflex, dizziness, drowsiness, edema, hypotension—orthostatic, myalgia, nausea/ vomiting, palpitations, psyche—delirium/disorientation/dysphoria/euphoria/insomnia/restlessness, respiratory depression,* sexual function—reduced libido/potency (long use), syncope, tremor, vision—blurred/diplopia/miosis. Overdosage: arrhythmias—bradycardia/cardiac arrest,* coma,* edema*—pulmonary, hypotension, severe respiratory depression*/arrest,* skeletal muscle flaccidity, deep sleep, visual—marked miosis.

Endocrine System: (Pregnancy Category B) anorexia, flushing—face/neck/upper thorax, dry mouth, porphyria, sweating, elevated transaminase. Labor: prolonged. Overdosage: hypothermia, skin—cold, clammy.

Immune System: anaphylaxis,* pruritus, urticaria/ hemorrhagic urticaria, rash.

Dosage: PO 10–30 mg q4h prn. This form is less effective than the parenteral. SC, IM 5–20 mg q4h prn. IV 2.5–15 mg in 4–5 mL of water for injection over 4–5 min. Epidural: 5 mg. If relief is insufficient in 1 h, increase slowly by 1–2 mg to a maximum of 10 mg/24 h. Intrathecal: Use approximately 1/10 of the epidural dose. Rectal: 10–20 mg q4h prn.

<u>Oxycodone</u> is a Schedule II narcotic, a semisynthetic derivative of opium alkaloid thebaine, with no antitussive action. It alters perception of and emotional responses to pain. Ten to 12 times more potent than codeine, it relieves moderate to moderately severe pain typical of orthopedic conditions. It is also of benefit in postoperative, postextraction, and postpartum pain. It is often given in combination with acetaminophen or aspirin.

Drug Interactions:
CNS depressant action is increased with other CNS depressants.

Side Effects

Nervous System: arrhythmias—bradycardia, bladder—dysuria/frequency/retention, bowel—constipation, dizziness, lightheadedness, nausea/vomiting, psyche—dysphoria/euphoria, respiratory depression,* sedation, shortness of breath.

Endocrine System: (Pregnancy Category B; D with prolonged use) anorexia.

Immune System: bleeding or bruising, hepatotoxicity* (with combinations containing acetaminophen), jaundice, pruritus.

Oxycodone 5 mg with acetaminophen 325 mg [Percocet-5] has the typical opiate side effects and may cause deadly hepatotoxicity in the acetaminophen combination.

Dosage: PO 1 tab q6h prn.

Oxycodone hydrochloride 4.5 mg and oxycodone terephthalate 0.38 mg combined with ASA 325 mg [Percodan]

Dosage: PO 1 tab q6h prn.

Propoxyphene hydrochloride [Darvon, others], propoxyphene napsylate [Darvon-N], Schedule IV drugs, have chemical structures similar to that of methadone. Though less effective than codeine, they can depress respiration and have negligible antitussive activity.

Drug Interactions: Alcohol and other CNS depressants add to CNS depression; fatalities reported with alcohol. May increase hypoprothrombinemic effects of warfarin. May increase carbamazepine toxicity through decreased metabolism. Orphenadrine increases CNS stimulation, anxiety, tremors, confusion.

Side Effects

Nervous System: bowel—constipation, dizziness, drowsiness, fatigue/weakness, headache, lightheadedness, liver dysfunction, nausea/vomiting, pain—abdominal, psyche—dysphoria/euphoria/paradoxical excitement/restlessness, respiratory depression,* sedation, tremor, vision—minor disturbances. Overdosage: arrhythmias—ECG abnormalities, circulatory collapse,* coma,* convulsions,* dilated pupils with advancing hypoxia, psyche—confusion/toxic psychosis.

Endocrine System: (Pregnancy Category C; D with prolonged use) hypoglycemia (with renal dysfunction). Overdosage: acidosis, nephrogenic diabetes insipidus.

Immune System: allergy, liver dysfunction. Hypersensitivity: skin eruptions. Overdosage: pulmonary edema.

Dosage: PO (tablets and suspension) HCl form 65 mg q4h prn; napsylate form 100 mg q4h prn.

▶ MIXED NARCOTIC AGONIST–ANTAGONISTS

This group of analgesics was created in the ongoing search for the still-undiscovered nonaddictive analgesic. Chemically combining narcotic agonists with antagonists results in drugs that are agonist on specific opioid receptors and compete as receptor blockers at others. Their weak narcotic antagonist action can cause withdrawal in a patient who has been on narcotics.

Buprenorphine hydrochloride [Buprenex], a Schedule V drug, has opiate agonist activity approximately 30 times that of morphine and antagonist action equal to or up to 3 times greater than that of naloxone. It treats moderate to severe postoperative pain, cancer, trauma, ureteral calculi, and MI pain, and trigeminal neuralgia.

Off Label: To reduce opiate use in opiate addiction and reverse fentanyl-induced anesthesia.

Drug Interactions: CNS depression increases with other CNS depressants. Possible respiratory or cardiovascular collapse with diazepam.

Side Effects

Nervous System: dizziness, drowsiness, headache, hyperventilation, hypotension, nausea/vomiting, psyche—amnesia/euphoria, respiratory depression,* vertigo, vision—miosis.

Endocrine System: (Pregnancy Category C) sweating.

Immune System: pruritus, injection site reactions.

Dosage: IM, IV 0.3 mg q6h or 0.6 mg q4h. Also per continuous IV infusion 25–50 mcg/h or per patient-controlled infusion device or epidurally 60–180 mcg over 48 h.

Butorphanol tartrate [Stadol] is used to relieve moderate to severe pain, preoperative or preanesthetic sedation and analgesia, obstetric analgesia during labor, cancer pain, renal colic, burns.

Off Label: musculoskeletal and postepisiotomy pain.

Drug Interactions: CNS depressant action is increased by other CNS depressants.

Side Effects

Nervous System: arrhythmias—bradycardia, biliary spasm, bladder—difficulty urinating, dizziness, drowsiness, floating feeling, headache, nausea, lethargy, lightheadedness, palpitations, psyche—confusion/insomnia/nervousness, respiratory depression,* sedation, skin—cyanosis in the extremities/ tingling, vertigo, weakness.

Endocrine System: (Pregnancy Category C) diaphoresis, skin—clammy/flushing/sensitivity to cold/warmth.

Immune System: pruritus, urticaria.

Dosage: IM 1–4 mg q3–4h prn. IV 0.5–2 mg q3–4h prn.

Nalbuphine hydrochloride [Nubain] is used to provide analgesia and weak antagonist action in moderate to severe pain. It also provides preoperative sedation analgesia and is a supplement to surgical anesthesia.

Drug Interactions: CNS depression compounded by other CNS depressants.

---

*Life-threatening side effect.

Incompatibilities

Solution/Additive: diazepam, pentobarbital, promethazine, thiethylperazine.

Y-site: nafcillin.

Side Effects

Nervous System: arrhythmias—bradycardia/tachycardia, bladder—urgency, cramps—abdominal, dizziness, dyspnea, headache, hypertension/hypotension, nausea/vomiting, paresthesias, psyche—confusion/crying/depression/distortion of body image/dysphoria/euphoria/hallucinations/insomnia/nervousness/restlessness, respiratory depression,* sedation, speech—difficult, taste—bitter, vertigo, vision—blurred/miosis.

Endocrine System: (Pregnancy Category B) flushing, dry mouth, skin—sweating/clammy.

Immune System: asthma, burning sensation, pruritus, urticaria.

Dosage: SC, IM, IV 10–20 mg q3–6h prn to maximum of 160 mg/d.

Pentazocine hydrochloride [Talwin], a Schedule IV drug, has one-third the potency of morphine, but is more potent than codeine. Weak antagonist action.

Drug Interactions: CNS depressants compound pentazocine's CNS depression action. Narcotic analgesics may precipitate narcotic withdrawal syndrome.

Incompatibilities

Solution/Additive: aminophylline, barbiturates, sodium bicarbonate, glycopyrrolate, heparin, nafcillin.

Y-site: glycopyrrolate, heparin, nafcillin.

Side Effects

Nervous System: arrhythmias—bradycardia/tachycardia, bladder—retention, bowel—constipation, dizziness, headache, lightheadedness, nausea/vomiting, psyche—euphoria, taste changes, vision disturbances. High doses: arrhythmias—tachycardia, hypertension, palpitations, psyche—anxiety/disturbed dreams/euphoria/hallucinations/mood changes, respiratory depression,* shock.*

Endocrine System: (Pregnancy Category C) flushing, dry mouth, sweating.

Immune System: anemia, anaphylaxis,* angioedema,* leukopenia, rash, thrombocytopenia.

Dosage: PO 50–100 mg q3–4h to maximum of 600 mg. SC, IM, IV 30 mg q3–4h to maximum of 360 mg. In labor: 20–30 mg IM, then 20 mg q2–3h for 1 or 2 doses.

*Life-threatening side effect.

Tramadol hydrochloride [Ultran, Zydol] is used to relieve moderate to severe pain by weak opiate receptor activity and also by blocking reuptake of norepinephrine and serotonin.

Drug Interactions: Carbamazepine significantly decreases tramadol levels (may need up to twice usual dose). Tramadol may increase adverse effects of MAOIs.

Side Effects

Nervous System: bladder—retention, bowel—constipation/diarrhea/flatulence, coordination—disturbed, dizziness, drowsiness, dyspepsia, fatigue, headache, nausea/vomiting, pain—abdominal, palpitations, psyche—anxiety/confusion/euphoria/restlessness/sleep disturbances, somnolence, vasodilation, vertigo, visual disturbances.

Endocrine System: (Pregnancy Category C) anorexia, menopausal symptoms, dry mouth, sweating.

Immune System: rash.

Dosage: PO 50–100 mg q4–6h prn to maximum of 400 mg/d. Decrease to 50–100 mg q12h in patients with Cl$_{cr}$ < 30 mL/min or with cirrhosis.

SYNTHETIC OPIATES (OPIOIDS)

The following analgesics were created in the 1920s and 1930s in Europe to improve on morphine. The synthetic opiates are Schedule II drugs.

Hydromorphone hydrochloride [Dilaudid], a Schedule II drug, is used to treat moderate to severe pain.

Drug Interactions: Alcohol and other CNS depressants compound sedation and CNS depression.

Incompatibilities

Solution/Additive: prochlorperazine, sodium bicarbonate, thiopental.

Y-site: minocycline, prochlorperazine, tetracycline.

Side Effects

Nervous System: arrhythmias—bradycardia/tachycardia, bowel—constipation, dizziness, drowsiness, hypotension, nausea/vomiting, psyche—euphoria, respiratory depression,* sedation, vision—blurred.

Endocrine System: (Pregnancy Category C) none noted.

Immune System: none noted.

Dosage: Moderate to severe pain: PO, SC, IM, IV 1–4 mg q4–6h prn. Rectal: 3 mg suppositories q4–6h prn for pain.

<u>Levorphanol tartrate [Levo-Dromoran]</u>, a Schedule II drug, is used to treat severe to moderate pain. The isomer of levorphanol, dextromethorphan, became an antitussive.

Drug Interactions: Alcohol and other CNS depressants compound sedation and CNS depression.

Incompatibilities

Solution/Additive: aminophylline, ammonium chloride, barbiturates, chlorothiazide, heparin, methicillin, phenytoin, sodium bicarbonate.

Side Effects

Nervous System: arrhythmias—bradycardia/tachycardia, bladder—frequency/retention, bowel—constipation, cramps, drowsiness, hypertension/hypotension, nausea/vomiting, physical dependence, psyche—confusion/euphoria/nervousness, respiratory depression,* sedation, vision—blurred.

Endocrine System: (Pregnancy Category B): dry mouth.

Immune System: none noted.

Dosage: PO, SC 2–3 mg q6–8h prn.

<u>Meperidine hydrochloride [Demerol]</u> was synthesized in Germany in 1937 in a search for atropine analogs. Found to have one-tenth the potency of morphine, but with no chemical resemblance to morphine, it was mistakenly thought to be nonaddictive (Sneader, 1985). It is addictive, of course (Schedule II). Like morphine, meperidine does depress respirations; however, it does not depress the cough reflex, to the degree that morphine does—an important benefit postoperatively when coughing is encouraged.

Drug Interactions: Alcohol and other CNS depressants, cimetidine cause additive sedation and CNS depression. Amphetamines may potentiate CNS stimulation. MAOIs, selegiline, furazolidone may cause excessive and prolonged CNS depression, convulsions, cardiovascular collapse. Phenytoin may increase toxic meperidine metabolites.

Incompatibilities

Solution/Additive: aminophylline, barbiturates, heparin, methicillin, morphine, phenytoin, sodium bicarbonate.

Y-site: cefoperazone, heparin, mezlocillin, minocycline, tetracycline.

Side Effects

Nervous System: arrhythmias—bradycardia/cardiovascular collapse*/tachycardia, bladder—oliguria/retention, bowel—constipation, arthralgia, biliary tract spasm, bronchoconstriction* (large doses), convulsions,* cough reflex—depressed, dizziness, headache, hyperactive reflexes, hypersensitivity to external stimuli, hypotension, lightheadedness, muscles—twitching/uncoordinated movements, nausea/vomiting, pain, palpitation, psyche—agitation/confusion/disorientation/dysphoria/euphoria/excitement/hallucinations, respiratory depression,* sedation, syncope, tremors, vision—corneal anesthesia/dilated pupils/miosis, weakness. Toxic dose: cardiac arrest*

Endocrine System: (Pregnancy Category B; D at term) bilirubin, BSP retention, facial flushing, dry mouth, profuse perspiration, increased levels of serum amylase.

Immune System: ALT/AST—elevated, pruritus, rash, urticaria. IV: flare/weal over IV site, phlebitis, tissue irritation, induration.

Dosage: PO, IM, IV 50–150 mg q3–4h prn for pain. Preoperative: IM, SC 50–150 mg 30–90 min before surgery. Obstetric analgesia: IM, SC 50–100 mg when pains become regular; may repeat q1–3h.

▶ PATIENT-CONTROLLED ANALGESIA

Pain interferes with healing, making the patient reluctant to move, breathe deeply, or cough. But fear of causing addiction makes some medical professionals wary of giving sufficient narcotic analgesia to relieve pain. Due to this fear, some doctors prescribe less medication than is needed and many nurses delay the administration of the medication, believing they are protecting the patient. This practice increases suffering and slows healing. The analgesic needs to be given on a regular basis to prevent or stay ahead of pain rather than as needed (prn) after the patient is in agony.

Patient-controlled analgesia (PCA) empowers the patient and prevents suffering postoperatively. As the patient heals, less medication is needed. This method requires evaluating and educating the patient prior to surgery. Preset dosages are prepared by the nurse and administered as needed by the patient into an open IV line.

▶ TRANSDERMAL ANALGESIA

Transdermal analgesia can provide pain relief without the risks or inconvenience of parenteral routes. It provides safe and prolonged administration and can be terminated simply by removing the transdermal patch. The site should be cleansed first and also should be dry, hairless, and free of cuts, abrasions, and infections. If hair is present, it should be clipped off, not shaved (DiPiro et al., 1997).

*Life-threatening side effect.

Fentanyl citrate [Duragesic] is used for continuous analgesia for up to 72 hours.

Drug Interactions: Alcohol and other CNS depressants potentiate effects. MAOIs may precipitate hypertensive crisis.

Incompatibilities

Solution/Additive: pentobarbital, thiopental.

Side Effects

Nervous System: arrhythmias—bradycardia/cardiac arrest*/circulatory depression,* bladder—retention, bowel—constipation, bronchoconstriction,* convulsions with high doses,* dizziness, hypotension, nausea/vomiting, psyche—delirium/euphoria, respiratory arrest*/depression/laryngospasm, sedation, vision—blurred/miosis. IV: muscle rigidity, especially muscles of respiration after IV infusion.

Endocrine System: (Pregnancy Category B; D for prolonged use or use of high doses at term) diaphoresis.

Immune System: contact dermatitis from patch, rash.

Dosage: Available for chronic pain: 25, 50, 75, and 100 µg/h in 10, 20, 30, and 40 cm² sizes. Patch circumference determines dosage per hour. To apply first cleanse the site with water and allow it to dry. Also PO 400 µg lozenge. Postoperative pain: IM 50–100 µg q1–2h prn.

▶ OPIATE ANESTHESIA

Narcotics play a major role in surgical procedures, usually as preoperative adjuncts to anesthesia, helping to calm the patient, or postoperatively to relieve the pain of a surgical wound. Some opiate drugs are given during the procedure itself to help provide balanced anesthesia, a practice that involves the use of agents for specific purposes, for example, regional anesthesia for analgesia and muscle relaxation, barbiturates for loss of consciousness, inhalants for continued unconsciousness, neuromuscular blockers for paralysis, and nitrous oxide and the opioids for analgesia. The side effects of opiate anesthesia include laryngospasm, apnea, depressed respirations, brady- and tachyarrhythmias, hiccups, hyper- and hypotension, muscle rigidity, priapism, and vertigo. Beta blockers increase the possibility of bradycardia. Because both fentanyl and sufentanil are unlikely to stimulate histamine release that can cause subsequent fluid loss from peripheral vessels, they are less likely to cause hypotension. During anesthesia with either fentanyl or sufentanil, large doses are used in conjunction with oxygen and neuromuscular blockers. If, under anesthesia, the patient becomes hypertensive and tachycardic, the condition can be countered by adding a gas anesthetic to decrease vascular constriction.

*Life-threatening side effect.

Usually, however, the opioids tend to decrease heart rate. The exception is meperidine [Demerol], which was discovered in a quest for an anticholinergic.

Alfentanil hydrochloride [Alfenta], a Schedule II drug, is used for brief surgical procedures, but also for long procedures in multiple injections where its duration is 30 minutes or continuous infusion where its duration is over 45 minutes. It is also used for anesthesia induction when mechanical ventilation will be needed.

Drug Interactions: Beta-adrenergic blockers increase incidence of bradycardia. CNS depressants such as barbiturates, tranquilizers, neuromuscular blocking agents, opiates, and inhalation general anesthetics may enhance the cardiovascular and CNS effects of alfentanil in both magnitude and duration when administered with alfentanil. Enhancement or prolongation of postoperative respiratory depression also may result from concomitant administration of any of these agents with alfentanil.

Incompatibilities: None noted.

Side Effects

Nervous System: arrhythmias—bradycardia/tachycardia, bowel—constipation, cramps, dizziness, drowsiness, dyspnea, extremities feel heavy and warm, hypertension/hypotension, nausea/vomiting, psyche—euphoria, respiratory—apnea*/depression,* thoracic muscle rigidity.

Endocrine System: (Pregnancy Category C) anorexia, diaphoresis, flushing.

Immune System: none noted.

Dosage: IV or multiple injection, 8–75 µg/kg. Maximum dosage dependent on procedure duration.

Fentanyl citrate [Sublimaze], a Schedule II drug, is used for preoperative and postoperative analgesic as well as for anesthesia induction and balanced anesthesia.

Drug Interactions: Alcohol and other CNS depressants potentiate effects. MAOIs may precipitate hypertensive crisis.

Incompatibilities

Solution/Additive: pentobarbital, thiopental.

Side Effects

Nervous System: arrhythmias—bradycardia/cardiac arrest*/circulatory depression,* bladder—retention, bowel—constipation, convulsions with high doses,* dizziness, hypotension, nausea/vomiting, psyche—delirium/euphoria, respiratory—arrest*/bronchoconstriction/ depression*/laryngospasm,* sedation, vision—blurred/ miosis. IV: muscle rigidity, especially muscles of respiration after rapid IV infusion.

Endocrine System: (Pregnancy Category B; D for prolonged use or use of high doses at term) diaphoresis.

Immune System: rash.

Dosage: Adjunct to regional anesthesia: IM 50–100 µg; IV 2–20 µg/kg over 1–2 min up to 50 µg/kg. General anesthesia: IV 50–150 µg/kg as needed. Pre-op: IM 50–100 mcg 30–60 min before surgery. Lozenge 400 mcg: suck on until sedated.

Remifentanil [Ultiva] is a potent, very-short-acting anilidopiperidine with affinity for mu opioid receptors. It has rapid onset and peak effect (±1 min) and a short half-life of 10–20 min. It is used as analgesia during induction and maintenance of general anesthesia for inpatient and outpatient procedures; continued analgesia into the immediate postoperative period under the direct supervision of an anesthetist in a postoperative anesthesia care unit or intensive care setting; and analgesia during monitored anesthesia care. Recovery is rapid and the effects noncumulative.

Drug Interactions: none noted.

Side Effects

Nervous System: apnea, arrhythmias—bradycardia/tachycardia, dizziness, headache, hypoxia,* hypertension/hypotension, nausea/vomiting, pain, psyche—agitation, respiratory depression, skeletal muscle rigidity, vision disturbances.

Endocrine System: (Pregnancy Category C) fever, shivering.

Immune System: pruritus.

Dosage: IV 0.5–1 µg/kg/min along with a hypnotic or volatile agent for anesthesia induction. Postoperative analgesia: 0.1 µg/kg/min. Adjust rate to balance patient's level of analgesia and respiratory rate.

Sufentanil citrate [Sufenta], a Schedule II drug, has an action similar to fentanyl, but it is more potent and has a more rapid onset (1.5–3 min) and recovery (40 min for low doses). Note: Discard if the contents are discolored or cloudy.

Drug Interactions: Beta-adrenergic antagonists increase incidence of bradycardia. Alcohol and other CNS depressants such as barbiturates, tranquilizers, opiates, and inhalation general anesthetics add to CNS depression. Cimetidine increases risk of respiratory depression.

Incompatibilities: none noted.

Side Effects

Nervous System: arrhythmias—bradycardia/tachycardia, bladder—retention, bowel—constipation, bron-

chospasm, hypertension/hypotension, nausea/vomiting, respiratory—apnea*/depression,* skeletal muscle rigidity (especially of trunk), spasms of sphincter of Oddi.

Endocrine System: (Pregnancy Category C) chills.

Immune System: itching.

Dosage: As with fentanyl. Dosage: Primary anesthetic: IV 8–30 µg/kg with oxygen and a muscle relaxant. Anesthetic adjunct: IV 1–8 µg/kg with oxygen and nitrous oxide, based on the duration of the procedure.

▶ THE OPIATE ANTAGONISTS OR BLOCKERS

The opiate blockers compete with opiates for receptor sites in opiate overdose and are used to reverse respiratory depression. The opiate blockers compete with opiate molecules and displace them from the receptors in the presence of sodium ions. Opiate blockers reverse overdose and are used to rule out opiate overdose as the cause of coma. The action of opiate antagonists is immediate and brief. Frequent administrations may be necessary before the overdosed patient is past the crisis.

Naloxone hydrochloride [Narcan], with no agonist properties, is used to treat narcotic overdose and to completely or partially reverse respiratory depression.

Off Label: To treat septic shock by blocking endorphin-mediated hypotension and also to reverse alcohol-induced or clonide-induced coma or respiratory depression.

Drug Interactions: none noted.

Incompatibilities: none noted.

Side Effects

Nervous System: excessive dosage in narcotic depression: analgesia reversal, BP increase, drowsiness, hyperventilation, tremors. Too rapid reversal: arrhythmias—tachycardia, nausea/vomiting.

Endocrine System: (Pregnancy Category B) Too rapid reversal: sweating.

Immune System: Excessive dosage in narcotic depression: elevated PTT.

Dosage: IV (the preferred route) 0.4–2.0 mg q2–3 min prn. SC, IM q2–3 min to a maximum of 10 mg. Postoperative opiate depression: IV 0.1–0.2 mg; may be repeated q2–3 min for up to 3 doses if necessary.

Naltrexone hydrochloride [Trexan] competes for opiate receptors, thereby helping to enhance the resolve of

---

*Life-threatening side effect.

detoxified addicts to stay opiate-free and to decrease the compulsive consumption syndromes of alcoholism. Unlabeled use for self-inflicted pain in the developmentally disabled, in whom such pain may be inflicted for the release of endorphins, and for obesity.

Drug Interactions: none noted.

Incompatibilities: none noted.

Side Effects

Nervous System: bowel—constipation, cramps—abdominal, dizziness, energy—decrease/increase, headache, nausea/vomiting, pain—muscle/joints, psyche—anxiety/depression/insomnia/irritability/nervousness.

Endocrine System: (Pregnancy Category C) chills, dry mouth, thirst.

Immune System: hepatotoxicity,* rash.

Dosage: PO. Start with 25 mg; an additional 25 mg may be given if there are no withdrawal signs within 1 h. Maintenance: 50–800 mg q24h. Alcohol dependence: PO 50 mg qd.

▶ ANTIDIARRHEALS

Our endogenous endorphins enhance digestion and slow it down to obtain maximum nutrients from the intestinal tract. Sometimes worry or disease speed up peristalsis, causing diarrhea. Opiates can help treat diarrhea. Opiates inhibit the GI tract, causing constipation. On the other hand, opiate withdrawal causes rebound diarrhea. Before the advent of refrigeration and more reliable food preservation, opiates, by their ability to slow peristalsis, saved lives that would have been lost to food poisoning, dysentery, and other diarrheal diseases.

Diphenoxylate hydrochloride with atropine sulfate [Lomotil, others], a Schedule V drug, is used to treat diarrhea. Atropine is added to discourage abuse.

Drug Interactions: MAOIs may precipitate hypertensive crisis. CNS depressants increase CNS depression.

Atropine Interactions: Amantadine, antihistamines, tricyclic antidepressants, quinidine, disopyramide, procainamide increase anticholinergic effects. Levodopa effects decreased. Phenothiazines' antipsychotic effects decreased by decreased absorption.

Side Effects

Nervous System: arrhythmias—tachycardia, bladder—retention, bowel—discomfort/distension/paralytic

ileus/toxic megacolon,* dizziness, drowsiness, headache, lethargy, malaise, nausea/vomiting, numbness of extremities, palpitations, psyche—depression/euphoria/restlessness, sedation, weakness, vision—blurred/miosis/mydriasis/nystagmus.

Endocrine System: (Pregnancy Category C) anorexia, flushing, dry mouth.

Immune System: angioedema,* gums swelling, pruritus, rash, giant urticaria.

Dosage: PO 1–2 tabs or 1–2 tsp (5 mL) tid or qid. Each dose contains 2.5 mg diphenoxylate hydrochloride and 0.025 mg atropine sulfate.

Loperamide [Imodium, Imodium AD] is chemically related to diphenoxylate and meperidine. An OTC drug.

Side Effects

Nervous System: abdominal—discomfort/distention/pain, bowel—constipation/toxic megacolon* (patients with ulcerative colitis, CNS depression, dizziness, drowsiness, fatigue), nausea/vomiting.

Endocrine System: (Pregnancy Category B) anorexia, fever, dry mouth.

Immune System: rash.

Dosage: PO 4 mg. Follow with 2 mg after each unformed BM to maximum of 16 mg/d.

Opium tincture (Laudanum) is a Schedule II drug. At one time this ancient mixture was sold without prescription. It contains morphine, codeine, and papaverine to treat diarrhea.

Drug Interactions: CNS depressants add to its CNS depressant action.

Side Effects

Nervous System: GI disturbances. Acute toxicity: CNS depression.

Endocrine System: (Pregnancy Category B) none noted.

Immune System: none noted.

Dosage: PO 0.6–1.0 mL qid. Maximum 6 mL/d.

Paregoric (Camphorated Opium Tincture) contains 2 mg anhydrous morphine, alcohol, benzoic acid, camphor, and anise oil. It is an ancient treatment for diarrhea and a Schedule III drug.

Drug Interactions: Increased CNS depression with other CNS depressants.

*Life-threatening side effect.

Side Effects

Nervous System: bowel—constipation, nausea/vomiting, pain—abdominal. High doses: dizziness, drowsiness, physical dependence.

Endocrine System: (Pregnancy Category B; D with prolonged use or high doses at term) High doses: facial flushing, sweating.

Immune System: none noted.

Dosage: PO 5–10 mL after loose stool. May administer q2h up to qid prn.

▶ ANTITUSSIVES

The medulla contains an area devoted to coughing. Opiates can suppress this center. The classic antitussive is codeine, but over the years scientists have created nonnarcotic antitussives.

Codeine as an antitussive. See codeine sulfate in the analgesic section of this chapter for side effects.

Dosage: PO 10–20 mg q4–6h prn cough. Maximum 120 mg/d.

Hydrocodone bitartrate [Dicodid], a Schedule III drug, is a synthetic codeine for the relief of hyperactive or nonproductive cough. For information about its use as an analgesic and about its side effects, refer to the analgesic section of this chapter.

Dosage: PO 5–10 mg q4h prn cough.

▶ NONNARCOTIC ANTITUSSIVES

The nonnarcotic antitussive dextromethorphan was developed in a quest for cough medications that did not suppress respirations or invite abuse as did opiate antitussives. It is the main ingredient in the numerous antitussive preparations available without prescription.

Dextromethorphan hydrobromide [Romilar, others], is an OTC antitussive derived from levorphanol. Though dextromethorphan is related to morphine, it has no analgesic or hypnotic effect. Unlike the opiate antitussives, it does not depress respiration.

Drug Interactions: High risk of excitation, hypotension, and hyperpyrexia with MAOIs.

Side Effects

Nervous System: abdominal discomfort, bowel—constipation, CNS depression with very large doses, dizziness, drowsiness, GI upset, psyche—excitability.

Endocrine System: (Pregnancy Category C) none noted.

Immune System: none noted.

Dosage: PO 10–20 mg q4h or 30 mg q6–8h. Maximum 120 mg/d, or 60 mg sustained action liquid bid.

Benzonatate [Tessalon], is related to tetracaine. Whereas it, too, suppresses the cough reflex in the medulla, benzonatate also has topical anesthetic effect on stretch receptors in the airways, lungs, and pleura. It is also used in bronchoscopy, thoracentesis, and other procedures when coughing must be avoided.

Side Effects

Nervous System: bowel—constipation, dizziness—mild, drowsiness, headache, nausea.

Endocrine System: (Pregnancy Category C) none noted.

Immune System: pruritus, rash.

Dosage: PO 100 mg tid to daily maximum of 600 mg.

 Chapter Highlights

- Opiates rank among the most ancient of all medical remedies to treat pain, diarrhea, and cough.

- No analgesic surpasses morphine for relief of severe pain.

- Codeine in combination with NSAIDs relieves moderate to severe pain.

- Opiates are subject to abuse by people seeking relief from emotional pain, making them controlled drugs.

- The search continues for a synthetic opioid that does not cause addiction.

- Severe pain impedes healing, and diarrheal diseases can kill.

- The opiate-derived drugs save lives.

The Endocrine System and Drugs

▶ PHARMACOLOGY OF THE ENDOCRINE SYSTEM

Pharmacology in the endocrine system consists of drugs that replace or supplement a lack of naturally occurring hormones, stimulate hormone production, treat body responses to hormone imbalance, create mineral balance, counter the inflammations of the immune system, lower blood pressure, and cause diuresis. Pharmacology takes into account the slow nature of the endocrine system. For example, in treating an asthma attack in progress, nervous system catecholamines help to counter the immune response and open the airway immediately. Glucocorticoids administered simultaneously are expected to manifest in 45 minutes and prevent relapse. The endocrine system is the slow but steady team member.

▶ ENERGY

Everything a cell does in following its genetic program takes energy. The endocrine system must make sure that billions of cells that make up a body have the necessary fuel to function. Cells wear out and must be replaced. The endocrine system repairs and replaces. And should a male and female sex cell fuse and attach to the wall of the uterus, the endocrine system focuses on the tremendous demands of gestation and birthing. At birth the endocrine system's hypothalamus helps create the mother–child bond and provides the milk that will nourish the infant.

▶ THE ENDOCRINE MASTER SYSTEM

If each of the three Master Systems could be said to have a personality, the nervous system would be nimble,

jumpy, and judgmental. The immune system would be rapidly responsive, pugnacious, and prejudiced against anything foreign, fighting for survival. The endocrine system would be seen as stable, slower to respond than the other two, and striving to keep the body in balance. The endocrine system might seem almost sluggish when compared with the lightning fast responses of the nervous system and the immune system.

However, the functions of the endocrine system do not depend on speed. Its cells speak gland language. Its functions require steadiness in maintaining routine rhythms and critical balances of elements, hormones, fuel, and water. It responds slowly and its actions cease slowly; for example steroid hormones take a characteristic 45 minutes to manifest an effect. Other hormones, such as thyroxine or growth hormone, may take months before the full effect can be completed. Traveling at the speed of the blood's circulation, endocrine hormone molecules are carried in the bloodstream to target glands. In turn, target glands spill their hormones into the circulation and the hypothalamus monitors their production levels.

▶ NEGATIVE FEEDBACK AND TARGET GLANDS

Through negative feedback the hypothalamus monitors hormone levels in the blood from faraway target glands. As those levels drop (become negative) below specific set points the hypothalamus sends releasing hormones downstream on the stalk that connects it to its servant the pituitary or master gland. In turn, the pituitary pours tropic hormones into the bloodstream. Depending on their shapes, these hormones lock into specific receptors on target glands and stimulate them to produce and release their own hormones. In this manner, the thyroid, the gonads, and the adrenal cortices produce the hormones essential to fueling, maintaining water and mineral balance, and reproducing.

In response to the stimulating hormones, the target glands produce and release their hormones into the bloodstream. When production reaches a satisfactory blood level, the hypothalamus stops sending down releasing hormones to the pituitary, and the pituitary ceases production and release of its stimulating hormones.

▶ HYPOTHALAMIC HORMONES

In addition to producing releasing hormones, the hypothalamus also produces two hormones that it sends as tiny, dewy drops down gossamer strands of the pituitary stalk for storage in the posterior pituitary. One of the hormones, antidiuretic hormone (ADH), regulates the kidneys' release and retention of water. The other, oxytocin, is essential to getting pregnant, birthing, and milk letdown. The hypothalamus regulates their release from the pituitary (Fig. II–1).

▶ HORMONE IMBALANCE

There are times when the target gland cannot respond, for instance, when ovaries stop functioning because of menopause or the thyroid fails because of a lack of iodine. In these situations the hypothalamus keeps sending down releasing hormones and the pituitary keeps sending ever larger amounts of stimulating hormones. In the case of the thyroid gland, goiter can result as the gland grows larger and larger in response to the thyroid-stimulating hormone (TSH). Blood tests can reveal the rising levels of stimulating hormones, reflecting the hypothalamus's attempt to get hormonal production underway in a target organ.

▶ THE MIND–BODY CONNECTION

Nestled in and under the emotional limbic system, the hypothalamus is the "mind–body" connection between the nervous system and the endocrine system. While some scientific arguments put it below the limbic system in the diencephalon and some in the limbic system, its position, connected to the pituitary and tucked under the thalamus of the limbic system, makes it a transitional structure connecting its functions for emotion to the production of glandular hormones. The hypothalamus is involved in pain, responding to both physical pain and the emotional pain of depression, pleasure, and reproduction, in addition to its monitoring duties. It makes us

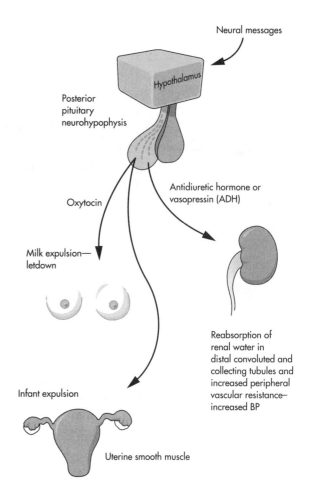

Figure II–1. Neurohypophysis (posterior pituitary): vasopressin (ADH—antidiuretic hormone) and oxytocin.

hunger and thirst. The paired amygdalae in the limbic system send out intense signals when the olfactory nerves sense pleasant or noxious smells, responds to threat with fear or rage, adds an ineffable quality to living.

Limbic and cortical information have an influence on the hypothalamus and its control over the release of hormones from the pituitary. Intimately involved with the nervous system, the endocrine turns nerve language, that is, neurotransmitter-mediated language, into gland or hormone language. Thus, the mind and body are inseparable, connected as they are by the endocrine system. The hypothalamus responds to pain signals from upstream with increased production of adrenocorticotropic hormone to stimulate the release of glucocorticoids from the adrenal cortex.

This connection of emotions to endocrine functions makes clear the impact of emotions on body functions outside the nervous system. The hypothalamus controls mammalian functions of internal temperature maintenance and live births with subsequent milk production by the mother. Not only does the endocrine link mind and body, it links generations through time and space.

8 Drugs for Lipid Control

▶ FAT: THE MOST POWER PER CALORIE

The endocrine system provides the fuel for all cells, and the most power-packed fuel, molecule for molecule, is fat. Whereas carbohydrates produce 4.1 kcal/g of energy and proteins 4.35 kcal/g of energy, when metabolized, a gram of fat releases 9 kcal/g of energy. Fats, or lipids, are compounds of glycerol with backbones of fatty acids that fuel the cell. In addition to fueling the cell, fats create the two lipid layers that make up every cell membrane that protects the cell from the watery extracellular environment. Fats also provide subcutaneous insulation, insulation around nerves, and the oil on the skin's surface. Fats help form the lipoproteins that carry fat in the blood.

ESSENTIAL FATTY ACIDS

Though the body can produce some fats, others need to be part of the diet. Fatty acids necessary for health or which cannot be made by the body are called **essential fatty acids.** Linoleic acid, one of those essential fatty acids, protects the integrity of skin and membranes and helps to metabolize cholesterol. In the immune system linoleic acid transports cholesterol in the blood to create prostaglandins, to increase clotting time, and to assist in the breakdown, or lysis, of fibrin, which forms the net or web of a clot.

CHOLESTEROL

Cholesterol is a high-molecular-weight cyclic alcohol, also called a sterol or steroid. Plants do not produce cholesterol. We make our own cholesterol or get it by eating other animals or their products. In health, cholesterol production drops when cholesterol intake increases and vice versa so that cholesterol levels remain fairly constant. However, a diet high in carbohydrates, fats, and proteins increases the liver's production of cholesterol.

Production of steroid hormones depends on fat. Women who do not have enough body fat may not be able to produce adequate amounts of the female steroid hormones. Young girls need to have stored fat to reach menarche. In another example of the importance of cholesterol, sunlight on skin reacts with the steroid 7-dehydrocholesterol to create vitamin D, a hormone that pulls dietary calcium from the alimentary channel. The liver synthesizes cholesterol and stores in it the gallbladder as bile salts, which, when released into the small intestine, break up dietary lipids. Cholesterol also packs itself in between the hydrocarbon tails that create the center of the two-layered lipid or fat sandwich that forms the cell membrane.

LIPOPROTEINS

Lipoproteins, as the name suggests, are molecules of fat wrapped in protein for transport in the watery bloodstream. Each of the several different kinds of lipoproteins carries a specific cargo of fat. The ratio of protein to fat determines the density of the lipoprotein—more protein equals higher density. Lipoproteins carry fatty acids, cholesterol, triglycerides, phospholipids, traces of steroid hormones, and fat-soluble vitamins. Chylomicrons transport dietary fat to liver cells. They consist mostly of triglycerides (90%) and have little protein. Very-low-density lipoproteins (VLDL) transport endogenous triglycerides to cells. Their work is supplemented by intermediate-low-density lipoproteins (ILDL). Low-density lipoprotein cholesterol (LDL-C) transports cholesterol to cells of the periphery. High-density lipoprotein cholesterol (HDL-C) transports unneeded cholesterol to the liver for breakdown and removal. The liver excretes cholesterol via the gallbladder in bile, which aids digestion of fat. The villains in atherosclerosis appear to be the LDLs and VLDLs.

HYPERLIPIDEMIA: ELEVATED BLOOD CHOLESTEROL

Though elevated cholesterol levels may not necessarily be a result of diet, diet is a good place to start if blood cholesterol levels are too high, that is, 200 mg/dL and above. The danger in elevated cholesterol levels is that cholesterol collects on blood vessel walls and calcifies. This hardening of the arteries causes the vessels to narrow, lose resiliency, and become rough enough to damage passing blood cells. Damaged blood cells trigger clotting, which can result in stroke or myocardial infarction. The narrowed, hardened vessels also contribute to hypertension, forcing the heart to work against greater resistance. Some patients with elevated blood cholesterol have the genetic predisposition called familial hypercholesterolemia, which cannot be altered by diet and puts the patient at high risk for coronary heart disease in the early decades of life. In addition to being a risk factor in cardiovascular disease, high cholesterol is associated with gallbladder disease because gallstones are composed of crystallized cholesterol.

▶ DRUGS TO LOWER CHOLESTEROL LEVELS

Because elevated cholesterol levels are linked to CAD, it is essential to keep cholesterol levels below 200 mg/dL to help prevent MI. Other risk factors that must be addressed include diabetes, hypertension, and smoking. Decreased intake of cholesterol, calories, and saturated fats is a good place to start to decrease cholesterol levels; however, when diet alone fails to lower cholesterol levels, drugs may help.

<u>Atorvastatin calcium [Lipitor]</u> lowers plasma cholesterol by inhibiting liver synthesis of 3-hydroxy-3-methylglutaryl coenzyme A (HMG-CoA) reductase and cholesterol and increasing the number of hepatic LDL receptors to increase uptake and catabolism of LDL.

Drug Interactions: Increased risk of myopathy with other lipid-lowering agents, cyclosporine, fibric acid derivatives, nicotinic acid, erythromycin, azole antifungals. Decreased plasma concentrations with Maalox, but no alteration in LDL-C reduction. Decreased plasma concentrations with colestipol, but LDL-C reduction is greater. Increased digoxin levels. Increased norethindrone and ethinyl estradiol levels with oral contraceptives.

Side Effects

Nervous System: arthralgia, asthenia, bowel—constipation/diarrhea/flatulence, dyspepsia, headache, myalgia, pain—abdominal/back.

Endocrine System: (Pregnancy Category X) none noted.

Immune System: allergic reaction, infection, sinusitis, pharyngitis, rash.

Dosage: PO 10 mg qd. Maximum of 80 mg/d.

<u>Clofibrate [Atromid-S]</u> decreases triglyceride production and VLDLs and shrinks xanthomas. It increases ADH release from posterior pituitary and excretion of neutral sterols in stool.

Drug Interactions: Oral anticoagulants increase hypoprothrombinemia and increase risk of bleeding. Probenecid increases clofibrate effects, and sulfonylureas increase hypoglycemic effects.

Side Effects

Nervous System: angina—decrease/increase, arrhythmias, bowel—diarrhea/distress/flatulence/loose stools,

CHF, dizziness, drowsiness, headache, nausea/vomiting, sexual function—impotence/libido decrease.

Endocrine System: (Pregnancy Category C) cholelithiasis, renal insufficiency.

Immune System: agranulocytosis,* allergy, ALT/AST—elevated, anemia, anticoagulant potentiation, eosinophilia, flu-like symptoms, leukopenia, neutropenia, rash, pruritus, urticaria, xanthoma sites—phlebitis/swelling.

Dosage: PO 2 g/d in divided doses. Diabetes insipidus: PO 1.5–2 g/d in 2–4 divided doses.

<u>Colestipol [Colestid]</u> reduces cholesterol by binding with bile acids in the GI tract for excretion in the stool.

Off Label: Digitoxin overdose and hyperoxaluria; control of postoperative diarrhea caused by excess bile acids.

Drug Interactions: Decreases GI absorption of oral anticoagulants, digoxin, iron salts, penicillins, phenobarbital, tetracyclines, thiazide diuretics, thyroid hormones, vitamins A, D, E, K.

Side Effects

Nervous System: belching, bowel—constipation/diarrhea/pain/distension/flatulence, nausea/vomiting, pain—joint/muscle, shortness of breath.

Endocrine System: (Pregnancy Category C) increases serum phosphorus/chloride, decreases serum sodium/potassium.

Immune System: arthritis, dermatitis, increased liver enzymes, urticaria.

Dosage: PO 15–30 g/d bid or qid ac and hs. Digitalis toxicity: PO 10 g followed by 5 g q6–8h as needed.

<u>Dextrothyroxine sodium [Choloxin]</u> increases cholesterol breakdown via increased catabolism and excretion of cholesterol by the liver. Most of its side effects are due to the increase in metabolism.

Drug Interactions: Decreased absorption with cholestyramine, colestipol. Increased blood glucose possible, requiring insulin or sulfonylurea adjustment. Increased risk of hypoprothrombinemia with warfarin. Increased myocardial stimulation with digoxin possible. Increased thyroid effects with other thyroid drugs.

Side Effects

Nervous System: angina, arrhythmias, bowel—constipation/diarrhea, dizziness, ECG—ischemic myocar-

dial changes, heart—size increase, insomnia, nausea, palpitations, paresthesias, psyche—changes/nervousness, taste—bitter, tinnitus, vision—disturbances/lid lag/retinopathy. Iodism: brassy taste.

Endocrine System: (Pregnancy Category C) exophthalmos, iodism metabolism increase, weight loss.

Immune System: hoarseness, MI,* peripheral vascular disease—worsened. Iodism: acneiform rash, bronchitis, conjunctivitis, coryza, laryngitis, pruritus, stomatitis.

Dosage: PO. Start 1–2 mg qd for 1 mo. Then increase monthly until therapeutic level is reached. Maximum: 8 mg/d.

<u>Gemfibrozil [Lopid]</u> decreases liver production of triglycerides, decreases VLDLs, and increases HDLs.

Drug Interactions: Increase in hypoprothrombinemic effects of oral anticoagulants. Increased risk of myopathy and rhabdomyolysis with lovastatin.

Side Effects

Nervous System: bowel—diarrhea/flatulence, arthralgia, cramps, dizziness, headache, myalgia, nausea/vomiting, pain—abdominal/back/epigastric/extremities, vision—blurred.

Endocrine System: (Pregnancy Category B) hyperglycemia—moderate, hypokalemia.

Immune System: dermatitis, eosinophilia, Hct/Hb—mild decreases, joint swelling, rash, pruritus, urticaria.

Dosage: PO 600–1500 mg/d, 30 min ac breakfast and dinner.

<u>Lovastatin [Mevacor, Mevinolin]</u> is derived from the fungus *Aspergillus terreus.* Lovastatin blocks the liver's production of a coenzyme necessary for its creation of cholesterol. It crosses the BBB and the placenta.

Drug Interactions: Increased risk of myopathy and rhabdomyolysis with cyclosporine, erythromycin, gemfibrozil.

Side Effects

Nervous System: abdominal cramps/pain, bowel—constipation/diarrhea/flatus, dizziness, fatigue, GI upset, headache, insomnia, nausea, vertigo, visual disturbances

Endocrine System (Pregnancy Category X) increased serum transaminase and creatine phosphokinase.

Immune System: pruritus, rash.

Dosage: To start PO 20 mg at dinner; then 20–40 mg daily with a meal.

---

* Life-threatening side effect.

<u>Niacin Vitamin B_3 (Nicotinic acid) [Niac, Nicobid, others]</u> decreases production and increases breakdown of triglycerides, cholesterol, LDL, and VLDL. Creates energy from proteins, carbohydrates, and fats and prevents pellagra.

Drug Interactions: May increase hypotensive effects of antihypertensives.

Side Effects

Nervous System: arrhythmias, bloating/flatulence/GI disorders, headache, hypotension—postural, nausea/vomiting, syncope, vasovagal attacks. With chronic use: psyche—nervousness/panic, vision—amblyopia/blurred/central vision loss/proptosis.

Endocrine System: (Pregnancy Category A, C) dry mouth, flushing—general with sensation of warmth, glycosuria, hyperglycemia, hyperuricemia, hypoalbuminemia, sebaceous gland activity increase, dry skin.

Immune System: hepatic function test abnormalities, keratitis nigricans, peptic ulcer activation, pruritus, rash.

Dosage: Hyperlipidemia: PO 1.5–6 g/d with meals or pc. RDA: 20 mg qd.

<u>Simvastatin [Zocor]</u> is derived from *Aspergillus terreus*. More potent than lovastatin, simvastatin inhibits HMG-CoA to increase HDL cholesterol and decrease LDL cholesterol and total cholesterol synthesis. It may be used alone or with bile acid sequestrants.

Drug Interactions: May increase PT with warfarin.

Side Effects

Nervous System: angina, asthenia, bowel—constipation/diarrhea/flatulence, dizziness, dyspepsia, fatigue, headache, insomnia, loss of balance, nausea/vomiting, nerve damage, pain/cramps—stomach, psyche—anxiety/depression/memory loss, altered taste, tingling, tremor, vision—blurred/eye muscle weakness.

Endocrine System: (Pregnancy Category X) anorexia, fatty changes in the liver.

Immune System: allergic reactions, hepatitis, liver cancer,* pancreatitis, pruritus, rash.

Dosage: PO 5–40 mg qd.

▶ GALLSTONES

The liver produces bile salts and cholesterol and stores them in the gallbladder in solution to be secreted into the small intestine to emulsify dietary fat. Gallstones are calcified biliary cholesterol in the gallbladder. A diet high in cholesterol may, over time, result in gallstones due to

cholesterol precipitation, or low-grade, chronic infections of the gallbladder may also cause stone formation. Gallstones can obstruct the cystic duct that leads from the gallbladder to the common bile duct. Gallstones may also form in the liver and may obstruct the common bile duct. Pancreatitis may occur when stones block the papilla of Vater, obstructing the passage of pancreatic enzymes into the intestine. Pancreatitis can result in the autodigestion of the pancreas by its proteolytic enzymes.

<u>Chenodiol (chenodeoxycholic acid) [Chenix]</u> is used to treat cholesterol (but not bile pigment) gallstones by suppressing hepatic production of cholesterol and cholic acid and decreasing biliary cholesterol secretion. The latter aids dissolution of uncalcified stones.

Drug Interactions: Increased biliary cholesterol secretion with estrogens. Oral contraceptives may counteract chenodiol effects. Decreased absorption of chenodiol with aluminum-containing antacids, anion exchange resins, cholestyramine, colestipol.

Side Effects

Nervous System: bowel—abdominal cramps/diarrhea/decreased fluid absorption in the colon/increased fluid secretion, dyspepsia, flatulence, nausea/vomiting.

Endocrine System: (Pregnancy Category X) serum total cholesterol/LDL—elevated, triglycerides—slight reduction.

Immune System: hepatitis,* ALT/AST—elevated.

Dosage: PO 250 mg bid for 2 wk; then 250 mg/wk to maximum of 13–16 mg/kg/d bid for up to 2 y.

▶ EMOLLIENTS: OIL AND THE SKIN

When weather, aging, bathing, or disease decreases the skin's natural oils, emollients are used in the form of creams, lotions, ointments, oils, and bath oils. They are applied topically during or after a bath, daily or more often. They should not be used on moist or seeping lesions.

▶ VITAMIN A, RETINOIDS, ACNE
 VULGARIS, AND PSORIASIS

The oil-soluble vitamin A is stored in and released from the liver as part of a retinol-binding protein that eventually binds to prealbumin. Epithelial cells require vitamin A. Without it those cells become keratinized; mucous linings fill with the tough, fibrous keratin, lose their water content, and become hard and dry. In the eye keratinization can result in blindness. Retinoids are forms of

---

* Life-threatening side effect.

vitamin A (retinol) which stimulate mitotic activity and increase follicular epithelial cell turnover, resulting in extrusion of the comedones, the basic lesions of acne.

Sebum, the oily secretion of the sebaceous glands in the skin, combines with sweat to form a mildly antibacterial and antifungal film that protects the skin against drying and infection. However, sometimes the bacterial breakdown of sebum into fatty acids irritates the subcutaneous tissue causing acne vulgaris, which can result in inflammation and scarring which can lead to emotional distress. Treatment consists of antibiotics (see Chapter 16) and the retinoids. The retinoids are also used to treat psoriasis and some forms of cancer.

Acitretin [Soriatane] is used to treat severe psoriasis in patients unresponsive to other therapies or whose clinical condition contradicts the use of other treatments.

Drug Interactions: May form the retinoid, etretinate, with concurrent ingestion of acitretin and ethanol. Increased risk of hepatotoxicity with etretinate and methotrexate.

Side Effects

Nervous System: arthralgia, hyperesthesia, paresthesia, rigors.

Endocrine System: (Pregnancy Category X) dry eyes, mouth, skin.

Immune System: alopecia, epistaxis, infection of nail margin, progression of existing lesions, rash, rhinitis, skin atrophy.

Dosage: PO. Start at 25 or 50 mg qd with main meal; maintain at 25–50 mg qd after initial response to treatment. Terminate when lesions have resolved sufficiently.

Isotretinoin [Accutane] is used to decrease sebum secretion in cystic acne.

Off Label: Lamellar ichthyosis, oral leukoplakia, hyperkeratosis, acne rosacea, scarring gram-negative folliculitis; adjuvant therapy for basal cell carcinoma of lung and cutaneous T-cell lymphoma, mycosis fungoides, psoriasis, chemoprevention for prostate cancer.

Caution: Not for use during pregnancy. Its side effects are dose related and reversible when the drug is discontinued.

Drug Interactions: Increased toxicity with vitamin A supplements.

Side Effects

Nervous System: arthralgia, dizziness, drowsiness, fatigue, headache, GI complaints, lethargy, nausea/vomiting, pain—abdominal/bone/chest/joint/muscle, paresthesias, vision—disturbances/dryness/night/papilledema/reduction.

Endocrine System: (Pregnancy Category X) anorexia, dry mouth/nose, hyperostosis, hyperuricemia, elevated triglycerides/VLDL/cholesterol/LDL.

Immune System: ALT/AST—increased, brittle nails, bruising, skin—cheilitis/erythema/granulation/infections/peeling/petechiae/photosensitivity/urticaria.

Dosage: PO 0.5–1 mg/kg/d divided bid for 4–5 mo. A second course is sometimes needed. Keratinization disorders: PO up to 4 mg/kg/d in divided doses.

Tazarotene gel [Tazorac] is a topical retinoid for the treatment stable-plaque psoriasis and mild to moderate acne vulgaris.

Drug Interactions: Increased photosensitivity with other drugs that cause photosensitivity.

Side Effects

Nervous System: none noted.

Endocrine System: (Pregnancy Category X) none noted.

Immune System: photosensitivity.

Dosage: Topical. Apply hs to clean, dry skin.

Tretinoin [Retin-A], a topical preparation containing retinoid acid and vitamin A acid, stimulates mitosis of follicular epithelial cells and causes the keratinocytes in the sebaceous follicle to be less adherent. It makes the follicular epithelium more fragile. Tretinoin is used for acne vulgaris and flat warts.

Off Label: Treatment of other skin conditions such as ichthyosis vulgaris, keratosis palmaris and plantaris, psoriasis, senile keratosis, basal cell carcinoma.

Drug Interactions: Potential increased inflammation with topical acne medication. Possible stinging with alcohol or menthol.

Side Effects

Nervous System: none noted.

Endocrine System: (Pregnancy Category B) none noted.

Immune System: all skin reactions: blistering, crusting, erythema, hyper-/hypopigmentation, peeling, redness, scaling, stinging.

Dosage: Acne: Topical: apply at hs. Acute promyelocytic leukemia: PO 45 mg/m²/d.

Vitamin A [Aquasol A, Del-Vi-A] is a fat-soluble vitamin essential to bones, teeth, epithelial and mucosal surfaces, and rhodopsin synthesis. It stimulates healing in topical form for cortisone-retarded wounds.

Drug Interactions: Decreased absorption with cholestyramine, mineral oil.

Side Effects

Nervous System: abdominal discomfort, headache, bulging fontanelles, intracranial hypertension, increased intracranial pressure, lethargy/malaise, vision—miosis/nystagmus, vomiting.

Endocrine System: (Pregnancy Category A; X if over RDA) anorexia, exophthalmos, growth—slowed, hypercalcemia, hypomenorrhea, polydipsia, polyuria, skin—dry/cracked/pigmented, subperiosteal thickening—radius/tibia/occiput, sweating.

Immune System: alopecia, anemia—hypoplastic, gingivitis, hepatosplenomegaly, jaundice, leukopenia, lip fissures, pruritus. Plasma levels over 1200 IU/dL: increased sedimentation rate and PT. IV: anaphylaxis,* death*.

Dosage: Severe deficiency: PO 500,00 IU/d for 3 d followed by 50,000 IU/d for 2 wk, then 10,000–20,000 IU/d for 2 mo. IM 100,000 IU/d for 3 d, then 50,000 IU/d for 2 wk. RDA: 10,000 IU.

Vitamin E [Aquasol E, Vita-Plus E, Vitec] is a group of fat-soluble molecules, called tocopherols, that prevent peroxidation, a cause of free radicals that result in cell damage. These tocopherols are essential to the digestion and metabolism of polyunsaturated fats. They decrease platelet aggregation and enhance vitamin A utilization, normal growth, and muscle health.

Off Label: muscular dystrophy and other conditions, though without empirical evidence.

Side Effects

Nervous System: bowel—cramps/diarrhea, fatigue, headache, muscle weakness, nausea, vision—blurred.

---

* Life-threatening side effect.

Endocrine System: (Pregnancy Category A) creatinuria, gonadal dysfunction, serum thyroxine/triiodothyronine—decreased, serum creatine kinase/cholesterol/triglycerides—increased, urinary androgens/estrogens—increased.

Immune System: sterile abscess, contact dermatitis, thrombophlebitis.

Dosage: Vitamin E deficiency: PO/IM 60–75 IU/d. Vitamin E deficiency prophylaxis: PO 12–15 IU/d.

Chapter Highlights

- Lipids play a major role in providing the calories that fuel the cell.

- Lipids form the hydrophobic cell membranes and protect the skin.

- Cholesterol is essential to steroid hormone and prostaglandin production and the digestion of dietary fats.

- In the immune system cholesterol plays a role in creating and breaking down clots.

- Cholesterol is a culprit in atherosclerosis, resulting in CAD and hypertension.

- Drugs to keep cholesterol blood levels below 200 mg/dL are used when diet is ineffective.

- Lipids play an important role in maintaining the integrity of the skin through sebum production.

- The oil-soluble vitamin A (retinol) is also essential to healthy cell development.

- Retinoids are used to treat a range of skin disorders, including acne, psoriasis, and basal cell carcinoma, as well as some other forms of cancer.

- Oil-soluble vitamin E helps to prevent the production of the free radicals, which cause cell damage.

9

Drugs to Treat Disorders
of the Islets of Langerhans

- acarbose [Precose]
- acetohexamide [Dymelor]
- bromocriptine mesylate [Parlodel]
- chlorpropamide [Diabinese]
- diazoxide [Hyperstat I.V., Proglycem]
- extended insulin zinc suspension [Humulin U]
- glipizide [Glucotrol, Glucotrol XL]
- glucagon
- glyburide [DiaBeta, Micronase]
- insulin injection [Humulin R, Novolin R, Regular Insulin, Pork Regular Iletin II, Regular Purified Pork Insulin, Velosulin, Velosulin BR, Velosulin Human]
- insulin lispro [Humalog]
- insulin zinc suspension [Humulin L, Lente Purified Pork Insulin, Lente Iletin I, Lente Iletin II, Novolin L]
- insulin zinc suspension, Prompt [Semilente, Semilente Purified Pork Insulin]
- isophane insulin suspension [NPH Iletin I, NPH, Insulatard NPH, Iletin II, Humulin N, Humulin 70/30, Novolin N, Novolin 70/30]
- metformin [Glucophage]
- prompt insulin [Semilente, Semilente Iletin I, Semitard]
- protamine zinc insulin (PZI) [Protamine + zinc + Iletin II]
- purified preparation of extended insulin zinc suspension [Humulin U, Ultralente]
- purified PZI [Protamine + zinc + Iletin II]
- repaglinide [Pradin]
- somatotropin or growth hormone [Bio-Tropin, Nutropin, others]
- tolazamide [Tolinaze]
- tolbutamide [Orinase]
- tolbutamide sodium [Orinase Diagnostic]
- troglitazone [Rezulin]

The pancreas contains little clusters, or triads, of specialized cells referred to as the islets of Langerhans. These islets, little islands, or islands consist of alpha cells, which make glucagon to turn glycogen back into glucose; beta cells, which produce insulin; and delta cells, creators of somatostatin, which suppresses secretions of the alpha and beta cells and slows digestion. At the junctures of the triads of these varied cells, a blood glucose sensor monitors blood sugar levels in much the way the hypothalamus monitors hormonal blood levels. Working together the alpha, beta, and delta cells of the pancreas maintain the blood

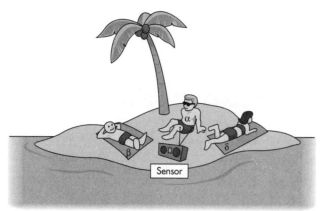

Beta, alpha, delta cells, and an Islet of Langerhans. A blood glucose sensor is found where these three types of cells form a junction. Beta cells make insulin. Alpha cells make glucagon. Delta cells make somatostatin.

Figure 9–1. An Islet of Langerhans.

sugar levels necessary to fuel the body's activities (Fig. 9–1).

All cells with a nucleus need fuel to carry out their genetically programmed activities. In fact, energy holds together the very structures that compose a cell. Adenosine triphosphate, formed from the food we eat, energizes cell functions. Carbon dioxide and water are the end products of the breakdown of fuel for energy.

Though cells of the heart and renal cortex may prefer fat to sugar, most cells thrive on glucose, and neurons prefer glucose. During prolonged starvation the brain can adapt to other fuel, but, normally, it must have sugar, in the form of glucose, or it will die. Brain cells, almost without exception, use sugar directly from the bloodstream and do not require insulin for transport through the cell membrane. Sugar is vital in maintaining adequate blood sugar levels in the diabetic to prevent brain damage or death when sugar intake is not adequate to the amount of insulin administered.

▶ INSULIN

Unlike brain cells, other cells cannot utilize the glucose that flows past in the bloodstream without a shuttle to help glucose pass through the cell membranes. Insulin, the name comes from the Latin word *insula* meaning island, acting at the membrane receptors of cells, triggers sugar shuttles, or transporter molecules inside the cells that require insulin to allow glucose to pass through the lipid cell membrane. Simultaneously, insulin causes the cell membrane to become more permeable to potassium, phosphate ions, and many amino acids.

THE FAT AND PROTEIN SPARER

Because insulin helps cells to use glucose rather than fat or protein, it is said to "spare" fat and protein. After a high-carbohydrate meal, glucose enters the blood, triggering insulin release from the pancreas. Insulin helps almost all cells to store and use glucose. Even fat cells need insulin to get needed glucose so that they can do their job of storing fat. In the liver insulin turns glucose into glycogen for liver storage. Glycogen storage halts without insulin, and an absence of insulin triggers an enzyme that splits up glycogen. Insulin promotes fatty acid production and fat stroage.

Insulin also helps resting muscle cells store glycogen. Muscle glycogen is stored power, useful later for short bursts of extreme energy in which the glycogen breaks down into lactic acid, even in the absence of oxygen. In addition, during heavy exercise contracting muscle cells become permeable to glucose and do not need insulin as a shuttle. Thus, the individual may need more glucose before exercise, and, more importantly, the diabetic may need less insulin if he or she exercises regularly.

Naturally occurring, or endogenous, insulin is removed from the blood and broken down rapidly after a meal—in about 10 minutes. This short duration of action is different from that of the injectable insulin that replaces the missing hormone in the treatment of diabetes. Insulin that replaces what is missing in diabetes is altered with crystals to extend its action for varying lengths of time and peak actions. The diabetic must have circulating glucose for the insulin to work on at those critical moments.

GLUCAGON: THE HYPERGLYCEMIC HORMONE

When the blood glucose drops to fasting levels, insulin production ceases and the sensors in the islets of Langerhans trigger the release of glucagon from alpha cells. Called the hyperglycemic factor or hormone because its job is to increase glucose in the blood stream, glucagon turns the stored liver glycogen back into glucose in an eight-step process. First glucagon activates adenyl cyclase in the hepatic cell membrane. This enzyme (1) causes the formation of cyclic adenosine monophosphate; which (2) activates protein kinase regulator protein; which (3) activates protein kinase; which (4) activates protein β kinase; which (5) converts phosphorylase β into phosphorylase α; which (6) promotes the degradation glycogen into glucose-1-phosphate; which (7) is dephosphorylated; (8) finally, glucose is released from the liver cells. Even after liver glycogen has been depleted, if more glucose is needed, glucagon continues its hyperglycemic function by increasing uptake of amino acids in the liver and converting them to glucose.

Glucagon [no trade names] may be given to counteract hyperinsulism. It is used to counter insulin shock when the unconscious diabetic cannot take sugar by mouth.

Side Effects

Nervous System: nausea/vomiting.

Endocrine System: (Pregnancy Category B) hyperglycemia, hypokalemia.

Immune System: hypersensitivity reactions, Stevens–Johnson syndrome.*

Dosage: Hypoglycemia: IM, IV, SC 0.5–1 U. May repeat q5–20min if no response for 1–2 more doses. Insulin shock therapy: IM, IV, SC 0.5–1 U usually 1 h after coma begins. If no response, may repeat in 25 min. Diagnostic aid to relax stomach or upper GI tract: IM, IV, SC 0.25–2 U 10 min before the procedure. Diagnostic aid for colon examination: IM, IV, SC 2 U 10 min before the procedure.

SOMATOSTATIN

Somatostatin, from the delta cells of pancreas, inhibits the secretions of the alpha and beta cells in the islets of Langerhans. Somatostatin also decreases the motility of the stomach, duodenum, and gallbladder and decreases the secretions and absorptions in the GI tract. The inhibitory actions of somatostatin may make nutrients available for a longer period of time (Guyton, 1996). Somatostatin is the same hormone that the hypothalamus secretes under the name growth hormone inhibitory hormone and that the upper gastrointestinal tract secretes. Somatostatin controls the levels of insulin and glucagon to maintain normal blood sugar levels. The hypothalamus and pituitary also produce somatotropin or growth hormone, which increases glucose levels.

BLOOD SUGAR LEVELS

Working together, alpha, beta, and delta cells and sensors normally maintain a blood glucose of 70–120 mg/dL. Some experts think that a healthy range is 60–100 mg/dL. A glucose tolerance test can reveal possible diabetes. In the test, a fasting blood sample is taken after the patient has ingested a 75-g glucose solution. A second blood sample is drawn in 2 hours and reveals the ability of pancreatic beta cells to produce the insulin necessary to utilize the 75 g of glucose. Impaired glucose tolerance is suspected if the result is between 140 and 200 mg/dL, and the individual is considered at risk for diabetes. Diabetes is diagnosed at 200 mg/dL and higher. On the other

hand, hypoglycemia is indicated by a glucose level of 20–50 mg/100 mL. A blood glucose level so low can cause irritability, fainting, convulsions, coma, and even death. Another method for diagnosing diabetes is the fasting blood sugar (FBS).

DIABETES AND INSULIN

As early as 1889 researchers understood that the pancreas was involved in diabetes mellitus. The name referred to the sweetness of the urine. One way to test for the amount of sugar in the urine was to taste it, and that was a task for nurses. Before the Canadians Banting and Best discovered insulin in the 1920s, diabetes mellitus, the failure of the pancreas to produce insulin, was usually fatal. The patient would experience intense hunger, thirst, copious voiding, body wasting (cachexia), and exhaustion and would die with blood full of sugar that the cells could not absorb through their membranes.

EDUCATION AND THE DIABETIC

Even with the advances in the treatment of diabetes, the disease is still a serious one, requiring thorough education and participation of the patient and the family. In essence, the patient must become his own pancreas, monitoring his blood sugar levels, a more immediate and accurate assessment than measuring the sugar in the urine, which is always a late indicator. Even with the best of care and compliance, the patient still runs great risks of generalized atherosclerosis and damage to retina and kidneys. Diabetes can lead to a host of resultant diseases including blindness, hypertension, stroke, myocardial infarction, nephropathy, impaired circulation, and gangrene. The patient is also more at risk to infections due to the impaired circulation (and possibly the increased blood glucose levels, though more likely the cause is some impairment of the immune system) (see box on page 132).

TYPE I DIABETES

Diabetes has different causes and forms. Type I diabetes, or "childhood-onset diabetes," may actually be an autoimmune disease to which its victims are genetically more vulnerable. According to this theory, damaged beta cells release factors normally never seen by the immune system because the normal beta cells keep them within the cell. The beta cells are tagged as foreign, and the immune system continues to destroy beta cells. Another possible cause of diabetes may be that growth hormone, which increases blood glucose levels, may simply burn out the beta cells. Yet another theory posits that viruses destroy beta cells. Whatever the cause, heredity is a factor either by causing beta cell degeneration or

---

* Life-threatening side effect.

What the Diabetic Needs to Know

1. Don't keep your condition a secret. Advise your friends and associates. Teach them the signs of hypoglycemia and hyperglycemia. Wear a Medic-Alert bracelet.
2. Insulin administration:
   a. Give insulin at room temperature to decrease chance of reactions.
   b. Do not shake the bottle to mix the contents. Instead, rotate gently.
   c. Inject at a 90° angle, using a ⅝ in. needle.
   d. Rotate injection sites to avoid lipodystrophy, which destroys potential injection sites.
   e. Insulin may be stored at room temperature for up to 1 month.
   f. For those who need it, the visiting nurse can draw up to a week's worth of syringes of insulin to be stored in the patient's refrigerator. (Novo Nordisk Pharmaceuticals produces a prefilled delivery system of cartridges and syringes.)
3. Exercise: Less insulin is needed with regular exercise.
4. Illness: Insulin requirements change with illness.
5. Pregnancy: Get immediate prenatal care.
6. Meals: Always keep in mind the risk of hypoglycemia and keep to a regular feeding schedule.
7. Stress: Can effect insulin needs.
8. Get regular eye examinations. Immediately report any vision changes.

making beta cells vulnerable to viral destruction or auto-immune antibodies (Guyton, 1996). Diabetes seems to come on rapidly, but only because the disease is not apparent until about 80% of the cells are damaged or destroyed. Type I diabetes usually begins in youth and requires insulin replacement for insulin-dependent and ketosis-prone individuals.

TYPE II DIABETES

After studying groups of Southwestern Indians whose ancestors had to adapt to eating and putting on weight in the summer when adequate rainfall provided food, and fasting during the months of yearly drought, some experts described a "thrifty gene" theory for type II diabetes. Obesity causes type II diabetes. Possibly when the body attains a "set point" of a genetically programmed weight or fat storage, the pancreas shuts down or slows

down insulin production. The body lives off of its fat until the weight loss reaches a point at which insulin production begins again.

Since type II, the maturity-onset form, is caused by obesity, it is usually treated by diet. Type II diabetics may require insulin when diet is not enough. Young people can also develop the latter, in which case the name is maturity-onset diabetes in the young (MODY).

ROUTES OF INSULIN ADMINISTRATION

The different forms of insulin are given subcutaneously. Only regular insulin can ever be given intravenously and for special circumstances since it is the only form that can be safely regulated on a minute-to-minute basis. Regular insulin is given IV in dextrose for life-threatening hyperkalemia, because insulin helps to shuttle potassium into cells along with glucose to decrease serum potassium.

The infusion pump delivers insulin subcutaneously and provides the best blood glucose control. (Humulin BR, the buffered form of regular insulin, is used to prevent insulin crystals from clogging the infusion pump catheter.) Otherwise, insulin is given with an insulin syringe that has a fine-gauge, ⅝-in. needle attached. The needle is short so that at a 90° angle it will deposit the insulin into the subcutaneous tissue, making it easier for patients to administer their own insulin.

COORDINATING MEALS WITH INSULIN

Insulin is given 15–30 minutes ac with a regular diet. The nurse must be sure that the hospitalized patient receives food on time and is able to eat it. Failure to eat on time can result in an insulin reaction, that is, hypoglycemia. **Caution: Give Lilly's new Humalog within 15 minutes of mealtime.**

INSULIN NEEDS AND STRESS

The amount of insulin needed is never stable. It varies in response to food intake, climate (heat and cold), illness, pregnancy, stress, growth needs, medications, and exercise. Stress increases the levels of glucocorticoids (steroids), which trigger the conversion of stored glycogen in the liver into glucose.

STEROIDS, OTHER HORMONES, AND DIABETES

All of the steroids—testosterone, progesterone, estrogen, and corticoids—tilt the body to hyperglycemia. Birth control pills, because they utilize the steroids, estrogen, and/or progesterone, may increase insulin needs. Other hormones that tilt the body toward gluconeogenesis include ACTH, growth hormone, thyroid hormones, epinephrine, and, of course, glucagon.

PREGNANCY-INDUCED DIABETES

Pregnancy-induced diabetes may also require insulin when diet is not sufficient for control. Maintaining a normal blood sugar level in the mother and bringing the pregnancy to a safe end are special challenges. The pregnant woman with diabetes is more apt to have complications such as toxemia. Insulin needs decrease for 24–72 hours postpartum, then slowly rise again. Nursing mothers may need less insulin.

Short Acting Insulin

Insulin injection [Humulin R, Novolin R, Regular Insulin, Pork Regular Iletin II, Regular Purified Pork Insulin, Velosulin, Velosulin BR, Velosulin Human] is the workhorse, the most commonly given, and the most predictable in terms of control. Regular insulin can be combined with the other longer acting forms for more accurate control of blood sugar. It may be given in combination with intermediate-acting or long-acting insulin to control blood glucose levels. Regular insulin is also used IV to stimulate growth hormone or to cause intracellular shift of potassium in treatment of hyperkalemia. Onset: 1/2–1 h. Peak: 2–3 h. Duration: 5–7 h.

Insulin lispro [Humalog], also a human DNA–derived insulin, is more rapid in onset and of shorter duration.

Drug Interactions

Nervous System: Beta blockers can mask the cardiovascular signs of hypoglycemia. Drugs like guanethidine, fenfluramine, alcohol, and the MAOIs can tilt the body toward hypoglycemia.

Endocrine System: Sulfinpyrazone also decreases blood sugar.

Immune System: Tetracycline, chloramphenicol, the salicylates, and phenylbutazone increase insulin's half-life.

Side Effects

Nervous System: aphasia, ataxia, arrhythmias—tachycardia, coma,* loss of consciousness,* convulsions,* fatigue, headache, mouth/tongue—circumoral pallor/numbness, nausea, palpitations, paresthesias, psyche—apprehension/confusion/inability to concentrate/incoherence/delirium/slurred speech/mania/personality changes, tremors/tremulousness, vision—blurred/diplopia/mydriasis/nystagmus/staring, weakness. Overdose: aphasia, psyche—mania/personality changes.

Endocrine System: (Pregnancy Category B) hunger, hypothermia, insulin resistance, negative for glucosuria, skin—cold/clammy/sweating, Somogyi effect—post-hyper/hypoglycemia. Injection sites: lipoatrophy/lipohypertrophy.

---

* Life-threatening side effect.

Immune System: anaphylaxis*—rare, insulin resistance, lymphadenopathy, urticaria. Injection site: allergic reaction, lipoatrophy/hypertrophy.

Dosage: SC 5–10 U 15–30 min ac and hs; adjust dose relative to blood glucose levels. Ketoacidosis (diabetic coma): IV 2.4–7.2 U loading dose; follow with 2.4–7.2 U/h continuous infusion based on close blood sugar monitoring (see box below).

OTHER FORMS OF INSULIN

Many refinements have been made on the original regular insulin. Longer acting forms were created to give the individual a more normal lifestyle, and purer forms help to prevent the immune system responses of allergy and reaction. Through genetic engineering, the human gene for insulin was inserted into *E. coli* bacteria, which now produce human insulin [Humulin], a form less likely to trigger the immune system to attack than insulin proteins of another species.

Insulin zinc suspension, Prompt [Semilente Purified Pork Insulin] is a suspension of small, rapidly absorbed zinc–insulin crystals. Onset: 1/2–1 1/2 h. Peak: 4–6 h. Duration: 12–16 h.

Dosage: Based on the individual's needs. Start with SC 10–20 U qd or bid.

Regular insulin combined with intermediate-acting insulin [Humulin 70/30, Novolin 70/30] are trade names that indicate a combination of 70% Neutral Protamine Hagedorn (NPH), Human Insulin Isophane and 30% Regular Human Insulin, which gives the individual the benefit of the rapid onset of action of regular insulin and the maximum effect at 2–12 h of the isophane with its potential duration of 24 h.

Intermediate-acting Insulins

Isophane insulin suspension [NPH Iletin I, NPH, Insulatard NPH, Iletin II, Humulin N, Novolin N] is an intermediate-

Facts Unique to Regular Insulin

Only regular insulin is clear in solution. All other forms are cloudy. When mixing insulins, always draw up the regular insulin first (Fast First). Regular insulin is the only form compatible with all the other forms. Only regular insulin is used in emergency situations like ketoacidosis (diabetic coma), or when the patient must have surgery or is under unusual stress. **Caution:** Only regular insulin should ever be given IV.

acting insulin. Onset: 1–1½ h. Peak: 8–12 h. Duration: 18–24 h.

Dosage: Based on individual needs. Start with SC 7–26 U qd or bid.

Long-acting Insulins

Insulin zinc suspension (Lente) [Humulin L, Lente Purified Pork Insulin, Lente Iletin II, Novolin L] is composed of 30% short-acting [Semilente] and 70% long-acting [Ultralente] insulin. The small [Semilente] crystals give immediate coverage; the large [Ultralente] crystals are more slowly utilized. The result is round-the-clock coverage. Hypoglycemia may occur in the afternoon. Onset: 1–2 h. Peak: 8–12 h. Duration: 18–24 h.

Dosage: Based on individual needs. Start with SC 7–26 U qd or bid.

Protamine zinc [Insulin (PZI), Iletin II], a long-acting insulin meant to last up to and beyond 36 hours. This duration may be too much of a good thing, since such long action increases the risks of hypoglycemia, especially during sleep, when the individual can least help himself.

Caution: Whereas some authorities believe regular insulin is compatible with all other insulins, others state it cannot be combined with this group of long-acting products.
Onset: 4–8 h. Peak: 14–24 h. Duration: 36 or more h.

Dosage: Based on the individual's needs. Start with SC 7–26 U qd.

Caution: Protamine zinc insulin and NPH isophane are incompatible with each other and with the lente insulins.

Extended insulin zinc suspension [Humulin U], purified preparation [Ultralente] is a group that is seldom used alone, but may be combined with [Lente] or [Semilente]. Onset: 4–8 h. Peak: 10–30 h. Duration: 36 or more h.

Dosage: Based on individual's needs. Start with SC 7–26 U qd.

Note: All insulin is supplied as U 100 and drawn up in the corresponding U 100 syringe. However, the nurse must be aware that there is a concentrated form of insulin—Insulin Injection Concentrated 500 U/mL—formulated for people whose diabetes has become resistant to the lower concentrations (see box on giving insulin safely).

▶ THE SULFONYLUREAS

For type II diabetes the best treatment is diet and weight loss, and the usefulness of or necessity for this group of drugs is debatable. However, the sulfonylureas may be prescribed for symptomatic type II, non-insulin-dependent, non-ketosis-prone diabetes uncon-

Giving Insulin Safely

As a safety precaution double-check the dosage drawn up with another nurse, with both nurses comparing the order to the amount drawn up, the unit strength of the syringe, and the unit strength of the supplied bottle. In addition, remember to use the Five Rights of Drug Administration: Right patient, Right drug, Right dose, Right route, Right time.

trolled by diet in people who cannot or will not take insulin. The sulfonylureas suppress glucagon secretion and cause the pancreas to secrete insulin in response to glucose. Unlike insulin, this drug group does nothing to control the vascular complications of diabetes. In addition, the sulfonylureas have long half-lives and can cause prolonged hypoglycemia.

Hypoglycemia is a problem in the age group most apt to get type II diabetes, the elderly. In the elderly hypoglycemia is not always easy to recognize. The prolonged hypoglycemia may require days-long IV dextrose infusion to parallel the drugs' long half-life. Tolazamide and tolbutamide are short-lived and safer. Women must not use the sulfonylureas during pregnancy because of the danger of fetal hypoglycemia. The sulfonylureas interact with some other drugs to increase the risk of hypoglycemia. Here they are classified by Master System.

Drug Interactions

Nervous system: alcohol, fenfluramine guanethidine, MAOIs. Chlorpropamide and tolbutamide can cause a disulfiram-like response with alcohol.

Endocrine System: anabolic steroids, clofibrate, insulin.

Immune System: chloramphenicol, dicumarol, phenylbutazone, salicylates, sulfonamides.

Acetohexamide [Dymelor] stimulates pancreatic beta cells to secrete insulin over a duration of 8–12 h.

Drug Interactions: Possible disulfiram-like reaction with alcohol. Possible increase in hypoglycemic response with chloramphenicol, clofibrate, fenfluramine, guanethidine, MAOIs, oxytetracycline, phenylbutazone, probenecid, salicylates, sulfonamides, sulfinpyrazone, warfarin. Possible hyperglycemia with thiazide diuretics. Decreased effect of both acetohexamide and diazoxide in combination. Decreased effect possible with phenytoin. Beta blockers may mask signs of hypoglycemia.

Side Effects

Nervous System: diarrhea, dizziness, dyspepsia, epigastric fullness, headache, nausea/vomiting, pain/discomfort—stomach.

Endocrine System: (Pregnancy Category C) anorexia, hypoglycemia*—severe.

Immune System: aplastic anemia,* agranulocytosis,* erythema, photosensitivity, pruritus, rash, thrombocytopenia, urticaria.

Dosage: PO 250 mg ac breakfast. Maximum 1.5 g/d. Doses >1 g should be given ac breakfast and dinner.

Chlorpropamide [Diabinese] can have an antidiuretic effect and is sometimes used for diabetes insipidus. Duration: 24–72 h.

Drug Interactions: Possible disulfiram-like reaction with alcohol. Possible increase in hypoglycemic response with MAOIs, probenecid. Possible hyperglycemia with thiazide diuretics. Increased adverse effects for chlorpropamide and phenytoin, NSAIDs, oral anticoagulants possible. Beta blockers may mask signs of hypoglycemia.

Side Effects

Nervous System: alcohol intolerance, bladder—oliguria, bowel—constipation/diarrhea, cramps—muscle, diarrhea, drowsiness, nausea, paresthesias, weakness.

Endocrine System: (Pregnancy Category C) anorexia, antidiuretic effect (SIADH), cholestatic jaundice, flushing, hypoglycemia,* hyponatremia, water intoxication.

Immune System: agranulocytosis,* leukopenia, photosensitivity, pruritus, rash, thrombocytopenia.

Dosage: PO 100–750 mg/d. Antidiuretic: PO 100–250 mg/d to maximum of 500 mg/d.

Glipizide [Glucotrol, Glucotrol XL] is a second-generation sulfonylurea hypoglycemic agent. It stimulates beta cells and increases insulin receptor sensitivity. Duration: 12 h.

Drug Interactions: Possible disulfiram-like reaction with alcohol. Possible increase in hypoglycemic response with chloramphenicol, clofibrate, MAOIs, phenylbutazone, probenecid, salicylates, sulfonamides, warfarin. Possible hyperglycemia with thiazide diuretics. Cimetidine may increase glipizide levels and hypoglycemia. Beta blockers may mask signs of hypoglycemia.

Side Effects

Nervous System: ataxia, arrhythmias—tachycardia, bowel—constipation/diarrhea, coma,* convulsions,* drowsiness, dyspepsia, fatigue, headache, nausea, pain—stomach, psyche—anxiety/confusion, vision disturbances.

Endocrine System: (Pregnancy Category C) anorexia, cholestatic jaundice, hunger, hypoglycemia,* porphyria.

---

* Life-threatening side effect.

Immune System: eczema, erythema, pruritus, rash, urticaria.

Dosage: PO 2.5–40 mg/d. SR 5–10 mg qd.

Glyburide [DiaBeta, Micronase] is a second-generation sulfonylurea hypoglycemic agent with 200 times the potency of first-generation drugs. Duration: 16 h.

Drug Interactions: Possible disulfiram-like reaction with alcohol. Possible increase in hypoglycemic response with chloramphenicol, clofibrate, MAOIs, phenylbutazone, probenecid, salicylates, sulfonamides, warfarin. Possible hyperglycemia with thiazide diuretics. Cimetidine may increase glyburide levels and hypoglycemia. Beta blockers may mask signs of hypoglycemia.

Side Effects

Nervous System: epigastric fullness, heartburn, nausea.

Endocrine System: (Pregnancy Category B) hypoglycemia,* cholestatic jaundice.

Immune System: erythema, pruritus, rash, urticaria.

Dosage: PO 1.25–20 mg/d.

Metformin [Glucophage] is a biguanide, not a sulfonylurea, and appears to increase insulin-receptor binding and to potentiate insulin action.

Drug Interactions: Increased hypoglycemia possible with captopril. Reduced clearance with cimetidine. Severe hypoglycemia with oral hypoglycemic drugs and azole antifungal agents, ie, fluconazole, ketoconazole, itraconazole.

Side Effects:

Nervous System: bowel—bloating/diarrhea, dizziness, fatigue, headache, nausea/vomiting, pain—abdominal, psyche—agitation, taste—bitter/metallic.

Endocrine System: (Pregnancy Category B) lactic acidosis, possible malabsorption of amino acids/vitamin B_{12}/folic acid.

Immune System: allergy.

Dosage: Start with PO 500 mg qd to tid. May increase by 500 mg/d q1–3wk to maximum of 3 g/d.

Repaglinide [Prandin] is an oral blood glucose–lowering drug of the meglitinide class to treat type II diabetes mellitus. Repaglinide lowers blood glucose levels by stimulating the release of insulin from functional beta cells in the pancreas.

Drug Interactions: Beta blockers mask the signs of hypoglycemia.

Side Effects

Nervous System: arrhythmias, bowel—constipation/diarrhea, dyspepsia, headache, nausea/vomiting, pain—back/chest, paresthesia. With severe hypoglycemia: coma,* neurologic impairment, seizure,* death.*

Endocrine System: (Pregnancy Category C) hypoglycemia.*

Immune System: allergy, anaphylaxis,* bronchitis, rhinitis, sinusitis, tooth disorder, URI, UTI.

Dosage: New patients: PO 0.5 mg 15–30 ac. Patients who have been treated previously with blood glucose–lowering drugs and with a HbA$_1$ of ≤ 8%: Start with PO 1–2 mg 15–30 min ac. Range: 0.5–4 mg with meals to maximum of 16 mg/d.

Tolazamide [Tolinase] is a sulfonylurea with a potency 5 times that of tolbutamide. Duration: 10–18 h.

Drug Interactions: Possible disulfiram-like reaction with alcohol. Possible increase in hypoglycemic response with chloramphenicol, clofibrate, MAOIs, phenylbutazone, probenecid, salicylates, sulfonamides, warfarin. Possible hyperglycemia with thiazide diuretics. Increased levels with cimetidine possible. Beta blockers may mask signs of hypoglycemia.

Side Effects

Nervous System: nausea/vomiting, vertigo.

Endocrine System: (Pregnancy Category C) cholestatic jaundice, hypoglycemia.*

Immune System: agranulocytosis,* photosensitivity.

Dosage: PO 100 mg–1 g/d to bid ac.

Tolbutamide [Orinase], tolbutamide sodium [Orinase Diagnostic] are sulfonylureas that act on beta cells to stimulate insulin release. Duration 6–12 h.

Drug Interactions: Possible disulfiram-like reaction with alcohol. Possible increase in hypoglycemic response with phenylbutazone. Possible hyperglycemia with thiazide diuretics. Beta blockers may mask signs of hypoglycemia.

Side Effects

Nervous System: ataxia, arrhythmias—tachycardia, bowel—constipation/diarrhea, coma,* convulsions,* drowsiness, dyspepsia, fatigue, headache, nausea, paresthesias, psyche—anxiety/confusion, taste changes, tremulousness, vision disturbances.

Endocrine System: (Pregnancy Category C) anorexia, cholestatic jaundice, hypoglycemia without loss of consciousness or neurologic symptoms, hunger, porphyria—cutanea tarda/hepatic, sweating.

Immune System: agranulocytosis,* anemia—aplastic*/hemolytic, erythema, leukopenia, photosensitivity, rash, urticaria, thrombocytopenia.

Dosage: PO 250 mg–3 g/d in 1–2 divided doses.

Troglitazone [Rezulin] is active in the presence of insulin for type II diabetes only when hyperglycemia is inadequately controlled with insulin.

Drug Interactions

Nervous System: none reported.

Endocrine System: birth control pills may not prevent pregnancy; cholestyramine reduces absorption; insulin: possible hypoglycemia. Take with food.

Side Effects

Nervous System: bowel—diarrhea, headache, pain.

Endocrine System: (Pregnancy Category B) anovulatory premenopausal women may begin to ovulate, elevated serum lipids.

Immune System: allergies, ALT/AST—elevated, Hb/Hct—increased, hepotoxicity, infections.

Dosage: PO start with 200 mg/d. Maximum dose 600 mg/d.

Note: The FDA is reviewing incidence of liver failure.

▶ A NOVEL WAY TO DECREASE BLOOD SUGAR

The following drug acts to prevent sugars from the diet from being absorbed into the bloodstream.

Acarbose [Precose] is an α-glucosidase inhibitor that interferes with the absorption of sugars from the GI tract, thus lowering sugar intake to decrease blood sugar. Inhibition depends on the enzymes involved on a continuum from least to most inhibited: glucoamylase, sucrase, maltase, and isomaltase; lactase is not affected. It can be used alone or with a sulfonylurea in treating type II diabetes (NIDDM).

Off Label: Adjunct for treatment of type I diabetes (IDDM).

Drug Interactions: none noted.

Side Effects

Nervous System: bowel—borborygmi/distension/diarrhea/flatulence, dizziness, headache, sleepiness, vertigo, weakness.

Caution: CNS signs may be due to poor diabetic blood sugar control.

---

* Life-threatening side effect.

Endocrine System: (Pregnancy Category B) hypoglycemia, especially in conjunction with sulfonylureas and insulin.

Immune System: anemia, especially iron deficiency, erythema, exanthema, liver function tests—increased, urticaria.

Dosage: PO. Start with 25 mg tid with meals. May increase q4–8wk up to 50–100 mg tid with meals to maximum of 150 mg/d for ≤ 60 kg and 300 mg/d for > 60 kg.

▶ **HYPOGLYCEMIA**

The diabetic who experiences hypoglycemia does so because the insulin he or she has administered is circulating with no sugar to transport into cells. This amounts to an insulin overdose and poses an immediate emergency because brain cells, even though they take in glucose without assistance from insulin, have no blood sugar available and may die.

Symptoms of hypoglycemia may rapidly advance from nausea, rapid, shallow breathing, circumoral numbness, and tingling to diplopia, seizures, and psychosis. The antidote for insulin is glucose given immediately by mouth if the person is conscious or can be roused. Even a little sugar placed on the tongue or in the buccal pouch can be helpful. Orange juice followed by crackers is a common intervention. If the person is unconscious, glucagon, given IM, makes the liver turn stored glycogen into glucose for release into the bloodstream. The individual may have to be taken to the emergency room for intravenous glucose if the early measures are not available or are administered too late.

A DRUG TO ELEVATE GLUCOSE

The following drug is used orally in hypoglycemia due to hyperinsulinism after unsuccessful medical or surgical interventions.

<u>Diazoxide [Hyperstat I.V., Proglycem]</u> is a glucose-elevating drug similar in structure to thiazide diuretics, though it is not a diuretic. It inhibits insulin release. Serious side effects limit its use. It can precipitate CVA, angina, MI, diabetes, hyperglycemia, and hyperuricemia, and can cause sodium and, thus, water retention. It is also given to restore salt balance in adrenal insufficiency when hydrocortisone replacement is not enough, in salt-losing forms of congenital adrenal hyperplasia, or in severe orthostatic hypotension caused by autonomic neuropathy. Diazoxide lowers blood pressure by possible competition with calcium for receptors. A diuretic is commonly used with it to counter the sodium retention. Dietary sodium should be restricted, and the patient may need potassium supplement.

Drug Interactions: Increased hyperglycemia and antihypertensive effects with thiazide diuretics. Increased risk of hyperglycemia with phenytoin and increased phenytoin metabolism possible with loss of seizure control. Sulfonylureas antagonize effects.

Side Effects

Nervous System: abdominal discomfort, ataxia, arrhythmias—atrial/ventricular, bladder—nocturia, bowel—constipation/diarrhea/ileus, CHF, cramps—muscle, dizziness, drowsiness, EPS, headache, hearing—transient loss/tinnitus, hypertension—transient, hypotension—orthostatic, insomnia, malaise, nausea/vomiting, pain—back/chest, palpitations, paresthesias, psyche—agitation/anxiety/euphoria, sensation of burning/itching/warmth, shock,* taste—loss, vision—blurred/ diplopia/lacrimation/papilledema/ scotoma, weakness.

Endocrine System: (Pregnancy Category C) anorexia, azotemia, breast lump enlargement, edema, fever, flushing, galactorrhea, glycosuria, hirsutism, hyperglycemia, hyperuricemia, nephrotic syndrome—reversible, proteinuria, retention—sodium/water, sweating, urinary output—decrease. Labor inhibited.

Immune System: bone age advance (children), Hb/Hct/IgG—decrease, eosinophilia, hair loss, hematuria, hepatic impairment, herpes, immunoglobinemia—decrease, leukopenia, monilial dermatitis, neutropenia—transient, rash, vision—subconjunctival hemorrhage/transient cataracts.

Dosage: PO for hypoglycemia 3–8 mg/kg divided q8–12h. IV for severe hypertension IV 1–3 mg/kg up to 150 mg. Repeat q 5–15 intervals if necessary.

▶ **KETOACIDOSIS OR DIABETIC COMA**

Unlike the abrupt onset of an insulin reaction, ketoacidosis, caused by the lack of insulin to help transport sugar into cells, comes on gradually. The individual becomes drowsy, thirsty; the breath smells like acetone; vision dims; respirations deepen. There may be vomiting and abdominal pain. The skin feels dry and appears flushed, the pulse is rapid and weak, and the eyeballs are soft.

In diabetes the absence of insulin causes fat cells to break down stored triglycerides into fatty acids and glycerol. The liver captures what fat it can. The remaining fatty acids and glycerol circulate in the bloodstream. In the liver fatty acids burn faster and faster, releasing acetoacetic acid into the blood as ketone bodies (β-hydroxybutyric acid and acetone). These products tilt the body

---

* Life-threatening side effect.

into acidosis. To balance the acidic condition, respirations increase as the lungs blow off excess CO_2. In an extreme situation, acidosis results in coma or death, and one of the most frequent causes of death in diabetes is acidosis. In addition, when fat supplies are scarce, the body must turn to protein for fuel. In prolonged, poorly controlled diabetes, the body is unable to synthesize proteins. The result is weight loss, weakness, and illness. The therapeutic goal in managing diabetes is to keep tight control on the blood sugar. Doing so requires commitment from the patient and family and the care providers.

▶ SOMATOTROPIN (GROWTH HORMONE) AND SOMATOSTATIN

Growth hormone and the pancreas have an intimate relationship. The anterior pituitary secretes growth hormone in response to growth hormone–releasing hormone from the ventromedial nucleus in the hypothalamus. The ventromedial nucleus, sensitive to hypoglycemia, causes the sensation of hunger. Other names for growth hormone include somatotropic hormone (SH) and somatotropin. Growth hormone diverts glucose to its own purpose, the increased metabolic demands of growth and repair. Growth hormone may precipitate diabetes by overtaxing the pancreas. The hypothalamus secretes growth hormone on a minute-by-minute basis in response to nutrition and the stresses of exercise, excitement, and physical and emotional trauma. Catecholamines from the nervous system also increase growth hormone secretion.

Cells respond to growth hormone by increasing in size and/or increasing mitosis, which results in more cells. Growth hormone shuttles amino acids through the cell membrane. Ribosomes in the cell synthesize protein from the amino acids. Long bones lengthen in response to growth hormone until the epiphyses unite, after which long bones simply get thicker. However, other bones and cartilage can respond indirectly as growth hormone stimulates production of the protein somatomedin in the liver, and possibly in the kidneys and muscles. In turn, somatomedin makes bones and cartilage grow by spurring the deposit of chondroitin and collagen. The hypothalamus produces growth hormone throughout life, as evidenced by the enlarged noses, ears, and chins of the elderly.

In the course of protein synthesis, growth hormone increases the release of fatty acids stored in adipose cells. By tilting the body to the use of fat for energy, growth hormone spares protein for growth and repair. However, a fatty liver can result when too much fat is released.

ACROMEGALY

Acromegaly is a continued growth of other than long bones. This disease is caused by overproduction of growth hormone in middle age and manifests in the gradual, marked growth of facial bones, jaw, and extremities. It is treated by resection of the pituitary with X-rays or surgery. Bromocriptine may help reduce production of growth hormone.

<u>Bromocriptine mesylate [Parlodel]</u>, the same drug used to treat Parkinson's disease by increasing dopamine levels in the brain and to treat female infertility, amenorrhea, or galactorrhea, is also used for acromegaly.

Drug Interactions: Decreased tolerance to alcohol possible. Increased hypotensive effect with antihypertensive agents. Possible amenorrhea and galactorrhea with estrogen and progestins. Increased prolactin possible with phenothiazines, tricyclic antidepressants, methyldopa, and reserpine.

Side Effects

Nervous System: angina—exacerbation, arrhythmias—exacerbation, bladder—frequency/incontinence/retention, bowel—constipation/diarrhea, cramps—abdominal/legs/feet, fatigue, nausea/vomiting, paresthesia—fingers, psyche—anxiety/depression/mania/nervousness/nightmares, shock,* vision—blurred/diplopia

Endocrine System: (Pregnancy Category C) anorexia, precipitates diabetes (by taxing the pancreas), dry mouth.

Immune System: MI,* rashes, peptic ulcer/hemorrhage.

Dosage: Acromegaly: PO. Start with 1.25–2.5 mg qd for 3 d. Increase by 1.25–2.5 mg qd every 3–7 d until desired result is achieved. Maintenance: 30–60 mg qd in divided doses.

GROWTH HORMONE–INHIBITING HORMONE

Growth hormone is opposed by growth hormone–inhibiting hormone, or somatostatin, which is secreted by both the hypothalamus and the pancreas. Somatostatin also inhibits the release of insulin and glucagon. The greatest control over the secretion of growth hormone, however, remains growth hormone–releasing hormone from the hypothalamus.

---

* Life-threatening side effect.

DWARFISM

Lack of growth hormone in childhood results in dwarfism. The treatment consists of replacing the missing hormone. The source is recombinant DNA and the use of bacteria to manufacture the hormone. Treatment requires caution because growth hormone inhibits cell response to insulin. Ketogenesis and hyperglycemia may result. The greatest risk is the potential for diabetes and hypothyroidism.

Somatotropin or growth hormone [Bio-Tropin, Nutropin, others] is used only for children with inadequate secretion of growth hormone.

Drug Interactions: Accelerated epiphyseal closure possible with anabolic steroids, androgens, estrogens, thyroid hormone. Inhibited growth response possible with ACTH, corticosteroids.

Side Effects

Nervous System: myalgia. Injection site: pain.

Endocrine System: (Pregnancy Category D) cholesterol oversaturation of bile, hypercalcuria, hyperglycemia, ketosis.

Immune System: accelerated growth of brain tumor,* GH antibodies (a cause of treatment failure).

Dosage: IM/SC up to 0.06 mg/kg 3 ×/wk with 48 h between doses for 6 mo. If no response, double the dose and give for another 6 mo. Nutropin: For inadequate hormone secretion. SC 0.3 mg/kg q wk.

---

* Life-threatening side effect.

 Chapter Highlights

- Insulin, glucagon, and somatostatin perform a delicate balancing act to maintain blood glucose levels necessary for health.
- When the pancreas cannot produce sufficient levels of insulin, diabetes results.
- The diabetic must, in effect, become his or her own pancreas, conscious of monitoring blood sugar levels, eating the right foods, and providing adequate insulin coverage in health and illness.
- Type I diabetes mellitus results from a failure of the beta cells to produce adequate supplies of insulin and requires insulin replacement.
- Type II diabetes results from obesity and can often be controlled by weight loss.
- The oral hypoglycemic drugs used in the management of type II diabetes spur the beta cells to secrete insulin.
- Somatostatin from the delta cells of the pancreas inhibits production of insulin from the beta cells of the pancreas and glucagon from the alpha cells and slows down digestion to possibly extend the time that nutrients are absorbed into the blood stream.
- Somatotropin or growth hormone from the hypothalamus tilts the body to the production of proteins for cell building and can tilt the body toward hyperglycemia and ketosis.
- Working together these hormones from the alpha, beta, and delta cells of the pancreas provide the cells with energy.

10

Adrenocorticotropic Hormone and the Glucocorticoids

- beclomethasone dipropionate [Beclovent, Beconase Nasal Inhaler, Vancenase Nasal Inhaler, Vanceril]
- betamethasone [Celestone]
- betamethasone acetate + betamethasone sodium phosphate [Celestone Soluspan]
- betamethasone benzoate [Benisone, Uticort]
- betamethasone dipropionate [Alphatrex, Diprogen, others]
- betamethasone sodium phosphate (pH 8.5) [Betameth, Celestone Phosphate, Celestone S, Cel-U-Jec, Selestoject]
- betamethasone valerate [Betacort, Valisone, Valisone Scalp Lotion, Valnac]
- budesonide [Rhinocort]
- corticotropin (ACTH) [Acthar, Cortigel-40, Cortigel-80]
- corticotropin repository [ACTH Gel, Acthron, Cortigel, others]
- corticotropin zinc hydroxide [Cortrophin-Zinc]
- cortisone acetate [Cortone]
- dexamethasone [Aeroseb-Dex, Decaderm, Decadron, Decaspray, Dexameth, Dexamethasone Intensol, others]
- dexamethasone acetate [Dalalone D.P., Decadron-LA, Decaject-LA, others]
- dexamethasone sodium phosphate [Ak-Dex, Alba Dex, Dalalone, Decadrol, Decadron Phosphate, Decaject, Dex-4, Dexacen-4, Dexasone, Dexon, Dexone, Hexadrol Phosphate, Maxidex ophthalmic, Savacort-D, Solurex]
- flunisolide [Nasalide (25 µg per spray), AeroBid (250 µg per spray)]
- fluorometholone [Fluor-Op, FML Forte, FML Liquifil Ophthalmic]
- fluticasone [Flonase]
- glucocorticoids
- hydrocortisone [Aeroseb-HC, Alphaderm, Cetacort, Cortaid, Cort-Dome, Cortenema, Cortril, DermaCort, Dermolate, Hydrocortone, Hytone, Proctocort, Synacort]
- hydrocortisone (cortisol) [Cortef, Hydrocortone]
- hydrocortisone acetate [Anusol HC, CaldeCort, Carmol HC, Colifoam, Cortaid, Cortamed, Cort-Dome, Cortef Acetate, Corticaine, Cortifoam, Epifoam, Hydrocortone Acetate]
- hydrocortisone cypionate [Cortef Fluid]
- hydrocortisone sodium phosphate [Hydrocortone Phosphate]

- hydrocortisone sodium succinate [Cortef, Solu-Cortef]
- hydrocortisone sodium succinate [Solu-Cortef]
- hydrocortisone valerate [Westcort]
- methylprednisolone [Medrol]
- methylprednisolone acetate [Depoject, Depo-Medrol, Depopred, Duralone, M-Prednisol, Rep-Pred]
- methylprodnisolone sodium succinate [A-methaPred, Solu-Medrol]
- mometasone furoate [Elocon]
- prednisolone [Delta-Cortef, Inflamase Forte, Prelone]
- prednisolone acetate [Econopred, Key-Pred, Pred Forte, Predcor]
- prednisolone sodium phosphate [AK-Pred, Hydeltrason, Inflamase, Inflamase Mild, Pred Mild]
- prednisolone tebutate [Hydeltra-TBA, Prednisol TBA]
- prednisone [Deltasone, Meticorten, Orasone, Panasol, Prednicen-M, Sterapred]
- triamcinolone [Aristocort, Atolone, Kenacort, Kenalog E]
- triamcinolone acetonide [Azmacort, Cenocort A_2, Kenalog, Triam-A, Triamonide, Tri-kort, Trilog]
- triamcinolone diacetate [Amcort, Aristocort Forte, Articulose LA, others]
- triamcinolone hexacetonide [Aristospan]

Dealing with life's highs and lows requires energy. The endocrine system deals with the daily stresses of life in a cyclical nature with a daily production of steroid hormones called glucocorticoids, which ebbs and flows over 24 hours, reaching its peak in the morning. In communication with the nervous system and the immune system, the endocrine system can also respond to added stresses of illness, injury, pain, and emotional turmoil.

Using its negative feedback loop, the hypothalamus monitors glucocorticoid levels and increases them in response to such stresses as fever or pain. It sends down corticotropin-releasing hormone (CRH) to the pituitary, which secretes adrenocorticotropic hormone (ACTH) to the cortex or "bark" of the adrenal glands via the bloodstream. In response to ACTH, the adrenals can release up to 20 times their normal amount of cortisol, the most abundant glucocorticoid.

▶ THERAPEUTIC USES FOR ADRENOCORTICOTROPIC HORMONE

ACTH, or corticotropin, stimulates release not only of glucocorticoids, but also catecholamines and beta-endorphins. ACTH can disrupt the negative feedback axis between the adrenals and the hypothalamus, decrease stress response, unbalance electrolytes, and cause an androgen effect in women. The most direct way to increase glucocorticoid levels is simply to give the glucocorticoids themselves. However, ACTH is sometimes used in adrenocorticoid-responsive diseases, such as multiple sclerosis, to shorten the episodes by decreasing edema in the areas of demyelination. The decision to use either IV methylprednisolone or IM or IV ACTH is simply the choice of the clinician. ACTH is also used diagnostically to test adrenocortical function and as an adjunct to the treatment of adrenal insufficiency.

Corticotropin (ACTH) [Acthar, Cortigel-40, Cortigel-80], corticotropin repository [ACTH Gel, Acthron, Cortigel, others], corticotropin zinc hydroxide [Cortrophin-Zinc] is an animal extract (pork) used to stimulate functional adrenal cortex to secrete cortical steroids: corticosterone, cortisol (hydrocortisone), androgen, and aldosterone.

Drug Interactions: Increased potential for hypoprothrombinemia with NSAIDs due to enzyme induction. Decreased effects with barbiturates, phenytoin, rifampin. Increased binding and effects possible with estrogens. Increased potassium loss with amphotericin B.

Incompatibilities

Solution/Additives: aminophylline, sodium bicarbonate.

Side Effects

Nervous System: abdominal distension, convulsions,* headache, nausea/vomiting, psyche—depression/euphoria/insomnia/mood swings, vision—glaucoma.

Endocrine System: (Pregnancy Category C) amenorrhea, calcium/potassium loss, cushingoid state, latent diabetes—activation, hirsutism, hyperglycemia, muscle mass loss, negative nitrogen balance, fragile skin, sodium/water—retention, wound healing impairment.

Immune System: acne, cataract, ecchymosis, hypersensitivity, osteoporosis, papilledema, peptic ulcer—hemorrhage/perforation, petechiae, latent tuberculosis—activation, vertebral compression fracture.

Dosage: IM, SC 40–80 U/d. Dosage highly individualized. Repository: 40–80 U q24–72h. Zinc hydroxide: IM 40 U q12–24h. Acute multiple sclerosis: IM 80–120 U/d for 2–3 wk. Repository: 80–120 U/d for 2–3 wk. Diagnostic for adrenal insufficiency: IV 10–25 U in 500 mL 5% dextrose in water solution over 8 h.

▶ GLUCOCORTICOIDS AND SUGAR

Glucocorticoids are part of the steroid family of hormones that includes the sex hormones—testosterone, progesterone, and estrogen—and the mineralocorticoid aldosterone (Fig. 10–1). These steroids all take about 45 minutes to exert their influence on the DNA of target cells. All of them cause sodium retention and can cause edema.

The purpose of glucocorticoids is to increase available sugar for energy in response to stress. Insulin stores extra sugar in the liver as glycogen; glucagon converts it back to sugar as needed. Glucocorticoids supply additional sugar during stress to fuel the body by stimulating gluconeogenesis in the liver, taking amino acids from extracellular fluids to use for glucose production, and increasing the liver cell enzymes needed to convert the amino acids into glucose. Glucocorticoids also stabilize lysosomal membranes and suppress the rampages of the immune system when one is injured or under attack by foreign matter or one's own immune system.

When necessary, cortisol slowly mobilizes fatty acids from the adipose cells for additional energy, sparing glucose and glycogen. If even more energy is needed after stored fat has been depleted, the glucocorticoids can convert cell storage of protein into energy in all but the liver cells, decreasing protein production and increasing protein breakdown to support glucose production.

---

*Life-threatening side effect.

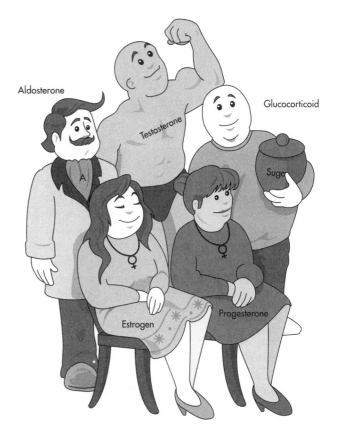

Clockwise from the top—testosterone, glucocorticoid (cortisone), progesterone, estrogen, and aldosterone. All can penetrate the cell membrane and make genetic changes in the nucleus. All take about 45 minutes to act.

Figure 10–1. The steroid family.

Protein catabolism interferes with wound healing. Glucocorticoids may help early wound healing by decreasing inflammation, but when used in long-term therapy, they disrupt protein synthesis and suppress fibroblast formation and the collagen deposits necessary for healing.

▶ THERAPEUTIC USES FOR GLUCOCORTICOIDS

The glucocorticoids are used in the treatment of Addison's disease (adrenal insufficiency), congenital adrenal hyperplasia, allergic rhinitis, asthma, rashes, repetitive use injury, rheumatoid arthritis, rheumatic fever, spinal cord injuries, acute glomerulonephritis, pericarditis, trauma, and as an adjunct to chemotherapy for cancer. Glucocorticoids help prevent transplanted organ rejection when given in conjunction with immunosuppressants. They may be used as an adjunct to treatment for some cancers because they have some "tumor-killing" ability. Glucocorticoids can prevent fat emboli in long bone fractures. Glucocorticoids also make the cardiovascular system receptors more responsive to catecholamines in circulation so that the heart and vessels can react more strongly to the stimulating neurotransmitters during stress. Like all steroids, the glucocorticoids also have a weak mineralocorticoid action and retain sodium ions, causing edema. Though they have been promoted as of some benefit in toxic shock, they have not yet proven to be of value, and therefore that use will not be covered in this text.

Because natural levels of glucocorticoids increase in the morning, the daily dose in replacement therapy is given in the morning too. Like ACTH, the glucocorticoids can disrupt the negative feedback system and must be withdrawn slowly by decreasing dosage over 7 days or more. Glucocorticoids can prevent full growth in children. Because they suppress the inflammation and fever of the immune response, these hormones mask infection, making their use of special concern in latent TB.

Cortisol is the most active of the glucocorticoids; only about 5% of glucocorticoid activity is carried on by the other glucocorticoids, corticosterone and cortisone. Cortisol has the ability to redistribute body fat, often causing a characteristic formation of fat deposit concentrations around the head and chest, accounting for the "moon face" and "buffalo chest" of patients on glucocorticoids. The adrenals produce up to 25 mg of cortisol and 4 mg of corticosterone each day. During stress the amount increases up to 10 times normal. Thus, a patient in crisis would need 10 times the normal daily production. In general, the systemic glucocorticoid preparations have the following side effects.

Side Effects

Nervous System: CHF, headache, insomnia, muscle, weakness, nausea/vomiting, psyche—confusion/euphoria/psychosis. Signs of adrenal insufficiency during the tapering period include depression, fatigue, hypotension, nausea/vomiting, pain—joint/muscle, vertigo, weakness.

Endocrine System: (Pregnancy Category C) carbohydrate intolerance, cushingoid syndrome, edema, hyperglycemia, hypokalemia, muscle wasting, sodium retention, wound healing delay. Children: growth suppression.

Immune System: bone—aseptic necrosis/osteoporosis/spontaneous fractures, cataracts, leukocytosis.

ROUTES OF GLUCOCORTICOID ADMINISTRATION

Glucocorticoids can be administered by injection, enema, topical, eye drops, and inhalation. Topically, they should be applied in a thin film. In using the inhaler, the patient must shake the inhaler; exhale completely; close lips tightly around the mouthpiece; activate inhaler while inhaling slowly; hold breath before exhaling slowly; and wait 1 minute before next inhalation. Because of the corticoid suppression of the immune system, use of the inhaler may cause a fungal infection in the oral cavity. Rinsing the mouth and gargling after inhaler use may prevent candidal infection.

NOTE: ABOUT OPHTHALMIC CORTICOIDS

Steroids for ophthalmic inflammation prevent scarring because they block fibrin and collagen deposits. However, they can raise intraocular pressure. Use only ophthalmic strength agents for the eyes, because hydrocortisone topicals for the body are too strong for use near the eyes—even the lids.[†]

ALLERGIC RHINITIS

Allergic rhinitis is the inflammation of the nasal mucosa caused by seasonal pollens, animal dander, dust mites, and molds. Glucocorticoids stabilize mast cell membranes. Nasal inhalers provide measured doses. The side effects are minimal.

ARTHRITIS

Glucocorticoids are used to treat the inflammation of rheumatoid arthritis (RA) and many other inflammatory conditions. Oral corticoids may be used in continuous low-dose therapy with short-term high dose bursts to control flares of RA (DiPiro, 1997). The IM route might be used for noncompliant patients for severe flareups. Intraarticular injections of the depot forms are used to treat synovitis and pain when small joints are involved.

ASTHMA

Once thought to be an innocuous, emotional response, asthma is an immune response that can be fatal. During an asthma attack the contents of lysosomes cause inflammation and trigger production of slow-reacting substance of anaphylaxis (SRSA). SRSA causes the bronchoconstriction that occurs during allergic reactions. The treatment for asthma includes drugs from the nervous system: adrenergics and xanthines to dilate the bronchi, anticholinergics to relax bronchial muscle, and cromolyn sodium or nedocromil sodium to stabilize mast cells. In the immune system drugs that inhibit leukotriens call off the immune response. Glucocorticoids in the endocrine system suppress the immune response. For the purposes of this chapter, only the use

---

[†]Eye related.

of corticoids of the endocrine system in treating asthma will be discussed.

In treating asthma, glucocorticoids decrease airway inflammation, mucosal edema, and mucus viscosity. Corticosteroids make the airway muscles more receptive to beta-2 adrenergics, increasing the affinity of epinephrine for its receptors. Given in conjunction with epinephrine or xanthines, their value is in preventing relapse. Glucocorticoids take effect in about 45 minutes and reach peak effectiveness within 4–8 hours. To prevent relapse, the patient must taper off the oral form of steroids over 10–12 days as he or she begins to use the inhaled form of steroids. Due to the slow onset of action (all steroids have a slow onset of action), steroids cannot stop an asthma attack in progress.

ORGAN TRANSPLANT

Glucocorticoids block transplant rejection by decreasing the numbers of antibodies and sensitized leukocytes at the organ site, hindering phagocytosis and stabilizing lysosome membranes inside cells so they won't rupture and release their toxic substances, (including the neurotransmitters histamine and bradykinin). Glucocorticoids are given in conjunction with other immunosuppressant drugs.

TRAUMA

Each year about 10,000 people, usually male, usually under 30 years of age, suffer from spinal cord injuries in diving accidents and car wrecks. As a result many wind up as paraplegics. In spinal cord injury, the immune system immediately causes local swelling. Increasing pressure decreases blood supply to the cord; the nerve cells begin to starve and die, resulting in a rift in the cord. What is often only a crushing or bruising, and not a severing, of the cord escalates and can result in paraplegia. Immediate, aggressive use of methylprednisolone may improve an otherwise bleak outlook for the patient.

▶ THE SYSTEMIC FORMS OF GLUCOCORTICOIDS

The systemic forms of glucocorticoids include the following: betamethasone, dexamethasone, hydrocortisone, methylprednisolone, prednisolone, prednisone, and triamcinolone.

Betamethasone [Celestone], betamethasone acetate and betamethasone sodium phosphate [Celestone Soluspan], betamethasone benzoate [Benisone, Uticort], betametha-

sone dipropionate [Alphatrex, Diprogen, others], betamethasone sodium phosphate (pH 8.5) [Betameth, Celestone Phosphate, Celestone S, Cel-U-Jec, Selestoject], betamethasone valerate [Betacort, Valisone, Valisone Scalp Lotion, Valnac] are synthetic, long-acting glucocorticoids that have weak mineralocorticoid activity and strong immunosuppressive, antiinflammatory, and metabolic actions. For side effects, see *hydrocortisone.*

Dosage: PO 0.6–7.2 mg/d. IM, IV 0.5–9 mg/d as sodium phosphate. Topical: Thin film to affected area 1–3 ×/d. Respiratory distress syndrome: IM 2 mL of sodium phosphate to mother qd 2–3 d before delivery.

Cortisone acetate [Cortone] is used for hormone replacement or inflammatory disorders.

Drug Interactions: Decreased effects with barbiturates, phenytoin, rifampin.

Side Effects

Nervous System: CHF, hypertension, muscle weakness, nausea, psyche—euphoria/insomnia, vertigo, vision—blurred/glaucoma/nystagmus.

Endocrine System: (Pregnancy Category D) edema, hyperglycemia, osteoporosis, wound healing impaired.

Immune System: acne, cataracts, compression fracture, ecchymosis, pancreatitis, peptic ulcer, petechiae, thrombocytopenia.

Dosage: Individualized dosage. PO, IM. Start with 20–300 mg/d, divided or not; then reduce 10–25 mg/d to lowest therapeutic dose. Topical: 0.25–2.5 mg in ointment form for skin allergy. It can mask infection and is not used for the lesions of infectious diseases.

Dexamethasone [Aeroseb-Dex, Decaderm, Decadron, Decaspray, Dexameth, Dexamethasone Intensol, and others], dexamethasone acetate [Dalalone D.P., Decadron-LA, Decaject-LA, and others], dexamethasone sodium phosphate [Ak-Dex, Alba Dex, Dalalone, Decadrol, Decadron Phosphate, Decaject, Dex-4, Dexacen-4, Dexasone, Dexon, Dexone, Hexadrol Phosphate, Maxidex ophthalmic, Savacort-D, Solurex] are forms of a long-acting synthetic glucocorticoid used to treat allergic conditions, collagen diseases, blood disorders, cerebral edema, and addisonian shock. Palliative use in cancer. For short-term use in rheumatic diseases. Diagnostic for Cushing's syndrome and differential diagnosis of adrenal hyperplasia and adrenal adenoma.

Off Label: Antiemetic in cancer chemotherapy; diagnostic for endogenous depression; to prevent hyaline membrane disease in premature infants.

Side Effects

Nervous System: CHF, convulsions,* dyspepsia, headache, hypertension, muscle weakness, nausea, psyche—euphoria/insomnia, vertigo.

Endocrine System: (Pregnancy Category C) appetite increase, atrophy—SC/cutaneous, cushingoid state, edema, hirsutism, hyperglycemia, ICP, menstrual irregularities, muscle mass loss, pigmentation—hypo/hyper, sweating, vision—exophtalmos/glaucoma/IOP, wound healing—impaired. Child: growth suppression.

Immune System: acne, allergy—dermatitis, bowel perforation,* candidiasis—oral, cataract—posterior subcapsular, ecchymoses, pancreatitis, pathologic fracture of long bones, peptic ulcer with possible perforation, petechiae, tendon rupture, vertebral compression fracture.* Aerosol: anosmia, asthma—bronchial, congestion—rebound, epistaxis, nasal septum—perforation, nares—dryness/irritation. IV: perineal area burning/tingling.

Dosage: Allergies, inflammation, neoplasias: PO 0.25–4 mg bid–qid. IM 8–16 mg q1–3wk or 0.8–1.6 mg intralesional q1–3wk. Cerebral edema: IV 10 mg; follow with 4 mg q4h; reduce dose after 2–4 d; taper over 5–7 d. Shock: IV 1–6 mg/kg as a single dose or 40 mg repeated q2–6h if necessary. Diagnosis of endogenous depression; dexamethasone suppression test: PO 0.5 mg q6h for 48 h. Inflammation: inhalation 1–3 inhalations tid or qid to a maximum of 12/d. Intranasal 2 sprays per nostril bid of tid up to 12/d. Ophthalmic: 1–2 gtt in conjunctival sac 4–6 × d.† Hourly for severe disease. Topical: thin film tid or qid.

Hydrocortisone [Aeroseb-HC, Alphaderm, Cetacort, Cortaid, Cort-Dome, Cortenema, Cortril, DermaCort, Dermolate, Hydrocortone, Hytone, Proctocort, Synacort], hydrocortisone acetate [Anusol HC, CaldeCort, Carmol HC, Colifoam, Cortaid, Cortamed, Cort-Dome, Cortef Acetate, Corticaine, Cortifoam, Epifoam, Hydrocortone Acetate], hydrocortisone cypionate [Cortef Fluid], hydrocortisone sodium phosphate [Hydrocortone Phosphate], hydrocortisone sodium succinate [Cortef, Solu-Cortef], hydrocortisone valerate [Westcort] constitute a group that has the typical corticoid side effects in addition to the following.

Side Effects

Nervous System: ataxia, arrhythmias—tachycardia, bladder—enuresis/frequency/urgency, bowel—cramping, flatulence, hypertension, malaise, palpitations, vision—blurred/decreased/nystagmus, syncope. IV: site pain, perineal burning/tingling.

Endocrine System: (Pregnancy Category C) amenorrhea, hunger, hyperglycemia, latent diabetes manifestations, moon facies, obesity, negative nitrogen balance, vision—exophthalmos/glaucoma/IOP, sweating, vitamins A, C—decreased serum concentrations.

Immune System: anaphylaxis,* angioedema,* esophagitis—ulcerative, infection*—aggravated/masked, melena, pancreatitis, peptic ulcer—perforation/hemorrhage, rash, thrombocytopenia, vision—corneal fungal infections. Intraarticular: Charcot-like arthropathy.

Dosage: PO 10–320 mg/d tid or qid. IM, IV 15–800 mg/d tid or qid to maximum of 2 g/d. Intraarticular, intralesional (acetate salt): IM 5–50 mg q3–5d for bursae and q1–4wk for joints. Topical: Apply 1–4 ×/d. Rectal: 1% cream, 10% foam, 10–25 mg suppository, or 100-mg enema hs.

Hydrocortisone (cortisol) [Cortef, Hydrocortone] is a cortisone analog.

Dosage: PO. Start with 10–320 mg/d tid or qid. IM 10–25 mg q12h.

Hydrocortisone Sodium Phosphate [Hydrocortone Phosphate] is a cortisone analog.

Dosage: IM, IV 15–240 mg/d q12h in divided doses.

Hydrocortisone Sodium Succinate [Solu-Cortef] is a cortisone analog.

Dosage: IM, IV. Start with 100–500 mg. Shock: 50 mg/kg stat; then q4h and/or q24h as needed; or start with IV 0.5–2 g and q2–6h as needed.

Methylprednisolone [Medrol], methylprednisolone acetate [Depoject, Depo-Medrol, Depopred, Duralone, M-Prednisol, Rep-Pred], methylprednisolone sodium succinate [A-methaPred, Solu-Medrol] are intermediate-acting corticoids with a half-life of 18–36 h and the typical uses of corticosteroids. Methylprednisolone may be used to prevent fat emboli in long-bone fractures. It is also palliative in neoplastic disease. The acetate form can be injected into lesions and joints to treat RA. Methylprednisolone has activity similar to hydrocortisone, but with less sodium and water retention.

Drug Interactions: Effectiveness decreased with isoniazid, phenobarbital, phenytoin, rifampin due to increased steroid metabolism. Increased potassium loss with amphotericin B, furosemide, thiazide diuretics. May enhance virus replication or increase vaccine side effects with attenuated virus vaccines.

---

*Life-threatening side effect.

† Eye related.

Incompatibilities

Solution/Additive: calcium gluconate, glycopyrrolate, metaraminol, nafcillin, penicillin G sodium, doxa-pram.

Side Effects

Nervous System: CHF, headache, edema, nausea/vomiting, muscle weakness, psyche—confusion/euphoria/insomnia/psychosis.

Endocrine System: (Pregnancy Category C) carbohydrate intolerance, cushingoid features, edema, hyperglycemia, hypokalemia, wound healing delay. Children: growth suppression.

Immune System: aseptic necrosis of bone, cataracts, spontaneous fractures, leukocytosis, muscle wasting, osteoporosis.

Dosage: PO 2–60 mg/d in 1 dose or divided doses. Acetate: IM 4–80 mg/wk for 1–4 wk. IV 1–250 mg q6h. Succinate: IV 10–250 mg q6h. Organ transplant: Precede first dose of muromonab-CD3 with IV 1 mg/kg methylprednisolone sodium succinate and follow first dose of muromonab-CD3 in 30 min with another 100 mg IV of the methylprednisolone to prevent the adverse effects of fever and respiratory distress. Acute spinal cord injury (must be given within 8 h of the injury): IV. Start with 30 mg/kg over 15 min; follow in 45 min with 5.4 mg/kg qh over the next 23 h.

Prednisolone [Delta-Cortef, Inflamase Forte, Prelone], prednisolone acetate [Econopred, Key-Pred, Pred Forte, Predcor], prednisolone sodium phosphate [AK-Pred, Hydeltrasol, Inflamase, Inflamase Mild, Pred Mild], prednisolone tebutate [Hydeltra-TBA, Prednisol TBA] have the common corticoid side effects. The tebutate, acetate, and phosphate forms are used for injection into lesions, joints, and the synovia of bursa or tendon sheaths.

Side Effects

Nervous System: prednisolone may cause hypotension*/shock reactions, vasomotor symptoms.

Endocrine System: heat sensitivity, altered sperm development.

Immune System: the topical form may cause perforation of the cornea.

Dosage: PO 5–60 mg/d in single or divided doses. Acetate/phosphate: IM 6–60 mg/d. Tebutate: 2–60 mg qwk. Phosphate: IV 4–60 mg/d. Ophthalmic 1–2 gtt in conjunctival sac qh during day; q2h at night; may decrease to 1 gtt tid or qid.†

---

*Life-threatening side effect.
† Eye related.

Prednisone [Deltasone, Meticorten, Orasone, Panasol, Prednicen-M, Sterapred] and prednisolone are two oral forms of glucocorticoids often used in autoimmune diseases and rheumatoid arthritis. The liver metabolizes prednisone into prednisolone. To spare a diseased liver the extra work, prednisolone is used.

Dosage: PO 5–60 mg q24h in single or divided doses.

Triamcinolone [Aristocort, Atolone, Kenacort, Kenalog-E], Triamcinolone acetonide [Azmacort, Cenocort A₂, Kenalog, Triam-A, Triamonide, Tri-kort, Trilog] triamcinolone diacetate [Amcort, Aristocort Forte, Articulose LA, others], triamcinolone hexacetonide [Aristospan] are more potent than hydrocortisone and are long-acting; with a half-life of 36–54 h.

Dosage: For inflammation, immunosuppression: PO, IM, SC 4–48 mg/d in divided doses. Intraarticular/intradermal: 4–48 mg/d. Inhaled 2–4 puffs qid. Topical: sparingly bid or tid. Acetonide: IM 60 mg. May repeat with 20–100 mg q6wk. Intradermal 1 mg per injection site to maximum of 30 mg total. Intraarticular 2.5–4.0 mg. Inhalation 2 puffs tid or qid to maximum of 16 puffs/d. Diacetate: PO 4–48 mg/d in 1–4 divided doses. IM 40 mg qwk. Intradermal 5–48 mg to maximum of 75 mg/wk. May repeat q1–2wk if needed. Intraarticular 2–40 mg q1–8wk. Hexacetonide: Intralesional up to 0.5 mg/in.² of skin. Intraarticular 2–20 mg q3–4wk.

▶ THE INHALANT FORMS OF GLUCOCORTICOIDS

The inhalant forms of glucocorticoids include beclomethasone, budesonide, flunisolide, fluticasone, and triamcinolone. They are used in the treatment of rhinitis and asthma.

Beclomethasone dipropionate [Beclovent, Beconase Nasal Inhaler, Vancenase Nasal Inhaler, Vanceril] suppresses the immune response of hayfever. The patient should gently clear the nares before use.

Side Effects

Nervous System: headache, sneezing, throat discomfort.

Endocrine System: (Pregnancy Category C) symptoms of increased cortisone.

Immune System: epistaxis, nasal congestion/irritation.

Dosage: Nasal inhaler 1 spray in each nostril bid–qid. Asthma: Oral inhaler 2 inhalations tid or qid up to 20 inhalations/d. Try reducing concomitant therapy after 1 wk.

Budesomide [Rhinocort] is a topical nasal spray to treat hayfever.

Side Effects

Nervous System: dysphonia, headache, sneezing, throat discomfort.

Endocrine System: (Pregnancy Category C) symptoms of hypercorticism.

Immune System: contact dermatitis, epistaxis, nasal congestion/irritation, wheezing.

Dosage: Intranasal 2 sprays per nostril bid, or 4 sprays per nostril qd.

Flunisolide [Nasalide (25 µg per spray), AeroBid (250 µg per spray)] treats rhinitis. It has the antiinflammatory action of hydrocortisone, to which it is related, plus vasoconstricting action. About 50% enters systemic circulation. In addition to typical corticoid nasal spray side effects, it can cause loss of the sense of taste/smell and vertigo and support conditions for candidal infections of the airway.

Side Effects

Nervous System: headache, loss of smell sense, sneezing, throat discomfort.

Endocrine System: (Pregnancy Category C) symptoms of hypercorticism.

Immune System: epistaxis, nasal congestion/irritation.

Dosage: Inhaled, intranasal 2 sprays orally, or intranasal per nostril bid. May increase to tid if needed.

Fluticasone [Flonase] is used to treat skin and mucous membrane inflammation. The topical may actually cause local skin allergy, and the spray may cause bronchospasm.

Side Effects

Nervous System: paradoxical bronchospasm, light-headedness, numbness/burning with the cream.

Endocrine System: (Pregnancy Category C) HPA axis suppression, dry skin, hirsutism.

Immune System: increased erythema, hives, irritation with the ointment.

Dosage: Intranasal 100 µg (1 puff) per nostril 1–2 ×/d to a maximum of qid. Topical: thin film to affected area bid.

Triamcinolone acetonide [Azmacort, others] is an immediate-acting synthetic flourinated corticoid, is 7–13 times more potent than hydrocortisone, causes little sodium and water retention.

Side Effects

Nervous System: muscle weakness.

Endocrine System: (Pregnancy Category C) hypopigmentation, hypotrichosis.

Immune System: burning, folliculitis, itching.

Dosage: Inhalation 2 puffs tid–qid.

▶ OPHTHALMIC GLUCOCORTICOIDS

Fluorometholone [Fluor-Op, FML Forte, FML Liquiflil Ophthalmic] is used to treat ocular inflammation. It can cause typical corticoid ocular side effects. IOP, caused by glucocorticoid sodium retention, is more common in the elderly.†

Side Effects

Nervous System: Excessive use: diminished visual field.

Endocrine System: (Pregnancy Category C) increased IOP. Excessive use: glaucoma exacerbation.

Immune System: corneal pathology. Excessive use: cataracts, optic nerve damage.

Dosage: Start with 1–2 gtt q1h and q2h at night for the first day or two; then 1–2 gtt bid or qid. Or apply a thin strip of ointment q4h for the first 24–48 h; then 1–3 ×/d.

Mometasone furoate [Elocon] is a topical synthetic corticosteroid used to relieve the inflammation and pruritus of corticosteroid-responsive dermatoses. Corticosteroids induce phospholipase A_2 inhibitory proteins (lipocortins), which control synthesis of inflammation mediators, eg, leukotrienes and prostaglandins, by inhibiting release of their common precursor, arachidonic acid, which is released from membrane phospholipids by phospholipase A_2.

Drug Interactions: none noted.

Side Effects

Nervous System: burning.

Endocrine System: (Pregnancy Category C) none noted.

Immune System: furunculosis, pruritus, rosacea, secondary infection, skin atrophy.

Dosage: Topical to affected skin qd in a thin film.

---

†Eye related.

Chapter Highlights

- Adrenocorticotropic hormone from the pituitary stimulates the secretion of glucocorticoids from the adrenal cortex on a daily basis and to produce extra glucose in times of stress or injury.

- As part of the steroid family, the glucocorticoids act slowly inside the target cells and have the characteristic sodium retention that produces edema.

- Glucocorticoids are invaluable in suppressing the destruction caused by the immune system in inflammatory conditions such as asthma and arthritis.

- Glucocorticoids are used in the emergency of spinal cord injury to prevent unwanted pressure on the cord caused by swelling as the immune system responds to the injury.

- In conjunction with immunosuppressant drugs, glucocorticoids make organ transplantation possible.

- Because glucocorticoids disrupt the feedback loop with the hypothalamus and the pituitary, they are used sparingly and gradually withdrawn.

11

Drugs for the Thyroid and Parathyroid Glands

- alendronate sodium [Fosamax]
- calcifediol [Calderol]
- calcitonin (human) [Cibacalcin]
- calcitonin (salmon) [Calcimar, Miacalcin]
- calcitriol [Calcijex, Rocaltrol]
- calcium acetate [Phos-Ex, PhosLo]
- calcium carbonate [BioCal, Calcite-500, Cal-Sup, Chooz, Dicarbosil, Nu-Cal, Os-cal, Oystercal]
- calcium chloride
- calcium citrate [Citracal]
- calcium gluceptate
- calcium gluconate [Kalcinate]
- calcium lactate
- dihydrotachysterol [DHT, DHT Intensol, Hytakerol]
- ergocalciferol [Activated Ergosterol, Calciferol, Deltalin, Drisdol, Dvisol, Vitamin D$_2$]
- iodine 131
- iodine drops [Pima, SSKI, Lugol's Solution]
- levothyroxine (T$_4$) [Levothroid, Synthroid]
- liothyronine (T$_3$) [Cytomel]
- liotrix (T$_3$, T$_4$) [Euthroid, Thyrolar]
- methimzaole [Tapazole]
- plicamycin [Mithracin, Mithramycin]
- propylthiouracil (PTU)
- thyroid [Armour Thyroid, Thyrar]
- tiludronate disodium [Skelid]

The thyroid gland produces hormones that stimulate cell metabolism and the parathyroids produce a hormone that increases calcium levels. However, the thyroid also produces the hormone calcitonin, which reduces blood calcium and increases bone resorption. Calcitonin also decreases kidney reabsorption of calcium, phosphate, and sodium.

The metabolic functions of the thyroid gland were understood earlier than the parathyroids' role in securing calcium because thyroid conditions such as goiter and cretinism were more obvious and the gland was easily palpable. The parathyroids were discovered only after surgical advancements made surgery possible on the thyroid and the patients became ill and died after removal of the thyroid. Research revealed the presence of the parathyroids located on and posterior to the thyroid.

▶ THE THYROID GLAND

The hypothalamus monitors the thyroid gland's hormone (T_3 and T_4) levels in the blood using the negative feedback loop. When thyroid hormone levels drop or we are stressed by our environment, illness, or other conditions, the hypothalamus sends thyroid-releasing hormones (THRH) down the stalk of the pituitary. In response, the pituitary secretes thyroid-stimulating hormones (TSH) into the bloodstream. TSH causes the thyroid to produce its hormones, given there is sufficient iodine for production. In response to the TSH, the thyroid "traps" iodine. The iodine is oxidized inside the gland and combined with the amino acid tyrosine.

The combination of oxidized iodine and tyrosine forms a molecule called thyroglobulin. Inside the thyroglobulin molecule the iodine and tyrosine become tightly bound, forming a molecule called monoiodotyrosine. The monoiodotyrosine molecules keep linking up, forming pairs called diiodotyrosine. In turn, the diiodotyrosine molecules begin linking together, forming the most abundant of the thyroid hormones, tetraiodothyronine—thyroxine or T_4. Simultaneously, additional monoiodotyrosine molecules are linking up with diiodotyrosine molecules, forming triiodothyronine, T_3, the more active of the thyroid hormones. T_3 is more potent than T_4, and even binds to the T_4 receptors better than T_4 (Fig. 11–1).

In addition to releasing hormones into the blood, the thyroid gland stores several months' worth of hormones. Thyroid hormones speed oxygen consumption and increase heat production in all cells but those of the spleen, adult brain, and gonads. Thyroid hormones increase levels of the enzymes that catalyze the breakdown of fats, glucose, and proteins. Thyroid hormones act like steroids in their ability to cross cell membranes and bind with receptors within the cells' nuclei. Some cells, for example, the liver's, contain thousands of thyroxine receptors; however, other cells may have few or no receptors, and thus do not respond. Thyroxine is essential for growth, though it is not clear if the hormone directly causes growth or simply spurs enzymes to cause growth. Lack of thyroid hormones causes a rise in blood lipids and contributes to atherosclerosis.

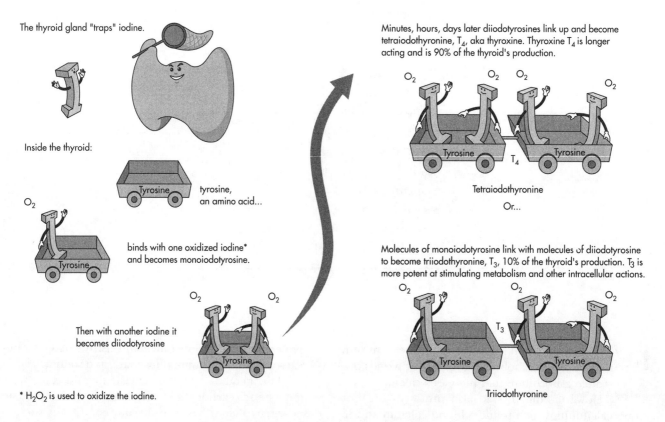

The thyroid gland "traps" iodine.

Inside the thyroid:

Tyrosine

tyrosine, an amino acid...

O_2 Tyrosine

binds with one oxidized iodine* and becomes monoiodotyrosine.

O_2 O_2

Then with another iodine it becomes diiodotyrosine

Tyrosine

* H_2O_2 is used to oxidize the iodine.

Minutes, hours, days later diiodotyrosines link up and become tetraiodothyronine, T_4, aka thyroxine. Thyroxine T_4 is longer acting and is 90% of the thyroid's production.

O_2 O_2 O_2 O_2

Tyrosine T_4 Tyrosine

Tetraiodothyronine

Or...

Molecules of monoiodotyrosine link with molecules of diiodotyrosine to become triiodothyronine, T_3, 10% of the thyroid's production. T_3 is more potent at stimulating metabolism and other intracellular actions.

O_2 O_2 O_2

Tyrosine T_3 Tyrosine

Triiodothyronine

Figure 11–1. The iodine–thyroid connection, parts I and II.

CRETINISM AND GOITER

Though both cretinism and goiter are the result of a lack of thyroid hormones, they are caused by different factors. Cretinism is the congenital lack of a thyroid gland. Prompt postnatal diagnosis and treatment are necessary to prevent permanent mental retardation during this critical period in brain development.

Goiter is the result of a dietary deficiency of iodine and can occur at any time in the patient's life. When the thyroid lacks iodine it cannot produce thyroid hormones in response to TSH. The hypothalamus reads these inadequate blood levels of thyroid hormones and sends down more releasing hormones to the pituitary. More TSH is released by the pituitary; and the thyroid enlarges in response. The resulting enlarged, ineffective gland is referred to as a goiter.

▶ DRUGS FOR AN UNDERACTIVE THYROID

Treatment of a sluggish thyroid with thyroid hormones carries the risk of stressing an unprepared body. For example, if a patient has both hypothyroid and hypoadrenal conditions, the adrenals would have to be treated first so that he or she can respond to the stress of increased thyroid hormone stimulation. Overdosage causes the side effects of hyperthyroidism.

Levothyroxine (T₄) [Levothroid, Synthroid] is used to replace the missing hormone. It is usually given PO, but may be administered IV for rapid replacement in coma of myxedema, when rapid replacement is necessary, or when the patient is not responding to the oral form.

Drug Interactions: Decreased absorption possible with cholestyramine, colestipol. Increased risk of cardiac insufficiency with epinephrine, norepinephrine. Increased hypoprothrombinemia possible with oral anticoagulants.

Side Effects

Nervous System: angina, arrhythmias—tachycardia/others, bowel—diarrhea, CHF, cramps—abdominal/leg, fatigue, headache, hypertension, nausea, palpitations, psyche—insomnia/irritability/nervousness, tremors, vision—staring expression, vomiting.

Endocrine System: (Pregnancy Category A) appetite changes, fever—as high as 106°F, heat intolerance, hyperglycemia—usually offset by increased cell oxidation of sugar, hyperthyroidism, menstrual irregularities, skin—warm/moist, sweating, thyroid storm, weight loss. The diabetic may need more insulin.

Immune System: none noted.

Dosage: PO. Start with 25–50 μg qd; increase by 50–100 μg q1–4 wk until the desired response is attained. Maintenance: 100–400 μg qd. The elderly require slower increments. Myxedema coma: IV 250–500 μg in one dose; next day 100–300 μg if necessary; then 50–200 μg/d until patient can take PO drug.

Liothyronine (T₃) [Cytomel] has a rapid onset and decrease in action as a synthetic T₃, making fast dosage adjustment possible.

Drug Interactions and Side Effects: See *levothyroxine.*

Dosage: PO 25 μg qd. Increase 12.5–25 μg q1–2wk until desired response is attained to maximum of 75 μg qd. Older patient: PO 2.5 μg qd for 3–6 wk; then double q6wk until desired response is attained. Myxedema: PO 5–100 mcg/d.

Liotrix (T₃, T₄) [Euthroid, Thyrolar] is used to replace the missing hormones.

Drug Interactions: Decreased absorption with cholestyramine, colestipol. Increased risk of cardiac insufficiency with epinephrine, norepinephrine. Increased hypoprothrombinemia possible with oral anticoagulants.

Side Effects

Nervous System: angina arrhythmias—tachycardia/others, bowel—diarrhea, CHF, cramps—abdominal/leg, fatigue, headache, hypertension, nausea, palpitations, psyche—insomnia/irritability/nervousness, tremors, vision—staring expression, vomiting.

Endocrine System: (Pregnancy Category A) appetite changes, fever—as high as 106°F, heat intolerance, hyperglycemia—usually offset by increased cell oxidation of sugar, hyperthyroidism, menstrual irregularities, skin—warm/moist, sweating, thyroid storm, weight loss. The diabetic may need more insulin.

Immune System: none noted.

Dosage: PO. Start with 12.5–30 μg qd; then increase slightly q1–2wk until desired response is attained. Older patient, cardiac patient, or long-standing hypothyroid patient: PO ¼ to ½ the adult dose, then double q8wk until desired response is attained.

Thyroid [Armour Thyroid, Thyrar] is used to replace missing hormone. It may be given as adjunct to antithyroid drugs to limit thyrotropic hormone release to prevent goitrogenesis and hypothyroidism.

Drug Interactions: Increased hypoprothrombinemia possible with oral anticoagulants. Increased need for insulin or sulfonylureas possible. Coronary insufficiency possible with epinephrine. Decreased absorption possible with cholestyramine.

Side Effects

Nervous System: angina, arrhythmias—various/tachycardia, bowel—diarrhea/cramps, coma,* CHF, cramps—legs, headache, palpitations, psyche—insomnia/nervousness, shock,* tremors, visual—staring expression, vomiting.

Endocrine System: (Pregnancy Category A) appetite changes, fever, heat intolerance, hyperglycemia, menstrual irregularities, skin—warm/moist, weight loss.

Immune System: none noted.

Dosage: PO 60 mg/d; increase q30d to 60–180 mg/d. Severe hypothyroidism: PO 15 mg/d; increase q2wk to 60 mg; then increase q30d if needed.

▶ DRUGS FOR A HYPERACTIVE THYROID

Hyperthyroidism, or Graves' disease, results in the overproduction of thyroid hormones. The symptoms may include exophthalmus and myxedema, in addition to the signs of thyroid hormone toxicity.

Propylthiouracil (PTU) prevents tyrosine from binding with iodine so no hormones can be made.

Drug Interactions: none noted.

Side Effects

Nervous System: arrhythmias—bradycardia, bowel—diarrhea/decreased GI motility, arthralgia, cramps—muscle (nocturnal), dizziness, drowsiness/sleepiness, dyspepsia, fatigue, headache, myalgia, nausea/vomiting, paresthesias, psyche—depression, taste—loss, vertigo, vision—ophthalmopathy worsened.

Endocrine System: (Pregnancy Category D) hair—lightening/loss, edema—hands/feet/periorbital, hyperpigmentation, hypothyroidism, liver—impaired function, menstrual changes, skin—cool/pale, thyroid—enlarged, weight gain.

Immune System: agranulocytosis,* hepatitis, hypoprothrombinemia, lymphadenopathy, leukopenia, lupus-like syndrome, myelosuppression, neuritis, ototoxicity, pruritus, rash, thrombocytopenia, urticaria, vasculitis.

Dosage: hyperthyroidism: PO. Start with 300–450 mg in divided doses q8h; may need 600–1200 mg/d initially. Thyrotoxic crisis: PO 200 mg q4–6h until the crisis resolves.

Methimazole [Tapazole] is a thioamide 10 times more potent that propylthiouracil, but with the same side effects.

* Life threatening side effect.

Drug Interactions: none noted.

Dosage: PO. Start with 5 mg tid–q8h. Moderate hyperthyroid: 10–15 mg tid–q8h. Severe hyperthyroid: 20 mg tid–q8h. Euthyroid: Maintenance 5–15 mg tid.

Iodine drops [Pima, SSKI] (SS means "saturated solution"), [Lugol's Solution] are used preoperatively to shrink the gland and decrease the amount of surgery needed. They are also used for thyrotoxic crises, after nuclear exposure, and in goiter-prone locations. Iodine inhibits production and release of thyroid hormones and decreases gland vascularity. In case of nuclear accidents in which iodine-131, a cancer-causing radioactive isotope, is released into the air, those exposed can protect against thyroid cancer by ingesting iodine or topically applying it to an area the size of one's hand. The saturated gland then will not trap the radioactive iodine.

Side Effects

Nervous System: arrhythmias, arthralgias, diarrhea, pain—stomach, paresthesias, productive cough, psyche—confusion, pulmonary edema, salivation, weakness. Poisoning: frontal headache/sneezing/nausea/metallic taste/vomiting—blue or yellow.

Endocrine System: (Pregnancy Category D) fever, goiter, hypothyroidism, pulmonary edema.

Immune System: acne, angioedema,* collagen disease-like syndromes, periorbital edema, eosinophilia, hemorrhage—cutaneous/mucosal, hyperthyroid adenoma, lymph node enlargements, small bowel lesions—nonspecific. Poisoning: coryza/bloody diarrhea, salivary glands—tender/swollen, stomatitis.

Dosage: PO 300–650 mg (1–2 tsp) pc bid or tid.

Iodine 131, a radioactive isotope, is used to destroy excess thyroid tissue as well as to test for thyroid function. This treatment is not without risk; hypothyroidism or thyroid cancer can result.

Drug Interactions: Iodine is synergistic with lithium, with the potential for hypothyroidism.

Other Side Effects: See *iodine.*

Dosage: PO or IV as prescribed and administered by the radiologist.

▶ THE THYROID GLAND AND CALCIUM

The thyroid gland monitors and reduces calcium levels. It secretes the hormone calcitonin, which increases kidney excretion of calcium in addition to potassium and sodium. These three elements are essential to the electrochemical conduction of neuronal impulses and muscle contraction.

▶ DRUGS FOR HYPERCALCEMIA

The most common causes for hypercalcemia are cancers and primary hyperparathyroidism. Cancers appear to increase reabsorption of calcium from the bone. Paget's disease, possibly the result of viral infection, causes resorption of bone, followed by rapid overgrowth.

<u>Calcitonin (human) [Cibacalcin], calcitonin (salmon) [Calcimar, Miacalcin]</u>, block the parathyroid hormones' actions on bone and kidneys by decreasing calcium levels. Keep refrigerated.

Drug Interactions: none noted.

Side Effects

Nervous System: bladder—nocturia, bowel—diarrhea, headache, nausea/vomiting, pain—abdominal/eye. Overdose—tetany caused by the inability of the sodium channels to close adequately during hypocalcemia. Human: bladder—frequency, chest pressure, dizziness, paresthesias, tenderness—palms/soles.

Endocrine System: (Pregnancy Category C) anorexia, diureses, edema—pedal, fever, flushing, urine—abnormal sedimentation. Human: chills.

Immune System: Human: nasal congestion. Salmon: anaphylaxis*/antibody formation, pruritus—ear lobes, rash.

Dosage: Paget's: Human: SC 0.5 mg qd or 2–3 ×/wk or 0.25–0.5 mg qd. Salmon: SC, IM. Start with 100 IU/kg. Maintenance: 50–100 IU qd or qod. Hypercalcemia: Salmon. SC, IM 4 IU/kg q12h; if response is poor after 1–2 d, increase to 8 IU/kg q6h; if needed, 2 d later, 8 IU/kg q6h. Postmenopausal osteoporosis: Salmon. SC, IM 100 IU qd. Miacalcin: 1 spray (200 IU) qd, alternate nostrils.

<u>Plicamycin [Mithracin, Mithramycin]</u> is used to treat the hypercalcemia secondary to malignancy or Paget's disease when the patient has not responded to IV hydration, PO phosphates, or steroids. Possibly by its action on DNA, it inhibits osteoclasts and blocks bone resorption.

Drug Interactions and Side Effects: See Chapter 17, Antineoplastics.

Dosage: Neoplasia: IV 25–30 μg/kg over 6h qd for 8–10 d or until toxicity requires dc. Maximum: 30 μg/kg/d for

10 d. Malignant hypercalcemia: IV 25 μg qd for 3–4 d; may repeat after 1 wk.

▶ DRUGS FOR THE PARATHYROIDS

The element calcium is essential in the nervous system to thought, other neuron activities, and muscle movement. The immune system uses it to help form clots. Calcium is stored in the bones, giving them strength, and is regulated by the four parathyroid glands, positioned on the back of the thyroid.

When calcium levels are low (normal: 8.5–10.5 mg/dL), the parathyroids sense this and secrete their hormone, parathyroid hormone (PTH). The parathyroids also trigger calcium reuptake in the kidneys and the release of calcium from bones into the bloodstream. Dietary vitamin D, sometimes called the sunshine vitamin, becomes D₃ in the skin in ultraviolet light. Parathyroid hormone activates vitamin D that has been stored in the kidneys and liver. The activated vitamin D becomes a hormone that moves into the gut, where it creates a calcium-binding protein in the epithelial cells of the intestine. The calcium-binding protein increases calcium absorption from the gut (Fig. 11–2).

The parathyroids enlarge during pregnancy and with rickets, a calcium deficiency in children that results in poor bone formation. In adults hypocalcemia is called osteomalacia and causes decreased bone density and strength. The parathyroids and the thyroid work together to balance calcium levels. In the thyroid, the hormone calcitonin decreases calcium levels.

▶ THE PARATHYROIDS AND PHOSPHATE

The parathyroids also regulate phosphate, an element essential to storing and using energy, as well as transmitting genetic information within a cell and beyond to

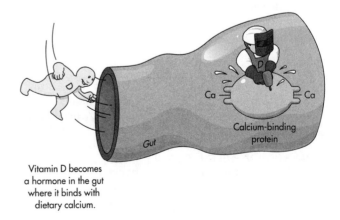

Vitamin D becomes a hormone in the gut where it binds with dietary calcium.

Figure 11–2. Inactive vitamin D becomes a hormone in the gut.

---

* Life threatening side effect.

other cells. Phosphate levels are balanced inversely to calcium, so that when calcium levels are up, phosphate levels (normal: 3–4.5 mg/dL) are down and vice versa.

Tiludronate disodium [Skelid] is a bisphosphonate used in the treatment of Paget's disease of the bone, in patients whose level of serum alkaline phosphatase is at least twice the upper limit of normal or who are symptomatic or may be at risk of complications.

Drug Interactions: Calcium or mineral supplements and aluminum or magnesium-containing antacids may interfere with absorption. Indomethacin and aspirin should not be taken within 2 h of tiludronate. Tiludronate should be taken within 2 h of food.

Side Effects

Nervous System: diarrhea, dysphagia, dyspepsia, edema, pain—chest, paresthesia.

Endocrine: (Pregnancy Category C) edema, hyperparathyroidism.

Immune System: esophagitis, ulcer—esophageal/gastric.

Dosage: PO 400 mg qd with 6–8 oz of plain water only ×3 mo.

▶ DRUGS FOR HYPOCALCEMIA

Hypocalcemia can be caused by dietary deficiencies, damage to the parathyroids, or disruption of its feedback loop. Owing to their location on the back of the thyroid gland, the parathyroids can be damaged during thyroid surgery. The kidneys assist in calcium balance by reabsorbing calcium in the tubules in response to PTH. Kidney dialysis disrupts calcium regulation, and the dialysis patient may suffer hypocalcemia.

Calcifediol [Calderol] is a Vitamin D analog that regulates serum calcium. It is used for metabolic bone disease when the patient has chronic renal failure.

Drug Interactions: Hypercalcemia possible with thiazide diuretics; hypercalcemia may cause digitalis arrhythmias with digitalis glycosides.

Side Effects

Nervous System: bladder—polyuria, bowel—constipation/diarrhea/cramps—abdominal, headache, lethargy, nausea/vomiting, pain—bone/muscle, vertigo, weakness.

Endocrine System: (Pregnancy Category C) anorexia, calcification of soft tissue, fever, hypercalcemia, hypercalciuria, hyperphosphatemia, dry mouth, thirst.

Immune System: none noted.

Dosage: PO 50–100 µg qd.

Calcitriol [Calcijex, Rocaltrol] is a synthetic metabolite of ergocalciferol (vitamin D$_2$) used to retrieve calcium from the kidney.

Drug Interactions and Side Effects: See *calcifediol.* In addition calcitriol may cause metallic taste, photophobia, blurred vision.

Dosage: PO. Start with 0.25 µg qd; adjust to serum levels. Maintenance: 0.5–1 µg. IV 0.5 µg 3 ×/wk at the end of dialysis.

Calcium acetate [Phos-Ex, PhosLo] is used to replace missing calcium.

Drug Interactions and Side Effects: See *calcium carbonate.*

Dosage: Hyperphosphatemia: PO 2–4 tabs with meals.

Calcium carbonate [BioCal, Calcite-500, Cal-Sup, Chooz, Dicarbosil, Nu-Cal, Os-cal, Oystercal] is used to replace missing calcium.

Drug Interactions: Increased inotropic and toxic effects of digoxin possible. Decreased absorption of tetracyclines, quinolones. Magnesium may compete for GI absorption.

Side Effects

Nervous System: acid rebound, bowel—constipation/diarrhea/flatulence, eructations, nausea. High doses, prolonged use: vomiting, psyche—mood/mental changes.

Endocrine System: (Pregnancy Category C) hypercalcemia with alkalosis, hypomagnesemia, hypophosphatemia (with low phosphate intake), hypercalciuria, metastatic calcinosis, renal calculi.

Immune System: none noted.

Dosage: PO 1–2 g bid or tid with meals to daily maximum of 8 g. As antacid: PO 0.5–2 g 4–6 ×/d. Hypophospatemia: PO 2–4 tabs with meals.

Calcium citrate [Citracal] is used to replace missing calcium.

Dosage: PO 1–2 g bid or tid.

Calcium chloride is an intravenous form of calcium used to replace missing calcium.

Drug Interactions: May increase inotropic and toxic effects of digoxin. Antagonizes verapamil and possibly other calcium channel blockers.

Side Effects

Nervous System: arrhythmias—bradycardia/others, cardiac arrest,* fainting, hypotension. IV site: pain/burning, peripheral vasodilation.

---

*Life threatening side effect.

Endocrine System: (Pregnancy Category C) hypercalcemia.

Immune System: with extravasation—necrosis/sloughing/thrombosis.

Dosage: IV 0.5–1 g slow injection. Cardiac arrest: IV 2.7–3.7 mEq × 1. Hypocalcemic tetany: IV 4.5–16 mEq prn.

Calcium gluceptate is an intravenous calcium replacement.

Drug Interactions and Side Effects: See *calcium chloride.*

Dosage: IM 0.5–1.1 g/d. IV 1.1–4.4 g/d.

Calcium gluconate [Kalcinate] is a calcium replacement. **Caution:** IV requires slow administration to avoid cardiac arrest.

Drug Interactions: See *calcium chloride.*

Side Effects

Nervous System: constipation, tingling. Rapid IV: arrhythmias—bradycardia and others, cardiac arrest,* hypotension, syncope, vasodilation.

Endocrine System: (Pregnancy Category C) increased gastric acid secretion.

Immune System: IV: cellulitis, tissue burning/irritation, soft tissue calcification. IV extravasation: necrosis/sloughing.

Dosage: PO 1–2 g bid to qid. IV 1–7 mEq q1–3d. Hypocalcemic tetany: IV 4.5–16 mEq prn. CPR: IV 2.3–3.7 mEq 1 dose. Hyperkalemia with cardiac toxicity: IV 2.25–14 mEq q1–2min. Exchange transfusion with citrated blood: IV 1.35 mEq for each 100 mL of blood.

Calcium lactate is a calcium supplement or replacement.

Drug Interactions and Side Effects: See *calcium carbonate.*

Dosage: PO 325 mg–1.3 g tid with meals.

Dihydrotachysterol [DHT, DHT Intensol, Hytakerol] is used to treat hypoparathyroidism.

Drug Interactions: none noted.

Side Effects

Nervous System: ataxia, atonia, bowel—constipation/diarrhea, drowsiness, headache, nausea/vomiting, nocturia/polyuria, pain—abdominal, psyche—depression, taste—metallic, tinnitus, vertigo, weakness.

Endocrine System: (Pregnancy Category A) anorexia, hypercalcemia, dry mouth, renal calculi.

Immune System: none noted.

Dosage: PO 0.75–2.5 mg qd. Adjust to serum levels. Maintenance: 0.2–1.0 mg/d.

Ergocalciferol [Activated Ergosterol, Calciferol, Deltalin, Drisdol, Dvisol, Vitamin D$_2$] mobilizes calcium to treat rickets/osteomalacia.

Drug Interactions: Decreased absorption of vitamin D with cholestyramine, colestipol, mineral oil possible.

Side Effects

Nervous System: ataxia, arrhythmias, bowel—constipation/diarrhea, convulsions,* cramps—abdominal, drowsiness, fatigue, headache, hypertension, nausea/vomiting, pain—joint/muscle, photophobia, taste—metallic, tinnitus, weakness.

Endocrine System: (Pregnancy Category C) anorexia, calcification—soft tissues, dry mouth, nephrotoxicity, osteoporosis, renal failure, thirst, weight loss. Children: mental and physical retardation.

Immune System: nephrotoxicity.

Dosage: PO, IM 25–125 µg/d. Vitamin D-dependent rickets; PO, IM 250 µcg–1.5 mg/d.

▶ OSTEOPOROSIS

Osteoporosis is a decreased bone mineral density that occurs in millions of older American women. The loss of calcium is most rapid between the ages of 45 and 59. Lack of calcium causes the bones to become fragile and may contribute to the risk of hip fractures, a leading cause of hospitalization and death in elderly women. Decreased bone density may also cause tiny spinal fractures that result in kyphosis, the humped back sometimes seen in elderly women.

Alendronate sodium [Fosamax] is used to treat bone loss, especially after menopause.

Drug Interactions: Decreased absorption with calcium, as in dairy products.

Side Effects

Nervous System: arthralgia, bowel—constipation/diarrhea/flatulence, dyspepsia, headache, myalgia, nausea/vomiting, pain—abdominal.

Endocrine System: (Pregnancy Category C) hypocalcemia.

Immune System: rash.

Dosage: Osteoporosis: PO 10 mg q AM with a full glass of water and remain upright for at least 30 min. Paget's disease: PO 40 mg qd × 6 mo.

---

*Life threatening side effect.

Chapter Highlights

- Using a negative feedback loop, the hypothalamus monitors the thyroid gland's hormones to maintain the optimum level of metabolism for the body.

- The thyroid "traps" iodine circulating in the blood to produce its hormones.

- A person's diet must be adequate in iodine for healthy thyroid functioning.

- Drugs for the thyroid gland consist of replacement thyroid hormones, iodine, and drugs to reduce hormone production or to destroy part of the overactive gland.

- The thyroid also produces calcitonin, which reduces calcium levels in the blood.

- The parathyroids increase calcium levels.

- Drugs for the parathyroid include calcium replacements.

12

Drugs That Maintain Mineral and Fluid Balance

- acetazolamide [Diamox]
- amiloride [Midamor]
- benazepril hydrochloride [Lotensin]
- bumetanide [Bumex]
- captopril [Capoten]
- chlorothiazide [Diachlor, Diuril, SK Chlorothiazide]
- chlorothiazide sodium [Sodium Diuril]
- chlorthalidone [Hygroton, Hylidone, Thalitone]
- desmopressin acetate [Stimate]
- dextran 40 [Gentran 40, others]
- dextran 70 [Macrodex]
- dextran 75 [Gentran 75]
- diazoxide [Hyperstat I.V., Proglycem]
- enalapril [Vasotec]
- enalaprilat [Vasotec IV]
- ethacrynic acid [Edecrin]
- furosemide [Lasix]
- hetastarch [HES, Hespan, Hydroxyethyl Starch]
- hydrochlorothiazide [Diqua, Esidrix, Hydro-Chlor, HydroDIURIL, Hydromal, Hytro-T, Oretic, SK-Hydrochlorothiazide, HCTZ]
- hydrochlorothiazide + triamterene [Dyazide]
- irbesartan [Avapro]
- isotonic (0.9%) sodium chloride
- lisinopril [Prinivil, Zestril]
- losartan potassium [Cozaar]
- losartan potassium hydrochlorothiazide [Hawser]
- mannitol [Osmitrol]
- methazolamide [Neptazane]
- metolazone [Diulo, Mykrox, Zaroxolyn]
- perindopril erbumine [Aceon]
- potassium chloride [K 10, Kaochlor, Kao-chlor-20 Concentrate, Kaon-Cl, Kato, Kay Ciel, KCl 5% and 20%, Klor, Klor-10%, Klor-Con, Kloride, Klorvess, Klotrix, Kdur, Klyte/Cl, K-tab Micro-K Extentabs, Rum-K, SK-Potassium Chloride, Slow-K]
- potassium gluconate [Kaon, Kaylixir, K-G Elixir]

▶ RULE: WATER FOLLOWS SODIUM

Water molecules have an affinity for sodium. To maintain necessary water levels for body functions, the mineralocorticoid aldosterone, a steroid, retains sodium. Aldosterone influences the kidneys to retain sodium, and the water follows (Fig. 12–1). On the other hand, aldosterone causes potassium excretion by the kidneys, thus maintaining the sodium–potassium balance. Aldosterone in the distal tubule, where most sodium is reabsorbed, influences how much of the last 5% of the excreted sodium will be reabsorbed.

▶ A BRIEF HISTORY OF DIURETICS

Originally edema was treated directly by bleeding the patient with leeches or scalpels. Medicinal herbs were used to make the patient sweat or urinate. However, modern diuretics are, in part, the result of careful intake and output records kept by nurses at the Wenckebach Clinic in Vienna. There, in 1919, a medical student, Arthur Vogl, treated a woman with a series of mercury injections for her syphilis. The charting revealed an increase in urine output from a low of 200 mL/d to 1200 mL/d. On the third day the patient voided 2000 mL/d. Another syphilitic patient, in congestive heart failure, voided more than 10 L (Sneader, 1985). However, it was discovered that mercury damages kidneys. Nearly 30 years passed until modern sulfa-based diuretics were created.

▶ DIURETICS

Most diuretics simply get rid of sodium. In the process water follows (Fig. 12–2). By decreasing blood volume, diuretics are first-line drugs in the treatment of hypertension and congestive heart failure. They are used in

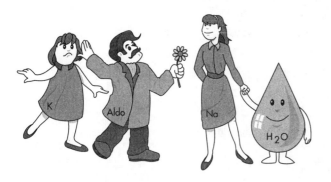

The word "aldosterone" contains an Italian sounding name, Aldo Sterone. Here is an imaginary love story or triangle to help the reader remember aldosterone's action.

In the love triangle Aldo is smitten by sodium who is always followed by water. On the other hand, Aldo hates potassium and keeps trying to get rid of what he sees as a pest. The result is that Aldo Sterone gets rid of potassium, and keeps sodium, and water follows sodium.

Figure 12–1. The story of Aldo Sterone.

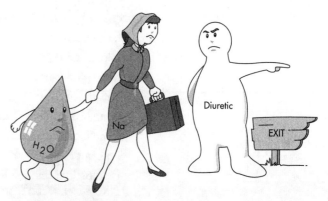

The diuretics basically cause kidneys to excrete sodium, and water follows. Diuretics are used to decrease blood volume in hypertension, CHF, and hepatic cirrhosis. They are also used for kidney dysfunction and for elevated calcium.

Figure 12–2. Diuretics.

the emergency treatment of intracranial pressure to relieve cerebral edema, and sometimes to relieve intraocular pressure.

Note: *Because of the large amounts of urine produced, it is best to give diuretics in the morning so that the patient will not be up all night voiding. Because diuretics create electrolyte imbalance, they must be used with caution when the patient is on cardiac glycosides. This is of special concern with the sulfonamide diuretics, which typically require potassium supplementation.*

CARBONIC ANHYDRASE INHIBITORS

The kidneys' ability to reabsorb water in the renal tubule depends on sodium reabsorption. In the distal end of the tubule, where bicarbonate is excreted, carbonic anhydrase exchanges hydrogen ions for sodium, thus retaining sodium. Carbonic anhydrase inhibitor diuretics block the action of carbonic anhydrase, causing the kidneys to excrete sodium, and water follows the sodium.

These diuretics are also used to treat glaucoma. In the eye they decrease the rate of aqueous humor formation and lower intraocular pressure. They may also be used as anticonvulsants by inhibiting CNS carbonic anhydrase, thus slowing abnormal discharges in vulnerable neurons.

Acetazolamide [Diamox] competes with carbon dioxide for its receptor on carbonic anhydrase. Unwanted systemic side effects make it a less-than-ideal diuretic, but it is used for glaucoma because, as a carbonic anhydrase inhibitor, it decreases the secretion of aqueous humor. In addition, because it binds with carbonic anhydrase, it raises CO_2 levels in the brain and raises the seizure threshold in epilepsy. This occurs because increased O_2 levels are associated with seizure activity.

Drug Interactions: Decreased excretion of amphetamines, ephedrine, flecainide, procainamide, quinidine, tricyclic antidepressants is possible. Increased excretion of lithium. Possible increased excretion of phenobarbital. Possible accelerated potassium loss with amphotericin B and corticosteroids. Potassium loss increases risk of toxicity with cardiac glycosides. Possible salicylate toxicity with high doses of salicylates.

Side Effects

Nervous System: bladder—dysuria/polyuria, bowel—diarrhea, fatigue, malaise, nausea/vomiting, paralysis/flaccidity, parathesias, psyche—depression/disorientation, sedation, muscle weakness.

Endocrine System: (Pregnancy Category C) anorexia, calcium/magnesium/potassium/sodium — increased excretion, crystalluria, glycosuria, hyperglycemia, hyperuricemia, metabolic acidosis, dry mouth, polyuria, thirst, weight loss.

Immune System: aplastic anemia,* bone marrow depression,* hematuria, hepatic dysfunction, hypersensitivity to sulfonamides.

Dosage: Glaucoma PO 250 mg qid. SR 500 mg bid. IM, IV 500 mg; may repeat in 2–4 h. Epilepsy PO 8–30 mg/kg/d in 1–4 doses. Edema: PO 250–375 q AM. High-altitude sickness: PO 250 mg q8–12h. SR 500 mg q12–24h; start 24–48 h before climb and continue for 48 h at high altitude.

Methazolamide [Neptazane] is used as an adjunct to treat chronic simple glaucoma and secondary glaucoma and as a preoperative treatment for acute angle-closure glaucoma to lower intraocular pressure.

Drug Interactions: See *acetazolamide.*

Side Effects

Nervous System: drowsiness, dyspepsia—mild, fatigue, headache, paresthesias, psyche—confusion/depression, vertigo.

Endocrine System: (Pregnancy Category C) anorexia.

Immune System: allergy

Dosage: PO 50–100 mg bid or tid.

LOOP DIURETICS

The sulfonamide diuretics are also referred to as **loop diuretics** because they act in the loop of Henle in the renal tubule. By inhibiting chloride reuptake, they cause sodium chloride loss. Water, by following sodium, is lost with the sodium. The loop diuretics also cause potassium loss and usually require potassium supplementation.

Bumetanide [Bumex] is more powerful than furosemide, but shorter acting. It causes magnesium and potassium loss and may inhibit phosphate and bicarbonate reabsorption.

Drug Interactions: Increased risk of ototoxicity with aminoglycosides, cisplatin. Increased risk of hypokalemia may cause digoxin toxicity. Weakened diuretic and hypotensive action with NSAIDs, and weakened diuretic action with probenecid possible. Possible decreased lithium excretion.

Incompatibilities

Solution/Additive: dobutamine.

Side Effects

Nervous System: bowel—diarrhea, cramps—muscle, dizziness, ECG changes, fatigue, headache, hearing—

---

* Life-threatening side effect.

discomfort/impairment/tinnitus, hyperventilation, hypotension, nausea/vomiting, muscle—pain/tenderness/stiffness, pain—arthritic/chest/stomach, weakness.

Endocrine System: (Pregnancy Category C) electrolyte imbalance, hypovolemia, glycosuria, dry mouth, sweating.

Immune System: allergy, ototoxicity.

Dosage: PO 0.5–10 mg/d. IM, IV 0.5–1 mg per dose; IV 1–2 min. Repeat q2–3h if needed. Maximum: 10 mg/d.

Ethacrynic acid [Edecrin] is used to treat the severe edema of CHF, cirrhosis, lymphedema, ascites of malignancy, nephrotic syndrome, and renal disease.

Off Label: nephrogenic diabetes insipidus, hypercalcemia, mild to moderate hypertension, adjunct therapy for hypertensive crisis complicated by pulmonary edema.

Side Effects

Nervous System: bowel—diarrhea, dysphagia, headache, hearing—deafness (temporary or permanent)/sense of fullness in ears/tinnitus, hypotension—postural, fatigue, nausea/vomiting, pain/discomfort—abdominal, psyche—apprehension/confusion, vertigo.

Endocrine System: (Pregnancy Category B) BUN/creatinine/urate levels—elevated, chills, electrolyte imbalance, fever, glycosuria, gynecomastia, gout—acute, hyperglycemia, hyperuricemia, hypovolemia.

Immune System: agranulocytosis,* hematuria, liver function tests—abnormal, neutropenia,* pruritus, rash, thrombocytopenia. IV: GI bleeding, local irritation/thrombophlebitis.

Dosage: Edema: PO 50–100 mg qd or bid; maximum of 400 mg/d. IV 0.5–1 mg/kg or 50 mg up to 100 mg; may repeat if necessary.

Furosemide [Lasix] is possibly the most commonly used of the loop diuretics. It can oppose antidiuretic hormone. Potassium loss requires replacement.

Drug Interactions: Increased diuresis with other diuretics and decreased with NSAIDs. Hypokalemia increases risk of digoxin intoxication. Prolonged blockage with nondepolarizing neuromuscular blocking agents. Hypokalemia potentiated by amphotericin B. Decreased lithium elimination and increased toxicity. Hypoglycemic effects altered by sulfonylureas/insulin.

Incompatibilities

Solution/Additive: ciprofloxacin, diphenhydramine, dobutamine, doxapram, doxorubicin, droperidol, gen-

tamicin, meperidine, metoclopramide, milrinone, netilmicin, pancuronium, quinidine thiamine.

Y-site: amrinone, ciprofloxacin, diazepam, diphenhydramine, doxorubicin, droperidol osmolal, fluconazole, gentamicin, methocarbamol, metoclopramide, morphine, netilmicin, ondansetron, quinidine, tobramycin, vinblastine, vincristine, vitamin B complex with C.

Side Effects

Nervous System: bladder—frequency, bowel—constipation/diarrhea, circulatory collapse,* cramps—abdominal, dizziness with excessive diuresis, hearing—feeling of fullness in ears/hearing loss, hypotension—acute episodes/postural, nausea/vomiting, paresthesia, photosensitivity, tetany (with hypocalcemia), vision—blurred, weakness.

Endocrine System: (Pregnancy Category C) alkalosis—metabolic, anorexia, BUN elevated, dehydration, glycosuria, hyperglycemia, hyperuricemia, hypo—calcemia/chloremia/kalemia/magnesemia/natremia, porphyria cutanea tarde, sweating.

Immune System: agranulocytosis,* allergic interstitial nephritis, anemia, aplastic anemia,* exfoliative dermatitis, leukopenia, ototoxicity, pancreatitis, purpura, renal failure—irreversible, SLE activation, thrombocytopenia, urticaria.

Dosage: Edema: PO 20–80 mg in 1 or more divided doses up to 600 mg/d if needed. IM, IV 20–40 mg (do not exceed 4 mg/min IV). May increase by 20 mg increments q2h if necessary. Hypertension: PO 10–40 mg bid to maximum of 480 mg/d.

THIAZIDE DIURETICS

The thiazide diuretics, by-products of saccharin production, inhibit sodium reabsorption in the distal tubule. Potassium and magnesium are also lost and potassium supplement is needed unless the thiazide is combined with a potassium-sparing chemical. If the patient is also on corticosteroids, the potassium loss may be greater, because of the steroid family trait of ridding the kidneys of potassium. In addition, because steroids tilt the body toward glucogenesis, the diabetic may need more insulin. The thiazides are not for use with lithium.

Chlorothiazide [Diachlor, Diuril, SK Chlorothiazide], chlorothiazide sodium [Sodium Diuril] are common thiazide duiretics.

Drug Interactions: Increased hypokalemia with amphotericin B, corticosteroids. Blunted hypoglycemic effects of sulfonylureas and insulin possible. Decreased thiazide absorption with cholestyramine, colestipol. Increased

* Life-threatening side effect.

hypoglycemic and hypotensive effects of diazoxide. Increased potassium and magnesium loss may cause digitoxin intoxication. Decreased lithium excretion may cause lithium toxicity. Increased risk of NSAID-induced renal failure and attenuated diuresis.

Incompatibilities

Y-site: amikacin, chlorpromazine, codeine phosphate, hydralazine, insulin, levorphanol, methadone, morphine, multivitamins, norepinephrine, polymyxin B, procaine, prochlorperazine, promazine, promethazine, streptomycin, tetracyclines, triflupromazine, vancomycin.

Side Effects

Nervous System: arrhythmias/weak pulse, bowel—diarrhea, dizziness, fatigue, headache, hypotension—postural, psyche—changes, respiratory distress, vertigo, vomiting.

Endocrine System: (Pregnancy Category B) fever, cholesterol/triglyceride—elevated, glycosuria, hyper—calcemia/glycemia/uricemia, hypochloremic alkalosis, hypo—kalemia/natremia, SIADH secretion.

Immune System: agranulocytosis,* anaphylaxis,* pancreatitis, photosensitivity, rash, urticaria.

Dosage: Hypertension and edema: PO. Start with 250 mg–1 g/d in divided doses. Maintenance: According to BP. IV 250 mg–1 g/d in 1 or 2 divided doses.

Chlorthalidone [Hygroton, Hylidone, Thalitone] is a sulfonamide derivative, chemically different from thiazides, but with similar characteristics. It may elevate blood lipids.

Drug Interactions: Increased hypokalemia with amphotericin B, corticosteroids. Blunted hypoglycemic effects of sulfonylureas and insulin possible. Decreased thiazide absorption with cholestyramine. Increased potassium and magnesium loss may cause digitoxin intoxication. Decreased lithium excretion may cause lithium toxicity. Decreased diuresis with NSAIDs.

Side Effects

Nervous System: bowel—constipation/cramping/diarrhea, dizziness, headache, hypotension—orthostatic, impotence, nausea/vomiting, paresthesias, vertigo.

Endocrine System: (Pregnancy Category B) anorexia, glycosuria, gout exacerbation, hyper—calcemia/glycemia, hypo—chloremia/kalemia/natremia, jaundice.

Immune System: agranulocytosis,* aplastic anemia,* photosensitivity, rash, thrombocytopenia, urticaria, vasculitis.

Dosage: Edema: PO 50–100 mg/d or 100–200 mg qod or qd 3 d/wk. Hypertension: PO 12.5–25 mg qd. May be increased to 100 mg/d if needed.

Hydrochlorothiazide [Diqua, Esidrix, Hydro-Chlor, Hydro-DIURIL, Hydromal, Hydro-T, Oretic, SK-Hydrochlorothiazide, HCTZ] is a thiazide diuretic whose action takes place in the cortical dilution segment of the nephron.

Off Label: Nephrogenic diabetes insipidus, hypercalciuria, electrolyte unbalance of renal tubular acidosis.

Drug Interactions: Increased hypokalemia with amphotericin B, corticosteroids. Blunted hypoglycemic effects of sulfonylureas and insulin possible. Decreased thiazide absorption with cholestyramine, colestipol. Increased hypoglycemic and hypotensive effects with diazoxide. Increased potassium and magnesium loss may cause digitoxin intoxication. Decreased lithium excretion may cause lithium toxicity. Increased risk of NSAID-induced renal failure and attenuated diuresis.

Side Effects

Nervous System: arrhythmias/weak pulse, bowel—diarrhea, dizziness, hypotension, lightheadedness, nausea/vomiting, paresthesias, psyche—mood changes, spasms—muscle, vision—blurred, weakness/tiredness.

Endocrine System: (Pregnancy Category B) anorexia, hyper—glycemia/uricemia, hypokalemia, glycosuria, dry mouth, thirst.

Immune System: agranulocytosis,* aplastic anemia,* hypersensitivity, leukopenia, jaundice, pancreatitis, photosensitivity, thrombocytopenia.

Dosage: Edema: PO 25–200 mg/d (tablets or liquid) in divided doses. Hypertension: PO 12.5–100 mg/d in 1 dose or 2 divided doses.

Metolazone [Diulo, Mykrox, Zaroxolyn] is similar to chlorothiazide, though a quinazoline, and may be more effective than thiazides in severe renal failure.

Drug Interactions: Increased hypokalemia with amphotericin B, corticosteroids. Blunted hypoglycemic effects of sulfonylureas and insulin possible. Decreased thiazide absorption with cholestyramine, colestipol. Increased hypoglycemic and hypotensive effects with diazoxide. Increased potassium and magnesium loss may cause digitoxin intoxication. Decreased lithium excretion may cause lithium toxicity. Increased risk of NSAID-induced renal failure and attenuated diuresis.

Side Effects

Nervous System: hypotension—orthostatic, vertigo.

---

* Life-threatening side effect.

Endocrine System: (Pregnancy Category D) cholestatic jaundice, dehydration, hyperuricemia, hyperglycemia, hypokalemia.

Immune System: allergy, leukopenia, venous thrombosis.

Dosage: PO 5–20 mg qd. Hypertension: PO 2.5–5 mg qd. Mykrox: 0.5–1 mg/d.

POTASSIUM-SPARING DIURETICS

The potassium-sparing diuretics were developed to avoid the potassium loss that accompanies sodium loss with most diuretics, a potential hazard when the patient is also on digitalis. Potassium supplements should not be given with these drugs.

<u>Amiloride [Midamor]</u> is a weak, potassium-sparing diuretic that can be given in combination with thiazide diuretics.

Drug Interactions: Hyperkalemia with arrhythmias possible with ACE inhibitors, blood from blood banks, potassium supplements, spironolactone, triamterene. Decreased lithium excretion may cause toxicity. Decreased antihypertensive effects possible with NSAIDs.

Drug–food Interactions: Potassium-containing salt substitutes may cause hyperkalemia.

Side Effects

Nervous System: arrhythmias, bladder—dysuria/frequency/spasms, bowel—constipation/diarrhea, cramps—abdominal/muscle, dizziness, drowsiness, dyspnea/SOB, fatigue, headache, dry mouth, nausea/vomiting, psyche—confusion/nervousness, sexual function—impotence/libido decrease, tinnitus, visual disturbances, weakness.

Endocrine System: (Pregnancy Category B) anorexia, eye—IOP, hyperkalemia,* hyponatremia, polyuria, thirst.

Immune System: aplastic anemia,* Coombs test positive, nasal congestion, photosensitivity, pruritus, rash.

Dosage: PO 5–20 mg/d in divided doses.

<u>Hydrochlorothiazide with triamterene [Dyazide]</u> is useful when hypokalemia cannot be risked. The addition of triamterene spares potassium loss caused by hydrochlorothiazide. No potassium supplements are used with this drug. The compound contains hydrochlorothiazide 25 mg and triamterene 37.5 mg.

Hydrochlorothiazide Side Effects and Drug Interactions: See *hydrochlorothiazide.*

Triamterene Side Effects and Drug Interactions: See *triamterene.*

Dosage: PO 1–2 capsules qd.

<u>Spironolactone [Aldactone]</u> competes with aldosterone for the receptor sites where sodium and potassium are exchanged. Sodium is excreted and potassium is spared. Spironolactone lowers blood pressure in primary hyperaldosteronism and essential hypertension, but acts too slowly for use in hypertensive crisis.

Off Label: Hirsutism with polycystic ovary syndrome or idiopathic hirsutism. Adjunct to treatment for myasthenia gravis and familial periodic paralysis.

Drug Interactions: Systemic acidosis possible in combination with acidifying doses of ammonium chloride. Decreased diuresis possible with NSAIDs. Decreased cardiac glycoside activity possible. Hyperkalemia with potassium supplements.

Side Effects

Nervous System: ataxia, bowel—diarrhea, cramps—abdominal, drowsiness, fatigue, headache, hypertension—postsympathectomy, lethargy, nausea/vomiting, psyche—confusion, sexual function—impotence.

Endocrine System: (Pregnancy Category D) acidosis—mild, androgenic effects, anorexia, BUN elevated, electrolyte imbalance, fever, glucose tolerance—decreased, gynecomastia, parathyroid changes.

Immune System: agranulocytosis,* rash, SLE, urticaria.

Dosage: Edema: PO 25–200 mg/d in divided doses for at least 5 d adjusted to response; add a loop or thiazide diuretic if needed. Hypertension: PO 25–100 mg/d in single or divided doses for at least 2 wk adjusted for response. Primary aldosteronism: PO 100–400 mg/d in divided doses.

<u>Triamterene [Dyrenium]</u>, a pteridine derivative structurally related to folic acid, prevents sodium reabsorption in the distal tubule, while allowing potassium reabsorption.

Drug Interactions: Decreased renal elimination of triamterene with indomethacin possible. Hyperkalemia possible with ACE inhibitors, other potassium-sparing diuretics. Decreased lithium excretion may cause toxicity.

Side Effects

Nervous System: bowel—diarrhea, cramps—muscle, dizziness, headache, hypotension, nausea/vomiting/other GI disturbances, weakness.

Endocrine System: (Pregnancy Category B) BUN elevated, folic acid reduced, hyperchloremic acidosis,

---

* Life-threatening side effect.

hyperkalemia/other electrolyte imbalances, dry mouth, uric acid elevated in patients predisposed gouty arthritis.

Immune System: anaphylaxis,* anemia—megaloblastic, blood dyscrasias, eosinophilia, granulocytopenia, photosensitivity.

Dosage: PO 100 mg/d in divided doses, to maximum of 300 mg/d. Maintenance: 100 mg qd or qod.

AN OSMOTIC DIURETIC

Water shifts from a place of lower solute concentration to a place of greater solute concentration. Osmotic diuresis is caused by the presence of particles (solutes) that the kidneys cannot reabsorb from the tubules, such as glucose, urea, or the drug mannitol.

Mannitol [Osmitrol], an important emergency drug made from dextrose, causes diuresis by raising the osmotic pressure of glomerular filtrate. Water and electrolyte reabsorption is inhibited. This drug is used for acute renal failure. Because its action is global, it can be used for elevated intraocular and intracranial pressures, where increasing the osmotic gradient causes a therapeutic fluid shift.

Drug Interactions: none noted.

Side Effects

Nervous System: angina-like pain, bladder—retention, CHF, convulsions,* dizziness, edema, headache, hyper-/hypotension, muscle—transient rigidity, nausea/ vomiting, vision—blurred.

Endocrine System: (Pregnancy Category C) acidosis, chills, dehydration, diuresis—marked, edema—local, fever, electrolyte imbalance (especially hyponatremia*), dry mouth, nephrosis, uricosuria.

Immune System: allergy. Extravasation: allergy, necrosis, thrombophlebitis.

Dosage: Acute renal failure. Test with IV 0.2 g/kg or 12.5 g as a 15–20% solution over 3–5 min. Use only if response is positive, ie, 30–50 mL of urine over 2–3 h. Then 50–100 g 15–20% solution over 90 min to several hours. Edema, ascites: IV 100 g as a 10–20% solution over 2–6 h. Relieve intracranial pressure: IV 1.5–2.0 mg/kg in solution over 30–60 min. Relieve intraocular pressure: As for intracranial pressure in 30 min. Acute chemical toxicity: IV 100–200 g depending on urine output. Measurement of glomerular filtration rate (GFR): IV 100 mL of 20% solution diluted with 180 mL NaCl injection infused at a rate of 20 mL/min.

▶ A DRUG TO RETAIN SODIUM

Though sodium is a leading culprit in edema, it is also essential to health. When restoration of sodium balance is required, the following drug can be of value.

Diazoxide [Hyperstat I.V., Proglycem] is a glucose-elevating drug similar in structure to thiazide diuretics, but it is not a diuretic; it inhibits insulin release. Serious side effects limit its use. It can precipitate angina, CVA, diabetes, hyperglycemia, hyperuricemia, and MI, and can cause sodium, and thus, water retention. It is also given to restore salt balance in adrenal insufficiency when hydrocortisone replacement is not enough, in salt-losing forms of congenital adrenal hyperplasia, or in severe orthostatic hypotension caused by autonomic neuropathy. Diazoxide lowers blood pressure by possible competition with calcium for receptors. Usually a diuretic is used with it to counter the sodium retention. Restrict sodium in diet. The patient may need potassium supplement.

Drug Interactions: Decreased effects with sulfonylureas. Increased antihypertensive effects and hyperglycemia with thiazide diuretics. Increased hyperglycemia with phenytoin possible. Increased phenytoin metabolism may decrease seizure control.

Side Effects

Nervous System: abdominal discomfort, ataxia, arrhythmias—atrial/ventricular, bladder—nocturia, bowel—constipation/diarrhea/ileus, CHF, sensation of burning/itching, cramps—muscle, dizziness, drowsiness, EPS, headache, hearing—transient loss/tinnitus, hypertension—transient, hypotension—orthostatic, insomnia, malaise, nausea/vomiting, pain—back/chest, palpitations, paresthesias, psyche—agitation/anxiety/euphoria, shock, taste—loss, vision—blurred/diplopia/lacrimation/papilledema/scotoma, weakness.

Endocrine System: (Pregnancy Category C) anorexia, azotemia, breast lump enlargement, edema, fever, flushing, galactorrhea, glycosuria, hepatic impairment, hirsutism, hyperglycemia, hyperuricemia, nephrotic syndrome—reversible, proteinuria, sodium/water—retention, sweating, urinary output—decrease, sensation of warmth. Labor inhibited.

Immune System: bone age advance (children), eosinophilia, hair loss, hematuria, Hb/Hct/IgG—decrease, herpes, immunoglobinemia—decrease, leukopenia, monilial dermatitis, neutropenia—transient, rash, vision—subconjunctival hemorrhage/transient cataracts.

Dosage: Severe hypertension: IV push 1–3 mg; repeat q5–15min until BP is at a desirable level.

---

* Life-threatening side effect.

► KIDNEY STONES, URIC ACID, AND GOUT

While the tasks of the kidneys include mineral and water balance, sometimes those abilities can be overwhelmed and stones can form. Kidney stones (renal calculi) are the result of several factors, including diet and inadequate hydration. The chemical analysis of a passed stone will reveal its composition so that therapeutic measures can be taken to prevent the continued formation of calculi. When proteins and purines in the diet are the cause, dietary changes are in order. In addition to renal calculi, the patient may have gouty deposits throughout the body, especially in the joints, resulting in gouty arthritis. The uricosuric drugs probenecid and sulfinpyrazone can reduce the serum urate concentration by increasing uric acid excretion and decreasing synthesis of uric acid. These agents prevent renal tubular reabsorption of uric acid.

URICOSURIC DRUGS

Probenecid [Benemid, Probalan, SK-Probenecid] is derived from sulfonamides and inhibits renal tubular reuptake of uric acid. If dosage is high enough, it will shrink old gouty tophi. It is not for use in the acute gout attack, nor combined with colchicine. Salicylates antagonize its renal action. However, it can be used to increase blood levels of penicillin, cephalosporin, rifampin, sulfonylureas, and also methotrexate, naproxen, indomethacin, clofibrate, and pantothenic acid.

Drug Interactions: Decreased uricosuric activity possible with salicylates. Decreased methotrexate elimination possible. Decreased nitrofurantoin effect and increased toxicity possible.

Side Effects

Nervous System: bladder—frequency, dizziness, headache, nausea/vomiting, respiratory depression (in overdose).

Endocrine System: (Pregnancy Category B) anorexia, calculi—uric acid, fever, flushing, gout exacerbations.

Immune System: anaphylaxis,* anemia, aplastic anemia,* dermatitis, hemolytic anemia,* hepatic necrosis,* pruritus, sore gums.

Dosage: Gout: PO 250 mg bid for 1 wk; then 500 mg bid to maximum of 3 g/d. Penicillin or cephalosporin therapy: PO 500 mg qid or 1 g with single-dose therapy.

Sulfinpyrazone [Anturane], like probenecid, inhibits renal tubular reuptake of uric acid in addition to other organic anions; however, it can be used with colchicine. Sulfinpyrazone also has immune system activity. It interferes with platelet aggregation due to its ability to inhibit prostaglandin production.

Drug Interactions: Increased risk of hypoglycemia by displacing sulfonylureas from protein binding. Increased prothrombin time with warfarin. Decreased absorption with cholestyramine. Decreased effect of nitrofurantoin for UTI and increased drug toxicity. The patient must be advised to push fluids and keep urine alkaline.

Side Effects

Nervous System: ataxia, bowel—diarrhea, colic—renal, coma,* convulsions,* dizziness, dyspnea, nausea/vomiting, pain—epigastric, tinnitus, vertigo.

Endocrine System: (Pregnancy Category C) fever, urolithiasis.

Immune System: precipitation of acute gout, blood loss, jaundice, rashes, peptic ulcer reactivation.

Dosage: PO 100–200 mg bid with meals for 1 wk; then increase to 200–400 mg bid; then decrease to 200 mg/d after serum urate levels are controlled to maximum of 800 mg/d. Inhibition of platelet aggregation: PO 200 mg tid or qid.

► CHELATION

Sometimes minerals accumulate in toxic amounts in the blood. Chelating agents are organic molecules which form a bond with the metal. The kidneys excrete the bonded metal-organic molecules.

Penicillamine [Cuprimine, Depen] is a chelating agent used when other treatments for rheumatoid arthritis have failed. It is also used to increase kidney excretion of excess copper in Wilson's disease and to treat cystinuria.

Off Label: Primary biliary cirrhosis, porphyria cutanea tarda, lead poisoning.

Drug Interactions: Possible increased adverse hematologic and renal effects with antimalarials, cytotoxics, gold therapy. Decreased absorption with iron possible.

Side Effects

Nervous System: arthralgia, bowel—diarrhea, nausea/vomiting, pain—epigastric, ptosis, taste—loss/metallic/reduction (salt and sweet), tingling—feet, weakness.

Endocrine System: (Pregnancy Category D) alopecia, anorexia, fever, hyperpyrexia, mammary hyperplasia, pyridoxine deficiency.

Immune System: agranulocytosis,* alveolitis, aplastic anemia,* hemolytic anemia,* hematuria, leukopenia, lymphadenopathy, membranous glomerulopathy, myasthe-

---

* Life-threatening side effect.

nia gravis syndrome, optic neuritis, pancreatitis, peptic ulcer, proteinuria, pruritus, thrombotic thrombocytopenic purpura—activation, pemphigus-like rash, rashes—early/late, skin—friability/excessive wrinkling, SLE-like syndrome, thyroiditis, thrombocytopenia, thrombophlebitis, urticaria.

Dosage: Rheumatoid arthritis: PO 125–250 mg/d. May increase at 1- to 3-mo intervals to a maximum of 1–1.5 g/d. Cystinuria: PO 250–500 mg qid. Calibrate doses to limit urinary excretion of cystine to 100–200 mg/d. Wilson's disease: PO 250 mg qid with 3 doses 1 h ac, and the last dose at least 2 h after the last meal.

PLASMA EXPANDERS

Normally the body maintains a balance between blood and tissue. This oncotic pressure gradient is the pressure difference between the colloid osmotic pressure or osmotic pressure of lymph and that of blood. Edema disrupts that balance, and diuretics help reestablish it. Whereas diuretics are used to remove extra volume from circulation, some conditions require volume expansion. Burns, surgery, sepsis, hemorrhage, or other trauma pose the danger of hypovolemic shock by disrupting the osmotic pressure gradient. Massive fluid shifts are life threatening and require plasma expanders.

<u>Dextran 40 [Gentran 40, others]</u> is a plasma expander of low molecular weight. This synthetic polysaccharide has colloidal properties similar to those of human plasma. It decreases blood viscosity and cell aggregation, making it useful to prime heart–lung equipment, and as prophylaxis against deep vein thrombosis (DVT) and pulmonary emboli (PE) in high-risk surgical procedures.

Drug Interactions: none noted.

Side Effects

Nervous System: none noted.

Endocrine System: (Pregnancy Category C) osmotic nephrosis/stasis/blocking, oliguria, renal failure.*

Immune System: anaphylaxis,* angioedema,* ALT/AST—increased, clotting disorders, interference with platelet function, pruritus, urticaria.

Dosage: Shock: IV 500 mL administered rapidly within 15–30 min; then if necessary, 20 mL/kg slowly in first 24 h; if still needed, doses up to 10 mL/kg/d for an additional 4 d. Prophylaxis for thromboembolic complications: IV 500–1000 mL (10 mL/kg) on the day of surgery; follow with 500 mL/d for 2–3 d; if necessary, continue with 500 mL q2–3d for up to 2 wk. Prime extracorporeal circulation: 10–20 mL/kg added to perfusion circuit.

---

* Life-threatening side effect.

<u>Dextran 70 [Macrodex], dextran 75 [Gentran 75]</u> are plasma expanders for emergency use in hypovolemic shock or impending shock due to hemorrhage, burns, surgery, trauma when whole blood or blood products are unavailable or there is no time to crossmatch blood.

Off Label: DVT prophylaxis, nephrosis, toxemia of pregnancy.

Side Effects

Nervous System: arthralgia, GI disturbances, hypotension, vomiting, wheezing.

Endocrine System: fever, low plasma protein levels.

Immune System: anaphylaxis*—severe, urticaria.

Dosage: Shock: IV 500 mL rapid over 15–30 min. Additional doses more slowly up to 20 mL/kg in the first 24 h. Doses up to 10 mL/kg/d for 4 d if needed.

<u>Hetastarch [HES, Hespan, Hydroxyethyl Starch]</u> is used, in addition to expanding plasma volume, to increase erythrocyte sedimentation rate and to increase granulocyte harvesting for leukapheresis. This colloidal preparation impedes the clotting mechanisms. The kidneys excrete the low-molecular-weight molecules, and the heavier ones are broken down by the reticuloendothelial system and blood amylases for eventual excretion by both kidneys and liver.

Drug Interactions: none noted.

Side Effects

Nervous System: headache, heart failure,* muscle pains, vomiting, wheezing.

Endocrine System: (Pregnancy Category C) calcium—decrease, chills, circulatory overload,* edema—periorbital/peripheral, fever, hyperbilirubinemia, plasma proteins—dilution.

Immune System: anaphylaxis,* clotting disorders—increased bleeding and clotting time/decreased fibrinogen/Hct/Hb/platelets, flu-like symptoms, sedimentation rate—increase, swelling—submaxillary/parotid glands.

Dosage: Shock: IV 500–1000 mL to maximum rate of 20 mL/kg/h. Maximum 1500 mL/d. Leukapheresis (continuous flow centrifugation): IV 250–750 mL infusion at a constant fixed ratio of 8:1 to venous whole blood.

▶ POTASSIUM

Potassium is one the elements essential to the electrochemical depolarization of neurons that make thought and movement possible. Use of non–potassium-sparing diuretics cause the excretion of potassium by the kidneys and may necessitate the use of potassium supplements. In addition, the steroid aldosterone causes potassium excretion by the kidneys to maintain sodium–potassium balance.

Potassium chloride [K 10, Kaochlor, Kao-chlor-20 Concentrate, Kaon-Cl, Kato, Kay Ciel, KCl 5% and 20%, Klor, Klor-10%, Klor-Con, Kloride, Klorvess, Klotrix, Kdur, Klyte/Cl, K-tab Micro-K Extentabs, Rum-K, SK-Potassium Chloride, Slow-K], Potassium gluconate [Kaon, Kaylixir, K-G Elixir] are all potassium supplements.

Drug Interactions: Hyperkalemia with ACE inhibitors, potassium-sparing diuretics.

Incompatibilities

Solution/Additive: amphotericin B, dobutamine (potassium phosphate only).

Y-site: diazepam, ergotamine, methylprednisolone, phenytoin, promethazine.

Side Effects

Nervous System: arrhythmias—bradycardia/arrhythmias*/cardiac depression*/arrest,* bowel—diarrhea, flaccid paralysis,* hypotension, limbs—heaviness, listlessness, muscle weakness, paresthesias, psyche—confusion/irritability, respiratory—arrest*/distress, sensitivity to digitalis glycosides—altered, swallowing difficulties.

Endocrine System: (Pregnancy Category A) hyperkalemia (serum potassium > 5.5 mEq/L), anuria, oliguria.

Immune System: none noted.

Dosage: Hypokalemia: PO 10–100 mEq in divided doses. IV 10–40 mEq diluted (always dilute potassium) in 1 L dextrose or sodium chloride IV solution to 10–20 mEq/100 mL of solution to maximum of 200–400 mEq/d. Monitor carefully.

Potassium iodide [Pima, SSKI] is used as an expectorant and an antithyroid agent. Potassium decreases mucus viscosity and the iodide temporarily inhibits thyroid hormone.

Drug Interactions: Increased hypothyroid and goiterogenic actions with lithium. Increased risk of hyperkalemia with ACE inhibitors, potassium-sparing diuretics, potassium supplements.

Side Effects

Nervous System: arrhythmias, bowel—diarrhea/small bowel lesions with enteric coated, cough—productive, nausea/vomiting, pain—stomach, paresthesias, psyche—confusion, weakness. Iodine poisoning: frontal headache, metallic taste, vomiting.

Endocrine System: (Pregnancy Category D) goiter, hyperthyroidism, hyperthyroid adenoma, periorbital edema. Hypersensitivity: fever.

Immune System: acneiform skin lesions (long use), adolescent acne flareup, pulmonary edema. Hypersensitivity: angioneurotic edema,* arthralgias, eosinophilia, hemorrhage—cutaneous/mucosal, lymph node enlargement. Iodine poisoning: coryza, sneezing, salivary glands—swollen/tender. Collagen disease-like syndromes.

Dosage: Expectorant: PO 300–650 mg pc, bid, or tid. Reduce thyroid vascularity: PO 50–250 mg tid for 10–14 d before surgery. Thyroid blocking in radiation emergency: PO 130 mg/d for 10 d. Adjunct to management of thyroid crisis: IV 500 mg q4h.

▶ SODIUM

Sodium is essential to normal nerve conduction—so essential that the body has one steroid, aldosterone, dedicated to sodium retention in the kidneys. Sodium is a frequent component of intravenous solutions. Normal saline or isotonic sodium chloride, the solution that bathes the body cells, contains 154 mEq of sodium and chloride. Intravenous solutions include varied amounts of sodium and are administered according to the patient's condition and requirements. The solutions include normal saline, 154 mEq/L; lactated Ringer's, 130 mEq/L; Normosol, 140 mEq/L; 5% albumin, 145 mEq/L; and hetastarch, 154 mEq/L.

Isotonic (0.9%) sodium chloride is used IV to replace fluids and restore electrolyte balance, and as a solution for irrigations and enemas. It is also a diluent to reconstitute parenteral drugs. NaCl also comes in 3% and 5% solutions, but these are not often used, and then, only in small amounts to avoid circulation overload. At 20% solution NaCl is an intraamniotic abortifacient.

Side Effects

Nervous System: none noted.

Endocrine System: (Pregnancy Category A) none noted.

Immune System: none noted.

Dosage: Isotonic saline: IV 2–8 mL/kg/h based on extent and severity of the surgery to counter third-space shift hypovolemia not due to blood loss. Oliguria, hypotension, or other signs of decreased cardiac output or hypovolemia: IV in a rapid infusion of 2–6 mL/kg.

Sodium bicarbonate (NaHCO₃) can be used as an emergency drug to counter metabolic acidosis in diabetes mellitus, shock, cardiac arrest, and vascular collapse. Sometimes sodium bicarbonate is used as a home rem-

---

* Life-threatening side effect.

edy soak or bath for minor skin irritations. Some OTC antacids like Alka-Seltzer, Bi-So-Dol, Bromo-Seltzer, Fizrin, and Gaviscon have sodium bicarbonate as a major ingredient. Sodium bicarbonate is not recommended as a gastric antacid due to CO_2 release and ensuing gastric distention, systemic alkalosis, and possible acid rebound.

Side Effects

Nervous System: belching, flatulence, gastric distension, tetany—with hypocalcemia.

Endocrine System: (Pregnancy Category C) dehydration, edema, pulmonary edema, hypocalcemia, metabolic alkalosis, milk–alkali syndrome, renal calculi/crystals, impaired renal function, sodium overload.

Immune System: severe tissue damage after extravasation of IV solution.

Dosage: Cardiac arrest: IV bolus 1 mEq/kg 7.5–8.4% solution; then 0.5 mEq/kg q10min based on arterial blood gas levels; give over 1–2 min. Metabolic acidosis: IV 2–5 mEq/kg for 4–8 h. Urinary alkalizer to lower uric acid crystallization during treatment with uricosuric drugs, raise sulfonamide solubility, aminoglycoside antimicrobial effect; raise barbiturate and salicylate excretion by kidneys following an overdose: PO 4 g initially; then 1–2 g q4h. Antacid: PO 0.3–2 g 1–4 ×/d or 1/2 tsp of powder in glass of water.

► ANTIDIURETIC HORMONE

In addition to sodium retention, the endocrine system has another way to retain fluid. When the hypothalamus detects an increase in the concentration of electrolytes in neurons in the lateral hypothalamus, it triggers the sensation of thirst. In addition, another part of the hypothalamus responds to a concentrated blood consistency by releasing ADH, or vasopressin, down the pituitary stalk, through the posterior pituitary and into the bloodstream. In the collecting ducts of the kidneys, ADH causes reabsorption of up to 90% of the water. In addition, vasopressin is also a powerful vasoconstrictor of arterioles and capillaries and raises blood pressure and pulmonary arterial pressure. Unofficially, vasopressin can be used as an adjunct vasopressor in massive GI bleeding. As a drug, antidiuretic hormone, or vasopressin, can cause cardiac arrhythmias, angina, or, if the dose is great enough, an MI. It increases peristalsis and contracts gallbladder and urinary bladder smooth muscles. Closely related to oxytocin, vasopressin can, if the dose is great enough, stimulate uterine muscle. Vasopressin also stimulates the release of corticotropins, FSH, and growth hor-

mone. The nurse must monitor BP, output (and specific gravity), and weight during treatment. Because ADH increases water absorption by the kidneys, water intoxication is a possibility. Signs of water intoxication include anuria, weight gain, headache, confusion, and drowsiness. Other side effects include pounding in the head and allergic reactions ranging from rashes to anaphylaxis.

Diabetes insipidus, the lack of antidiuretic hormone, is treated with replacement of the hormone, as is the polyuria caused by the antidiuretic hormone deficiency resulting from head trauma (Fig. 12–3). ADH is also used in radiology to propel flatus that might cloud the x-ray picture. Because it increases peristalsis, it is used to prevent or relieve postoperative abdominal distention, though this action is better achieved with cholinergics.

Desmopressin acetate [Stimate] is a synthetic analog of ADH used to treat diabetes insipidus and the polydipsia and polyuria resulting from trauma in the area of the pituitary. Its action is longer and more specific than that of ADH, with less chance of allergic reaction. Though it acts like ADH on the renal tubules, it does not have the side effects of stimulating production of other hormones

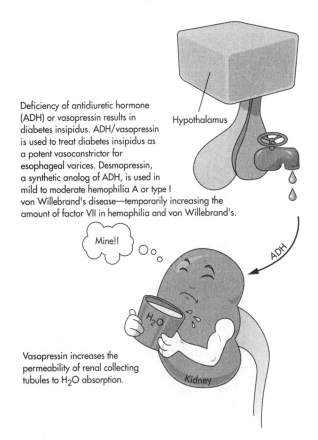

Deficiency of antidiuretic hormone (ADH) or vasopressin results in diabetes insipidus. ADH/vasopressin is used to treat diabetes insipidus as a potent vasoconstrictor for esophageal varices. Desmopressin, a synthetic analog of ADH, is used in mild to moderate hemophilia A or type I von Willebrand's disease—temporarily increasing the amount of factor VII in hemophilia and von Willebrand's.

Mine!!

Vasopressin increases the permeability of renal collecting tubules to H_2O absorption.

Figure 12–3. Hypothalamus produces antidiuretic hormone and sends it to the posterior pituitary.

such as ACTH. Desmopressin also is used to temporarily increase factor VIII in some cases of hemophilia and in type I von Willebrand's disease, which is manifested by abnormally slow blood clotting.

Side Effects

Nervous System: cramps—abdominal, BP—slight rise, drowsiness, headache, heartburn, listlessness, nausea, pain—vulva, SOB.

Endocrine System: (Pregnancy Category B) flushing—facial.

Immune System: nasal—congestion/irritation, rhinitis. Injection site: swelling/pain.

Dosage: Diabetes insipidus: PO 0.2–0.4 mg/d. Intranasal 0.1–0.4 mL qd or divided bid or tid. SC, IV 2–4 μg/d divided in 2 doses. Von Willebrand's disease: IV, SC 0.3 μg/kg 30 min preop; IV over 15–30 min. May repeat in 48 h if needed. Enuresis: Intranasal: 5–40 μg hs.

Vasopressin injection [Pitressin] is an animal extract with the actions described above.

Drug Interactions: Decreased antidiuretic effects possible with alcohol, demeclocycline, epinephrine, heparin, lithium, phenytoin. Decreased antidiuretic effects with guanethidine, neostigmine. Increased antidiuretic effect possible with chlorpropamide, clofibrate, carbamazepine.

Side Effects

Nervous System: angina in coronary artery disease, arrhythmias—cardiac arrest,* bronchoconstriction,* belching, bowel—flatulence, cramps—uterine, nausea/vomiting, pallor—circumoral/facial, pounding in head, tremor. Intraarterial: arrhythmias—bradycardia/others, pulmonary edema. Intranasal: abdominal cramps, BM—increased, headache, heartburn. Large doses: arrhythmias—heart block/bradycardia/minor/premature atrial contractions, blanching, coronary insufficiency, cramps—abdominal, nausea, peripheral vascular collapse.

Endocrine System: (Pregnancy Category X) sweating, uterine cramps, water intoxication.

Immune System: anemia, anaphylaxis,* angioedema,* leukopenia, rash, urticaria. Intraarterial: injection site gangrene. Intranasal: congestion, conjunctivitis, irritation, mucosal ulceration, postnasal drip, pruritus, rhinorrhea. Large doses: MI.*

Dosage: SC, IM, intranasal. Diabetes insipidus: IM, SC 5–10 U aqueous solution 2–4×/d. Intranasal: Apply with cotton plegit/intranasal spray. X-ray: IM, SC 5–15 U 2 h and 1/2 h before x-ray. Abdominal distention: IM. Start

with 5 U; increase to 10 U q3–4h if needed. Rectal: Insert tube (if ordered) and leave in place for 1 h.

Note: Monitor infusion site qh for blanching—a sign of impending gangrene. Intraarterial infusion: 0.2–0.4 U/min for massive GI bleeding. Use for this condition can cause ischemic colitis.

Vasopressin tannate in oil is never given IV.

Dosage: Diabetes insipidus: SC, IM 1.25–2.5 U q36–72h.

▶ RENIN, ANGIOTENSIN-CONVERTING ENZYME, BLOOD VOLUME, AND HYPERTENSION

When the nervous system triggers blood vessel constriction with its catecholamine neurotransmitters, the effect on blood pressure is immediate and short-lasting. The endocrine system also constricts blood vessels, but in the endocrine system's steady, deliberate manner, with a slow onset of longer duration. Thus, hypertension is also an endocrine condition, and the endocrine system offers another avenue of treatment—the ACE inhibitors.

As blood flows through the glomerulus, in Bowman's capsule in the kidneys, cells in the entering, or afferent, arteriole detect any drop in blood flow volume. In response to such a drop, the arteriole cells secrete renin into the blood. Renin then splits the end off of a plasma protein called renin substrate, releasing angiotensin I. The bloodstream carries angiotensin I to the lungs where angiotensin-converting enzyme (ACE) splits angiotensin I into angiotensin II. Angiotensin II is the molecule that ultimately and powerfully constricts arterioles (Fig. 12–4). In addition, angiotensin II signals the release of more aldosterone, which in turn retains more sodium. Water follows sodium, and blood volume is increased.

ACE INHIBITORS

ACE inhibitors prevent the conversion of angiotensin I into angiotensin II. ACE inhibitors interfere with aldosterone and its reduction of potassium and disrupt the sodium-retaining mechanism. ACE inhibitors occasionally cause a first-dose hypotension, and the full therapeutic antihypertensive effect may not occur for weeks. A thiazide diuretic may also be needed to control blood pressure.

Benazepril hydrochloride [Lotensin] is used to treat hypertension by preventing the conversion of angiotensin I into angiotensin II.

Drug Interactions: Increased risk of hyperkalemia with potassium-sparing diuretics. Increased lithium levels possible.

---

* Life-threatening side effect.

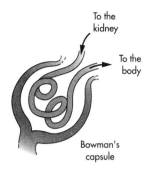

To the kidney

To the body

Blood flow to the afferent arteriole drops: cells in the afferent arteriole secrete renin into the blood.

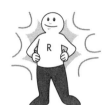

Bowman's capsule

Renin is an enzyme. It splits the end off of a plasma protein called renin substrate.

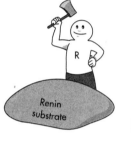

Renin substrate

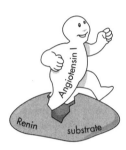

Renin substrate

Renin may continue doing this for an hour.

Angiotensin I is cleaved to form angiotensin II in the lungs by a "converting enzyme."

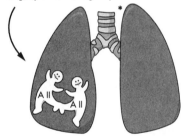

Angiotensinase will break down angiotensin II quickly.

* ACE inhibitor drugs work here.

Angiotensin II constricts arterioles and, to a degree, veins. This constriction increases arterial pressure and venous flow to the heart.

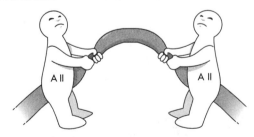

Figure 12–4. Angiotensin-converting enzyme (ACE).

Side Effects

Nervous System: bowel—constipation/diarrhea, cough, dizziness, fatigue, headache, hypotension, nausea, pain—back, weakness.

Endocrine System: (Pregnancy Category D) azotemia, hyperkalemia, oliguria, renal failure in patients with CHF.

Immune System: bronchitis, gastritis.

Dosage: PO 10–40 mg/d in 1 dose or 2 divided doses.

Captopril [Capoten], an ACE inhibitor, is given 1 h after meals for maximum absorption. It may cause a metallic or salt taste, even loss of taste. If the patient is hyponatremic before the start of therapy, discontinue any diuretic therapy and increase sodium intake 7–10 d before captopril therapy begins.

Side Effects

Nervous System: arthralgia, cough, dizziness, fainting, heart rate—slight increase, first dose hypotension, taste—metallic/salt.

Endocrine System: (Pregnancy Category D) azotemia, hyperkalemia, nephrotic syndrome, impaired renal function,* weight loss.

Immune System: agranulocytosis,* angioedema,* antinuclear antibody positive, membranous glomerulonephritis, pruritus, rash, serum sickness–like syndrome, urticaria.

Dosage: PO 6.25–25 mg tid 1 h after meals for maximum absorption; may increase to maximum of 450 mg/d. Resistant hypertension: increase to 100 mg tid; maximum 450 mg/d. Congestive heart failure: Start with 6.25–12.5 mg tid in addition to a diuretic; maximum 450 mg/d.

Enalapril [Vasotec], enalaprilat [Vasotec IV] are ACE inhibitors activated when hydrolyzed by the liver. They are 10–20 times more potent than captopril, act longer, and have fewer side effects. Diabetics may experience hyperglycemia. Enalapril may be given with meals.

Drug Interactions: Decreased antihypertensive activity possible with NSAIDs. Hyperkalemia possible with potassium supplements, potassium-sparing diuretics. Increased lithium levels and toxicity possible.

Side Effects

Nervous System: asthenia, bowel—diarrhea, cough, dizziness, dyspepsia, fatigue, headache, hypotension, pain—abdominal/chest, palpitations, paresthesias, psyche—insomnia/nervousness/somnolence, syncope, taste—loss.

---

* Life-threatening side effect.

Endocrine System: (Pregnancy Category D) hyperkalemia, renal function—deterioration/acute failure.*

Immune System: agranulocytosis,* angioedema,* erythema, Hb/Hct—decrease, pruritus, rash.

Dosage: Hypertension: PO 5 qd or 2.5 mg qd for patients on diuretics, and when creatinine clearance is less than 30. Maintenance: 10–40 mg qd or divided bid. IV 1.25 mg q6h; may give up to 5 mg q6h in hypertensive crisis. Congestive heart failure: PO 2.5 mg 1–2 ×/d; may increase up to 5–20 mg/d in 1 dose or 2 divided doses to maximum of 40 mg/d.

Note: Normal creatinine clearance is 150–180 mL/min.

Lisinopril [Prinivil, Zestril] is an ACE inhibitor used to treat hypertension.

Drug Interactions: Decreased antihypertensive activity possible with NSAIDs. Hyperkalemia possible with potassium supplements, potassium-sparing diuretics. Increased lithium levels and toxicity possible.

Side Effects

Nervous System: bowel—constipation/diarrhea, cough, dizziness, dyspnea, fatigue, headache, nausea/vomiting, pain—chest.

Endocrine System: (Pregnancy Category D) anorexia, azotemia, BUN/creatinine—increase, hyperkalemia.

Immune System: rash.

Dosage: PO 10 mg qd. May increase up to 20–40 mg qd to maximum of 80 mg/d.

Perindopril erbumine [Aceon] inhibits ACE, resulting in decreased angiotensin II and lowered blood pressure.

Drug Interactions: Excessive reduction of blood pressure with diuretics. Increased potassium with potassium-sparing diuretics and potassium supplements. Increased lithium levels.

Side Effects

Nervous System: cough, dyspepsia, hypertonia, palpitation, pain—back/upper extremities.

Endocrine System: (Pregnancy Category C in first trimester; D in last two) fever, proteinuria.

Immune System: ear infection, viral infection, sinusitis.

Dosage: PO 4 mg qd to maximum of 16 mg qd.

ANGIOTENSIN II INHIBITORS

Angiotensin II is the final product in the cascade of reactions that result in powerful vasoconstriction of

the arterioles and, to some extent, the veins. Angiotensin II inhibitors block angiotensin to relieve hypertension.

Irbesartan [Avapro] is used to treat hypertension alone or in combination with other hypertensive drugs.

Drug Interactions: none noted.

Side Effects

Nervous System: arrhythmias—tachycardia, bowel—diarrhea, dizziness, dyspepsia/heartburn, fatigue, headache, nausea/vomiting.

Endocrine System: (Pregnancy Category C first trimester; D in last two) edema.

Immune System: rash, upper respiratory infection.

Dosage: PO 150 mg qd to maximum of 300 mg qd.

Losartan potassium [Cozaar], an angiotensin II receptor antagonist, works in vascular smooth muscle and adrenal glands to block vasoconstriction and aldosterone secretion of angiotensin II.

Drug Interactions: Decreased serum levels of losartan and metabolites with phenobarbital.

Side Effects

Nervous System: bowel—diarrhea, cough, cramps—muscle, dizziness, dyspepsia, headache, insomnia, myalgia, pain—back/legs.

Endocrine System: (Pregnancy Category C first trimester; D last two) none noted.

Immune System: congestion—nasal, infection—upper respiratory, sinusitis.

Dosage: PO 25–50 mg in 1 dose or 2 divided doses to maximum of 100 mg/d. Start with 25 mg/d if on diuretics.

Losartan potassium hydrochlorothiazide [Hawser] has side effects similar to those of losartan potassium.

Dosage: PO 25–50 mg qd.

Ramipril [Altace] inhibits angiotensin II formation to decrease peripheral vascular resistance and lower BP. Inhibiting ACE also decreases serum aldosterone levels.

Drug Interactions: Decreased antihypertensive activity possible with NSAIDs. Hyperkalemia possible with potassium supplements, potassium-sparing diuretics. Increased lithium levels and toxicity possible.

---

* Life-threatening side effect.

Side Effects

Nervous System: belching, bowel—diarrhea, cough, dizziness, fatigue, headache, nausea/vomiting.

Endocrine System: (Pregnancy Category D) hyperkalemia, hyponatremia.

Immune System: angioedema,* erythema, pruritus.

Dosage: CHF, hypertension: PO 2.5–5 mg qd to maximum of 20 mg/d in 1 dose or 2 divided doses.

Valsartan [Diovan] lowers blood pressure by blocking angiotensin II from binding with its receptors in vascular smooth muscle and the adrenals.

Drug Interactions: none noted.

Side Effects

Nervous System: arthralgia, dizziness, headache, bowel—diarrhea, cough, nausea.

Endocrine System: (Pregnancy Category C in first trimester; D in last two) edema.

Immune System: pharyngitis, rhinitis, sinusitis.

Dosage: PO 80 mg qd to maximum of 320 mg qd.

---

* Life-threatening side effect.

 Chapter Highlights

- The endocrine system maintains fluid and electrolyte balance to keep blood volume at an optimal range.
- Aldosterone retains sodium and excretes potassium.
- Most diuretics work on the basis of the rule that water follows sodium—they cause the kidneys to lose sodium and water follows.
- The kidneys can produce calculi as the result of diet and inadequate hydration.
- Chelating agents are organic molecules that bind with toxic metals in the blood and are excreted by the kidneys.
- The endocrine system also prevents water loss with the hormone antidiuretic hormone or ADH.
- While maintaining blood volume, the endocrine system also maintains blood pressure by producing angiotensin, a hormone that constricts arterioles and, to a lesser degree, veins.
- The ACE inhibitors work as antihypertensives by blocking angiotensin, with the result that blood vessels are more relaxed and blood pressure is lower.

13

Sex Hormones

- bromocriptine mesylate [Parlodel]
- clomiphene citrate [Clomid]
- danazol [Danocrine]
- diethylstilbestrol (DES)
- estradiol [Climara, Estrace, Estraderm]
- estradiol cypionate [Depo-Estradiol Cypionate, others]
- estradiol valerate [Delestrogen, Dioval, others]
- estrogenic substance aqueous suspension [Estroject-2]
- estrogens, conjugated [Premarin, Progens]
- estrogens, esterified [Estratab, Menest, Menrium]
- estrone aqueous suspension [Estronol, Kestrone-5, Theelin Aqueous]
- estropipate [Ogen]
- finasteride [Propecia]
- hormone contraceptives
- human chorionic gonadatropin (HCG) [Antuitrin, A.P.L., Chorex, Chorigon, Choron 10, Corgonject-5, Follutein, Glukor, Gonic, HCG, Pregnyl, Profasi HP]
- medroxyprogesterone acetate [Amen, Cycrin, Depo-Provera, Provera]
- menotropins (FSH + LH) [Pergonal]
- methylergonovine maleate [Methergine]
- nilutamide [Nilandron]
- norethindrone [Micronor, Norlutin, Nor-Q.D.]
- oxytocin injection [Pitocin, Syntocinon, Syntocinon Nasal Spray]
- progesterone [Gesterol 50, Progestaject, Progestasert]
- ritodrine hydrochloride [Yutopar]
- testosterone [Andro 100, Histerone, Testoderm]
- testosterone cypionate [Andro-Cyp, Andronate, depAndro, Depo-Testosterone, Depotest, Duratest]
- testosterone enanthate [Andro L.A., Delatest, Delatestryl, Everone, Testone L.A., Testrin PA]
- testosterone propionate [Testex]

Each of us is the result of the random throw of genetic dice. Created by genes, we become the vehicles that carry them over space and time. We think possessively about our genetic endowment; we have our mother's eyes or our father's nose. But perhaps the genes could be said to own us. Made of molecules of nucleic acids formed from a nitrogenous base, phosphoric acid, and a sugar into ladder-like strands of DNA, then tightly coiled and packed into chromosomes, genes control the cells we are made of. The three Master

Systems work together to move the genes that made us into the future.

The nervous system influences what Shakespeare called the "organs of increase," the genitalia, both external and internal. The brain, however, is the primary sexual organ. In the limbic system, just upstream from the endocrine system's hypothalamus, the amygdalae, which also create fear and rage, cause ejaculation or ovulation in some animals. Reward and pleasure centers in the limbic system make reproductive behavior attractive. The endocrine system's hypothalamus regulates the sex hormones that prepare sperm, egg, uterus, and breasts. It supports gestation and prepares the breasts to produce milk. At the end of birthing, the hypothalamus triggers the mother's bonding with the infant and the flow of milk. The immune system lets down its barriers in the woman to make pregnancy possible. The mucus created by the immune system as a barrier to protect against foreign invasion can help or hinder the sperm's path to the egg, depending on its viscosity. Pregnancy can take place only if the woman's immune system response is suppressed by the fertilized egg, which is, of course, a foreign substance to her body.

► SEX HORMONES

Sex hormones, both male and female, are steroids, oil-soluble molecules that slip through cell membranes and cause changes in the DNA of cells. All steroids tilt the body chemistry toward increased glucose and help to retain sodium in an effort to maintain life.

► THE SEX CYCLE

What is called the menstrual cycle is actually a reproductive or sex cycle. Menstruation only signals the end of the cycle. The negative feedback loop of the hypothalamus monitors gonadal production of hormones. In the female the drop in ovarian hormones causes the plush uterine lining that they created to deteriorate and shed. Sensing the low level of ovarian hormones in circulation, the hypothalamus sends down luteinizing hormone-releasing hormone (LHRH) to the pituitary. In response, the pituitary releases follicle-stimulating hormone (FSH) and luteinizing hormone (LH) into the bloodstream. FSH and LH lock into receptors in the ovarian cells; the ovaries respond by secreting estrogen and progesterone. Ova get larger. Layers of granulosa cells develop around the egg. The granulosa cell layers make progesterone. A capsule of theca cells develops and makes estrogen. About 20 of these follicles develop during a cycle. Estrogen-rich fluid fills the follicles and increases the number of FSH receptors on the granulosa

cells. After a week of growing, one follicle outpaces the rest while the other follicles begin to involute. Forty-eight hours before ovulation, LH and FSH levels surge. LH turns the granulosa and theca cells into lutein cells. Lutein cells secrete less estrogen and more progesterone. At this point enzymes dissolve the capsule wall (Fig. 13–1). Blood vessels form in the capsule walls; prostaglandins dilate the vessels; the follicle swells and ruptures, releasing the ovum. The empty follicle becomes a corpus luteum, secreting large amounts of progesterone and estrogen. In 5–7 days the corpus luteum involutes and becomes connective tissue. Even though LH is released by the pituitary, a still unknown local hormone delays luteinizing until after ovulation. The hypothalamus reads the high levels of estrogen and progesterone and does not send down releasing hormones to the pituitary.

When the corpus luteum degenerates after 12 days (26th day of the sex cycle), estrogen and progesterone levels drop. Without hormones to maintain it, the uterine lining sheds, causing menstruation and triggering the hy-

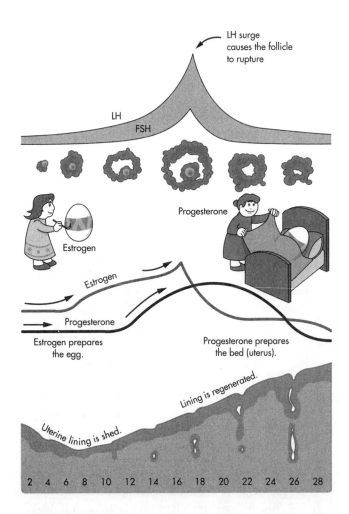

Figure 13–1. The sex cycle. LH = luteinizing hormone. FSH = follicle stimulating hormone.

pothalamus once more. If pregnancy does occur, the placenta will secrete a hormone, chorionic gonadotropin, which is very similar to LH, to keep the corpus luteum alive for 3–4 months longer.

FEMALE HORMONES

The female hormones of reproduction are estrogen, progesterone, and oxytocin. Estrogen develops the female form and prepares the egg. Progesterone prepares the bed (uterus). Oxytocin from the hypothalamus contracts the uterus to expel the fetus and let down milk.

Estrogen

Estrogen causes cell proliferation and thus the growth of tissues in the sex organs and breasts. In the fallopian tubes estrogen proliferates glandular tissue and increases the number of cilia as well as their fanning motion, which propels the fertilized ovum toward the uterus. Estrogen makes the breasts capable of producing milk, but other hormones complete the process. Estrogen makes bones grow rapidly by stimulating osteoblasts. It also helps the epiphyses join with the shafts of long bones, stopping growth in the female years before the male. Estrogen helps retain calcium and phosphate owing to its bone-growing ability. In protein building, estrogen is more selective than testosterone and is basically limited to organs of reproduction. It does create subcutaneous fatty deposits on thighs and buttocks. In creating the female shape, estrogen also makes skin soft and vascular.

The Forms of Estrogen

Estrogen is the most complex sex hormone, and testosterone is the least complex. Progesterone and testosterone are made first in the gonads and are then converted into estrogen. Of six different natural estrogens, three occur in significant amounts; beta-estradiol is 12 times more potent than estrone and 80 times more than estriol. The ovaries also produce testosterone, though only 1/15 as much as the testes do. The liver breaks down estrogens into glucuronides and sulfates, which go into bile or urine. Estrogen changes glucose metabolism, increases triglycerides, and decreases cholesterol and low-density lipoproteins. Estrogen tilts the body toward coagulation, increasing prothrombin and factors VII, IX, and X. However, estrogen protects women against heart attack, which is infrequent in nonsmoking women before menopause. Incidence of MI increases after menopause and eventually equals the rate in males.

THE FEMALE HORMONES AS DRUGS

Estrogen replacement during menopause relieves vaginal atrophy and "hot flashes" caused by vasomotor instability and conserves calcium and phosphorous to prevent the bone loss of osteoporosis. The hormone is also given to supplement or replace production in hypogonadism and oophorectomy. Estrogen is also used to counter excessive male hormones in women, as manifested by acne and hirsutism. Estrogen is a palliative in metastatic cancer of the breast (5 years postmenopausal) and in metastatic prostatic cancer. Some tumors are hormone dependent, but if receptors are blocked by a hormone slightly different in shape from the one the tumor needs, tumor growth process is slowed. Estrogen is sometimes given to male sex offenders in an attempt to curb unlawful sexual compulsions, though this use is debatable.

Estradiol [Climara, Estrace, Estraderm], estradiol cypionate [Depo-Estradiol Cypionate, others], estradiol valerate [Delestrogen, Dioval, others] are used to replace the missing hormone or for palliation in advanced prostatic carcinoma and in inoperable metastatic breast cancer in women at least 5 years postmenopause.

Drug Interactions: Decreased effect with barbiturates, phenytoin, rifampin. Increased hypoprothrombinemic effects with oral anticoagulants.

Side Effects

Nervous System: bloating, bowel—constipation/diarrhea/chorea, convulsions,* cramps—abdominal/leg, dizziness, headache/migraine, hypertension, nausea/vomiting, pain—abdominal, psyche—depression, sexual function—impotence/libido changes, vision—scotomas/astigmatism/myopia (worsened).

Endocrine System: (Pregnancy Category X) anorexia, appetite increase, breast secretions, carbohydrate tolerance—reduced, chloasma, edema, endometrial cystic hyperplasia, endometriosis—reactivation, folic acid deficiency, hair—hirsutism/loss, hyper—calcemia/glycemia, jaundice—cholestatic, mastodynia, menstrual changes, porphyria—acute/intermittent, premenstrual-like syndrome, weight changes. Males: feminization, gynecomastia, impotence, testicular atrophy.

Immune System: candidiasis—vaginal, cervical erosion, cervical secretions—altered, colitis, cystitis-like syndrome, dermatitis, existing fibromyomatas—increased size, hemolytic uremic syndrome, hepatoadenoma—benign, pancreatitis—acute, pruritus, seborrhea, thromboembolic disorders.* Injection site: flare/pain/sterile abscess.

Dosage: Menopause, atrophic vaginitis, kraurosis vulvae, female hypogonadism, female castration, primary ovarian failure: PO 1–2 mg/d in a cyclic regimen.

* Life-threatening side effect.

Topical: 2–4 g vaginal cream qd for 1–2 wk; then 1–2 g/d for 1–2 wk; then 1 g 1–3 ×/wk. Transdermal patch: Estraderm 2/wk. Climara q wk in cyclic regimen. IM. Cypionate: 1–5 mg once q3–4wk. Valerate: 10–25 mg once q4wk. Metastatic breast cancer: PO 10 mg tid. Prostatic cancer: PO 1–2 mg tid. Valerate: IM 30 mg once q1–2wk. Postpartum breast engorement: Valerate: IM 10–25 mg at end of first stage of labor.

Diethylstilbestrol (DES) is used to treat atrophic vaginitis, kraurosis vulvae, and abnormal bleeding, as well as female hypogonadism, primary ovarian failure, vasomotor symptoms associated with menopause, and as palliative therapy of prostatic carcinoma.

Drug Interactions: Decreased levels with carbamazepine, phenytoin, rifampin. Decreased anticoagulant effects with oral anticoagulants possible.

Side Effects

Nervous System: bloating, bowel—constipation/diarrhea, cramps—abdominal/leg, dizziness, headache, hypertension, nausea/vomiting, pain—abdominal, psyche—chronic depression, sexual function—libido changes, vision—intolerance to contacts/myopia (worsened).

Endocrine System: (Pregnancy Category X) anorexia, breakthrough bleeding, breast secretions, carbohydrate tolerance—reduced, chloasma, dysmenorrhea, edema, folic acid deficiency, gynecomastia, hair—hirsutism/loss, hyper—calcemia/glycemia, mastodynia, menstrual changes, weight changes.

Immune System: candidiasis—vaginal, erythema multiforme or nodosum, jaundice—cholestatic, thromboembolic disorders.*

Dosage: Breast carcinoma palliation: 15 mg/d. Prostate cancer: PO 1–3 mg/d; may increase for advanced cancers. Prostate carcinoma: PO 50 mg tid; may increase to 200 mg or more tid if tolerated. IV 0.5 g followed by 1 g/d for 5 or more days; then may reduce to 0.25–0.5 g 1–2 ×/week. Postcoital contraception: PO 25 mg bid within 72 h after intercourse and for 5 d.

Estrogens, conjugated [Premarin, Progens] are used to replace the missing hormone; to treat osteoporosis; as a palliative for breast and prostate carcinoma.

Off Label: postcoital contraceptive.

Drug Interactions: Decreased effect with barbiturates, phenytoin, rifampin. Increased hypoprothrombinemic effects with oral anticoagulants. Increased steroid effects with corticosteroids.

Side Effects

Nervous System: cramps—leg, dizziness, dysmenorrhea, headache, hypertension, nausea/vomiting, premenstrual tension, psyche—depression, sexual function—libido changes, vision—intolerance to contact lenses.

Endocrine System: (Pregnancy Category X) amenorrhea, carbohydrate tolerance—reduced, dysmenorrhea, fluid retention, gall stones, menstrual flow—changes/spotting.

Immune System: clotting disorders,* estrogen-dependent tumor, liver cancer.

Dosage: Breast cancer: PO 10 mg tid for at least 3 mo. Female hypogonadism: PO 2.5–7.5 mg qd–tid for 20 d. Stop for 10 days. If no bleeding by the end of 10 days, resume schedule. If bleeding does occur start a 20-d estrogen-progestin cyclic regimen of conjugated estrogens: 2.5–7.5 mg qd in divided doses. Add progestin to regimen for last 5 d. If bleeding begins before end of regimen DC and resume on day 5 of bleeding to start new cycle. Menopause, osteoporosis, atrophic vaginitis, kraurosis vulvae: PO 0.3–1.25 mg/d for 21 d q mo; adjust to lowest dose for symptom control. IM, IV 25 mg; repeat in 6–12 h if needed. Topical 2–4 g of cream/d. Postcoital contraception: PO 30 mg/d in divided doses for 5 consecutive days beginning within 72 h of coitus. Palliation of prostatic cancer: PO 1.25–2.5 mg tid.

Estrogens, esterified [Estratab, Menest, Menrium] are used to replace missing hormone and for palliatiation therapy in breast and prostatic carcinoma.

Drug Interactions: Decreased effect with carbamazepine, phenytoin, rifampin. Increased steroid effects with corticosteroids possible. Decreased anticoagulant effect of oral anticoagulants.

Side Effects

Nervous System: bloating, bowel—diarrhea, cramps—leg, dizziness, headache, hypertension, nausea/vomiting, psyche—depression, sexual function—libido changes, vision—intolerance to contact lenses.

Endocrine System: (Pregnancy Category X) amenorrhea, bloating, carbohydrate tolerance—reduced, fluid retention, cholestatic jaundice, mastodynia.

Immune System: clotting disorders.*

Dosage: Female hypogonadism, primary ovarian failure, female castration: PO 2.5–7.5 mg/d in 1–3 divided doses for 20 d followed by 10 d rest period. Give PO progesterone during last 5 d of estrogen. Breast cancer: PO 10 mg tid × 2–3 mo. Prostate cancer: PO 1.25–2.5 mg tid × 3 wk.

---

* Life-threatening side effect.

Estrone aqueous suspension [Estronol, Kestrone-5, Theelin Aqueous], estrogenic substance aqueous suspension [Estroject-2] is used to treat atrophic vaginitis, kraurosis vulvae, and abnormal bleeding, as well as female hypogonadism, primary ovarian failure, vasomotor symptoms associated with menopause, and as palliative therapy of prostatic carcinoma.

Drug Interactions: Decreased levels with carbamazepine, phenytoin, rifampin. Increased steroid effects of corticosteroids possible. Decreased anticoagulant effects with oral anticoagulants possible.

Side Effects

Nervous System: diarrhea, dizziness, hypertension, leg cramps, nausea/vomiting, psyche—depression, sexual function—libido changes.

Endocrine System: (Pregnancy Category X) bloating, carbohydrate tolerance—reduced, mastodynia, menstrual flow changes, spotting.

Immune System: cholestatic jaundice, clotting disorders.*

Dosage: Female hypogonadism, primary ovarian failure: IM 0.1–0.5 mg 2–3 ×/wk. Menopause: IM 0.1–0.5 mg 2–3 ×/wk. Palliation of inoperable prostatic cancer: IM 2–4 mg/d 2–3 ×/wk.

Estropipate [Ogen] is used to treat atrophic vaginitis, kraurosis vulvae, and abnormal bleeding, as well as female hypogonadism, primary ovarian failure, vasomotor symptoms associated with menopause, and as palliative therapy of prostatic carcinoma.

Drug Interactions: Decreased levels with carbamazepine, phenytoin, rifampin. Increased steroid effects of corticosteroids possible. Decreased anticoagulant effects with oral anticoagulants possible.

Side Effects

Nervous System: cramps—legs, dizziness, dysmenorrhea, headache, hypertension, nausea/vomiting, psyche—depression, sexual function—libido changes, vision—intolerance to contact lenses.

Endocrine System: (Pregnancy Category X) carbohydrate tolerance reduction, dysmenorrhea, mastodynia, menstrual flow changes.

Immune System: clotting disorders.*

Dosage: Female hypogonadism, primary ovarian failure, female castration: PO 1.5–9 mg/d in 1–3 divided doses for 21 d, follow with a 8–10 d drug-free period.

Menopause, atrophic vaginitis, kraurosis vulvae: PO 0.75–6 mg/d × 21 d qmo. Adjust to lowest dose possible. Intravaginal 2–4 g of cream qd in a cyclic regimen.

Progesterone

Progesterone, the major progestin, is broken down in minutes into other steroids by the liver. Ten percent is excreted by the kidneys. Progesterone helps make the endometrium more hospitable to the fertilized ovum so that it can implant. The corpus luteum produces most of the progesterone, but some is also made by the adrenals. After the fourth month of pregnancy, the placenta produces 10 times more progesterone than the corpus luteum. Progestins, via the negative feedback loop, signal the hypothalamus and the pituitary to stop releasing luteinizing hormones to the ovary. In the fallopian tubes progesterone helps create secretions to nourish the fertilized ovum before it implants. It helps breast lobules and alveoli develop, and the alveoli to secrete. However, it does not trigger milk letdown. That is the job of oxytocin. Progesterone has a protein catabolic effect as it breaks down protein from the mother's body for the fetus to use. Progestins can masculinize a fetus. They also are not for use in breast cancer and vaginal bleeding of unknown cause, or in patients with a tendency to form thrombi. In clinical application, progesterone helps regulate sex cycles, treats endometriosis, helps prevent threatened abortion in some forms of infertility, and it may help prevent endometrial cancer when used in replacement therapy with estrogen.

Medroxyprogesterone acetate [Amen, Cycrin, Depo-Provera, Provera] is used to treat nonovulating amenorrhea when there is estrogen production. It is given IM (after a pregnancy test) to cause endometrial growth, which is then sloughed off in a week's time as withdrawal bleeding. It is not used in breast cancer and vaginal bleeding of unknown cause or in patients with a tendency to form thrombi. The dosages are greater for such conditions as endometriosis, endometrial hyperplasia, palliative treatment of advanced or metastatic endometrial cancer, and to suppress menstruation in women at risk of hemorrhage when chemotherapy destroys platelets. As a contraceptive it interferes with cervical mucus and egg implantation and can suppress ovulation.

Off Label: Obstructive sleep apnea.

Drug Interactions: none noted.

Side Effects

Nervous System: cramps—abdominal, hypertension, nausea/vomiting, psyche—depression.

Endocrine System: (Pregnancy Category X) amenorrhea, breakthrough bleeding, breast changes/tenderness, edema, menstrual flow changes, weight changes.

---

* Life-threatening side effect.

Immune System: angioedema,* cholestatic jaundice, pulmonary embolism,* cerebral thrombosis*/hemorrhage, vaginal candidiasis.

Dosage: Secondary amenorrhea: PO 5–10 mg/d for 5–10 d any time after the endometrium is adequately estrogen primed; withdrawal bleeding starts 3–7 d after discontinuing therapy. Abnormal bleeding caused by hormone imbalance: PO 5–10 mg for 5–10 d beginning on the 16th or 21st calculated day of the sex cycle; if bleeding is controlled, administer 2 subsequent cycles. Carcinoma: IM 400–1000 mg/wk; continue at 400 mg/mo if improvement occurs and disease stabilizes. Contraception: IM 100 mg q3mo.

Norethindrone [Micronor, Norlutin, Nor-Q.D.] is used for hormone imbalance resulting in amenorrhea or abnormal bleeding and for endometriosis.

Drug Interactions: none noted.

Side Effects

Nervous System: cramps—abdominal, dysmenorrhea, hypertension, nausea/vomiting.

Endocrine System: (Pregnancy Category X) breakthrough bleeding, dysmenorrhea, edema, menstrual flow changes.

Immune System: cholestatic jaundice, pulmonary embolism,* cerebral thrombosis*/hemorrhage.

Dosage: Amenorrhea: PO 5–20 mg day 5 through day 25 of the cycle. Endometriosis: PO 10 mg/d for 2 wk; increase by 5 mg/d q2wk up to 30 mg/d; remain at this dose for 6–9 mo or until breakthrough bleeding.

Progesterone [Gesterol 50, Progestaject, Progestasert] is used to treat secondary amenorrhea, functional uterine bleeding, endometriosis, and premenstrual syndrome. In combination with estrogens for birth control.

Drug Interactions: none noted.

Side Effects

Nervous System: cramps—abdominal, dizziness, dysmenorrhea, fatigue/lethargy, headache—migraine, insomnia/somnolence, nausea/vomiting, psyche—depression, sexual function—decreased libido, vision—changes/diplopia/proptosis. Injection site: pain.

Endocrine System: (Pregnancy Category X) amenorrhea, breakthrough bleeding, cervical secretion changes, chloasma, cholestatic jaundice, dysmenorrhea, edema, excretion increase (transient)—sodium/chloride, fever, galactorrhea, gynecomastia, hair—hirsutism/loss, hyperglycemia, weight changes.

Immune System: acne, allergic rash, cervical erosion, clotting disorders,* hepatic disease, pulmonary emboli,* pruritus vulvae, retinal vascular lesions, urticaria, vaginal candidiasis, vision—papilledema/retinal vascular lesions.

Dosage: Amenorrhea: IM 5–10 mg for 6–8 d. Intrauterine contraceptive: Intrauterine insert in uterus for 1 y. Premenstrual syndrome: Rectal: 200–400 mg/d. Uterine bleeding: IM 5–10 mg/d for 6 d.

▶ HORMONE CONTRACEPTIVES

Because human reproduction has been enormously successful, with more than 5 billion humans now living, birth control is now more important than ever before. Oral contraceptives have proven successful in family planning. They are more convenient to use than mechanical devices and more reliable than any other method. Because so many companies manufacture hormone contraceptives, the trade names will not be listed in detail. A general overview of the actions of the two categories should suffice.

The hormone combinations suppress FSH and LH and thus prevent ovulation. They also make the cervical mucus less slippery and the endometrium less hospitable, impeding sperm and ultimate implantation. The hormonal form of birth control is safer than pregnancy and childbirth unless the woman smokes and is over 40.

Drug Interactions: The combination-hormone contraceptives can interfere with the effectiveness of anticonvulsants, tricyclic antidepressants, drugs for hypertension, sulfonylureas, warfarin, vitamins. May increase lorazepam, oxazepam metabolism. Decreased effectiveness of the combination-hormone contraceptives and breakthrough bleeding possible with analgesics, including drugs for migraines, antibiotics such as penicillin V, barbiturates, chloramphenicol, isoniazid, neomycin, phenytoin, rifampin, sulfonamides, tetracycline, major and minor tranquilizers.

Side Effects

Nervous System: CAD, headache, hypertension, vision—disturbances/even loss of vision.

Endocrine System: gallbladder disease, impaired glucose metabolism, pregnancy.

Immune System: CVA,* clotting disorders,* embolism,* gynecologic tumors, liver disease, neoplasms, UTIs.

▶ THE THREE TYPES OF COMBINATION HORMONAL BIRTH CONTROL

Combination oral contraceptives consist of three different strategies. Monophasic: In this group the dosages of

---

* Life-threatening side effect.

estrogen and progesterone are the same throughout the cycle. Biphasic: Estrogen dosage is unchanged through the cycle, but progesterone dosage is increased in the second half of the cycle to mimic normal proliferation and secretory phases. Triphasic: Estrogen dosage may remain the same or vary during the cycle. The progesterone amount varies. The dosage varies, with some packets having placebo pills so that the woman takes a pill every night. Other packets require the woman to take all the pills in sequence, to stop after the last one (20 or 21), and to begin again in one week.

PROGESTIN-ONLY ORAL CONTRACEPTIVES

The progestin-only BC pills make conditions unfavorable for sperm and for egg implantation. Sometimes they can also suppress ovulation. Though these pills have many of the same side effects as the combination pills, they can often be used by women who suffer from hypertension, migraines, PMT, and edema. (See Medroxyprogesterone acetate [Depo-Provera] in this chapter).

TOCOLYTICS

Tocolytics inhibit uterine contractions to prevent premature birth. They lock into beta-2 uterine smooth muscle receptors (and bronchial smooth muscle, too). The muscles relax. Tocolytics are not used if the fetus has died or is less than 20 weeks; if membranes have raptured; if there is eclampsia or severe preeclampsia or hemorrhage (must deliver); or if there is infection or other conditions such as pulmonary hypertension, cardiac arrhythmias, or asthma requiring beta adrenergics and glucocorticoids. The latter may cause pulmonary edema. This is a potential emergency and may require ICU for mother and child. Surgery may also be necessary.

Ritodrine hydrochloride [Yutopar] is used to manage premature labor in selected patients.

Drug Interactions: Possible pulmonary edema with corticosteroids. Increased cardiovascular adverse effects with beta agonists. Decreased effects of both ritodrine and beta blockers.

Side Effects

Nervous System: arrhythmias—various, maternal BP—altered, bowel—constipation/diarrhea/ileus, drowsiness, dyspnea, epigastric distress, headache, maternal and fetal heart rates—altered, hyperventilation, malaise, nausea/vomiting, pain—chest, palpitations, psyche—anxiety/nervousness, restlessness, tremors, weakness.

Endocrine System: (Pregnancy Category C) chills, glycosuria, hyperglycemia, hypokalemia, sweating.

Immune System: anaphylaxis,* pulmonary edema,* myotonic and muscular dystrophy, rash.

Dosage: PO. Start 30 min before terminating infusion; 10 mg q2h for first 24 h, then 10–20 mg q4–6h to maximum of 120 mg/d. IV 50–100 µg/min; may increase by 50 µg q10min until uterine relaxation is achieved; may continue for up to 12 h after contractions have ceased.

OXYTOCIN

Oxytocin from the posterior hypothalamus causes uterine contractions, starts or reinforces labor, and stimulates milk letdown. By contracting the uterus, oxytocin can help control postpartum hemorrhage. It can help induce or complete abortion. Oxytocin is also used to induce labor in maternal diabetes, preeclampsia, eclampsia, and erythroblastosis fetalis.

Oxytocin injection [Pitocin, Syntocinon, Syntocinon Nasal Spray] is used to initiate or improve uterine contractions at term. It stimulates milk letdown or relieves breast engorgement and controls postpartum hemorrhage and enhances postpartum uterine involution. It is also used to induce labor in maternal diabetes, erythroblastosis fetalis, preeclampsia, and eclampsia.

Drug Interactions: Severe hypertension with vasoconstrictors. Hypotension, maternal bradycardia, arrhythmias with cyclopropane anesthesia.

Side Effects

Nervous System: arrhythmias—ECG changes/PVCs, BP—hypertensive episodes/hypotension, cardiovascular spasm*/collapse,* cyanosis/redness, dyspnea, headache, nausea/vomiting, pain—precordial, psyche—anxiety, uterus—hypertonicity/tetanic contractions/rupture.* Fetus: bradycardia and other arrhythmias, death,* hypoxia, intracranial hemorrhage,* neonatal jaundice, trauma from too rapid expulsion.

Endocrine System: (Pregnancy Category X) ADH—severe water intoxication/hyponatremia.

Immune System: anaphylaxis,* blood flow—increase, fatal afibrinogenemia,* hematoma—pelvic, hemorrhage—postpartum/subarachnoid,* irritation—peribuccal.

Dosage: Induce labor: IV drip 1 mU/min; gradually increase by 1 mU/min q15min to maximum of 20 mU/min. Postpartum bleeding: IV drip 10 U in 1 L nonhydrating solution at rate to control uterine atony. Milk letdown: Nasal: 1 spray into one or both nares 2–3 min before emptying breasts.

---

* Life-threatening side effect.

Methylergonovine maleate [Methergine] is an ergot derivative that acts like oxytocin and is used to treat or prevent hemorrhage postpartum or after abortion when the uterus loses tonus and cannot contract.

Drug Interactions: Increased pressor effects and possible hypertension with parenteral sympathomimetics and other ergot alkaloids.

Side Effects

Nervous System: bowel—diarrhea, bradycardia, severe hypertensive episodes* (CVA), nausea/vomiting (with IV), tingling of toes and fingers, shock.*

Endocrine System: (Pregnancy Category C) thirst.

Immune System: allergic shock.*

Dosage: Prevent postpartum hemorrhage: IM, IV 0.2 mg q2–4h to maximum of 5 doses; then PO 0.2–0.4 mg q6–12h to maintain tonus to maximum of 1 wk.

▶ DRUGS TO TREAT INFERTILITY

The treatment of infertility begins with the search for the cause of infertility. Is the cause in the brain's production and release of releasing and stimulating hormones of the brains or in the gonads of the partners? What are the immune factors? If the mates are too close genetically, the fertilized egg cannot repel the mother's immune system strongly enough to gestate, and the mother will abort. The latter probably helps prevent inbreeding. Have infections or anatomy created obstructions in passages? When the cause is hormonal, the goal is to induce ovulation. Drugs to induce ovulation can cause multiple births, and the woman must be warned of this.

Bromocriptine mesylate [Parlodel] is used in Parkinson's disease to stimulate dopamine receptors in the corpus striatum; however, dopamine is also an important neurotransmitter in the hypothalamus, and stimulation of dopamine receptors there block prolactin release. Thus, bromocriptine can help treat the infertility resulting from increased prolactin release. In addition to infertility, bromocriptine can be used to help treat amenorrhea and galactorrhea.

Drug Interactions: Decreased alcohol tolerance possible. Increased hypotensive effects with antihypertensive agents. Decreased effect with oral contraceptives estrogen, progestins possible, causing amenorrhea and galactorrhea. Increased prolactin with phenothiazines. Tricyclic antidepressants, methyldopa, reserpine may interfere with bromocriptine activity.

Side Effects

Nervous System: exacerbation of angina, asthenia, constipation, dizziness, dyskinesia, dysphagia, fainting, fatigue, headache, hypotension—postural, intermittent ischemia of the extremities, acute MI,* nausea/vomiting, pain—epigastric, palpitations, psyche—anxiety/depression/mania/nervousness/nightmares, sedation, shock,* metallic taste, vision—blepharospasms/blurred/burning sensation in eyes/blepharospasms/diplopia.

Endocrine System: (Pregnancy Category C) anorexia, dry mouth,

Immune System: rash, urticaria, extremities—edematous/hot/red/tender, nasal congestion, peptic ulcers.

Dosage: Amenorrhea, galactorrhea, female infertility: PO 1.25–2.5 mg/d 2.5 mg bid or tid. Suppression of postpartum lactation: PO 2.5 mg bid starting 4 h postpartum for 14–21 d.

Note: Padding a bra with sanitary pads to create a tight fit will also suppress lactation, and without medication.

Note: For infertility get a pregnancy test if menses does not occur within 3 days of due date and stop the medication.

Menotropins (follicular stimulating hormone, FSH, luteinizing hormone, LH) [Pergonal] is used to stimulate follicle growth when the pituitary fails to stimulate ovulation; however, menotropins can be deadly if the ovaries are overstimulated and suddenly enlarge. Cysts can rupture, causing hemorrhage into the peritoneum.

Drug Interactions: none noted.

Side Effects

Nervous System: bowel—diarrhea, nausea/vomiting.

Endocrine System: (Pregnancy Category X) multiple births, ruptured cysts,* birth defects, hypovolemia,* multiple ovulations, ovarian hyperstimulation* (with ascites and possible pleural effusion).

Immune System: embolism, febrile allergic reaction, hemoperitoneum.

Dosage: For ovulation: IM 1 ampule daily for 9–12 d. For spermatogenesis: after HCG IM 1 ampule 3× wk ×4–6 mo. May increase to 2 ampules 3× wk.

Human chorionic gonadotropin (HCG) [Antuitrin, A.P.L., Chorex, Chorigon, Choron 10, Corgonject-5, Follutein, Glukor, Gonic, HCG, Pregnyl, Profasi HP] is used for prepubertal cryptorchidism without obstruction, for male hypogonadism due to pituitary deficiency, and, with menotropins, to induce ovulation in treating infertility.

Drug Interactions: none noted.

---

* Life-threatening side effect.

Side Effects

Nervous System: fatigue, headache, psyche—depression/irritability/restlessness.

Endocrine System: (Pregnancy Category X) ectopic pregnancy,* edema, increased urinary steroid excretion. With menotropins: ascites, multiple births, ovarian hyperstimulation,* pleural effusion.

Immune System: arterial thromboembolism.*

Dosage: Prepubertal cryptorchidism (child): 4000 U 3 ×/wk for 3 wk, or 5000 U qod for 4 doses, or 500–1000 U 3 ×/wk for 4–6 wk. Hypogonadotropic hypogonadism: IM 500–1000 U 3 ×/wk for 3 wk; then 2 ×/wk for 3 wk or 4000 U 3 ×/wk for 6–9 mo followed by 2000 U 3 ×/wk for 3 mo. Stimulation of spermatogenesis: IM 5000 U 3 ×/wk until normal testosterone levels are achieved (4–6 mo), then 2000 U 2 ×/wk with menotropins for 4 mo. Induction of ovulation: IM 500–1000 U when the follicles ripen 1 d after last dose of menotropins to mimic the natural LH surge that triggers ovulation.

Note: The process is repeated if no pregnancy results after ovulation. The dose is doubled if the woman does not ovulate in response to the lower dosage.

Clomiphene citrate [Clomid] is another drug used to induce ovulation. Clomiphene antagonizes estrogen, interfering with the negative feedback to the hypothalamus. In response to a perceived drop in estrogen, the hypothalamus and pituitary respond by stimulating the ovaries.

Off Label: Male infertility, gynecomastia, fibrocystic breast disease, menstrual abnormalities, regulation of cycles in patients using rhythm method of contraception, endometrial hyperplasia, persistent lactation.

Drug Interactions: none noted.

Side Effects

Nervous System: bladder—urgency/frequency, fatigue, headache, insomnia, nausea/vomiting, psyche—depression, vasomotor instability, vertigo, vision disturbances.

Endocrine System: (Pregnancy Category X) spontaneous abortion, increased appetite/weight gain, breast tenderness, hair loss, ovarian cysts, ovarian failure, vaginal dryness. Fetus: congenital deformities.

Immune System: bleeding—vaginal, dermatitis.

Dosage: PO 50 mg qd for 5 d; repeat for two cycles if needed.

---

* Life-threatening side effect.

If ovulation still does not occur, give double the dose for 5 d. Pregnancy usually occurs within 6 mo.

▶ TESTOSTERONE: THE MALE HORMONE

Testosterone causes the male form to develop and spurs production of sperm cells. Like the glucocorticoids—aldosterone, estrogen, and progesterone—testosterone is a steroid, and steroids tilt the body toward increased sodium retention and increased glucose levels. Without the randomness of the male's genetic contribution, each infant would be the mother's clone and vulnerable to the same disease hazards. The reason for males is to ensure a species' genetic variety and the hardiness of its genetic stock. Chromosomes XX equal a female. Chromosomes XY equal a male. Genes in the Y chromosome trigger the placenta's hormone, chorionic gonadotropin (similar to LH), to develop interstitial or Leydig cells in the fetal testes. In response, the fetal testes secrete testosterone, causing growth of the penis, scrotum, prostate, seminal vesicles, and seminiferous tubules, and suppressing female development. In the seventh month of gestation, the testes move into the scrotum. From birth to puberty little testosterone is secreted. At puberty testosterone enlarges the male sex organs, makes body hair grow (in females too), and causes increased skin oil and acne. In response to testosterone, protein anabolism develops the muscles. Bones get bigger. Testosterone as dihydrotestosterone enters cells and causes the cells to produce protein. LH from the pituitary stimulates sperm production. FSH starts the conversion of primary spermatocytes. Testosterone completes the conversion. The rate of testosterone production is based on the negative feedback of testosterone levels building up to suppress the production of LHRH in the hypothalamus. Without LHRH, the pituitary will not produce FSH. Male hormones are called androgens, from the word *andro,* meaning "man."

Anabolic steroids are now Schedule III Controlled Drugs, due to abuse by men who use them to build up their bodies. These steroids are made synthetically and used therapeutically to treat males for hypogonadism. In prepuberty this treatment develops secondary sex traits such as a deeper voice and facial and body hair. Postpuberty use helps to maintain or reestablish those traits, in addition to increasing sperm and treating impotence and cryptorchidism. In women, the anabolic steroids are used to treat estrogen-dependent breast cancer. Because anabolic steroids build tissue, they can be used in catabolic or wasting conditions, such as trauma and burns, and in debilitating disease where the body has tipped over into a negative nitrogen balance.

Danazol [Danocrine] is a synthetic androgen that suppresses FSH and LH, resulting in anovulation and associated amenorrhea. It is used for endometriosis when other therapies haven't worked or cannot be used, and for fibrocystic breast disease and hereditary angioedema.

Off Label: Used to treat precocious puberty, gynecomastia, menorrhagia, premenstrual syndrome, chronic immune thrombocytopenic purpura, autoimmune hemolytic anemia, hemophilia A and B.

Drug Interactions: none noted.

Side Effects

Nervous System: BP—elevated, dizziness, fatigue, headache, psyche—emotional lability/irritability/nervousness, sexual function—libido decrease, sleep disorders, tremors, voice—deepening/pitch breaks/weakness.

Endocrine System: (Pregnancy Category C) amenorrhea, breast-size decrease, edema, hot flushes, glucose tolerance—impaired, hair—hirsutism/loss, HDL decrease, LDL increase, menstrual patterns—irregular, skin/hair—oily, sweating, vision—conjunctival edema, weight gain.

Immune System: acne, congestion—nasal, gastroenteritis, hepatic damage,* rash, swelling/lock-up—joints, vaginitis—bleeding/burning/drying/itching.

Dosage: Do pregnancy test first or start during menstruation. Fibrocystic breast disease: PO 100–400 mg divided bid up to 6 mo. Endometriosis: PO 400 mg bid up to 6 mo. Hereditary angioedema: PO. Start with 200 mg bid–tid; if results are good, decrease by half or less over 1- to 3-month intervals according to the patient's need.

Note: Angioedema is a potentially deadly form of edema, especially of the face and neck, with the capability of closing the airway.

Finasteride [Propecia] is used to treat male pattern hair loss in men only. It is shown to be safe in men between 18 and 41 y of age with mild to moderate hair loss of the vertex and anterior mid-scalp area; however, pregnant women or women who may potentially be pregnant must not handle crushed or broken tablets or ingest finasteride owing to the potential risk of abnormalities to the external genitalia of male fetuses. Finasteride inhibits steroid type II 5α-reductase, an intracellular enzyme that converts the androgen testosterone into 5α-dihydrotestosterone (DHT).

Drug Interactions: None noted.

Side Effects

Nervous System: erectile dysfunction, decreased libido.

Endocrine System: (Pregnancy Category X) decreased volume of ejaculate.

Immune System: none noted.

---

* Life-threatening side effect.

Dosage: PO 1 mg qd.

Nilutamide [Nilandron] is an androgen specific for treating cancer. See Chapter 17.

Testosterone [Andro 100, Histerone, Testoderm], testosterone cypionate [Andro-Cyp, Andronate, depAndro, Depo-Testosterone, Depotest, Duratest], testosterone enanthate [Andro L.A., Delatest, Delatestryl, Everone, Testone L.A., Testrin PA], testosterone propionate [Testex], a Schedule III drug, is used for hormone replacement in delayed male puberty; it is also palliative for female breast cancer (1–5 y postmenopausal) and postpartum breast engorgement. It is available in fixed combination with estrogens in many preparations.

Drug Interactions: Increased hypoprothrombinemia with oral anticoagulants possible. Decreased insulin requirement possible.

Side Effects

Nervous System: bowel—diarrhea, insomnia, nausea/vomiting, pain—gastric, psyche—excitation, sexual function—impotence/libido increase/priapism.

Endocrine System: (Pregnancy Category X) anorexia, edema, flushing, hyper—calcemia/cholesterolemia/natremia, acute intermittent porphyria, renal calculi, retention—sodium/water (especially in the elderly), female and prepubescent male virilization. Hypoestrogenic female: flushing, menstrual irregularities, sweating. Prolonged use: decreased virilization.

Immune System: acne, anaphylaxis,* bladder irritability, leukopenia. Hypoestrogenic female: vaginitis with bleeding/drying/pruritus. Injection site: irritation/sloughing.

Dosage: Male hypogonadism: IM 10–25 mg 2–3 ×/wk. Propionate: 10–25 mg 3 ×/wk. Cypionate, enanthate: 50–400 mg q2–4 wk. Topical: 6 mg/d; if scrotum is inadequate, use 4 mg/d system. Delayed puberty: IM. Cypionate, enanthate: 50–200 mg q2–4wk. Metastatic breast cancer: IM. Short-acting testosterone: 50–100 mg 3 ×/wk. Cypionate, enanthate: 200–400 mg q2–4wk. Propionate: 100 mg 3 ×/wk. Postpartum breast engorgement: IM 25–50 mg/d for 3–4 d, Propionate: 25–50 mg/d for 3–4 d.

 Chapter Highlights

- The sex hormones are steroids used to replace missing hormones, prevent unwanted pregnancy, and enhance conception.

- The male hormones are also used as palliation for some hormone-dependent cancers in women.

- Estrogen may be used in treating hormone-dependent cancer in men.

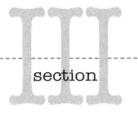

section **III**

The Immune System and Drugs

The immune system protects and defends the body in the constant battle to survive against the competition for life in the food chain. Life is full of potential for disease and injury in this great crowd of microscopic competition, because, as large as we are, we are still part of life's food chain. Not all threats to human life have teeth and claws. Most of them cannot even be seen by the unaided eye as they teem on familiar objects, lurk in food, swirl in the air, and live on our skin and mucous membranes.

Infectious and parasitic diseases result in about 17.5 million deaths annually, more deaths than any human war has ever caused in 1 year. Billions of humans suffer from infections of viruses, bacteria, and parasites. For example, two billion are infected with hepatitis B. Yearly, over two hundred million new sexually transmitted disease (STD) infections occur. Intestinal worms, though not necessarily microbial, infest billions of people. And even though new drugs are under scrutiny for HIV, the disease looms large in the future.

The immune system evolved out of this ancient, never-ending war, this constant combat for survival at the level of cellular life. Holistically, it works in tandem with the endocrine and the nervous systems. In its "take-no-prisoners" approach to infection, it creates much of the misery and suffering experienced as fever, pain, inflammation, swelling, coryza, and rashes.

▶ THE IMMUNE RESPONSE: ALWAYS PROPORTIONATE TO THE TRAUMA

The response of the immune system is always in proportion to the trauma or infection. A WBC will normally increase to a degree that reflects the extent of trauma suffered in any damage to the body, from a bone fracture to

an infection. The amount of redness and swelling around a localized infection will indicate the extent of the infection: Viruses and bacteria, however, develop strategies to counter the immune defenses. For example, while the staphylococcus bacterium, with its lethal toxins, triggers a rapid immune response, streptococcus slips into the body in small numbers and spreads without toxins, entrenching itself in and damaging vital organs like the heart or the kidneys before the immune system can respond.

▶ AUTOIMMUNE DISEASE

Sometimes the immune system is our own worst enemy. Diseases once thought to occur for other reasons are now seen, at least in part, as the result of the immune system's misdirected attack on the body when intracellular proteins become exposed to the immune system and the system responds by attacking the organ or structures involved. Diabetes mellitus type I, for example, seems to begin as an autoimmune disorder. What follows is a list of other autoimmune disorders and the involved organs or tissues:

- Addison's disease: adrenal gland.
- autoimmune hemolytic anemia: red blood cell membrane protein.
- Crohn's disease: gut.
- Goodpasture's syndrome: kidneys and lungs.
- Graves' disease: thyroid.
- Hashimoto's thyroiditis: thyroid.
- idiopathic thrombocytopenic purpura: platelets.
- lupus erythematosus: kidneys, nervous system, platelets, and, skin.
- multiple sclerosis: brain and spinal cord.
- myasthenia gravis: nerve and muscle synapses.
- pemphigus vulgaris: skin.

- pernicious anemia: gastric parietal cells.
- poststreptococcal glomerulonephritis: kidney.
- psoriasis: skin.
- rheumatoid arthritis: connective tissue.
- scleroderma: heart, gut, lungs, and kidney.
- Sjögren's syndrome: brain, kidney, liver, salivary glands, and thyroid.
- spontaneous infertility: sperm.

The culprit suspected of playing a role in exposing proteins to the immune system in such cases may often be viral.

▶ NOSOCOMIAL INFECTIONS

Clinics and hospitals contain some of the most virulent microbes, and sometimes otherwise healthy patients can be infected during therapeutic procedures. Such events are referred to as nosocomial infections. If the patient's immune system is strong enough, it can usually deal with the infection, but the weak, debilitated patient may not be able to cast off a nosocomial infection. Many medical and most surgical procedures may cause some trauma in the process of being therapeutic and also trigger the immune response. Interventions that present the risk of infection must be done with care to prevent damage and infection.

▶ DRUGS OF THE IMMUNE SYSTEM

The drugs used in this Master System either help the immune system fight disease and injury; relieve some of the distressing symptoms caused when the immune system engages the enemy; or suppress the immune response. The science of pharmacology has harnessed microbes to help the immune system, for example, in producing antibiotics and vaccines. Drugs counter or encourage clotting. Drugs can help loosen or eliminate mucus, when it fails to protect. Drugs from the nervous and endocrine systems can be used to tamp down or prevent destruction to self from a misguided immune system. Although drugs are meant to be therapeutic, if they cause changes in the cells' DNA, they have the potential to inhibit the immune system by suppressing bone marrow production in the cells that fight infection. Drugs as old and safe as phenytoin or as new as the ACE inhibitors can suppress the immune system's production of blood cells, a potentially deadly condition called agranulocytosis. Symptoms of damage to the immune system in agranulocytosis from drug therapy can include sore throat and bruising. Some drugs can also trigger the swift, deadly, and misguided anaphylaxis. The allergic response to drug therapy poses an immediate danger with circulatory collapse and airway obstruction in anaphylaxis. The catecholamines of the nervous system and the glucocorticoids of the endocrine system can save lives when the immune system flares up against a medication. Some drug therapies intentionally suppress the immune system. Chemotherapy for cancer, corticosteroids for inflammatory conditions, and immunosuppressants for organ transplant all put the patient at risk for lack of protection from the impaired immune system. And in this age of AIDS, opportunistic infections have an added edge. Administering drugs requires constant awareness and assessment of the patient's immune system's response to drug therapy.

▶ THE THREE MASTER SYSTEMS AND INFECTION AND TRAUMA

The three Master Systems are linked in the struggle for life. The struggle to survive infection or trauma takes a toll, not only on the immune system, but also on the emotions. The resulting stress raises the cortisol output of the endocrine system. The nurse's assessment, intervention, evaluation, and patient education regarding infection and trauma must always take into account all three Master Systems. Just as the immune response is always proportionate to the damage, the emotional response to infection or trauma is proportionate to the event and can range from mere annoyance to terror. The patient may withdraw in denial or try to scare away the threat with anger and rage. It is a mistake to say that humans "overreact" emotionally. We react to danger in a response that includes our history, our present condition, and the enormity of the trauma as we sense it. Fear can kill. Sometimes timely patient education can fill in gaps and reduce the fear.

▶ PREGNANCY AND THE IMMUNE SYSTEM

Pregnancy, though natural and normal, constitutes the invasion of the female by a foreign organism, the developing embryo. Conception suppresses the maternal immune response in a way not yet fully understood. Interestingly, sometimes maternal antibodies do destroy and reject the embryo when, oddly, the embryo too closely matches the mother's genetic makeup. Perhaps this is a function to prevent inbreeding. The exception to the rule of suppression of the maternal immune system occurs when an Rh negative mother becomes sensitized to Rh positive blood and aborts subsequent Rh positive pregnancies. Scientists are studying the phenomenon of immune suppression during pregnancy to see how it might be used therapeutically in other conditions.

▶ HOW THE IMMUNE SYSTEM FUNCTIONS

The immune system is comprised of many lesser systems with specific tasks all aimed at protecting the body. The systems within the immune system include cells of the myeloid and lymphoid branches of the pluripotent stem cells in bone marrow, which flow freely within their circulatory routes on guard against invasion or injury. The complement system, chemotaxis, clotting, and mucus constitute other elements of the immune system.

▶ BONE MARROW AND THE IMMUNE SYSTEM

The cells of the immune system are blood cells, the wandering offspring of bone marrow, which itself originally wandered to the bone from the fetal liver. All immune system cells descend from one type of cell, the pluripotent stem cell. From this primary cell come the two major branches of the immune system's cellular defense, the myeloid and the lymphoid.

▶ THE IMMUNE SYSTEM'S FIRST LINE OF DEFENSE: THE MYELOID BRANCH

The myeloid cells, produced in the bone marrow, create all the other blood cells: erythrocytes, neutrophils, monocytes (which become macrophages), eosinophils, basophils (which possibly become mast cells), and the giant megakaryocytes, which disintegrate into platelets—cell fragments essential to the clotting process. Basophils, eosinophils, and neutrophils are also called "granulocytes" because they contain cytoplasmic granules. Eosinophils are the parasite killers and, to a lesser degree, they also destroy bacteria. They detoxify an area after an allergic episode and limit the area of damage. Neutrophils are mature, ready-for-action white cells that give a fast response to inflammation and can also ingest infective microbes (Fig. III–1).

▶ THE IMMUNE SYSTEM'S MEMORY: THE LYMPHOID BRANCH

From the lymphoid branch come B cells and T cells, which do the basic work of detecting self and non-self. B cells are programmed in bones for their life's work of making antibodies to attach to mast cells and basophils. T cells receive their life's program in the thymus. They secrete hormones that trigger inflammation and the destruction of antigens. T cells, specifically the T_4 or CD_4 cell, are the ones compromised by the virus associated with AIDS (Fig. III–2).

▶ LYMPHATIC CIRCULATION

Immobility can kill. The lymphatic system's circulation depends on muscle activity, which is why movement and

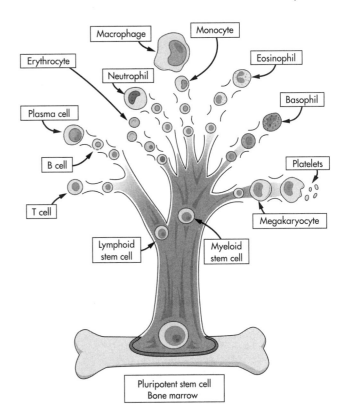

Figure III–1. The blood cell family tree.

ambulation are essential during convalescence. Valves in the lymphatics keep lymph flowing in one direction, propelled by pressure from exercise, movement, external pressures, and pulsing blood vessels. The valves in the lymph capillaries allow the fluid and particles to enter, but not exit. Lymph is dumped into the bloodstream at the vena cava after draining into the lymphatic circulation from interstitial spaces and carrying away proteins and large particles from the tissues that the venous capillaries cannot. Bacteria enter and are killed in the lymph nodes. Increased interstitial fluid proteins and increased capillary permeability increase lymph flow rate. Without lymphatic function, death would occur in a day.

▶ THE ANAPHYLAXIS SYSTEM AND THE ALLERGIC RESPONSE

Allergy is a function the anaphylactic system of sensitized basophils and mast cells, which explode, releasing destructive chemicals when antibodies on their surfaces are disturbed by antigens. The anaphylactic system is based on antibodies or, more precisely, immunoglobulins, antennae-like markers made by B cells when exposed to anything foreign from viruses to plastic products. The antibodies attach to explosive cells called mast cells, which lodge in tissue, and basophils, which float like mines in

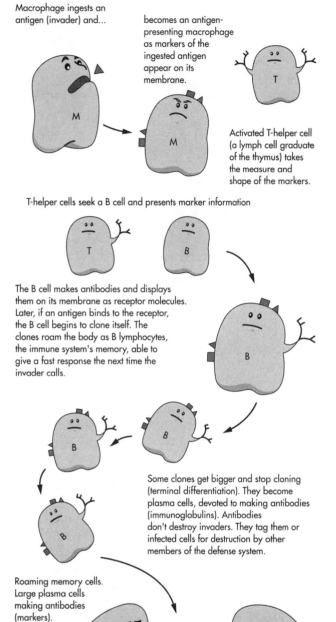

Macrophage ingests an antigen (invader) and...

becomes an antigen-presenting macrophage as markers of the ingested antigen appear on its membrane.

Activated T-helper cell (a lymph cell graduate of the thymus) takes the measure and shape of the markers.

T-helper cells seek a B cell and presents marker information

The B cell makes antibodies and displays them on its membrane as receptor molecules. Later, if an antigen binds to the receptor, the B cell begins to clone itself. The clones roam the body as B lymphocytes, the immune system's memory, able to give a fast response the next time the invader calls.

Some clones get bigger and stop cloning (terminal differentiation). They become plasma cells, devoted to making antibodies (immunoglobulins). Antibodies don't destroy invaders. They tag them or infected cells for destruction by other members of the defense system.

Roaming memory cells. Large plasma cells making antibodies (markers).

Plasma Cell

Plasma Cell

Figure III-2. B cells and T cells: educated lymphocytes.

the watery bloodstream. An antigen making contact with two of the protruding IgE antibody receptors draws the two together, exposing a reactive site. Toxic substances explode from the cell to destroy the antigen. This subsystem is not perfect, and the result, when it backfires, is anaphylaxis. The victim suffers immediate symptoms that can include hives, nausea, dizziness, seizures, or loss of consciousness. A precipitous drop in blood pressure results as the neurotransmitter histamine increases capillary permeability and great volumes of fluid escape from circulation. The drop in blood pressure may trigger a heart attack or deadly arrhythmias. The lips, tongue, and larynx may swell and obstruct the airway. The nurse must always be alert for anaphylaxis when administering drugs, such as the penicillins.

▶ THE COMPLEMENT SYSTEM

Complement refers to a chemical cascade meant to attract or draw the neutrophils and macrophages to an affected area and to neutralize and isolate damage. The complement mechanism consists of nine enzyme precursors plus other substances that attack antigens and protect the host. Some of the enzyme precursors lyse the invaders' membranes, making their cells rupture. Other enzymes make the invaders easier for macrophages to consume by agglutination, the clumping together of antigens. Complement enzymes also can neutralize viruses and cause inflammation, which heats up and coagulates protein to stop the invaders' progress. Heat also draws more white cells to the site (Fig. III-3).

CHEMOTAXIS

Chemotaxis occurs, in addition to the anaphylactic factors, when an antigen uncovers a reactive site on a mast cell or basophil. Enzyme precursors are released. Enzymes begin a cascading response to trauma or invasion.

LYSOSOMES: BAGS OF POISON

Lysosomes are minute pouches of poison within cells. Lysosomal enzymes released from the ruptured lysosomes during an allergy attack can go on destroying body tissues long after the antigen is gone, which is the case with reactions to poison ivy, oak, and sumac.

▶ PHAGOCYTOSIS: CLEANING UP AFTER THE BATTLE

After an infection or exposure to foreign matter, the site is littered with dead cells, proteins, the remains of dead white cells; what is referred to as pus. Phagocytes—the

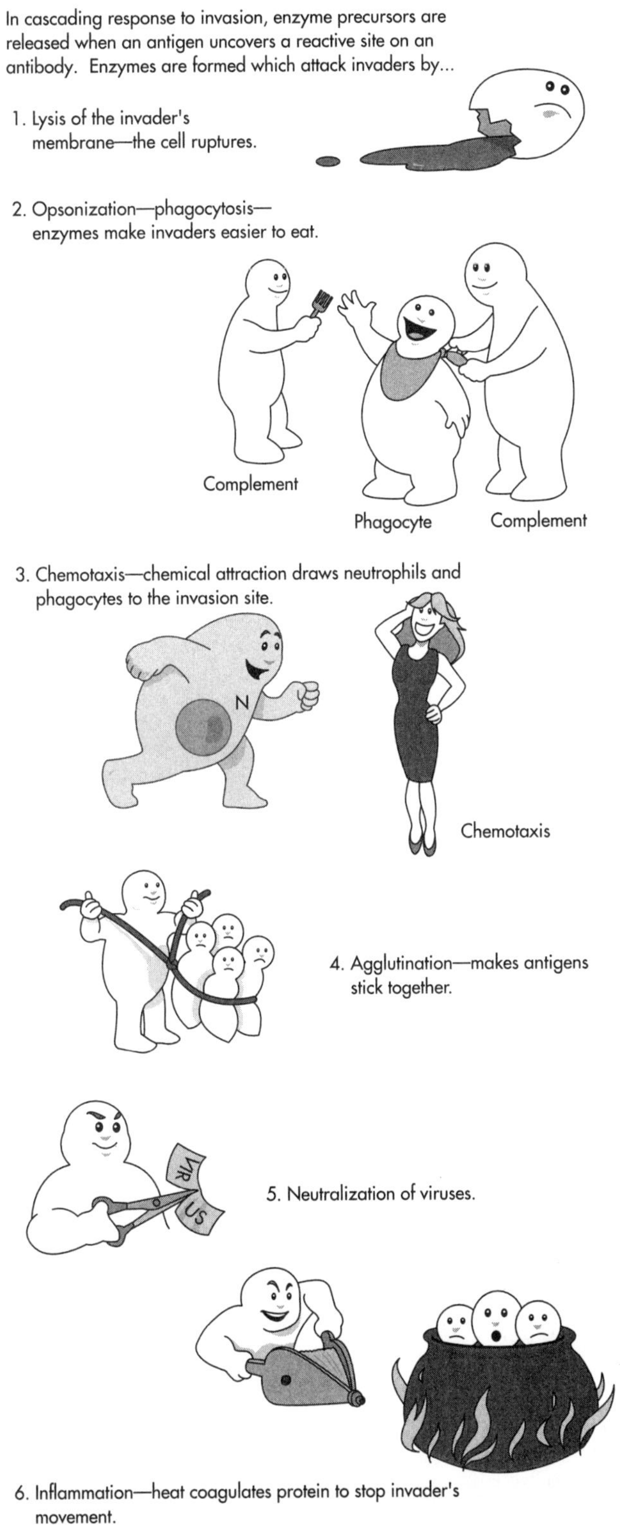

In cascading response to invasion, enzyme precursors are released when an antigen uncovers a reactive site on an antibody. Enzymes are formed which attack invaders by...

1. Lysis of the invader's membrane—the cell ruptures.

2. Opsonization—phagocytosis—enzymes make invaders easier to eat.

Complement

Phagocyte   Complement

3. Chemotaxis—chemical attraction draws neutrophils and phagocytes to the invasion site.

Chemotaxis

4. Agglutination—makes antigens stick together.

5. Neutralization of viruses.

6. Inflammation—heat coagulates protein to stop invader's movement.

Figure III–3. The complement system.

word means "cells that eat"—ingest the remains of the battle, as well as waste from wear and tear and degeneration of cells. They can also consume foreign material, not just life forms, but dust and oil particles, too. The macrophages, literally "big eaters," take days to come on the scene of an infection or trauma; however, they have an enormous appetite. Emerging from bone as immature monocytes, they drift in the bloodstream until they get lodged in organ tissues, where they mature into tissue macrophages. Bone, liver, skin, and lungs teem with macrophages for protection. Moving like amoebae, macrophages ooze pseudopods around the occasional invader and ingest it, or enter areas of damage and consume pus, clots, enzymes, even malarial parasites.

When a macrophage ingests foreign matter, it presents markers of that matter on its surface. T cells take the measure of these markers and present them to the B cells, which then make antibodies to the foreign matter. Should such foreign matter present itself again, the antibodies, or molecular memory, will trigger a rapid defense (see Fig. III–2).

▶ TURNING OFF THE IMMUNE RESPONSE

The immune system also has suppressor activity. This is probably a function of certain T cells and monocyte–macrophages to shut down the response when the enemy has been destroyed or sealed off, or the crisis has passed.

▶ AGRANULOCYTOSIS

Sometimes bone marrow goes out of business and stops producing the pluripotent stem cells. When this vital blood cell production ceases, a deadly condition called agranulocytosis occurs. Agranulocytosis cripples the immune system. Within days microbial life causes the mucous membranes of mouth and gut to ulcerate and the lungs to fill with infection. Without treatment, death comes within the week. Radiation exposure can cause agranulocytosis. This is one of the immediate risks of nuclear accident. Irradiation is also done therapeutically to kill immune system cells in preparation for such procedures as bone marrow transplant or to kill off lingering malignant cells after cancer therapy. Agranulocytosis can also be caused by drugs such as chloramphenicol, barbiturates, the sulfonamides, and thiouracil.

Side effects such as sore throat, fever, and bruising must be taken seriously as possible signs of agranulocytosis.

Agranulocytosis is the absence of the immune system. The disorder shows clearly how vital the immune system is in protecting and defending us against the sea of microbes that surrounds us.

14

Nonsteroidal Antiinflammatories (NSAIDs)

Until the end of the last century, fever was thought to be a disease in and of itself, rather than a symptom of infection and trauma. But even though medical practitioners saw fever as the disease, not as a sign, they did recognize it as part of the mnemonic—rubor, dolor, tumor, and calor (redness, pain, swelling, and heat)—that describes the signs of infection or injury. The four signs are the immune system's calling card, signaling the battle for survival. The immune system's response is always proportionate to the insult.

Fever is meant to destroy microbial invaders. At the site of the damaged tissue, cells release prostaglandins into the bloodstream. The endocrine system regulates body temperature in the hypothalamus and responds to the immune system's prostaglandin signals by increasing the temperature. In addition to the visible signs of damage or infection, the WBC count will indicate the extent of the injury in the healthy individual. Although we need the immune system responses, we also benefit from the drugs that relieve the misery caused by the release of prostaglandins.

▶ NONSTEROIDAL ANTIINFLAMMATORY DRUGS

The endocrine system's powerful steroidal glucocorticoids suppress inflammation, but are best used sparingly. Because body cells produce prostaglandins by way of microsomal enzymes whenever they are damaged, drugs called nonsteroidal antiinflammatory drugs (NSAIDs) that can interfere with prostaglandins offer a more specific approach to reducing their inflammatory actions and relieving the fever and pain associated with them. The first NSAID, willow bark, was used to treat fever since ancient times, but the Scottish doctor Thomas Mac Lagan is credited with the first use of the willow bark's active ingredient, salicin, to treat rheumatic fever in 1874 (Sneader, 1985). The body converts salicin into salicylic acid.

Healers also sought to ease the pain of "rheumatism," a term that has given way to the terms *arthritis* and *rheumatoid arthritis*. The drug salicylic acid tasted awful and caused vomiting, but did relieve pain. In Germany, the Bayer Company produced acetylsalicylic acid and named it "aspirin" from the "a" in acetyl and "spirin" from the plant source of salicylic acid, *Spirea ulmaria* (Sneader, 1985). Aspirin is possibly the most used drug in the world. Many refinements have been made on aspirin, producing the spinoff NSAIDs.

Acetylsalicylic acid (aspirin) [Alka-Seltzer, ASA, Aspergum, Bayer, Cosprin, Easprin, Ecotrin, Empirin, Halfprin, Measurin, ZORprin], the prototype of the NSAIDs, relieves pain by inhibiting prostaglandin production locally. It also appears to act on the nervous system at the level of the hypothalamus. Salicylates help relieve the pain of headache, muscle, and joints—structures outside the viscera. ASA (and acetaminophen) can be combined with the opiates, especially codeine, for a wider range of pain-killing effectiveness.

Drug Interactions: Increased toxicity possible with aminosalicylic acid. Decreased renal elimination with ammonium chloride and other acidifying agents. In-creased risk of bleeding with anticoagulants. Increased hypoglycemic activity with hypoglycemic agents when aspirin doses are over 2 g/d. Toxicity increased with carbonic anhydrase inhibitors. Increased ulcer activity with corticosteroids. Increased methotrexate toxicity. Low dose may antagonize uricosuric effects of probenecid and sulfinpyrazone.

Side Effects

Nervous System: bowel—diarrhea, bronchospasm, dizziness, drowsiness, hearing—loss/tinnitus, nausea/vomiting, stomach pain, psyche—confusion.

Endocrine System: (Pregnancy Category D) anorexia, prolonged pregnancy, impaired renal function.

Immune System: anaphylaxis,* increased bleeding—during delivery, bleeding—GI/occult, prolonged bleeding time, bruising, heartburn, laryngeal edema, petechiae, rash, thrombocytopenia, urticaria.

Dosage: Analgesic/antipyretic: PO, rectal 350–650 mg q4h to maximum of 4 g/d. Arthritis: PO 3.6–5.4 g/d in 4–6 divided doses. Thromboembolic disorders: PO 325–650 mg qd or bid. TIA prophylaxis: PO 650 mg bid. MI prophylaxis: PO 80–325 mg/d.

Acetaminophen, paracetamol [Acephen, ACINAL, Anacin-3, Anuphen, APAP, Datril Extra Strength, Dolanex, Halenol, Liquiprin, Panadol, Tapar, Tempra, Tylenol, Valadol] acts in the hypothalamus to control fever and pain with little or no effect on bleeding time. Acetaminophen is preferred over ASA when there is a risk of gastric bleeding and for children, in whom ASA may contribute to Reye's syndrome. Unlike ASA, it has no antiinflammatory activity and can damage the liver.

Drug Interactions: Decreased absorption with cholestyramine. Increased potential for chronic hepatotoxicity with chronic coadministration of barbiturates, carbamazepine, phenytoin, rifampin. Increased risk of hepatotoxicity with chronic alcohol abuse.

Side Effects

Nervous System: bowel—diarrhea, dizziness, chronic indigestion, nausea/vomiting, lethargy, pain—abdominal/epigastric.

Endocrine System: (Pregnancy Category B) anorexia, chills, hypoglycemia, acute renal failure,* sweating.

Immune System: hepatic coma*/toxicity, leukopenia, neutropenia, pancytopenia, thrombocytopenic purpura, elevated serum transaminases/bilirubin.

---

* Life-threatening side effect.

Dosage: PO 325–650 mg q4–6h, not to exceed 4 g/d in short-term treatment or 2.6 g/d in long-term therapy. Rectal 650 mg q4–6h to maximum of 4.g/d.

Note: For acetaminophen overdose, acetylcysteine [Mucomyst] can prevent hepatic necrosis.

▶ NEWER NONSTEROIDAL ANTIINFLAMMATORY AGENTS

A never-ending search for drugs that do not upset the stomach and cause GI bleeding, as aspirin can, led scientists to explore the carboxylic acid group in the aspirin molecule. Aspirin is the parent drug to the current generation of nonsteroidal antiinflammatory drugs (Fig. 14–1). All of the aspirin-related drugs share many of the same side effects.

Bromfenac sodium [DurAct] is used for short-term pain management, but not for osteoarthritis or rheumatoid arthritis.

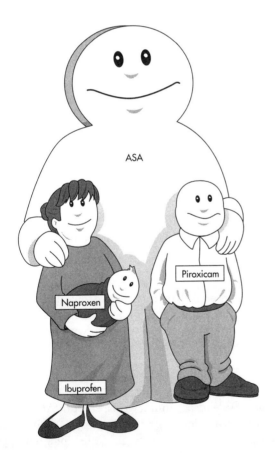

Aspirin's carboxylic acid group makes it antiinflammatory. Ibuprofen, in a way, is aspirin's child—the result of a quest for the carboxylic acid group. Naproxen [Naprosyn] is derived from ibuprofen. Another of aspirin's offspring is piroxicam.

Figure 14–1. The aspirin family.

Drug Interactions: Increase levels with cimetidine. Decreased levels with phenytoin. Increased clotting time with warfarin.

Food Interaction: A high-fat meal decreases plasma levels.

Side Effects

Nervous System: dizziness, dyspepsia, headache, nausea, pain—abdominal.

Endocrine System: (Pregnancy Category B) none noted.

Immune System: bleeding, GI—bleeding/ulceration/perforation, liver enzyme elevations.

Dosage: PO 25 mg q6–8h prn for pain.

Diclofenac sodium [Voltaren], diclofenac potassium [Cataflam] has analgesic and antipyretic activity.

Drug Interactions: Increased cyclosporin-induced nephrotoxicity. Increased methotrexate toxicity. Decreased antihypertensive effects of diuretics possible. Increased level/toxicity of lithium possible. Increased digoxin levels possible.

Side Effects

Nervous System: bowel—constipation/diarrhea/flatulence, cramps, abdominal distension, dizziness, drowsiness, dyspepsia, headache, indigestion, nausea/vomiting, pain—abdominal/back/leg/joint, tinnitus.

Endocrine System: (Pregnancy Category B) hyperglycemia, fluid retention.

Immune System: asthma, prolonged bleeding time, abnormal liver tests, liver enzymes/transaminases—increased, platelet aggregation—decreased.

Dosage: Ankylosing spondylitis: PO 25 mg qid and 25 mg hs. Cataract surgery: Ophthalmic 1 gtt of 1% solution in affected eye qid beginning 24 h postop and next 2 wk.[†] Osteoarthritis: PO 100–150 mg/d in 3–4 divided doses. Rheumatoid arthritis: PO 150–200 mg/d in 3–4 divided doses.

Etodolac [Lodine] may inhibit cyclooxygenase activity and prostaglandin synthesis. It may also suppress production of rheumatoid factor to treat osteoarthritis and acute pain, as well as rheumatoid arthritis.

Off Label: Temporal arteritis.

Drug Interactions: May increase digoxin and lithium levels and nephrotoxicity due to cyclosporin. Reduced effects of diuretics and hypertensive effects of beta blockers and other antihypertensives possible.

† Eye related.

Side Effects

Nervous System: bladder—frequency, bowel—diarrhea/flatulence, dizziness, drowsiness, dyspepsia, insomnia, nausea/vomiting, pain—abdominal, tinnitus, vision—blurred.

Endocrine System: (Pregnancy Category C) edema, fluid retention.

Immune System: asthma, bleeding time increase, gastritis, GI bleeding, hepatotoxicity, melena, peptic ulcer, pruritus, rash, thrombocytopenia.

Dosage: Acute pain: PO 200–400 mg q6–8h prn. Osteoarthritis: PO 600–1200 mg/d in 2–4 divided doses to maximum of 1200 mg or 20 mg/kg for patients ≤ 60 kg. Rheumatoid arthritis: PO 150–200 mg bid.

Fenoprofen calcium [Nalfon] is used to treat acute and chronic rheumatoid arthritis and osteoarthritis, giving relief for mild to moderate pain.

Drug Interactions: May prolong bleeding time. Should not be given with oral anticoagulants, heparin. Increased side effects of phenytoin, sulfonylureas, sulfonamides possible.

Side Effects

Nervous System: bladder—dysuria, bowel—constipation/flatulence, deafness, dizziness, drowsiness, dyspnea, fatigue, headache, hearing—decrease/tinnitus, insomnia, lassitude, malaise, nausea/vomiting, psyche—confusion/ depression/nervousness, tremor, vision—blurred.

Endocrine System: (Pregnancy Category B; D in third trimester) anorexia, anuria, azotemia, dry mouth, edema, oliguria, sweating.

Immune System: agranulocytosis,* anaphylaxis,* hematuria, hemolytic anemia,* cystitis, GI bleeding, allergic nephritis, nephrotoxicity, pancytopenia,* peptic ulcer, pruritus, purpura, rash, thrombocytopenia, urticaria, vision—papillary necrosis.

Dosage: Inflammatory disease: PO 300–600 mg tid or qid. Not to exceed 3200 mg/d. Mild to moderate pain: PO 200 mg q4–6h prn.

Ibuprofen [Advil, Haltran, Ibuprin, Medipren, Motrin, Nuprin, PediaProfen, Pamprin-IB, Rufen, Trendar] is the prototype of the propionic acid NSAIDs. It blocks prostaglandin synthesis to relieve fever and pain and is used to treat rheumatoid arthritis and osteoarthritis, to relieve mild to moderate pain, and to reduce fever.

Off Label: Gout, juvenile rheumatoid arthritis, psoriatic arthritis, ankylosing spondylitis, vascular headache.

---

* Life-threatening side effect.

Drug Interactions: Increased bleeding time with oral anticoagulants and heparin possible. Increased lithium and methotrexate toxicity possible.

Side Effects

Nervous System: bowel—constipation/diarrhea, bronchospasm,* CHF, drowsiness, fatigue, hearing impairment/tinnitus, nausea/vomiting, pain/discomfort—abdominal, psyche—anxiety/confusion/depression/emotional lability, vision—changes/nystagmus/scotomas.

Endocrine System: (Pregnancy Category B) anorexia, azotemia, creatine clearance—decreased, fluid retention, acute renal failure, serum alkaline phosphatase—transitory elevation.

Immune System: acne, anaphylaxis,* angioedema,* aplastic anemia,* AST/ALT—transitory increase, occult blood loss, cystitis, erythema, GI ulceration, hematuria, Hb/Hct—decreased, toxic hepatitis,* hypersensitivity reactions, nephrotoxicity, neutropenia, pruritus, rectal itching, serum sickness, skin eruptions, SLE, Stevens–Johnson syndrome,* thrombocytopenia, toxic hepatitis.

Dosage: Inflammatory disease: PO 400–800 mg tid or qid to maximum of 3200 mg/d. Mild to moderate pain/dysmenorrhea: PO 400 mg q4–6h to maximum of 1200 mg/d. Fever: PO 200–400 mg tid or qid to maximum of 1200 mg/d.

Naproxen [EC-Naprosyn, Naprosyn], naproxen sodium [Aleve, Anaprox, Anaprox DS] is used to treat acute and chronic rheumatoid arthritis, juvenile arthritis (naproxen only), and primary dysmenorrhea. It is also used to treat ankylosing spondylitis, osteoarthritis, and gout.

Off Label: Bartter's syndrome, Paget's disease of bone.

Drug Interactions: Prolonged bleeding time with oral anticoagulants, heparin possible. Increased lithium toxicity possible.

Side Effects

Nervous System: CHF, dizziness, drowsiness, dyspnea, edema—peripheral/pulmonary, headache, hearing—loss/tinnitus, indigestion, nausea/vomiting, palpitations, psyche—depression, vision—blurred.

Endocrine System: (Pregnancy Category B) anorexia, thirst.

Immune System: agranulocytosis,* serum ALT/AST—elevated, GI bleeding,* ecchymosis, eosinophilia, leukopenia, nephrotoxicity, inhibited platelet aggregation, pruritus, rash, thrombocytopenia.

Note: 250 mg naproxen = 275 mg naproxen sodium.

Dosage: Inflammatory disease: PO 250–500 mg bid. Not to exceed 1000 mg/d of naproxen or 1100 mg/d of naproxen sodium. Mild to moderate pain/dysmenorrhea: PO 500 mg followed by 200–250 mg q6–8h prn to maximum of 1250 mg/d.

Piroxicam [Feldene] provides analgesia and treatment for osteoarthritis and rheumatoid arthritis.

Off Label: Acute and chronic relief of mild to moderate pain.

Drug Interactions: Prolonged bleeding time with oral anticoagulants, heparin possible. Increased lithium toxicity. Increased risk of GI hemorrhage with alcohol, aspirin.

Side Effects

Nervous System: exacerbation of angina, bladder—dysuria, bowel—constipation/diarrhea/flatulence, bronchospasm,* CHF worsening, dizziness, dyspnea, dyspepsia, peripheral edema, hearing loss, hypertension, muscle cramps, nausea/vomiting, palpitations, psyche—depression/insomnia/nervousness, somnolence, syncope, tinnitus, vision—changes/scotomas.

Endocrine System: (Pregnancy Category C) anorexia, corneal deposits, fever, hyperglycemia, hyperkalemia, hypoglycemia, dry mouth, nephrotic syndrome, proteinuria, acute renal failure,* sweating, weight gain.

Immune System: anemia, angioedema,* aplastic anemia,* GI bleeding,* prolonged bleeding time, bruising, dermatitis, eosinophilia, hematuria, Hb/Hct—decrease, hepatitis, hypersensitivity reactions, jaundice, leukopenia, peptic ulceration, rash, allergic rhinitis, Stevens–Johnson syndrome,* thrombocytopenia, urticaria.

Dosage: Arthritis/pain: PO 10–20 mg qd or bid.

▶ SEROTONIN AND INFLAMMATION

Serotonin, a neurotransmitter in the nervous system, also plays a role in the immune system. Platelets release serotonin when damaged. Though the aspirin-derived NSAIDs were developed to block production of prostaglandins, the NSAID indomethacin was created with the knowledge that serotonin (5-HT), an indolic hormone, helps trigger platelet aggregation in the immune system's inflammatory process. Other drugs related to indomethacin include sulindac and tolmetin.

Indomethacin [Indameth, Indocin, Indocin SR] offers analgesic and antiinflammatory action to treat moderate to severe rheumatoid arthritis, ankylosing rheumatoid spondylitis, acute gouty arthritis, and osteoarthritis of the hip when patient is intolerant or unresponsive to salicylates and other therapy. It is also used IV to close patent ductus arteriosus in the premature infant.

Off Label: Biliary pain, dysmenorrhea, Paget's disease, athletic injuries, juvenile arthritis, idiopathic pericarditis.

Drug Interactions: Prolonged bleeding time with oral anticoagulants, heparin. Increased lithium toxicity possible. Increased effects of oral anticoagulants, phenytoin, salicylates, sulfonamides, sulfonylureas due to protein-binding displacement. Increased toxicity and GI bleeding with NSAIDs. Decreased effects of antihypertensives and diuretics possible.

Side Effects

Nervous System: arrhythmias—bradycardia/tachycardia, ataxia, bladder—frequency, abdominal—bloating/distention, elevated BP, rapid BP drop, bowel—diarrhea, CHF, coma,* convulsions,* dizziness, drowsiness, dyspnea, epilepsy aggravation,* fatigue, hearing disturbances/tinnitus, lightheadedness, nausea/vomiting, pain—chest/eye, parkinsonism, psyche—confusion/depersonalization/depression/hallucinations/insomnia/nightmares, syncope, vision—blurred/lacrimation/visual field changes.

Endocrine System: (Pregnancy Category B; D in third trimester) anorexia, breast changes, edema, flushing, glycosuria, hair loss, hyperglycemia/hypoglycemia, hyperkalemia/hypokalemia, renal function impairment, sweating, weight gain.

Immune System: agranulocytosis,* aplastic anemia,* asthma syndrome in aspirin-sensitive patients, bleeding per vagina/rectum, epistaxis, erythema nodosum, exfoliative dermatitis, hemolytic anemia, GI—ulceration*/perforation, hematuria, hemorrhage,* irritation/extravasation of tissue, leukopenia, platelet aggregation inhibition, proctitis, purpura, retinal/macular disturbances, stomatitis with ulceration, thrombocytosis.

Dosage: Bursitis: PO 25–50 mg tid or qid to maximum of 200 mg/d or SR 75 mg 1–2 ×/d. Gout: PO 50 mg tid during acute pain, then decrease quickly and end therapy course. Rheumatoid arthritis: PO 25–50 mg bid or tid to maximum of 200 mg/d or SR 75 mg 1–2 ×/d.

Sulindac [Clinoril] has a longer half-life than aspirin in treating acute and long-term symptoms of osteoarthritis, rheumatoid arthritis, ankylosing spondylitis, acute painful shoulder (acute subacromial bursitis or supraspinatus tendinitis), or acute gouty arthritis.

Drug Interactions: Bleeding time prolonged with oral anticoagulants, heparin. Increased lithium toxicity possible. Increased ulcer activity with aspirin and other NSAIDs. Increased methotrexate toxicity possible. Decreased effect with dimethylsulfoxide (DMSO).

---

* Life-threatening side effect.

Side Effects

Nervous System: bowel—diarrhea/flatulence, CHF, dizziness, drowsiness, peripheral edema, headache, hearing—decrease/tinnitus, nausea/vomiting, abdominal pain, palpitations, psyche—anxiety/nervousness, vertigo, vision—changes/amblyopia.

Endocrine System: (Pregnancy Category B; D in third trimester) anorexia, edema, fever, dry mouth, renal impairment.

Immune System: anaphylaxis,* angioedema,* aplastic anemia,* increased bleeding time, eosinophilia, toxic epidermal necrolysis syndrome, gastritis, GI bleeding, leukopenia, pruritus, rash, Stevens–Johnson syndrome,* stomatitis, ulceration.

Dosage: Arthritis, ankylosing spondylitis, gouty arthritis: PO 150–200 mg bid. Not to exceed 400 mg/d × 7–14 d.

Tolmetin sodium [Tolectin, Tolectin DS] is used to treat acute and chronic rheumatoid arthritis, alone or in combination with gold or corticosteroids.

Drug Interactions: Bleeding time prolonged with oral anticoagulants, heparin. Increased lithium toxicity possible. Increased ulcer activity with aspirin and other NSAIDs. Increased methotrexate toxicity possible.

Side Effects

Nervous System: bowel—constipation, dizziness, drowsiness, dyspepsia, edema, headache, hypertension—mild or moderate, insomnia, lightheadedness, nausea/vomiting, pain—epigastric or abdominal, psyche—depression/mood elevation/nervousness, tinnitus.

Endocrine System: (Pregnancy Category B; D in third trimester) BUN increase, edema, proteinuria.

Immune System: anaphylaxis*—especially after drug is discontinued and reinstituted, toxic epidermal necrolysis,* GI bleeding,* granulocytopenia, hematuria, Hb/Hct—transient/small decreases, leukopenia, morbilliform eruptions, petechiae, pruritus, purpura, urticaria.

Dosage: PO 400 mg tid to maximum of 1800 mg/d.

▶ OTHER ASPIRIN DERIVATIVES

The following drugs interfere with prostaglandin production and with their receptor sites to treat inflammatory conditions.

Meclofenamate sodium [Meclofen, Meclomen] competes with prostaglandin receptor sites to treat acute or chronic rheumatoid arthritis and osteoarthritis. It is also used in combination with gold salts or corticosteroids for rheumatoid arthritis.

* Life-threatening side effect.

Off Label: Psoriatic arthritis, mild to moderate postoperative pain, dysmenorrhea.

Drug Interactions: Bleeding time prolonged with oral anticoagulants, heparin. Increased lithium toxicity possible. Increases action and toxicity of phenytoin, sulfonylureas, sulfonamides, warfarin by protein-binding displacement.

Side Effects

Nervous System: bowel—constipation/diarrhea (severe and dose related)/flatulence, dizziness, dyspepsia, edema, eructation, headache, nausea/vomiting, pain—abdominal, psyche—lack of concentration/confusion, vision—blurred, tinnitus.

Endocrine System: (Pregnancy Category B; D in third trimester) anorexia, BUN/creatinine—elevated, edema, renal failure.

Immune System: bleeding*—GI, jaundice, pruritus, pyrosis, rash, urticaria.

Dosage: PO 200–400 mg tid or qid to maximum of 400 mg/d.

Mefenamic acid [Ponstan, Ponstel] is used to treat mild to moderate pain.

Drug Interactions: Bleeding time prolonged with oral anticoagulants, heparin. Increased lithium toxicity possible. Increased action and toxicity of phenytoin, sulfonylureas, sulfonamides, warfarin by protein-binding displacement.

Side Effects

Nervous System: bladder—dysuria, bowel—constipation/diarrhea/flatus, bronchoconstriction*—in aspirin-sensitive patients, cramps—abdominal, dizziness, drowsiness, dyspnea, headache, nausea/vomiting, pain—ear, palpitations, psyche—confusion/insomnia/nervousness, vision—blurred/reversible color loss.

Endocrine System: (Pregnancy Category C) albuminuria, BUN elevation, sweating.

Immune System: agranulocytosis,* megaloblastic anemia, anemia—severe autoimmune hemolytic with long-term use, asthma*—acute exacerbation, bone marrow hypoplasia, edema—facial, eosinophilia, eye irritation, hematuria, leukopenia, nephrotoxicity, pancytopenia, prolonged PT, purpura, rash, ulceration/bleeding,* urticaria.

Dosage: PO. Loading dose 500 mg, then 250 mg q6h prn.

▶ GOLD

Gold treatment started out in the misguided notion that gold was an antiseptic especially useful in treating tuberculosis. In a poorly constructed trial, patients suffering from rheumatic fever were given aurothioglucose [Solganal], which relieved their joint pain. By the 1940s the effect of gold compounds on the arthritic condition was recognized (Sneader, 1985). Gold compounds are sometimes used on selected cases of early rheumatic arthritis to halt or reverse the condition by some unknown process, perhaps by suppressing phagocytosis or inhibiting prostaglandin synthesis.

Aurothioglucose [Gold thioglucose, Solganal] is an adjunct to treatment of adult and juvenile active rheumatoid arthritis when NSAIDs are infective.

Off Label: Felty's syndrome, nondisseminated LE, pemphigus, psoriatic arthritis.

Drug Interactions: Increased risk of blood dyscrasias with immunosuppressant, antimalarials, penicillamine, phenylbutazone possible.

Side Effects

Nervous System: arrhythmias—bradycardia, bowel—diarrhea, cramps—abdominal, arthralgia—temporary, dysphagia, dyspnea, metallic taste, nausea/vomiting, syncope.

Endocrine: (Pregnancy Category C) anorexia, fever, nephrotic syndrome, proteinuria, thickening of tongue.

Immune: anaphylaxis,* agranulocytosis,* aplastic anemia,* eosinophilia, erythema, fibrosis—pulmonary, gold dermatitis, granulocytopenia, hematuria, interstitial pneumonitis, photosensitivity, Stevens–Johnson syndrome,* synovial fluid destruction, thrombocytopenia, urticaria, vaginitis. Injection site: irritation.

Dosage: IM (deep) 10 mg week 1; 25 mg weeks 2–3, 50 mg/wk to a cumulative dose of 1 g. If improved, 25–50 mg q2–3wk, then q3–4wk indefinitely or until side effects occur. Observe 20–30 min for immune reaction.

Gold sodium thiomalate [Myochrysine] is a water-soluble gold compound used to treat acute rheumatoid arthritis.

Off Label: Felty's syndrome, psoriatic arthritis.

Drug Interactions: Increased risk of blood dyscrasias with immunosuppressant, antimalarials, penicillamine, phenylbutazone possible.

Side Effects

Nervous System: arrhythmias—bradycardia, dizziness, dysphagia, dyspnea, nausea/vomiting, psyche—confusion/hallucinations, seizures,* syncope, metallic taste.

Endocrine System: (Pregnancy Category C) flushing, nephrotic syndrome, proteinuria, sweating.

Immune System: angioedema,* agranulocytosis,* anaphylaxis,* aplastic anemia,* exfoliative dermatitis with alopecia/nail loss, fibrosis—pulmonary, fixed drug eruption, eosinophilia, erythema, glomerulitis with hematuria, glossitis, hepatitis, peripheral neuritis, photosensitivity, interstitial pneumonitis, pruritus, stomatitis.

Dosage: IM 10 mg week 1; then 25 mg week 2; then 25–50 mg/wk to a cumulative dose of 1 g. If improved, maintain on 25–50 mg q2wk for 2–20 wk. Then q3–4wk thereafter.

Note: *Treat overdose with anabolic steroids and chelating agents, eg, dimercaprol and penicillamine.*

▶ QUININE FOR RHEUMATOID ARTHRITIS AND LUPUS ERYTHEMATOSUS

Quinine, the traditional antimalarial drug, benefits some patients with inflammatory illnesses.

Hydroxychloroquine sulfate [Plaquenil Sulfate], besides being a classic antimalarial, is also used to treat lupus erythematosus and rheumatoid arthritis.

Off Label: Porphyria cutanea tarda.

Drug Interactions: Decreased absorption with aluminum- and magnesium-containing antacids and laxatives. Give 4 h apart. May interfere with response to rabies vaccine.

Side Effects

Nervous System: bowel—diarrhea, cramps—abdominal, fatigue, headache, nausea/vomiting, psyche—anxiety/mood changes, vertigo.

Endocrine System: (Pregnancy Category C) anorexia, weight loss.

Immune System: agranulocytosis,* aplastic anemia,* hair—bleaching or loss, hemolysis in G6PD deficiency, itching, rash, retinopathy, thrombocytopenia.

Dosage: Rheumatoid arthritis: PO 400–600 mg/d with food. Decrease 5–10 d later to maintain optimum dose. Decrease in 4–12 wk to 200–400 mg/d. Lupus erythematosus: PO 310 mg qd or bid for weeks or months.

▶ DRUGS FOR GOUT

Whereas rheumatoid arthritis is an autoimmune disease in which the body attacks itself as foreign, gout has long been described as a disease of plenty, a rich person's disease. As the result of diet, uric acid crystals collect in various tissues, and when those deposits occur in the joints, inflammation and pain result.

---

* Life-threatening side effect.

<u>Allopurinol [Lopurin, Zyloprim]</u>, discovered in the 1960s, decreases synthesis of uric acid by inhibiting xanthine oxidase and, thus, prevents recurrent uric acid kidney stones in addition to treating gout attacks. This is not a first-line drug and is not used during the acute phase, when it may actually exacerbate the attack. The patient must push fluids to protect the kidneys and, in addition, avoid iron salts and thiazide diuretics.

Drug Interactions: Increased toxicity of azathioprine, cyclophosphamide, mercaptopurine (give only ⅓ the usual dosage). Extends the half-life of anticoagulants. Decreased renal excretion of uric acid with alcohol possible. Increased toxicity/hypersensitivity with thiazides possible. Increased risk of rashes with ampicillin, amoxicillin.

Side Effects

Nervous System: abdominal discomfort/indigestion, bowel—diarrhea, drowsiness, headache, malaise, nausea/vomiting, vertigo.

Endocrine System: (Pregnancy Category C) none noted.

Immune System: agranulocytosis,* aplastic anemia,* bone marrow depression,* toxic epidermal necrolysis, hepatotoxicity, nephrotoxicity, pruritus, rash.

Dosage: Hyperuricemia: PO 100 mg/d. May increase by 100 mg/wk to maximum of 800 mg/d. Divided doses over 300 mg/d. Secondary hyperuricemia: PO 200–800 mg/d for 2–3 d or longer. Divide doses over 300 mg/d. Prevent uric acid kidney stones during cancer therapy: PO 600–800 mg qd for 2–3 days.

<u>Colchicine,</u> the first gout medicine, came from the meadow saffron from the Colchis region of Asia Minor hundreds of years ago, where it was used by the Arabs. This ancient drug has lost favor only recently with the creation of allopurinol and ibuprofen, but may still be used in the acute stage, when it decreases the inflammatory response to the uric acid crystals.

Off Label: Sarcoid arthritis, chondrocalcinosis (pseudogout), arthritis of erythema nodosum, adenocarcinoma, acute calcific tendonitis, familial Mediterranean fever, leukemia, multiple sclerosis, mycosis fungoides, and in experimental studies of normal and abnormal cell division.

Drug Interactions: Decreased intestinal absorption of vitamin B_{12}.

Side Effects

Nervous System: diarrhea, muscle weakness, nausea/vomiting, pain—abdominal, psyche—confusion.

Endocrine System: (Pregnancy Category C) anorexia, azotemia, oliguria, serum creatine kinase elevation, sperm count depression, steatorrhea.

Immune System: agranulocytosis,* aplastic anemia,* bone marrow depression,* hemorrhagic gastroenteritis, hepatotoxicity, peripheral neuritis, neutropenia, pancreatitis, thrombocytopenia.

Dosage: Acute attack: PO 0.5–1.2 mg; then 0.5–0.6 mg q1–2h to maximum of 4 mg until pain relief or diarrhea or gastric distress occurs. IV 2 mg over 2–5 min, follow with 0.5 mg q6h to maximum of 4 mg in the attack. Prophylaxis: PO 0.5 or 0.6 mg hs or qohs prn. Severe attacks may require up to 1.8 mg/hs. IV 0.5–1 mg 1–2 ×/d.

<u>Phenylbutazone [Butazolidin]</u> is used for short-term treatment of rheumatoid and osteoarthritis, as well as ankylosing spondylitis and acute gout. Antiinflammatory, antipyretic, analgesic, and mildly uricosuric, it inhibits prostaglandin production, leukocyte attraction per chemotaxis, and the release of lysosomal enzymes, as well as platelet clumping. This drug is potentially fatal, especially for adults over 40, and must not be used frivolously or for patients over 60. It requires frequent CBCs. The patient must be taught to immediately report fever, sore throat, edema, black or tarry stools, and epigastric pain.

Drug Interactions: Increased activity and toxicity of warfarin, oral hypoglycemic agents, phenytoin, salicylates, sulfonamides. Increased digitoxin metabolism. Increased methotrexate toxicity.

Side Effects

Nervous System: abdominal distension/flatulence, bowel—constipation/diarrhea, cardiac decompensation, dyspepsia, edema, headache, hearing—loss/tinnitus, hypertension, nausea/vomiting, psyche—confusion/nervousness, taste changes, trembling, vision—blurred/oculomotor palsy/scotomas.

Endocrine System: (Pregnancy Category D) acidosis—metabolic, alkalosis, azotemia, calculi—renal, edema, hyperglycemia, dry mouth, hyperplasia—thyroid, toxic goiter, myxedema, NaCl—retention, nephrotic syndrome, rapid volume expansion with plasma dilution.

Immune System: agranulocytosis,* anaphylaxis,* aplastic anemia,* asthma, bone marrow depression,* bowel ulceration, conjunctivitis, drug fever, fixed drug eruptions, erythema nodosum and multiforme, esophagitis, glomerulonephritis, hepatitis—fatal*/nonfatal, leukemia, leukopenia, LE activation, Lyell's syndrome, neuritis, pancreatitis, pancytopenia, peptic ulcer reactivation, pericarditis, renal failure*—acute, retinal hemorrhage/detachment, salivary gland enlargement, serum sickness, Stevens–Johnson syndrome,* stomatitis—ulcerative, thrombocytopenia, urticaria.

Dosage: Ankylosing spondylitis, osteoarthritis, rheumatoid arthritis: PO 300–600 mg/d in 3–4 divided doses. Acute gouty arthritis: PO 400 mg once; then 100 mg q4h until relief.

---

* Life-threatening side effect.

Chapter Highlights

- The nonsteroidal antiinflammatory agents derived from aspirin are important in giving relief from the prostaglandin effects initiated by the immune response to injury or infection.

- NSAIDs all share in common the side effects of prolonged bleeding and gastric problems.

- Gold is also used for the treatment of arthritis, though its action is not clearly understood.

- Gout is treated with drugs that interfere with uric acid inflammation.

15

Drugs That Affect Clotting and Mucus

▶ BARRIERS TO FOREIGN INVASION: THE VALUE OF CLOTS AND MUCUS

The immune system uses clotting to seal off injured blood vessels and prevent blood loss and also to seal off microbial invasions. Lack of clotting factors, as seen in hemophilia, is life threatening and is treated by replacement of missing factors.

Mucus, formed in the mucous membranes that line all tissue having direct contact with the environment, is also meant to trap foreign matter. Mucus acts almost like fly paper, causing invading allergens and microbes to get stuck. Interestingly, the viscosity of mucus also plays a role in conception, either allowing the passage of sperm or impeding their progress. Clotting and mucus are essential protective strategies, but they can also pose a threat to health when they function improperly.

▶ WHEN CLOTTING IS A PROBLEM

Every moment one lives, the immune system tilts between clotting and dissolving clots. Though clotting is meant to protect, sometimes clots can injure and kill. The lungs and liver are especially vulnerable to clotting because the blood flows slowly through these organs and concentrates the substances that cause coagulation. Immobilization during long trips or bed rest of a week or more can slow circulation and trigger clotting. Dehydration, pressure, constrictive clothing and elastics, birth control pills, atherosclerosis, obesity, aging, diabetes, and hypertension can contribute to clotting. Drugs for this immune system process help to reestablish the critical balance between clotting and not clotting.

▶ ATHEROSCLEROSIS

Atherosclerosis, a disease of the arteries, especially the coronary arteries of the heart and arteries of the brain, develops when layers of a plaque collect on arterial walls. Calcium added to this mix hardens it. The process continues; hard and rough, the arteries get thicker and thicker, eventually occluding the vessels. Passing RBCs, damaged by the roughness of the vessel walls, trigger clot formation (Fig. 15–1).

   The clot, or thrombus, that forms blocks the artery. Cardiac muscle or brain cells downstream, dependent on oxygen, begin to die. The resulting myocardial infarction (MI) or acute ischemic stroke or cerebrovascular accident (CVA) require aggressive reversal of coagulation with thrombolytics, enzymes that lyse the thrombus. Thrombolytic treatment cuts the mortality rate, lowers the incidence and severity of congestive heart failure, decreases infarction size, and improves left ventricular function. In addition, timely intervention with thrombolytics prevents the devastation of brain damage when a clot occludes blood flow and neurons downstream are deprived of blood. However, CVA can also be caused by the rupture of a vessel in the brain, contraindicating the use of thrombolytics, which would only cause more bleeding and damage. Once the thrombolytic enzymes have reduced the clot and reperfusion is accomplished, anticoagulants prevent more clotting. The anticoagulant heparin and the oral anticoagulants are the second and third therapeutic agents.

STEP ONE

Prothrombin activator, a complex of substances forms in responses to...

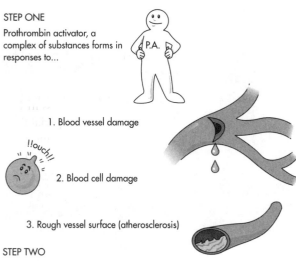

1. Blood vessel damage

!!ouch!!

2. Blood cell damage

3. Rough vessel surface (atherosclerosis)

STEP TWO

Prothrombin activator (thrombokinase) catalyzes prothrombin (factor II) into thrombin in the presence of calcium (factor IV) using intrinsic or extrinsic pathways.

Heparin interferes with the conversion of prothrombin to thrombin.

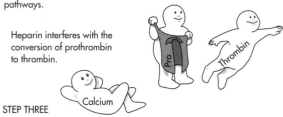

STEP THREE

Warfarin competes with vitamin K for receptors in the liver to block synthesis of clotting factors II (prothrombin), VII (serum prothrombin conversion accelerator "SPCA"), IX (plasma thromboplastin component "PTC" or Christmas factor or antihemophilic factor B) and, finally, X (Stuart factor or antihemophilic factor C)— all of which depend on vitamin K.

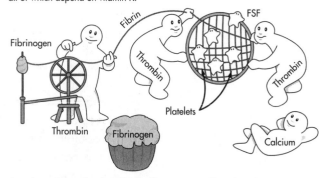

Thrombin is the catalyst that changes fibrinogen into fibrin threads to trap platelets, blood cells, and plasma to form a clot.

Finally—blood and trapped platelets release fibrin-stabilizing factor (FSF) (factor XIII) to link the fibrin threads together. In a few minutes it squeezes out the serum (plasma minus the clotting factors). Platelets continue to release FSF, securing the fibrin threads even more.

Aspirin works during this last step as an anticoagulant by making platelets "slippery."

Figure 15–1. The three steps of coagulation: steps 1, 2, 3 . . .

► DISSEMINATED INTRAVASCULAR
  COAGULATION (DIC)

Emboli from DIC frequently lodge in pulmonary arteries, especially in the right lung, and they constitute a serious threat to the patient's life. DIC can form in the pelvic area or the arms, but are most common in the deep veins of the legs, where they can cause local complications and emboli. Early signs of deep vein thrombi (DVT) include edema of the affected limb, warmth and redness in the calf, and cyanosis below the site of the clot. If arterial flow is slowed by edema, the leg will instead be cool and pale (Hickey, 1994); however, the opposite may be true if the clot is of great length, as may be the situation with the postpartum mother or the patient with a severe febrile condition. The resulting edema will cause the leg to be hot and appear white. The white appearance and its association with childbirth caused the condition to be called "milk leg." Homan's sign, which is pain upon forced dorsiflexion of the foot, is present only about 10–20% of the time (Hickey, 1994). Though exercise and activity can help prevent DIC, once a thrombus has formed, the patient's activities are restricted and bed rest becomes essential to prevent an embolus. Drug therapy is begun immediately with anticoagulants to tilt the clotting response away from forming new clots.

► DRUGS FOR THE TREATMENT OF CLOTTING

PLASMIN AND THE THROMBOLYTIC AGENTS

Just as the body forms clots, the body also dissolves clots. Clot dissolution involves plasmin or fibrinolysin. Plasmin "eats" fibrin threads, fibrinogen, factor V, factor VIII, prothrombin, and factor XII. Both tissue and blood contain activating factors: thrombin, activated factor XII, lysosomal enzymes, and four factors from vascular endothelium. These activators cause plasmin formation one to two days after trauma. Thrombolytic enzymes break up clots.

 Urokinase, a naturally occurring enzyme that breaks up clots in urine, is used for patients allergic to streptokinase. Streptokinase is derived from streptococcal bacteria, which can get past the immune system's protective clotting by dissolving clotted lymph and tissue that would otherwise wall off the invading bacteria. The third thrombolytic, tissue plasminogen activator (t-PA) is an emergency drug used early post-MI and CVA or stroke to reduce ischemia and prevent necrosis by producing early reperfusion; however, such early reperfusion of cardiac muscle may cause cardiac arrhythmias. As t-PA binds to the clot surface, it triggers the conversion of plasminogen to plasmin. During thrombolytic treatment, the nurse must monitor the patient for signs of hemorrhage.

Alteplase recombinant (t-PA) [Actilyse, Activase], a recombinant DNA–derived form of human tissue–type plasminogen activator (t-PA), is a thrombolytic agent promoting thrombolysis by forming the active proteolytic enzyme plasmin. It degrades fibrin, fibrinogen and factors V, VIII, and XII. It is used within 6 hours of MI for recanalization of the coronary artery in selective cases.

Off Label: Lysis of arterial occlusions in bypass and peripheral vessels.

Drug Interactions: none noted.

Side Effects

Nervous System: arrhythmias—bradycardia/idioventricular rhythms*/ventricular tachycardia.*

Endocrine: (Pregnancy Category C) cholesterol embolism.*

Immune System: anaphylaxis,* internal and superficial bleeding*—cerebral/retroperitoneal/GU/GI.

Dosage: Acute ischemic stroke (within 3 h and after CT scan): IV 0.9 mg/kg to maximum of 90 mg over 60 min with 10% of the total dose as an initial bolus over 1 min. Acute MI: IV 60 mg over first hour, with 6–10 mg bolus infused over first 1–2 min; then 20 mg/h over next 2 h (100 mg over 3 h). Accelerated administration: IV 15 mg bolus; then 0.75 mg/kg to maximum of 50 mg over 30 min; then 0.5 mg/kg to maximum of 35 mg over 60 min. Pulmonary embolism: IV 100 mg infused over 2 h.

Note: Follow with IV heparin therapy over 24 h.

Reteplase recombinant [Retavase] is a plasminogen activator that lyses the clot by degrading the matrix of the thrombus in the treatment of acute MI to improve ventricular function, reduce the incidence of CHF, and reduce mortality.

Drug Interactions: Increased risk of bleeding with ABCIXIMAB, aspirin, dipyridamole, heparin, or vitamin K antagonists.

Side Effects

Nervous System: arrhythmias—as seen in the course of an MI, ie, AV block/bradycardia/cardiac arrest*/accelerated idioventricular rhythm/PVC/SVT/ventricular tachycardia*/ventricular fibrillation,* cardiogenic shock*, electromechanical dissociation,* mitral regurgitation,* pulmonary edema.

Endocrine System: (Pregnancy Category C) cholesterol embolism.*

Immune System: anaphylaxis,* bleeding at cutdown/puncture/surgical wound sites, cardiac tamponade,*

* Life-threatening side effect.

hemorrhage,* ischemia,* myocardial rupture,* pericardial effusion,* pericarditis,* venous embolism*/thrombosis.

Dosage: IV 10 + 10 U double-bolus. Give first bolus over 2 min. Follow in 30 min after initiation of first bolus with second bolus over 2 min.

Streptokinase [Kabikinase, Streptase], derived from beta-hemolytic streptococci, converts plasminogen to plasmin to dissolve fibrin, fibrinogen, and other clotting proteins.

Drug Interactions: Increased risk of bleeding with anticoagulants. Reversed action with aminocaproic acid.

Side Effects

Nervous System: BP—unstable, bronchospasm, dysrhythmias—atrial/ventricular,* headache, nausea/vomiting, pain—musculoskeletal.

Endocrine System: (Pregnancy Category C) fever, flushing.

Immune System: anaphylaxis,* angioedema,* bleeding/oozing with percutaneous trauma, bleeding time prolonged systemically, spontaneous bleeding—GU/GI/retroperitoneal, phlebitis, swelling—periorbital.

Dosage: MI: IV 1.5 million IU over 60 min. Intracoronary 15,000–20,000 IU bolus. Then 2000–4000 IU/min for 60 min. DIC/pulmonary or arterial embolism: IV 250,000 IU over 30 min loading dose; then 100,000 IU/h × 48–72 h. Initial dose for AV cannula occlusion: 250,000 IU in 2 mL IV solution, slowly (25–35 min). Clamp cannula for 2 h. Aspirate and flush with saline.

Urokinase [Abbokinase, Open-Cath] is a kidney enzyme that interrupts conversion of plasminogen into plasmin, acting within and on the surface of the thrombus or embolus. It causes high plasma levels of fibrin and fibrinogen degradation products. It is most effective on newly formed clots and is used in lysis of acute massive pulmonary and peripheral emboli. It also restores patency in occluded IV catheters. It is used in acute MI, lysis of clot-occluded arteriovenous canulas, retinal vessel occlusion, and other clotting conditions.

Drug Interactions: none noted.

Side Effects

Nervous System: see *streptokinase.*

Endocrine System: see *streptokinase.*

Immune System: see *streptokinase.*

Dosage: Occluded coronary artery: IV. Precede with heparin bolus of 2500–10,000 U per IV; instill urokinase

6000 IU/min for periods up to 2 h. Continue until artery is maximally open; usually 15–30 min using about 500,000 IU. Administer through in-line 0.22 or 0.45 mcg filter using a constant infusion pump. Pulmonary embolus: IV 4400 IU/kg diluted in 0.9% NaCl or 5% dextrose infused over 10 min, followed by continuous infusion of 4400 IU/kg/h for 12 h. Administer through in-line 0.22 or 0.45 mcg filter using a constant infusion. Central venous catheter clearance: IV. Instill 5000 IU/mL solution into catheter port. After 5 min try to aspirate urokinase and clot. If no success after 30 min, cap port for 30–60 min and try again. Instruct patient to exhale and hold breath any time catheter is disconnected from syringe or IV tubing. Avoid excessive pressure of instillation to prevent rupture of catheter or forcing clot into circulation.

ANTICOAGULANTS

Anticoagulants prevent clotting. They cannot dissolve clots; that is the work of thrombolytics. The rapid-action anticoagulant is heparin. If the patient is to be on long-term anticoagulant therapy, heparin is given until the liver's store of clotting factors is depleted and oral anticoagulants can be effective. For centuries doctors used medicinal leeches to "reestablish" the balance of the four humors (yellow and black bile, blood, and phlegm) they believed caused illness. Leeches, like mosquitoes, use heparin to keep the blood they suck from coagulating. In fact, prior to heparin, powdered leech heads were used as anticoagulants. The liver makes heparin, named after the Greek word for liver because it was first discovered in dog livers. Mast cells all over the body constantly secrete heparin. The lungs and liver are loaded with mast cells because these organs have to fight great numbers of invader organisms. Heparin made possible kidney dialysis and extracorporeal circulation.

Ardeparin Na [Normiflo Injection] is a low-molecular-weight heparin from pork to prevent DVT, which may lead to pulmonary embolism after knee replacement surgery.

Drug Interactions: See *heparin.*

Side Effects

Nervous System: arthralgia, bowel—constipation, dizziness, nausea/vomiting, pain—chest, psyche—confusion.

Endocrine System: (Pregnancy Category C) fever.

Immune System: anemia, ecchymosis, hemorrhage at injection site, pruritus, rash, thrombocytopenia, urticaria.

Dosage: Deep SC 50 anti-Xa U/kg of body weight q12h. Begin treatment evening of the day of surgery or the following morning and continue for up to 14 d or until patient is fully ambulatory, whichever is shorter.

---

* Life-threatening side effect.

Danaparoid sodium [Orgaran] is an antithrombotic agent derived from pork intestinal mucosa.

Drug Interactions: Increased bleeding time with oral anticoagulants and/or platelet inhibitors.

Side Effects

Nervous System: asthenia, bladder—retention, bowel—constipation, dizziness, headache, insomnia, nausea/vomiting, peripheral edema. Injection site: pain.

Endocrine System: (Pregnancy Category B) edema, fever.

Immune System: anemia, joint disorders, pruritus, rash, urinary tract infection.

Dosage: SC 750 anti-Xa units bid beginning 1–4 h preop, and not sooner than 2 h postop. Continue treatment q12h until postop risk of DVT has decreased, usually 7–10 d, and up to 14 d.

Heparin calcium [Calciparine], heparin sodium [Heparin Sodium Lock Flush Solution, Hep-Lock, Lipo-Hepin, Liquaemin Dosium] can only be given intravenously or subcutaneously, because heparin is digested in the stomach. It must never be given intramuscularly, however, because of the danger of bleeding in muscles. The sodium form is used in the heparin lock, a device making it possible to leave intravenous catheters such as central venous, femoral, or dialysis catheter lines free of clots. It is used to prevent and/or treat venous thrombosis and pulmonary embolism and to prevent clotting complications arising from cardiac and vascular surgery, frostbite, and MI. It is also used to treat DIC and atrial fibrillation with emboli. It is used in blood transfusions, extracorporeal circulation, and dialysis.

Off Label: Prophylaxis in hip and knee surgery.

Note: The danger in giving heparin is hemorrhage. Heparin administration is a tightrope balancing act. The dosage is always calibrated according to the clotting system's production of thrombin, the catalyst that changes fibrinogen into fibrin threads to trap platelets, blood cells, and plasma to form a clot. The lab test used is called the partial thromboplastin time (PTT). The PTT must be done frequently to monitor dosage. The PTT must be kept below 30 sec. The specimen is drawn 30 min before scheduled SC injection or intermittent IV, and every 4 h for continuous IV administration. So important is the PTT to heparin administration that the nurse must always consult the up-to-date result to see whether or not to give heparin and if so, how much (see the box on this page).

Drug Interactions: Prolonged PT possible with oral anticoagulants. Increased risk of bleeding with NSAIDs. Decreased anticoagulant activity with IV nitroglycerin possible. The antidote is protamine.

Administering Heparin

Besides checking an up-to-date PTT and the corresponding amount of heparin to be given, other precautions in giving heparin include:
- Always double-check the amount of heparin drawn up with a second nurse to ensure accuracy.
- Use a tuberculin syringe for accurate measure.
- For subcutaneous administration: change needles after drawing up the heparin.
- Use universal precautions for handling blood.
- Advise the patient that the procedure is a slow one.
- Because the procedure is slow, the nurse can use this opportunity for therapeutic interaction with the patient and to assess how the patient is dealing with the stress of a serious illness.
- Because the needle on the tuberculin syringe is short, use a 90° angle of injection.
- Select and ice an area with an adequate layer of subcutaneous fat that the patient will not have to lie on.
- The most frequent site of injection is the fatty layer over the abdomen; usually in a 2-in. radius around the umbilicus or near the iliac crest.
- After cleansing the skin, do not pinch, but hold up skin with the underlying fat.
- Inject slowly into the fatty subcutaneous layer after releasing grasp.
- Never aspirate when injecting heparin.
- Pause a few seconds before withdrawing the needle to avoid trailing heparin up through the needle tract.
- Apply gentle pressure to the site.
- Reapply ice.
- Do not rub or massage the injection site.
- Rotate injection sites.
- Assess for objective and subjective signs of bleeding.

Note: Intravenous therapy with heparin should be preceded by insertion of the IV to prevent bleeding at the site.

Incompatibilities

Solution/Additive: amikacin, codeine, chlorpromazine, cytarabine, diazepam, dobutamine, doxorubicin, droperidol, erythromycin, gentamicin, haloperidol, hyaluronidase, hydrocortisone, kanamycin, levorphanol, meperidine, methadone, methicillin, methotrimeprazine, morphine, netilmicin, nitroglycerin, pentazocine, polymyxin B, promethazine, streptomycin, tetracycline, tobramycin, triflupromazine, vancomycin.

Y-site: amikacin, dacarbazine, diazepam, diphenhydramine, doxorubicin, doxycycline, droperidol, ergotamine, erythromycin, gentamicin, haloperidol, kanamycin, methotrimeprazine, netilmicin, nitroglycerin, phenytoin, polymyxin B, streptomycin, tobramycin, triflupromazine, vancomycin.

Side Effects

Nervous System: arthralgia, BP—elevated, bronchospasm, burning/itching sensation—feet, cyanosis, headache, lacrimation, numbness/tingling—hands/feet, pain—arms/legs/chest/injection site, sexual function— priapism, vasospasm.

Endocrine System: (Pregnancy Category C) chills, fever, hyperkalemia, rebound hyperlipidemia, hypoaldosteronism, suppressed renal function.

Immune System: alopecia, ALT/AST—increases, anaphylactoid reactions,* bleeding—spontaneous, ecchymoses, hypofibrinogenemia, nasal congestion, osteoporosis, pruritus, rashes, thrombocytopenia— transient, tissue irritation/sloughing, urticaria, white clot syndrome.

Dosage: IV bolus of 5000 U; then 20,000–40,000 U infused over 24 h. Adjust dose to maintain desired APTT; or 5000–10,000 U IV piggyback q4–6h. SC 10,000–20,000 U followed by 8000–20,000 U q8–12h. Open heart surgery: IV 150–300 U/kg. Use up to 400 U for procedures > 1 h. Device: Heparin Lock. Initial dose: IV 10 U/mL or 100 U/mL instilled into the lock.

THE ANTIDOTE FOR HEPARIN

Heparin is acidic. Its antidote is a base, protamine, which is made from fish sperm or testis. Protamine acts immediately to neutralize the heparin and lasts 2 h.

<u>Protamine sulfate</u> is the antidote for heparin calcium or heparin sodium.

Off Label: Antidote for heparin during extracorporeal circulation.

Drug Interactions: none noted.

Side Effects

Nervous System: abrupt BP drop with rapid IV infusion, arrythmia, bradycardia, dyspnea, lassitude, nausea/vomiting.

Endocrine System: (Pregnancy Category C) flushing, warm feeling.

Immune System: anaphylaxis,* angioedema,* pulmonary edema, heparin rebound, urticaria.

Dosage: Initial dose: Relative to heparin. IV 1 mg of protamine neutralizes 80–100 U of heparin. Give slowly. 1 mg neutralizes 90 U of beef-lung heparin, 115 U of intestinal mucosa–derived heparin, or 100 U of calcium heparin. Calculate approximate dose and give the first 25–50 mg by slow IV push and the rest by continuous infusion over 8–16 h. Caution: Do not exceed 50 mg in any 10-min period.

► LONG-TERM ANTICOAGULANT THERAPY: THE ORAL ANTICOAGULANTS

Some patients will require long-term anticoagulant therapy, and heparin simply is not the drug of choice for long-term use. The oral anticoagulants can be taken by patients at home as long as they follow the guidelines carefully—follow through on getting routine PT, avoid activities that cut or bruise, take the medication as prescribed, and report any signs of bleeding to the primary caretaker.

<u>Dicumarol [Bishydroxycoumarin]</u> is a long-acting coumarin derivative that prevents clotting by depressing hepatic synthesis of vitamin K–dependent coagulation factors II, VII, IX and X.

Drug Interactions: See *warfarin.*

Side Effects

Nervous System: bowel—diarrhea/flatulence, cramps— abdominal, nausea/vomiting, sexual function—priapism.

Endocrine System: (Pregnancy Category D) fever.

Immune System: agranulocytosis,* dermatitis, hair loss, hematuria, hemorrhage,* leukopenia.

Dosage: PO 200–300 mg on day 1. Maintenance: 25– 200 mg qd if PT is 1.5–2.5 times the control.

<u>Warfarin sodium [Coumadin Sodium, Panwarfin]</u> was discovered in red clover that killed the cattle that ate it by causing internal hemorrhage. The "warf" part of the name stands for Wisconsin Alumni Research Foundation. Originally, the product was used as rat poison until a young man tried to kill himself with it, and doctors realized its potential use in humans as an anticoagulant (Sneader, 1985). Warfarin acts in the liver, competing for vitamin K receptor sites in the production of vitamin K–dependent clotting factors (II, VII, IX, X). Because already present clotting factors take about 3–5 days to be depleted before warfarin can take effect, heparin is used initially as an anticoagulant. Warfarin is used for venous

---

* Life-threatening side effect.

thrombi and prosthetic heart valves, but is not used in arterial thrombi (platelet-produced conditions).

Drug Interactions: Decreased action with alcohol,* barbiturates, carbamazepine, chloral hydrate,* cholestyramine,* corticosteroids, corticotropin, diuretics, ethchlorvynol, glutethimide,* griseofulvin, laxatives, mercaptopurine, oral contraceptives containing estrogen,* rifampin, spironolactone, vitamin C, vitamin K (dietary). Increased action with alcohol,* chloral hydrate.* The addition or withdrawal of any drug requires more frequent PT testing and careful observation with dose adjustment as needed.

Incompatibilities

Solution/Additive: ammonium chloride, 5% dextrose, Ringer's lactate, aminoglycosides, ascorbic acid, epinephrine, metaraminol, oxytocin, promazine, tetracycline, vancomycin, vitamin B complex with C.

Side Effects

Nervous System: bowel—diarrhea, cramps—abdominal, nausea/vomiting, paralytic ileus.

Endocrine System: (Pregnancy Category D) anorexia, fever, steatorrhea.

Immune System: bleeding, dermatitis, hair loss, hemorrhage,* hepatitis, jaundice, necrosis—toes/tip of nose/buttocks/thighs/calves/female breast/abdomen/other fat-rich areas, pruritus, stomatitis, increased serum transaminase levels, urticaria.

Dosage: IV, PO 5–15 mg/d for 2–5 d; then 2–10 mg qd. Regulate per PT at 2–10 mg qd. Onset: 12–24 h. Duration: 2–5 d.

▶ VITAMIN K: WARFARIN ANTIDOTE

Vitamin K works in the liver to help form blood clotting factors II, VII, IX, and X. It does not reverse the action of heparin.

Phytonadione (vitamin K) [Aquamephyton, Konakion, Mephyton, Phylloquinone] is a fat-soluble naphthoquinone derivative chemically identical to and with similar degree of activity as naturally occurring vitamin K. The oral anticoagulants are metabolized, ie, changed or broken apart, in liver cells by microsomal enzymes.

Drug Interactions: Drugs that speed up the cells' microsomal metabolism decrease the effective duration of oral anticoagulant activity. Such drugs include alcohol, barbiturates (including the derivative phenytoin), carbamazepine, ethchlorvynol, griseofulvin, rifampin. In addition, when some drugs compete with oral anticoagulants that are protein-bound and dislodge them from the car-

rier proteins, the anticoagulant molecules are set free to compete for receptors with vitamin K. The result is increased anticoagulant activity. Some drugs that compete this way include aspirin (which also slows clotting through another process), chloral hydrate, clofibrate, diazoxide, ethacrynic acid, mefenamic acid, nalidixic acid, phenylbutazone, sulfonamides, sulfonylureas. Mineral oil decreases absorption of oral phytonadione.

Side Effects

Nervous System: bronchospasm,* cardiac arrest,* chest constriction sensation, convulsive-like movements, dizziness, dyspnea, gastric upset, headache, pain—cramping at injection site, respiratory arrest,* shock, taste changes, weakness.

Endocrine System: (Pregnancy Category C) chills, flushing, sweating.

Immune System: anaphylaxis,* erythematous skin eruptions, hematoma/nodule formation, hypoprothrombinemia.

Dosage: PO, SC, IM 2.5–10 mg. Rarely up to 50 mg/d. May repeat parenteral dose after 6–8 h if needed. May repeat PO dose after 12–24 h. Emergency: IV 10–15 mg ≤ 1 mg/min. Repeat in 4 h if needed.

▶ PROSTAGLANDINS AND CLOTTING

A prostaglandin, thromboxane A_2, causes platelets to become sticky and clump together. Aspirin inhibits production of the prostaglandin, causing the platelets to remain slippery so they cannot adhere to the fibrin web of a forming clot. Aspirin helps decrease the chance for clotting for post-MI, for TIA, and prosthetic heart valves. Dipyridamole [Persantine], a vasodilator and antiplatelet aggregate, is used with aspirin.

ABCIXIMAB (c7E3 Fab) [ReoPro] inhibits platelet aggregation by preventing fibrinogen, von Willebrand's factor, and other molecules from adhering to GPIIb/IIIa receptor sites of the platelets. It is produced from human–murine monoclonal antibody fragment antigen binding (Fab) and used as an adjunct to aspirin and heparin to prevent acute cardiac ischemic complications in percutaneous transluminal coronary angioplasty (PTCA).

Drug Interactions: Increased bleeding risk with oral anticoagulants, dextran, dipyridamole, NSAIDs.

Side Effects

Nervous System: none noted.

Endocrine System: (Pregnancy Category C) none noted.

Immune System: bleeding*—hematemesis/intracranial/retroperitoneal, thrombocytopenia.

* Avoid concurrent use if possible.

* Life-threatening side effect.

Dosage: IV: 0.25 mg/kg bolus. Follow by infusion of 10 mcg/min × 12 h.

Anagrelide hydrochloride [Agrylin] reduces platelets in essential thrombocythemia thus decreasing elevated platelet count and the risk of thrombosis. Anagrelide may interfere with megacaryocyte hypermaturation. Platelet counts are needed q2d during the first week of treatment and weekly thereafter until the maintenance dosage is reached.

Side Effects

Nervous System: bowel—diarrhea, headache, pain—abdominal, palpitations. In thrombocythemia: arrhythmia—atrial fibrillation/complete heart block, cardiomegaly/cardiomyopathy, CHF, pulmonary hypertension, seizure.*

Endocrine System: (Pregnancy Category C) none noted.

Immune System: MI,* CVA,* gastroduodenal ulceration, pancreatitis, pericarditis,* pulmonary infiltrates/fibrosis.

Dosage: PO. Start with 0.5 mg qid or 1 mg tid. Increase to 1.5 to 3 mg/d. Adjust to maintain platelet count at 500,000/mL. Not to exceed 10 mg/d or 2.5 in a single dose.

Aspirin (for trade names and side effects, see Chapter 14: Nonsteroidal Antiinflammatories), inhibits prostaglandin synthesis, thus interfering with platelet aggregation. High serum concentrations may impair liver synthesis of factors VII, IX, X by possibly inhibiting vitamin K action.

Drug Interactions: Increased risk of toxicity with aminosalicylic acid, carbonic anhydrase inhibitors. Decreased renal elimination and increased risk of toxicity with ammonium chloride and other acidifying agents. Increased risk of bleeding with anticoagulants. Increased hypoglycemic activity with oral hypoglycemic agents when aspirin doses are over 2 g/d. Increased ulcer activity with corticosteroids. Increased methotrexate toxicity. In low doses may antagonize uricosuric effects of probenecid and sulfinpyrazone.

Dosage: Thromboembolic disorders: PO 325–650 mg qd or bid. TIA prophylaxis: PO 650 mg bid.

Dipyridamole [Persantine, Pyridamole, IV Persantine] is a non-nitrate coronary vasodilator that selectively dilates coronary arteries to increase myocardial oxygen supply. It has a mild anatropic action, but little effect on blood pressure and blood flow in peripheral arteries. It is used to prevent postoperative clotting complications associ-

ated with prosthetic heart valves and as an adjunct for thallium stress testing.

Off Label: Reduces occurrence of post-MI reinfarction. Also prevents transient ischemic attacks and coronary bypass graft occlusion.

Drug Interactions: none noted.

Side Effects

Nervous System: bowel—diarrhea, dizziness, faintness, headache, nausea/vomiting, syncope, peripheral vasodilation, weakness.

Endocrine System: (Pregnancy Category C) flushing.

Immune System: pruritus, rash.

Dosage: Thromboembolic disorders: PO 75–100 mg qd in divided doses. Duration: 4 h. Thromboembolic prevention in cardiac valve replacement: PO 75–100 mg/d qid. Thallium stress test: IV 0.142 mg/kg/min for 4 min.

Ticlopidine [Ticlid] is a platelet aggregation inhibitor interfering with platelet membrane functioning. It reduces the risk of thrombolic stroke in patients intolerant to aspirin.

Off Label: Prevents venous thromboembolic disorders. Maintenance of bypass graft patency and of vascular access sites in hemodialysis. Improves exercise performance in patients with ischemic heart disease and intermittent claudication. Helps prevent postoperative DVT.

Drug Interactions: Decreased bioavailability with antacids. Increased risk of bleeding with anticoagulants. Decreased clearance with cimetidine. Decreased bleeding time with corticosteroids. May decrease cyclosporin levels. Increases theophylline half-life by 42%. Increased bioavailability possible with food.

Side Effects

Nervous System: bowels—flatulence, cramps—abdominal, dizziness, dyspepsia, nausea/vomiting.

Endocrine System: (Pregnancy Category B) anorexia.

Immune System: agranulocytosis,* erythema nodosum, hemorrhage—ecchymosis/epistaxis/menorrhagia/GI bleeding, leukopenia, abnormal liver function tests, neutropenia, pancytopenia,* thrombocytopenia, urticaria.

Dosage: Stroke prevention: PO 250 mg bid with food.

▶ A DRUG TO DECREASE BLOOD VISCOSITY

Many drugs in this chapter are commonly referred to as "blood thinners," even though they do not "thin" the blood. Viscosity does refer to thickness, however, making pentoxifylline a true blood "thinner."

Pentoxifylline [Trental] is a methylxanthine, like caffeine and theophylline, and increases RBC flexibility, de-

---

* Life-threatening side effect.

creases platelet and RBC aggregation, and decreases fibrinogen. Pentoxifylline is used to treat intermittent claudication of occlusive peripheral vascular disease and diabetic angiopathies.

Off Label: Helps improve psychopathologic symptoms associated with cerebral vascular insufficiency. Reduces incidence of stroke in recurring TIAs.

Drug Interactions: none noted.

Side Effects

Nervous System: angina, abdominal discomfort—belching/bloating/flatus, arrhythmias, chest pain, loss of consciousness, convulsions,* dizziness, drowsiness, dyspnea, earache, edema, headache, hypotension, insomnia, malaise, nausea/vomiting, palpitations, psyche—agitation/confusion/nervousness, excessive salivation, somnolence, unpleasant taste, vision—blurred/scotomas.

Endocrine System: (Pregnancy Category C) flushing, weight change.

Immune System: brittle fingernails, leukopenia, pruritus, rash, sore throat, swollen neck glands, urticaria.

Dosage: Intermittent claudication: PO 400 mg tid with meals × 8 wk. If side effects occur, decrease to 400 mg bid.

▶ HEMOPHILIA

Hemophilia is a genetic disorder passed on from mother to son on her X chromosome. Although the gene is carried by the female, she is protected by having two X chromosomes, since only one will carry the defect. Hemophilia became associated with European royalty when the female offspring of Queen Victoria carried it into the genetic lines of the royal houses of Russia and Spain. Hemophilia is a result of missing clotting factors (V, VIII, XI, or XIII). In addition, factors II, VII, IX, and X can also be deficient. The only treatment is replacement of missing factors. Factor VIII is produced in such minute quantities that numerous units of plasma are required to obtain it. The more units of plasma needed, the greater the risk of hepatitis or AIDS.

Factor IX complex [Konyne, Konyne-HT, Profilnine, Proplex, Proplex SX] is used to replace the missing clotting factor to control bleeding in factor IX deficiency. Proplex is used to control bleeding in patients with hemophilia A (who have factor VIII inhibitors).

Drug Interactions: none noted.

Side Effects

Nervous System: With rapid infusion: changes in BP/pulse rate, headache, lethargy, nausea/vomiting, somnolence, tingling.

Endocrine System: (Pregnancy Category C) With large doses: chills, fever. With rapid infusion: chills, fever, flushing.

Immune System: anaphylactic shock* (rare), viral hepatitis. With large doses: DIC,* MI,* thrombosis.*

Dosage: For bleeding in hemophilia A clients with factor VIII inhibitors. IV 75 IU/kg with second dose in 12 h. Hemophilia B clients prophylaxis of bleeding. IV 10–20 IU/kg 1–2 times per wk. (Check package insert for dosage guidelines for individual factor deficiencies.)

▶ HEMOSTATIC AGENTS

The following agents are sometimes used to inhibit bleeding caused by surgical procedures. The patient must be monitored for signs of thrombosis.

Aminocaproic acid [Amicar, EACA (epsilon-aminocaproic acid)] inhibits the substances that trigger plasminogen in systemic bleeding caused by hyperfibrinolysis and urinary fibrinolysis.

Drug Interactions: Anesthetics, skeletal muscle relaxants increase neuromuscular blocking effects. Increased risk of ototoxicity and nephrotoxicity with acyclovir, amphotericin B, bacitracin, capreomycin, cephalosporins, colistin, cisplatin, carboplatin, ethacrynic acid, furosemide, methoxyflurane, polymyxin B, vancomycin.

Incompatibilities

Solution/Additive: aminophylline, amphotericin B, cephalosporins, chlorothiazide, erythromycin, heparin, oxytetracycline, penicillins, phenytoin, thiopental, vitamin B complex with C, warfarin.

Y-site: amphotericin B, heparin, phenytoin, thiopental.

Side Effects

Nervous System: arrhythmias, bladder—frequency, bowel—diarrhea, convulsions,* cramps, dizziness, dysuria, faintness, headache, hypotension—orthostatic, malaise, muscle weakness, nausea/vomiting, sweating, tinnitus.

Endocrine System: (Pregnancy Category C) anorexia, oliguria, reddish-brown urine (myoglobinuria), prolonged menstruation with cramping, acute renal failure.*

Immune System: conjunctival erythema, nasal congestion, rash, thrombophlebitis,* thromboses.*

Dosage: PO, IV 4–5 g during first hour; then 1–1.25 g qh for 8 h or until bleeding is controlled to maximum of 30 g /24 h.

---

* Life-threatening side effect.

► THE IMMUNE SYSTEM'S MUCOUS MEMBRANES

As part of the immune system, the mucous membranes line the walls of the respiratory tract, the gastrointestinal system and the genitourinary system, secreting a clear, slightly sticky or viscous fluid. All these structures are vulnerable to invasion by microbes from the environment and are protected and defended by the secretions of the mucous membranes. The viscosity of mucus is a prime factor in maintaining health. Mucus must be just sticky enough to adhere to potentially disease-causing microscopic particles, but slippery enough to glide easily on the surface of the mucous membranes. Changes in color, consistency, and smell can indicate disease, for example, a yellow-green exudate is common in bronchiectasis and infections of the bronchi, the bronchioles, and also the nasopharynx. Drugs for this system help to create optimal viscosity of mucus.

The mucociliary blanket in the respiratory tract traps microbes and dust. Mucus is carried on top of the hair-like cilia that propel it with a waving, fanning action up from the bronchi and down from the nose to a point where the individual may then swallow it or cough and expectorate. Mucus is produced throughout the airway. The average adult moves approximately a cup of mucus up the airway with the help of the cilia and swallows it in the course of a day. Mucus must be slippery enough to be propelled out of the airway. When it is too thick and tenacious, as in asthma or cystic fibrosis, it becomes part of the problem by obstructing the airway. Thick mucus may also become a breeding ground for microbes. Tenacious, difficult-to-expectorate mucus may be a temporary problem as the respiratory system cleans up after an infection, or it may be a part of a patient's daily reality in dealing with chronic obstructive pulmonary disease (COPD).

CYSTIC FIBROSIS (CF) AND CHRONIC OBSTRUCTIVE PULMONARY DISEASE (COPD)

The young patient with CF must constantly keep tenacious mucus from clinging to the bronchial tree, thus creating an environment for infection. A genetic disease of the exocrine glands, cystic fibrosis results in a disruption of the flow of chloride ions out of cells, resulting in dry, tenacious mucus. Because the mucus is difficult to expectorate, it creates obstructions of the airway that eventually cause lung damage. Even with the best of care, the person with CF has a short life span.

Patients with COPD may require more assistance to move mucus out of the respiratory system so that it does not become a breeding ground for infection. For them, postural drainage and chest physiotherapy, which evolved from the technique of manual cupping, can give some relief.

The older adult suffering from COPD after years of smoking or working in conditions that are hazardous to the respiratory system has to adjust to a new reality of fighting for each breath with little energy left over for being social. Smoking destroys the cilia, leaving the patient with only mucus and a cough to protect him from infection.

ASTHMA

Thick, tenacious mucus can be terrifying to the person suffering an acute asthmatic attack in which, not only are copious amounts of thick mucus produced, but the airway is in spasm. Such an attack is a true emergency; though mucus is part of the problem, the first concern is to relieve the spasm and prevent recurrence with drugs of the nervous and endocrine systems—sympathomimetics and corticosteroids.

CORYZA

Coryza or rhinitis occurs when the mucous membranes of the nose and sinuses become inflamed and swollen due to allergy or infection. The capillaries dilate and become more permeable, leaking clear fluid from the bloodstream as mast cells release histamine. In addition, the mucous membranes increase their secretions (see the box on page 211).

ATELECTASIS

Though mucus is a protective secretion, sometimes it can impair health. A mucus plug in the bronchial tree can cause atelectasis when the blood passing through the lungs for reoxygenation picks up all the oxygen below the plug and the empty alveoli collapse like tiny deflated balloons. To prevent atelectasis, the postoperative or long-term bedridden patient needs to move, turn, take deep breaths, cough frequently, and get adequate hydration.

COUGH

Coughing helps to expel mucus. Mucolytic drugs do not suppress the cough reflex. Sometimes, however, a mucolytic such as guaifenesin may be combined with a cough suppressant such as dextromethorphan. But for the most part, conditions in which mucus is thick and obstructing the airway call for expelling the mucus, not suppressing the cough.

MUCUS AS A HEALTH HAZARD

At one time public buildings in this country had spittoons for the convenience of those who spit in public. Then public health concerns made spittoons obsolete. Spitting continues, however, and so does the health hazard. Bacteria and viruses trapped in the mucus are set free to blow

Chicken Soup and Coryza

Long considered folklore, chicken soup as a restorative agent for the misery of the flu and other upper respiratory infections makes sense in view of the fluid loss of coryza due to the immune response's shift of fluid from the bloodstream through the capillaries, where it mixes with mucus. In essence, this is a hemorrhage of the clear portion of the blood. Chicken soup contains the electrolytes lost in the watery discharge. It's a transfusion of sorts.

in the dust of a street once the mucus has dried. Passersby breathe them in. In fact, street sweepers have a high incidence of TB as an occupational hazard.

Adequate fluid intake and the mucolytics help decrease mucus viscosity and set the stage for expectorating the mucus. Sometimes a patient cannot easily cough up and expectorate mucus. Perhaps recent surgery makes such activity painful, or maybe opiate analgesics have suppressed the cough reflex.

DRUGS TO LOOSEN MUCUS

The drugs for making mucus less viscous are called mucolytics (mucus cutters) and make it less tenacious by lowering surface tension. Simply making mucus less tenacious helps the patient expectorate. Mucolytics are often sold OTC. Some cough syrup formulas are combinations of mucolytics and antitussives. Coughing is essential in cleansing the lower respiratory tract, and it may not be beneficial to suppress the cough in some conditions. The patient must be educated as to whether or not cough suppression is desirable. The patient needs to know that a persistent cough may signal a condition requiring medical intervention.

Acetylcysteine [Mucomyst, Mucosol, N-Acetylcysteine], the prototype mucolytic, is used via inhalation or direct installation to loosen abnormally thick mucus by breaking sulfur chains. It is an important drug for acute and chronic obstructive pulmonary diseases, including cystic fibrosis, atelectasis, and postoperative atelectasis, as well as for tracheostomy and acetaminophen overdose.

Drug Interactions: Though acetylcysteine can be mixed with some antibiotics and bronchodilators, it should never be combined with erythromycin lactobionate, oxytetracycline, sodium ampicillin, or tetracycline.

Side Effects

Nervous System: bronchospasm, burning sensation in upper respiratory passages, dizziness, drowsiness, nausea/vomiting.

Endocrine System: (Pregnancy Category B) none noted.

Immune System: epistaxis, rhinorrhea, stomatitis, urticaria.

Dosage: Mucus inhalation: 1–10 mL of 20% solution q4–6h or 2–20 mL of 10% solution q4–6h. Direct instillation: 1–2 mL of 10–20% solution q1–4h. Acetaminophen overdose: PO 140 mg/kg 5% solution followed by 70 mg/kg q4h for 17 doses.

Guaifenesin [Amonidrin, Anti-Tuss, Breonesin, Gee-Gee, GG-Cen, Glyceryl Guaiacolate, Glycotuss, Glytuss, Guaituss, Hytuss, Malotuss, Mytussin, Nortussin, Robitussin] is used to treat dry, nonproductive cough associated with colds and bronchitis.

Drug Interactions: May increase risk of hemorrhage in patients receiving heparin due to inhibition of platelet functions.

Side Effects

Nervous System: drowsiness, GI upset, nausea.

Endocrine System: (Pregnancy Category C) none noted.

Immune System: none noted.

Dosage: PO 100–400 mg q4h up to 2.4 g/d.

Potassium iodide, saturated solution [Pima, SSKI] eases bronchial drainage and cough in asthma, chronic bronchitis, bronchiectasis, emphysema, and respiratory tract allergies characterized by difficult-to-raise sputum.

Drug Interactions: Hypothyroid and goitrogenic actions may be potentiated with antithyroid drugs, lithium. Increased risk of hyperkalemia with ACE inhibitors, potassium-sparing diuretics, potassium supplements.

Side Effects

Nervous System: arrhythmias, arthralgias, diarrhea, pain—stomach, paresthesias, productive cough, pulmonary edema, salivation, weakness. With poisoning: coryza/sneezing, frontal headache, nausea/vomiting—blue or yellow, psyche—confusion.

Endocrine System: (Pregnancy Category D) fever, goiter, hypothyroidism, pulmonary edema,

Immune System: acne, angioedema,* collagen disease-like syndromes, bloody diarrhea, eosinophilia, hemorrhage—cutaneous/mucosal, hyperthyroid adenoma, lymph node enlargements, small bowel lesions—non-

* Life-threatening side effect.

specific. With poisoning: edema—periorbital/pulmonary, salivary glands—tender/swollen, stomatitis.

Dosage: PO 300–650 mg pc bid or tid.

Chapter Highlights

- Clotting and production of mucus are both functions of the immune system intended to form barriers.

- Clots form barriers to prevent more blood loss and to block the passage of infectious agents.

- Abnormal clotting conditions are treated with drugs that lyse clots, prevent them, or if clotting factors are missing, replace the factors.

- Mucus is meant to protect the mucous membranes from damage or infection.

- When mucus is too thick or tenacious, it cannot be easily expectorated and may become a problem.

- Mucolytics and expectorants help loosen mucus so that the patient can cough it up.

16

Antimicrobials: Antivirals, Antibiotics, Antifungals, and Antiparasitics

drug list

- acyclovir [Acycloguanosine, Zovirax]
- acyclovir sodium
- amantadine hydrochloride [Symmetrel]
- aminosalicylic acid [P.A.S.]
- amoxicillin [Amoxil, others]
- amoxicillin + potassium clavulanate [Augmentin]
- amphotericin B [Fungizone]
- amphotericin B lipid complex [ABELCET]
- ampicillim sodium + sulbactam sodium [Unasyn]
- ampicillin [various]
- atovaquone [Mepron]
- azithromycin [Zithromax]
- aztreonam [Azactam]
- butenafine [Mentax]
- capreomycin [Capastat Sulfate]
- cefamandole nafate [Mandol]
- cefazolin sodium [Ancef, Kefzol, others]
- cefepime hydrochloride [Maxipime]
- cefixime [Suprax]
- cefonicid sodium [Monocid]
- cefoperazone sodium [Cefobid]
- cefotaxime sodium [Claforan]
- cefotetan disodium [Cefotan]
- cefoxitin [Mefoxin]
- cefpodoxime [Vantine]
- cefprozil [Cefzil]
- ceftazidime [Ceptaz, Fortaz, Tazicef, Tazidime]
- ceftizoxime sodium [Cefizox]
- ceftriaxone sodium, [Rocephin]
- cefuroxime axetil [Ceftin]
- cefuroxime sodium [Kefurox, Zinacef]
- cephalexin [Keflex, others]

drug list

- cephalothin sodium [Keflin, Seffin]
- cephapirin sodium [Cefadyl]
- cepharidine [Anspor]
- chloramphenicol + salts [Chloromycetin, others]
- chloroquine hydrochloride [Aralen Hydrochloride]
- chloroquine phosphate [Aralen Phosphate]
- ciclopirox olamine [Loprox]
- cidofovir [Vistide]
- cinoxacin [Cinobac]
- ciprofloxacin hydrochloride [Cipro]
- clarithromycin [Biaxin]
- clindamycin salts [Cleocin, others]
- clotrimazole [Gyne-Lotrimin, Lotromin, Mycelex]
- cloxacillin [Tegopen, others]
- cycloserine [Seromycin]
- dapsone [DDS]
- delavirdine mesylate [Rescriptor]
- demeclocycline [Declomycin]
- dicloxacillin [Dynapen, others]
- didanosine (DDI) [Videx]
- dirithromycin [Dynabac]
- doxycycline hyclate [Vibramycin, others]
- econazole nitrate [Spectazole]
- emetine hydrochloride
- erythromycin [E-Mycin, others]
- erythromycin estolate [Ilosine]
- erythromycin ethylsuccinate [E.E.S., others]
- erythromycin gluceptate [Ilotycin Gluceptate]
- erythromycin stearate [Eramycin, others]
- ethambutol hydrochloride [Myambutol]
- ethionamide [Trecator-SC]
- fluconazole [Diflucan]
- flucytosine [Ancobon, others]
- foscarnet [Foscavir]
- fosfomycin tromethamine [Monurol]
- ganciclovir (DHPG) [Cytovene]
- gentamicin sulfate [Garamycin, Genoptic, others]
- griseofulvin [Fulvicin-U/F, Grifulvin V, Grisactin]
- griseofulvin ultramicrosize [Fulvicin P/G. Grisactin Ultra, Gris-PEG]
- haloprogin [Halotex]
- hydroxychloroquine sulfate [Plaquenil Sulfate]
- imipenem + cilastatin [Primaxin]
- indinavir [Crixivan]

- isoniazid [INH]
- itraconazole [Sporanox]
- kanamycin [Kantrex]
- ketoconazole [Nizoral]
- lamivudine (3TC) [Epivir]
- levofloxacin [Levaquin]
- lincomycin hydrochloride [Lincocin]
- lindane [Gemabenzene, Kwell, Scabene]
- malathion
- mefloquine hydrochloride [Lariam]
- methenamine hippurate [Hiprex, Urex]
- methenamine mandelate [Mandelamine, Mandameth]
- methicillin [Staphcillin]
- methylene blue [Urolene Blue]
- metronidazole [Flagyl, MetroGel, others]
- miconazole [Monistat IV]
- miconazole nitrate [Monistat, Micatin, others]
- nafcillini [Unipen]
- nalidixic acid [Neg Gram]
- nelfinavir mesylate [Viracept]
- neomycin [Mycifradin, Neosporin]
- netilmicin sulfate [Netromycin]
- nevirapine [Viramune]
- nitrofurantoin [Furadantin, Macrodantin, Macrobid, others]
- nitrofurazone [Furacin]
- nystatin [Mycostatin, Nilstat, others]
- oflaxacin [Floxin, Ocuflox]
- oxacillin sodium [Bactocill, Prostaphlin]
- paromomycin sulfate [Humatin]
- pecnicillin G salts [various]
- penicillin V [Pen-V, others]
- penicillin V potassium [Pen-V, others]
- pentamidine isethionate [NebuPent, Pentam 300]
- primaquine phosphate
- purified protein derivative (PPD) [Aplisol, Tubersol]
- pyrazinamide [Tebrazid]
- pyrimethamine [Daraprim]
- quinacrine [Atabrine]
- quinine sulfate [Quinamm]
- rifampin [Rifadin]
- ritonavir [Norvir]
- saquinavir mesylate [Invirase]
- silver sulfadiazine [Silvadene]

- sparfloxacin [Zagam]
- stavudine (d4T) [Zerit]
- streptomycin sulfate
- sulfamethoxazole [Gantanol]
- sulfisoxazole [Gantrisin]
- terbinafine cream [Lamisil]
- tetracycline hydrochloride [Achromycin, others]
- tobramycin sulfate [Nebcin, Tobrex]
- trimethoprim [Proloprim, others]
- trimethoprim + sulfamethoxazole (TMP-SMZ) [Bactrim, Septra, others]
- trimetrexate [Neotrexin]
- troleandomycin [Tao]
- valacyclovir hydrochloride [Valtrex]
- vancomycin hydrochloride [Vancocin, others]
- vidarabine [Adenine Arabinoside, ARA-A, Vira-A]
- zalcitabine (ddC, dideoxycytidine) [Hivid]
- zidovudine (azidothymidine, AZT) [Retrovir]

A s part of the food chain we eat other creatures and other creatures eat us. Voracious enemies range from microbes to worms and insects and have taken great tolls in human life and suffering, causing plagues throughout history. The struggle continues. Though germ theory has helped us conquer many infectious illnesses with aseptic technique, vaccines, and antiinfectives, new plagues loom. Infectious organisms keep adjusting and adapting to survive our defense strategies in this ongoing struggle to survive life in the food chain. Human behavior favors infection. Crowding, overpopulation, poverty, rapid long-distance travel, poor hygiene, and inadequate waste disposal all contribute to infection. Even health professionals contribute to infections with poor asepsis practices, long hair and nails, and inadequate hand washing.

▶ ANTIVIRALS

The name *virus* means "slime and poison," but the late Nobel Laureate scientist Peter Medawar described viruses best as "a piece of bad news wrapped up in protein." Viruses carry no baggage—no cell membranes, no organelles. Mere strands of DNA or RNA (retroviruses), bits of genetic messages wearing coats—they don't eat or breathe. As obligate intracellular parasites, these genetic

fragments cause misery, death, and disease seemingly out of proportion to such insignificant, incomplete bits and pieces, so small they can fit in the chains of DNA in a cell nucleus. Viruses enter cells through receptors they have the right fit for. Viruses have adapted to cell receptors on almost all species of life from bacteria to plants to vertebrates, entering receptor sites intended for passage of materials essential to the cells. Some viruses even become a permanent part of the host DNA and "contribute to the evolutionary changes of the host." Humans carry "vestiges of viral DNA" in the chromosomes and pass them on "from generation to generation as passengers in our genetic endowment" (Levine, 1992). Viruses can cause certain cancers, for example, liver cancer can follow hepatitis B infection. The Epstein–Barr virus is a DNA tumor virus associated with Burkitt's lymphoma and nasopharyngeal carcinoma. HTLV-I is linked to T-cell leukemia and HTLV-II to hairy-cell leukemia (Levine, 1992). The herpes virus in the smegma of uncircumcised men can cause penile cancer.

Once inserted into the DNA of the host cell, the infected cell becomes the virus's hostage and can no longer control its own growth and replication. To a virus, a cell represents nothing more than a copy machine to replicate itself, using the cell's genetic machinery. When the cell has served its purpose, the viral copies bud out from the cell membrane and move on to the next copy machine (*Scientific American,* 1993). Whereas DNA viruses tend to be stable replicators, retroviruses, consisting of RNA, make poor copies with frequent coding changes or mutations. This feature makes them a hard target for the immune system. Because viruses integrate into the genetic material of the infected cell, the only way the immune system can destroy them is to destroy the cell. The immune system does this by finding the clue to a virus's presence within a cell. As a virus enters a cell it sheds its coat on the cell surface. The helper-T cells find this protein clue and informs the B cells, which start creating antibodies to tag infected cells for destruction by the immune system. The antibodies will be ready for more rapid response in the event of future infections, tagging the viruses before they can enter cells (Fig. 16–1).

▶ ANTIVIRALS FOR INFLUENZA AND OTHER VIRAL INFECTIONS

Flu, the name commonly given to colds (and incorrectly to temporary GI upset), is far from trivial. The viruses responsible for the flu typically arise in the south of Asia and circle the earth yearly. Some years they cause epidemics, spotty, isolated outbreaks. Other years they cause massive, global pandemics that can kill large numbers of the vulnerable—the elderly, the very young, and people with impaired respiratory or immune systems—as they did in the pandemic of 1918. Though vaccines offer some temporary hope of prevention, they sometimes fail to protect. Antiviral drugs can help shorten the period of illness.

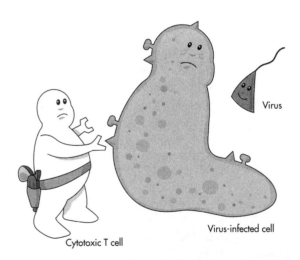

As a virus enters a cell it leaves viral proteins embedded in the cell's membrane. Cytotoxic T cells recognize the foreign molecules displayed in combination with the host's identifying protein markers. The cytotoxic T cell kills the infected cells.

Figure 16–1. Viral infection.

Amantadine hydrochloride [Symmetrel] is a prophylactic and symptomatic treatment for influenza A.

Drug Interactions: Increased CNS effects with alcohol. Increased effects of anticholinergics possible.

Side Effects

Nervous System: ataxia, convulsions,* dizziness, dyspnea, edema—peripheral, headache, hypotension—orthostatic, lightheadedness, nausea/vomiting, psyche—anxiety/concentration difficulties/confusion/hallucinations/insomnia/irritability/mood and mental changes/nervousness/nightmares, vision—blurring/loss.

Endocrine System: (Pregnancy Category C) edema—peripheral, dry mouth.

Immune System: leukopenia, rashes.

Dosage: PO 200 mg qd or 100 mg q12h.

NUCLEOSIDE ANTIVIRALS

This class of antivirals interfere with DNA synthesis to inhibit replication of herpes simplex virus types 1 and 2 (HSV-1 and HSV-2) and varicella zoster. Some of these antivirals are useful in treating HIV (Fig. 16–2).

Acyclovir [Acycloguanosine, Zovirax], acyclovir sodium reduces viral shedding and formation of new lesions and speeds healing time by interfering with DNA synthesis of herpes simplex virus types 1 and 2 (HSV-1 and HSV-2) and varicella zoster virus. It is also used to treat herpes virus simiae (B virus) and Epstein–Barr virus (infectious mononucleosis, varicella zoster, and cytomegalovirus). This drug requires adequate hydration to prevent kidney damage.

Drug Interactions: Decreased elimination with probenecid. Increased drowsiness, lethargy.

Incompatibilities

Solution/Additive: albumin, bacteriostatic water for injection, dopamine, dobutamine, hetastarch.

Y-site: foscarnet.

Side Effects

Nervous System: bowel—diarrhea, dizziness, fatigue, headache, lethargy, lightheadedness, nausea/vomiting, psyche—confusion, seizures,* sensation of burning/stinging, tremors.

Endocrine System: (Pregnancy Category C) acute renal failure.

---

* Life-threatening side effect.

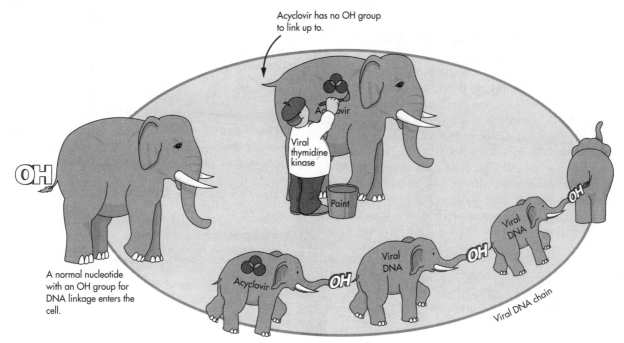

Acyclovir has no OH group to link up to.

Viral thymidine kinase

Acyclovir

Paint

OH

A normal nucleotide with an OH group for DNA linkage enters the cell.

Acyclovir

OH

Viral DNA

OH

Viral DNA

OH

Viral DNA

OH

Viral DNA chain

Unsuspecting viral thymidine kinase adds three phosphates to acyclovir (now acyclovir triphosphate), never realizing it has no OH group to which the next nucleotide must attach in the DNA chain. The DNA chain-building stops and the viral-infected cell cannot replicate.

Figure 16–2. Nucleus of a cell infected by a virus.

Immune System: glomerulonephritis, irritation, pruritus, rash, renal tubular damage, sensitization, urticaria. IV site: inflammation/phlebitis, sloughing with extravasation.

Dosage: Prophylaxis of genital herpes simplex: PO 200 mg 2–5 ×/d or 400 mg bid. Herpes zoster: PO 800 mg q4h 5 ×/d. Herpes simplex encephalitis: IV 10 mg/kg q8h. Varicella zoster, child/adolescent: PO 20 mg/kg to maximum of 800 mg qid for 5 d. Start within 24 h of rash onset.

<u>Cidofovir [Vistide]</u> is a nucleotide analog used to treat cytomegalovirus (CMV) and other herpes viruses. Cidofovir contains a phosphonate group that enables it to bypass initial virus-dependent phosphorylation. It is given with high-dose probenecid to decrease the risk of nephrotoxicity.

Drug Interactions: none noted.

Side Effects

Nervous System: asthenia, bowel—diarrhea, headache, nausea/vomiting, ocular hypotony/decreased IOP, pain—abdominal.

Endocrine System: (Pregnancy Category C) fever, proteinuria.

Immune System: alopecia, anemia, neutropenia, rash.

Dosage: Precede administration with probenecid PO 2 g 3h before and IV 1 L NS over 1 h just prior to cidofovir. If tolerated, another 1 L of NS with or after cidofovir. Follow in 2 h and 8 h with probenecid PO 1 g. CMV retinitis: IV 5 mg/kg over 1 h weekly for 2 wk. Maintenance: 5 mg/kg over 1 h qowk.

<u>Delavirdine mesylate [Rescriptor]</u> is a non-nucleoside reverse transcriptase inhibitor used to treat, but not to cure, HIV-1. It is used in combination with other appropriate antiretrovirals.

Drug Interactions: Increased levels of clarithromycin, dapsone, indinavir, rifabutin, saquinavir, warfarin possible and may increase or prolong their effects. Decreased levels with carbamazepine, phenobarbital, phenytoin, rifabutin, rifampin possible.

Side Effects

Nervous System: bowel—diarrhea, fatigue, headache, nausea/vomiting.

Endocrine System: (Pregnancy Category C) none noted.

Immune System: ALT/AST—elevated, pruritus, rash.

Dosage: PO 400 mg tid.

Didanosine (DDI) [Videx] inhibits replication of HIV. It is used to treat advanced HIV infection in patients who are intolerant to zidovudine (AZT) or who demonstrate significant clinical or immunologic deterioration during zidovudine therapy.

Drug Interactions: Increased aluminum- and magnesium-associated adverse effects possible with aluminum and magnesium antacids. Reduced effectiveness of dapsone in prophylaxis of *Pneumocystis carinii* pneumonia possible. Increased neuropathy with zalcitabine (ddC) possible.

Drug–Food Interactions: Decreased absorption with food. Take on empty stomach.

Side Effects

Nervous System: arrhythmias, bowel—constipation/diarrhea, poor coordination, cough, dizziness, dyspnea, headache, hypoventilation, insomnia, lethargy, myalgia, nausea/vomiting, neuropathy—peripheral, pain—abdominal, palpitations, photophobia, psyche—nervousness, seizures,* strength decrease, vasodilation, vision—blindness/blurred/diplopia.

Endocrine System: (Pregnancy Category B) depigmentation—retinal, dry mouth, hypocalcemia, hypokalemia, hypomagnesemia, hyperuricemia, hypertriglyceridemia, muscle atrophy, sweating.

Immune System: asthma, arthritis, congestion, ecchymosis, eczema, Hb—increased, hemorrhage, epistaxis, impetigo, increased liver enzymes—lymphocyte/platelet counts, optic neuritis, pancreatitis,* petechiae, pharyngitis, pruritus, rash, rhinitis, rhinorrhea, rhonchi/rales, sinusitis, stomatitis, thrombocytopenia, WBC/neutrophils—increased.

Dosage: PO. Weight 35–49 kg: 125-mg tab bid; 167 mg powder bid. Weight 50–74 kg: 200-mg tab bid; 250 mg powder bid. Weight ≥ 75 kg: 300 mg bid; 375 mg powder bid. Two tablets should be taken at each dose to ensure adequate buffering.

Foscarnet [Foscavir] is used to treat infections of all known herpes viruses resistant to acyclovir.

Drug Interactions: Increased risk of nephrotoxicity with aminoglycosides, amphotericin B, vancomycin. Increased hypocalcemia possible with etidronate, pamidronate, pentamidine (IV).

Side Effects

Nervous System: bowel—diarrhea, fatigue, headache, muscle twitching, nausea/vomiting, psyche—anxiety/confusion, tremor, twitching, weakness.

Endocrine System: (Pregnancy Category C) hyperphosphatemia, hypophosphatemia, hypocalcemia, acute renal failure.

Immune System: anemia, fixed drug eruption, leukopenia, nephrotoxicity with tubular necrosis,* rash, thrombocytopenia, thrombophlebitis if infused through a peripheral vein, ulceration—penal.

Dosage: CMV retinitis: IV. Induction 60 mg/kg infused over 1 h q8h for 2–3 wk; may be repeated if relapse occurs during maintenance therapy. Alternate induction therapies: 100 mg/kg q12h for 2–3 wk or 20–30 mg/kg infused over 30 min followed by a continuous infusion of 180–230 mg/kg/d for 2–3 wk. Maintenance: 90–120 mg/kg/d infused over 2 h. Herpes simplex infections in AIDS: IV 40–60 mg/kg q8h for 2–3 wk; may be followed by 50 mg/kg/d for 5–7 d/wk for up to 15 wk. Acyclovir-resistant HSV in immunocompromised patients: IV 40 mg/kg q8–12h for up to 3 wk or until lesions heal.

Note: See package insert for required dose adjustments for renal insufficiency.

Ganciclovir (DHPG) [Cytovene] is used to treat CMV retinitis and for prophylaxis and treatment of systemic CMV infection in immunocompromised patients, including HIV-positive and transplant patients.

Drug Interactions: Increased bone marrow suppression and other toxic effects with antineoplastic agents, amphotericin B, didanosine, trimethoprim-sulfamethoxazole (TMP-SMZ), dapsone, pentamidine, probenecid, and zidovudine possible. Increased risk of nephrotoxicity from cyclosporin. Increased risk of seizures with imipenem + cilastatin.

Incompatibilities

Solution/Additive: bacteriostatic water for injection, fludarabine, foscarnet, ondansetron.

Y-site: total parenteral nutrition (TPN).

Side Effects

Nervous System: ataxia, coma,* dizziness, edema, headache, nausea/vomiting, paresthesia, psyche—confusion/disorientation/mental status changes/nervousness, somnolence, tremor.

Endocrine System: (Pregnancy Category C) anorexia, edema, fever, hyperbilirubinemia, hyperthermia, hypoglycemia, infertility.

Immune System: bone marrow suppression,* eosinophilia, granulocytopenia, leukopenia, liver enzyme—elevated phlebitis, rash, thrombocytopenia.

Dosage: Induction therapy: IV 5 mg/kg over 1 h q12h for 14–21 d. Dose range: 2.5–5.0 mg/kg over 1 h q8–12h for

---

* Life-threatening side effect.

10–35 d. Maintenance: IV 5 mg/kg over 1 h qd or 6 mg/kg over 1 h qd 5 d/wk. PO 1000 mg tid or 500 mg 6 ×/d q3h while awake.

Lamivudine (3TC) [Epivir] is a synthetic nucleoside analog that inhibits the transcription of the HIV viral DNA chain. It is used to treat infection in combination with zidovudine.

Drug Interactions: Increased C_{max} of zidovudine. Increased serum levels of lamivudine with trimethoprim-sulfamethoxazole.

Side Effects

Nervous System: arthralgia, bowel—diarrhea, cough, dizziness, dyspepsia, fatigue, headache, malaise, myalgia, nausea/vomiting, neuropathy, pain—abdominal, psyche—depression/insomnia/sleep disorders.

Endocrine System: (Pregnancy Category C) anorexia, fever.

Immune System: ALT—increased, amylase, anemia, neutropenia, thrombocytopenia.

Dosage: HIV: PO 150 mg bid; Weight < 50 kg: 2 mg/kg bid.

Nevirapine [Viramune] is used to treat HIV-1 mutants resistant to nucleoside reverse transcriptase inhibitors. Oral absorption is not affected by food or antacids. Keep refrigerated.

Drug Interactions: Not available.

Side Effects

Nervous System: arthralgia, fatigue, myalgia, nausea/vomiting, somnolence.

Endocrine System: (Pregnancy Category C) fever.

Immune System: liver function test—elevated, rash.

Dosage: 200 mg/d for 2 wk. If no rash appears increase to 200 mg bid. Give in combination with additional antiviral agent.

Stavudine (d4T) [Zerit] is a synthetic analog of thymidine used to treat advanced HIV in patients who are intolerant of other antiretroviral agents or who have deteriorated on the other agents.

Drug Interactions: none noted.

Side Effects

Nervous System: cramping, headache, neuropathy—peripheral, pain—abdominal, paresthesias.

Endocrine System: (Pregnancy Category C) chills, fever.

Immune System: anemia, liver function test—elevated, rash.

Dosage: PO. Weight ≥60 kg: 40 mg q12h. Weight < 60 kg: 30 mg q12h. 50% dose reduction with peripheral neuropathy or creatinine clearance of 25–50 mL/min.

Valacyclovir hydrochloride [Valtrex] is changed in the intestinal wall into acyclovir. Because of its higher GI absorption, valacyclovir has a higher plasma level than acyclovir when both are taken orally. Treats herpes zoster (shingles) in immunocompetent adults.

Drug Interactions: Decreased elimination with probenecid, cimetidine. May cause increased drowsiness and lethargy.

Side Effects

Nervous System: bowel—diarrhea/flatulence, dizziness, dyspepsia, fatigue, headache, lethargy, nausea/vomiting, pain—abdominal, psyche—confusion, somnolence, weakness.

Endocrine System: (Pregnancy Category B) acute renal failure.

Immune System: glomerulonephritis, pruritus, rash, renal tubular damage, urticaria.

Dosage: PO 1 g tid for 7 d. Start within 48 h of zoster rash onset. Genital herpes: PO 500 mg bid.

Vidarabine [Adenine Arabinoside, ARA-A, Vira-A] is a pyrimidine nucleoside derived from *Streptomyces antibioticus* for treatment of HSV types 1 and 2, varicella zoster, vaccinia, cytomegalovirus, hepatitis B virus, and Epstein–Barr virus.

Drug Interactions: Increased risk for CNS side effects with allopurinol.

Side Effects

Nervous System: IV, high doses: ataxia, bowel—diarrhea, dizziness, malaise, nausea/vomiting, pain—injection site, psyche—confusion/hallucinations/psychosis, tremor, weakness. Ophthalmic: burning, foreign body sensation/itching/lacrimation/pain/photophobia.[†]

Endocrine System: (Pregnancy Category C) IV: fatal metabolic encephalopathy.[*]

Immune System: anemia, bilirubin/AST—elevated, neutropenia, pruritus, thrombocytopenia, WBC/Hb/Hct—decreased. Ophthalmic: superficial punctate keratitis, punctal occlusion, and plugged lacrimal glands.[†]

Dosage: Herpes simplex encephalitis, herpes zoster: IV 15 mg/kg/d infused over 12–24 h. Herpes keratitis:

[†] Eye related.
[*] Life-threatening side effect.

Ophthalmic: Instill 1 cm (1/2 in.) ribbon of ointment into lower conjunctival sac q3h 5 ×/d.[†]

<u>Zalcitabine (ddC, dideoxycytidine) [Hivid]</u> inhibits replication of HIV by inhibition of viral DNA synthesis to treat AIDS in combination with zidovudine. Second-line monotherapy for AIDS.

Off Label: May be used in children.

Drug Interactions: Increased peripheral neuropathy with didanosine possible.

Side Effects

Nervous System: bowel—diarrhea, arthralgia, exacerbation of preexisting cardiomyopathy/CHF—possible, malaise, neuropathy—peripheral, numbness.

Endocrine System: (Pregnancy Category C) fever.

Immune System: anaphylaxis,* cutaneous eruptions, possible exacerbation of preexisting hepatic dysfunction, neutropenia, pancreatitis,* thrombocytopenia, ulcers—mouth/esophagus.

Dosage: HIV: PO 0.01 mg/kg q8h. HIV: PO 0.75 mg q8h in combination with zidovudine 200 mg q8h.

<u>Zidovudine (azidothymidine, AZT) [Retrovir]</u> is the prototype of the thymidine analogs. It is converted in host cells into triphosphate by endogenous thymidine kinase. AZT was developed originally in 1964 to fight leukemia, but was ignored until the AIDS epidemic showed it to have antiviral properties. It is now being shown to be highly effective against breast tumors in rats and will be researched further (*Science News,* June, 1997). It is used in HIV-positive patients with a CD4 count < 500/mm³, asymptomatic HIV infection, and early and late symptomatic HIV disease and in prevention of perinatal transfer of HIV.

Off Label: Children, postexposure prophylaxis.

Drug Interactions: Increased bone marrow suppression with acetaminophen possible. Increased AZT toxicity with amphotericin B. Possible increased toxicity with aspirin, dapsone, doxorubicin, flucytosine, indomethacin, interferon alfa, pentamidine, vincristine. Decreased AZT elimination with probenecid.

Side Effects

Nervous System: bowel—diarrhea, dizziness, dyspnea, headache, insomnia, malaise, myalgia, nausea/vomiting, pain—GI, paresthesias, psyche—agitation/anxiety/confusion/restlessness, weakness.

Endocrine System: (Pregnancy Category C) anorexia, fever, sweating.

Immune System: anemia,* bone marrow depression,* granulocytopenia,* rash.

Dosage: Asymptomatic HIV infection/postexposure prophylaxis: PO 100 mg q4h while awake, 5 ×/d. Symptomatic HIV infection: PO 200 mg q4h (1200 mg/d). After 1 mo may reduce to 100 mg q4h (600 mg/d). IV 1–2 mg/kg q4h (1200 mg/d).

PROTEASE INHIBITORS

This class of antivirals cripples the enzyme protease, which is vital to the late stages of HIV reproduction, whereas older AIDS antivirals work at the onset of infection. The protease enzyme is less prone to mutations, and protease inhibitors are more readily absorbed into HIV-infected cells than earlier antivirals.

<u>Indinavir [Crixivan],</u> an HIV protease inhibitor, prevents cleavage of the viral polyproteins, causing formation of immature noninfectious viral particles.

Drug Interactions: Decreased metabolism of astemizole, cisapride, midazolam, triazolam with increased cardiac arrhythmias. Prolonged sedation possible. Decreased levels with fluconazole, ketoconazole, quinidine, rifampin. Increased levels of clarithromycin, indinavir, zidovudine. Increased levels of estrogen and progestin in oral contraceptives, isoniazid, rifabutin. Increased levels of trimethoprim without change in sulfamethoxazole. Food decreases absorption by about 75%.

Side Effects

Nervous System: asthenia, bladder—frequency/nocturia, bowel—constipation/diarrhea/flatulence, cough, dizziness, dyspnea, dysuria, headache, malaise, myalgia, nausea/vomiting, pain—abdominal/back/chest/eye/flank/musculoskeletal/shoulder, psyche—agitation/anxiety/disturbed dreams/depression/excitement/insomnia, (mental acuity decreased), renal colic, reflux, sleep disorders/somnolence, syncope, taste changes, vertigo, vision—blurred.

Endocrine System: (Pregnancy Category C) anorexia/appetite increase, body odor, chills, eye—swelling/orbital edema, fever, hyperbilirubinemia, dry mouth, renal calculi (push fluids to 1.5 L/d), dry skin, sweating/night sweats, urine sediments/urolithiasis, uterine abnormality.

Immune System: cholecystitis, contact dermatitis, flu-like illness, gastritis, gastroenteritis, gingival hemorrhage, gingivitis, hematuria, hepatic transaminases elevated—transient, herpes simplex, herpes zoster, liver cirrhosis, pharyngitis, pneumonia, pruritus, seborrhea, sinusitis, stomatitis, URI, urticaria.

---

* Life-threatening side effect.
[†] Eye related.

Dosage: PO 800 mg q8h. Mild to moderate hepatic insufficiency: 600 mg q8h. Give with water 1 h ac or 2 h pc.

Nelfinavir mesylate [Viracept] inhibits HIV protease in the treatment of HIV infection in combination with nucleoside analogs or alone for up to 24 weeks. To be taken with nonacidic food.

Drug Interactions: Cardiac arrhythmias or prolonged sedation possible with astemizole, cisapride, midazolam, rifampin, triazolam. Decreased levels with carbamazepine, phenobarbital, phenytoin, rifabutin. Increased levels with other HIV protease inhibitors. Decreased levels with oral contraceptives.

Side Effects

Nervous System: asthenia, bowel—diarrhea/flatulence, nausea.

Endocrine System: (Pregnancy Category C) none noted.

Immune System: bleeding (hemophilia type A and B may require additional factor VIII).

Dosage: PO 750 mg tid with meals

Ritonavir [Norvir] is an HIV protease inhibitor.

Drug Interactions: Increased levels of amiodarone, astemizole, bepridil, bupropion, cisapride, clozapine, encainide, erythromycin, flecanide, meperidine, methylphenidate, pentoxifylline, phenothiazines, piroxicam, propafenone, propoxyphene, quinidine, rifabutin, warfarin possible, with an increased risk of arrhythmias, hematologic complications, seizures. Decreased levels of atovaquone, clofibrate, daunorubicin, diphenoxylate, metaclopramide, sedative/hypnotics possible. Extreme sedation and respiratory depression with alprazolam, chlorazepate, diazepam, estazolam, fluorazepam, midazolam, triazolam, zolpidem.

Side Effects

Nervous System: arrhythmias—tachycardia, asthenia, bowel—constipation/diarrhea/flatulence, dizziness, dyspepsia, headache, hypotension, malaise, nausea/vomiting, pain—abdominal/neck, paresthesias, psyche—abnormal thinking/insomnia/somnolence, taste changes, vision—abnormal/ambylopia/blurred.

Endocrine System: (Pregnancy Category C) anorexia, chills, dehydration, edema, fever, flushing, glycosuria, gout, thirst, serum triglyceride levels elevated, sweating, vitamin deficiency, xerostomia.

Immune System: hepatic transaminases/CPK—elevated, pharyngitis, rash.

Dosage: PO taken with food. Start with 300 mg q12h and increase to 600 mg q12h over 1 wk. If patient cannot tolerate after 2 weeks, DC.

Saquinavir mesylate [Invirase] is an HIV protease inhibitor for advanced HIV infection usually in combination with zidovudine and zalcitabine.

Drug Interactions: Decreased levels with rifampin and rifabutin. Possible decreased levels with phenobarbital, phenytoin, dexamethasone, carbamazepine. Possible serum increase of terfenadine or astemizole.

Side Effects

Nervous System: asthenia, ataxia, bowel—diarrhea, headache, nausea/vomiting, pain—abdominal, psyche—confusion/suicide attempt,* seizures.*

Endocrine System: anorexia.

Immune System: anemia, liver disease exacerbations, rash, thrombophlebitis, transaminases—elevated.

Dosage: PO within 2 h after a meal for adequate absorption for advanced HIV disease in combination with nucleoside analogs: 600 mg q8h.

▶ ANTIBIOTICS

While fungi can hurt us, they can also help, as the story of penicillin demonstrates. *Penicillium notatum,* a rare mold that produces copious amounts of penicillin, floated in from another lab where such molds were being used to create allergy vaccines. It settled on a petri dish culture of *Staphylococcus.* First the weather turned cool, allowing the mold to grow. Then the weather warmed and the staph grew everywhere on the petri dish except where inhibited by the mold. When Alexander Fleming (1928) returned to his lab from vacation, he noticed the results of the mold-versus-bacteria battle. Although he knew that this was somehow worthwhile, he never harnessed penicillin's potential to cure infection. Limited by his experience of observing bacterial and mold colonies on culture media, he never realized penicillin's effect if ingested or injected. He used his mold "juice" only to isolate *Hemophilus influenzae* bacteria (Sneader, 1985).

As World War II heated up, the U.S. military eventually fostered penicillin research. After Boston's Coconut Grove nightclub fire, the death toll of 500 would have been higher had penicillin, a military secret, not been covertly used to prevent and treat infections in the burn survivors. Later, Giuseppe Brotzu discovered cephalosporin in the clear coastal water of Sardinia, where sewage was discharged and bacteria devoured by *Cephalosporium acremonium* (Sneader, 1985).

Penicillin and the cephalosporins are fairly similar, and a patient who is allergic to one will probably be allergic to the other. These antibiotic discoveries triggered

---

* Life-threatening side effect.

a massive, worldwide treasure hunt in soil and water for potential antibiotic microorganisms by pharmaceutical companies. From Caracas, Venezuela, came chloramphenicol. From Terre Haute, Indiana, came tetracycline [Terramycin]. Infections that once maimed and killed are no longer as fearsome, though maybe they ought to be. Infections once considered potentially deadly are now easily treated, for example, simple eye infections, now treated with antibiotic drops. However, out of complacency and ignorance, giving too little antibiotic too often in this battle of the food chains has given microbes time to develop strategies (like penicillinase) to resist destruction by these drugs. In addition, health care professionals are not as careful as they could be in keeping the patient's environment clean, in not considering hospital floors to be extremely pathogenic, in wearing scrub suits and lab coats to and from work, in not washing their hands before and after caring for a patient, and even in wearing uniforms into grocery stores to shop after leaving the hospital. When health professionals are not careful about the diseases they deal with, they are at risk and become vectors, as capable as any rat or insect of spreading disease. Certainly, we have antibiotics, but the best treatment is prevention of infection.

▶ ANTIBIOTIC CLASSIFICATIONS

Antibiotics are divided into aminoglycosides, beta-lactams (penicillins), beta-lactams (cephalosporins), lincosamides, macrolides, tetracyclines, quinolones, the miscellaneous antiseptics, sulfonamides, and drugs to treat mycobacterial infections such as tuberculosis.

AMINOGLYCOSIDES

Gentamicin sulfate [Garamycin, Genoptic, others], derived from *Micromonospora purpurea*, is a broad-spectrum aminoglycoside with bactericidal activity against the following gram-negative bacteria: *Citrobacter, E. coli, Enterobacter, Klebsiella, Proteus, Pseudomonas aeruginosa, Serratia*. It is also effective against some gram-positive organisms, especially penicillin-sensitive and some methicillin-resistant strains of *Staphylococcus aureus*. This parenteral antibiotic is restricted to treating serious infections.

Topical: For primary and secondary skin infections and external eye infections.

Off Label: Prophylaxis of bacterial endocarditis in patients undergoing operative procedures or instrumentation.

Drug Interactions: Increased risk of nephrotoxicity with amphotericin B, capreomycin, cisplatin, methoxyflurane, polymyxin B, and vancomycin. Increased risk of autotoxicity with ethacrynic acid and furosemide. Potentiated neuromuscular blockade with general anesthetics and neuromuscular blocking agents. Increased levels in neonates with indomethacin.

Incompatibilities

Solution/Additive: fat emulsion, TPN, amphotericin B, ampicillin, carbenicillin, cephalosporins, cytarabine, heparin.

Y-site: furosemide, iodipamide.

Side Effects

Nervous System: apnea, hearing impairment, hyper-/hypotension, muscle weakness, nausea/vomiting, neuromuscular blockade, respiratory paralysis—high doses.

Endocrine System: (Pregnancy Category C) fever, hypocalcemia, hypokalemia, hypomagnesemia.

Immune System: anaphylaxis,* granulocytopenia, laryngeal edema, nephrotoxicity,* SGOT/SGPT/serum LDH/bilirubin—transient increase, skin—allergic reactions, thrombocytopenia.

Dosage: IM/IV severe infection 2–2.5 mg/kg in divided doses. UTI 1.5 mg/kg in divided doses.

Ophthalmic: 1–2 gtt in eye q4h up to 2 gtt q1h or small amount ointment bid or tid.†

Kanamycin [Kantrex] is a broad-spectrum antiobotic that is also used in hepatic coma to reduce ammonia-producing GI tract bacteria. It is used to treat many gram-negative microorganisms.

Drug Interactions: Increased nephrotoxicity with amphotericin B, cisplatin, methoxyflurane, vancomycin possible. Increased neuromuscular blocking with general anesthetics, muscle relaxants. Increased autotoxicity, nephrotoxicity with capreomycin. Increased risk of autotoxicity with loop and thiazide diuretics.

Incompatibilities

Solution/Additive: ampicillin, carbenicillin, cephalothin, cephapirin, chlorpheniramine, colistimethate, heparin, hydrocortisone, methicillin, methohexital, mezlocillin, penicillin, piperacillin.

Y-site: heparin, methohexital.

Side Effects

Nervous System: similar to gentamycin.

Endocrine System: (Pregnancy Category D) serum creatinine/BUN—increased.

Immune System: similar to gentamycin.

---

* Life-threatening side effect.
† Eye related.

Dosage: Preop, intestinal antisepsis: PO 1 g q1h for 4 doses; then q6h for 36–72 h. Hepatic coma: PO 8–12 g/d in divided doses. Serious infection: IM, IV 15 mg/kg/d in equally divided doses q8–12h. Intraperitoneal 500 mg in 20 mL sterile water per wound catheter. Inhalation 250 mg in 3 mL NS per nebulizer q6–12h. Irrigation 0.25% solution prn.

Neomycin [Mycifradin, Neosporin] is poorly absorbed from the gut, making it good for bowel cleansing before procedures and surgery in the bowel. It is also good for eye, ear, and small skin area infections.

Side Effects: See *gentamycin*.

Drug Interactions: Decreased absorption of cyanocobalamin possible.

Dosage: For diarrhea PO 50 mg/kg in 4 divided doses × 2–3 d. Bowel cleansing PO 1 g q1h × 4, then 1 g q4h × 5. Hepatic coma PO 4–12 g/d in 4 divided doses × 5–6 d. Topical qd to tid.

Netilmicin sulfate [Netromycin] is one of the newest aminoglycosides.

Drug Interactions: Increased neuromuscular blocking effects with anesthetics, muscle relaxants. Increased risk of autotoxicity, nephrotoxicity with acyclovir, amphotericin B, bacitracin, capreomycin, carboplatin, cephalosporins, cisplatin, colistin, ethacrynic acid, furosemide, methoxyflurane, polymyxin B, vancomycin.

Incompatibilities

Solution/Additive: furosemide, heparin.

Y-site: furosemide.

Side Effects

Nervous System: drowsiness, headache, hearing—permanent loss, lethargy, nausea/vomiting, neuromuscular blockade,* psyche—disorientation, respiratory arrest,* seizures,* twitching, vision—blurred/nystagmus.

Endocrine System: (Pregnancy Category D) BUN/serum creatinine/creatinine clearance—decreased, oliguria, polyuria, proteinuria.

Immune System: agranulocytosis,* ALT/AST/alkaline phosphatase/bilirubin—increased, anemia, leukopenia, nephrotoxicity,* neutropenia, thrombocytopenia, thrombocytosis.

Dosage: IM, IV 1.5–2 mg/kg/d q8h or 4–7 mg/kg 8d.

Paromomycin sulfate [Humatin] is produced from *Streptomyces rimosus* and resembles kanamycin and neomycin. Paromomycin is both bactericidal and amebicidal, especially inside the GI tract, where it can also help eradicate tapeworms. Because it kills intestinal flora, paromomycin is used to kill nitrogen-forming bacteria during hepatic coma. Paromomycin has the potential to cause ototoxicity and nephrotoxicity, especially in patients with a history of GI ulcers.

Drug Interactions: none noted.

Side Effects

Nervous System: bowel—diarrhea/abdominal cramps, headache, nausea/vomiting and vertigo.

Endocrine System (Pregnancy Category C) steatorrhea.

Immune System: secondary enterocolitis, eosinophilia, exanthema, heartburn, nephrotoxicity (in patients with GI inflammation or ulcerations), ototoxicity, overgrowth of nonsusceptible organisms, pruritus, rash.

Dosage: Amebiasis: PO 25–35 mg/kg divided tid for 5–10 days. Hepatic coma: 4 g divided bid or qid for 5–6 d.

Streptomycin sulfate can damage the eighth cranial nerve (ear). It is combined with penicillin. For TB, it is combined with isoniazid, rifampin, and pyrazinamide.

Drug Interactions: Increased anticoagulant effects of warfarin possible.

Side Effects

Nervous System: encephalopathy, headache, lassitude, neuromuscular blockade, paresthesias—peripheral/facial, psyche—inability to concentrate, vision—scotomas, weakness—muscle. IM site: irritation/pain.

Endocrine System: (Pregnancy Category C) drug fever.

Immune System: anemia—hemolytic/aplastic,* anaphylaxis,* angioedema,* arachnoiditis, ear—auditory damage/labyrinthine damage, eosinophilia, exfoliative dermatitis,* hepatotoxicity, leukopenia, lymph nodes—enlarged, nephrotoxicity, neutropenia, pancytopenia, pruritus, rash, stomatitis, superinfections, vision—optic nerve toxicity.

Dosage: TB: IM 15 mg/kg to maximum of 1 g/d, 25–30 mg/kg × 2/wk, or 25–30 mg/kg × 3/wk. Tularemia: IM 1–2 mg/d in divided doses for 7–10 d. Plague: IM 2–4 mg/d in 2–4 divided doses.

Tobramycin sulfate [Nebcin, Tobrex] is more active than gentamicin against *Pseudomonas* and is also less toxic to the body. Tobramycin is combined with other antibiotics

---

* Life-threatening side effect.

for septicemia and burns, and for CNS, urinary tract, bone, and soft tissue infections. It has side effects similar to the other aminoglycosides.

Drug Interactions: Increased neuromuscular blocking with anesthetics, skeletal muscle relaxants. Increased risk of autotoxicity, nephrotoxicity with acyclovir, amphotericin B, bacitracin, capreomycin, carboplatin, cephalosporins, cisplatin, colistin, ethacrynic acid, furosemide, methoxyflurane, polymyxin B, vancomycin.

Incompatibilities

Solution/Additive: alcohol 5% in dextrose, cephalosporins, clindamycin, heparin, penicillins.

Side Effects

Nervous System: headache, lethargy, nausea/vomiting.

Endocrine System: (Pregnancy Category D) fever.

Immune System: AST/ALT/LDH—increased, hypersensitivity, increased serum bilirubin, nephrotoxicity, neurotoxicity, pruritus, rash, superinfections, urticaria. Ophthalmic: burning, stinging after drug installation; lid itching/edema.

Dosage: IM, IV 3–5 mg/kg/d in divided doses tid or qid. Ophthalmic: 1–2 gtt 0.3% q15–30 min until improvement, then reduce dosage slowly. Ophthalmic ointment: ½ in. line q3–4h until improvement, then bid–tid.[†]

BETA-LACTAMS: PENICILLINS

Even though some strains of bacteria have become resistant, the penicillins are still important antibiotics, and some have been developed to work against *Staphylococcus aureus,* while others can be effective in combination with other antibiotics. Though refinements have been made to decrease allergic reactions, severe allergic reaction still remains a life-threatening side effect for some patients. Penicillins kill bacteria by finding a receptor site in the bacterial cell membranes of rapidly multiplying bacteria and destroying their cell walls with beta-lactam. The prototype of penicillin is penicillin G. Aqueous penicillin is for intravenous use. IM penicillin contains procaine or benzathine. Penicillin V is the preferred oral form, because PO penicillin G requires higher doses.

Drug Interactions: Gentamicin increases penicillin potency. Ascorbic acid decreases activity. Erythromycin inhibits penicillin against most bacteria, but increases action against resistive *S. aureus.*

Note: Multiple-dose vials of penicillin, properly labeled by the person who reconstitutes them, are possibly the only exception to the rule of never giving a drug another nurse has prepared.

Amoxicillin [Amoxil, others] inhibits mucoprotein synthesis in the cell wall of rapidly multiplying bacteria. It is bactericidal and inactivated by penicillinase.

Drug Interactions: Decreased activity with tetracyclines. Prolonged activity with probenecid.

Side Effects

Nervous System: bowel—diarrhea, nausea/vomiting.

Endocrine System: (Pregnancy Category B) none noted.

Immune System: agranulocytosis,* anemia—hemolytic, colitis—pseudomembranous*, conjunctival ecchymosis, eosinophilia, pruritus, urticaria.

Dosage: PO 250–500 mg q8h. Gonorrhea: PO 3 g in a single dose with 1 g probenecid.

Amoxicillin and potassium clavulanate [Augmentin] The addition of potassium clavulanate expands the spectrum of treatable infections to include many strains of beta-lactamase-inhibiting bacteria in otitis media, integumentary infections, lower respiratory tract infections, and UTI.

Drug Interactions: Decreased activity with tetracyclines. Prolonged activity with probenecid.

Side Effects

Nervous System: bowel—diarrhea, nausea/vomiting.

Endocrine System: (Pregnancy Category B) none noted.

Immune System: agranulocytosis,* ALT/AST—moderate elevation, glomerulonephritis, vaginitis—candidal.

Dosage: PO 250–500 mg/125 mg clavulanic acid q8–12h.

Ampicillin [various] is a broad-spectrum semisynthetic aminopenicillin relatively stable in gastric acid. It is highly bactericidal even at low concentrations, but is sensitive to penicillinase.

Drug Interactions: Increased incidence of rash with allopurinol, impaired effectiveness in patients with severe end-stage renal disease. Reduced effects with chloramphenicol, erythromycin, tetracycline possible. May interfere with contraceptive action of oral contraceptives.

Drug–Food Interactions: Food may decrease absorption. Take 1 h before or 2 h after meals.

Incompatibilities

Solution/Additive: any dextrose-containing solution including parenteral nutrition solutions.

Y-site: aminoglycosides, clindamycin, erythromycin, lidocaine, verapamil.

[†] Eye related.

* Life-threatening side effect.

Side Effects

Nervous System: bowel—diarrhea, nausea/vomiting, seizures* (high doses).

Endocrine System: (Pregnancy Category B) none noted.

Immune System: anaphylaxis,* anemia—hemolytic, eosinophilia, interstitial nephritis, phlebitis—after IV, pseudomembranous colitis*, rash, superinfections.

Dosage: PO 250–500 mg q6h. IM 500 mg–1.5 g q4–6h. Meningitis: IV 150–200 mg/kg/d divided q4–6h. IV 500 mg–3 g q4–6 h to a maximum of 12 g/d.

Ampicillin sodium and sulbactam sodium [Unasyn] is used to treat infections resistant to cephalosporins and penicillin.

Drug Interactions: Increased risk of rash with allopurinol. Decreased effectiveness with severe end-stage renal disease. Reduced effectiveness with chloramphenicol, erythromycin, tetracycline possible. May interfere with oral contraceptive effectiveness.

Incompatibilities

Solution/Additive: any dextrose-containing solution, including parenteral nutrition.

Y-site: aminoglycosides, clindamycin, erythromycin, lidocaine, verapamil.

Side Effects

Nervous System: bladder—dysuria, bowel—diarrhea, distension, fatigue, headache, itching, nausea/vomiting.

Endocrine System: (Pregnancy Category B) none noted.

Immune System: anaphylaxis,* candidiasis, neutropenia, rash, thrombocytopenia.

Dosage: IM, IV 1.5–3 g q6–8h to a maximum of 12 g/d.

Penicillin V, penicillin V potassium [Pen-V, others]

Side Effects

Nervous System: bowel—diarrhea, dyspepsia, nausea/vomiting, neuropathy.

Endocrine System: (Pregnancy Category B) None noted.

Immune System: anaphylaxis,* anemia, eosinophilia, leukopenia, skin reactions, superinfections, thrombocytopenia.

Dosage: PO 125–500 mg q6–8h. Endocarditis prophylaxis: PO 2 g 30–60 min before procedure; then 1 g q6h for 8 doses.

---

* Life-threatening side effect.

Antistaphylococcal Penicillins

These drugs are used primarily for *S. aureus* infections. Their side effects are similar.

Side Effects

Nervous System: diarrhea, flatulence, nausea/vomiting.

Endocrine System: (Pregnancy Category B) none noted.

Immune System: anaphylaxis,* eosinophilia, pruritus, rash, urticaria, wheezing/sneezing (all but methicillin).

Cloxacillin [Tegopen, others] is used to treat infections caused by penicillinase-producing and penicillin-resistant staphylococci. It may be used to initiate therapy in suspected staphylococcal infections pending culture and sensitivity. Concentration is enhanced by probenecid.

Drug Interactions: Decreased elimination with probenecid.

Side Effects

Nervous System: bowel—diarrhea/flatulence, nausea/vomiting.

Endocrine System: (Pregnancy Category B) chills, fever.

Immune system: agranulocytosis,* ALT/AST—elevated, anaphylaxis,* eosinophilia, leukopenia, jaundice, pruritus, rash, sneezing, superinfections, urticaria, wheezing.

Dosage: PO 250–500 mg q6h.

Dicloxacillin [Dynapen, others] is used to treat penicillinase-resistant staphylococci. It is less potent than penicillin G against penicillin-sensitive microorganisms and is generally ineffective against methicillin-resistant staphylococci and gram-negative bacteria. It is used primarily in systemic infections.

Drug Interactions: Decreased elimination with probenecid.

Side Effects

Nervous System: diarrhea, flatulence, nausea/vomiting, pain—abdominal.

Endocrine System: (Pregnancy Category B) none noted

Immune System: ALT—increase, anaphylaxis,* eosinophilia, pruritus, rash, sneezing, superinfections, urticaria, wheezing

Dosage: PO 125–500 mg q6h.

Methicillin [Staphcillin] is used to treat infections caused by penicillinase-producing staphylococci. It may be used to initiate therapy in suspected staphylococcal infections pending culture and sensitivity results.

Incompatibilities

Solution/Additive: amikacin, chlorpromazine, codeine, heparin, hydrocortisone, levorphanol, meperidine, metaraminol, methadone, methohexital, morphine, tetracyclines, promethazine, sodium bicarbonate, streptomycin, vancomycin.

Side Effects

Nervous System: none noted

Endocrine System: (Pregnancy Category B) none noted

Immune System: anaphylaxis,* candidal superinfections—oral/rectal/vaginal, eosinophilia, acute interstitial nephritis, pruritus, skin rash, serum sickness, urticaria. IM site: irritation. IV site: thrombophlebitis.

Dosage: IM, IV 1–2 g q4h–6h up to 12 g/d.

Nafcillin [Unipen, others] treats penicillinase producing staphylococcal infections.

Drug Interactions: May antagonize warfarin effect.

Incompatibilities

Solution/Additive: aminophylline, ascorbic acid, aztreonam, bleomycin, cytarabine, hydrocortisone, methylprednisolone, promazine.

Y-site: droperidol, Innovar, labetalol, nalbuphine, pentazocine, verapamil.

Side Effects

Nervous System: bowel—diarrhea, nausea/vomiting, pain.

Endocrine System: (Pregnancy Category B) drug fever. High IV doses: hypokalemia.

Immune System: anaphylaxis* (particularly after parental therapy), eosinophilia, allergic interstitial nephritis, neutropenia (with long-term therapy), pruritus, rash, increased serum transaminase (IM), thrombophlebitis (post IV), tissue irritation, urticaria.

Dosage: IM, IV 500 mg–2 g q4–6h to maximum of 12 g/d. PO 250–1000 mg q4–6h.

Oxacillin sodium [Bactocill, Prostaphlin] is used to treat infections caused by penicillinase-producing staphylococci.

Incompatibilities

Solution/Additive: cytarabine, tetracyclines.

Y-site: verapamil.

Side Effects

Nervous System: bowel—diarrhea/flatulence, nausea/vomiting.

Endocrine System: albuminuria fever.

Immune System: agranulocytosis,* granulocytopenia, hepatitis, leukopenia, superinfections, thrombocytopenia.

Dosage: PO 500–1000 mg q4-6h. IM, IV 250 mg–2 g q4–6h to maximum of 12 g/d.

Aztreonam [Azactam] is used to treat gram-negative infections of the urinary tract, lower respiratory tract, and integumentary system, for intraabdominal and gynecologic infections, septicemia, and as adjunctive therapy for surgical infections. It is often used in combination with other antibiotics active against gram-positive and anaerobic bacteria in mixed infections.

Drug Interactions: Decreased action with cefoxitin, imipenem + cilastatin sodium possible. Slowed elimination with probenecid.

Incompatibilities

Solution/Additive: ampicillin, metronidazole, nafcillin.

Side Effects

Nervous System: bowel—diarrhea, dizziness, headache, insomnia, nausea/vomiting, pain—injection site, paresthesias, psyche—confusion, seizures,* sneezing, sweating, tinnitus, vision—diplopia.

Endocrine System: (Pregnancy Category B) none noted.

Immune System: anaphylaxis,* congestion—nasal, dermatitis, eosinophilia, erythema, liver function test—elevated, petechiae, purpura, superinfection—vaginal candidiasis/gram-positive cocci, thrombophlebitis (post IV), urticaria.

Dosage: IM, IV 1–2 g q6–8h to maximum of 8 g/24 h. UTI: IM, IV 0.5–1 g q8–12h.

Penicillin G salts [various] are used to treat gram-positive and gram-negative cocci. It is also effective against gram-positive bacilli, including gas gangrene and tetanus, and gram-negative bacilli. Parenteral penicillin is effective against some strains of salmonella, shigella, and spirochetes.

Drug Interactions: Renal elimination decreased with probenecid. May decrease efficacy of oral contraceptives. Decreased absorption with colestipol. Potential for hyperkalemia with potassium-sparing diuretics.

Drug–Food Interactions: Food increases breakdown in stomach.

---

* Life-threatening side effect.

Incompatibilities

Solution/Additive: aminophylline, amphotericin B, cephalothin, chlorpromazine, dextran 40, dopamine, fat emulsion, hydroxyzine, metaraminol, metoclopramide, pentobarbital, prochlorperazine, promazine, sodium bicarbonate, tetracyclines, thiopental.

Side Effects (occur immediately to within 72 h):

Nervous System: arrhythmias—cardiac arrest,* bowel—diarrhea, broncho-/laryngospasm,* circulatory collapse,* coma,* coughing, cramps—abdominal (severe), hyperflexia, lethargy, malaise, nausea/vomiting, pain—mouth/tongue, psyche—confusion/irritability, seizures,* sneezing, stupor, twitching, uneasiness.

Endocrine System: electrolyte imbalances, fever, flushing.

Immune System: anemia, angioedema,* anaphylaxis,* asthma, drug fever, Jarisch–Herxheimer reaction, Loeffler's syndrome, serum sickness, skin reactions—abscess/inflammation/phlebitis, Stevens–Johnson syndrome,* SLE-like syndrome, superinfections, thrombocytopenia.

Dosage: IM, IV 1.2–24 million U divided q4h.

Procaine penicillin: IM 600,00–4,800,000 U qd in divided doses. Uncomplicated gonorrhea: IM 4,800,000 U divided in 2 different injection sites. Give 1 g of probenecid 30 min before. Syphilis: IM 2–4 million U/d for 10–14 d. The preferred agent is penicillin G aqueous IV. Endocarditis IM 1.2 million U q6h × 2–4 wk.

Extended-Spectrum Penicillins

Imipenem and cilastatin [Primaxin], with the greatest spectrum of the beta-lactam antibiotics, is used for the serious infections.

Side Effects

Nervous System: bowel—diarrhea, dizziness, dyspnea, encephalopathy, headache, hearing loss—transient, heartburn, hyperventilation, myoclonus, nausea/vomiting, pain—abdominal/injection site, paresthesia, polyarthralgia, psyche—confusion, seizures,* somnolence, sweating, tremors, weakness.

Endocrine System: (Pregnancy Category C) chills, fever, flushing, electrolyte changes, urinary volume changes.

Immune System: edema—facial, colitis—hemorrhagic and pseudomembranous,* Hb/Hct—decrease, phlebitis—injection site, skin reactions, superinfections, WBC—increased.

---

* Life-threatening side effect.

Dosage: IM 500–750 mg q12h. IV 250–500 mg infused over 20–30 min q6–8h to maximum of 1 g infused over 40–60 min q6h.

BETA-LACTAMS: THE CEPHALOSPORINS— FOUR GENERATIONS AND A CEPHAMYCIN

The second generation of cephalosporins is used prophylactically for gynecologic and colorectal surgery and treatment of PID, diverticulitis, and abdominal wounds. The third generation is for bacteria resistant to the first or second generations. This generation has some forms resistant to beta-lactamase. Sometimes probenecid is used with cephalosporins to slow renal excretion.

Cefamandole nafate [Mandol] is used to treat serious infections of respiratory, genitourinary, and biliary tracts, skin and soft tissue, and bones and joints, as well as septicemia and peritonitis. It is also used for perioperative prophylaxis to reduce infections in patients undergoing potentially contaminated procedures.

Drug Interactions: Disulfiram-like reaction with alcohol. Decreased renal elimination with probenecid.

Incompatibilities

Solution/Additive: aminoglycosides, calcium gluconate, calcium gluceptate, cimetidine, metronidazole, magnesium, Ringer's lactate.

Y-site: aminoglycosides.

Side Effects

Nervous System: cramps—abdominal, diarrhea, pain—injection site.

Endocrine System: (Pregnancy Category B) vitamin K deficiency.

Immune System: colitis—pseudomembranous*, eosinophilia, skin changes—allergic, sterile abscess—injection site, superinfections.

Dosage: IM, IV 500 mg–1 g q4–8h to maximum of 2 g q4h. Surgical prophylaxis: IM, IV: 1–2 g 30–60 min before surgery; then q6h for 24–48 h.

Cefazolin sodium [Ancef, Kefzol, others] is a first-generation cephalosporin used to treat severe infections of urinary and biliary tracts, skin, soft tissue and bone, as well as septicemia and endocarditis. It is also used for perioperative prophylaxis in procedures with high risk of infection, such as open heart surgery.

Drug Interactions: Decreased renal elimination with probenecid.

Incompatibilities

Solution/Additive: aminoglycosides, amobarbital, ascorbic acid, bleomycin, calcium chloride, calcium gluceptate, calcium gluconate, cimetidine, colistin, erythromycin, lidocaine, pentobarbital, polymyxin B, tetracyclines, vitamin B complex with C.

Y-site: aminoglycosides.

Side Effects

Nervous System: cramps—abdominal, diarrhea, seizure* (high doses with renal insufficiency).

Endocrine System: (Pregnancy Category B) anorexia, fever.

Immune System: anaphylaxis,* eosinophilia, skin reactions, superinfections.

Dosage: IM/IV only. Mild to moderate infections: 250–500 mg q8h. Uncomplicated UTIs: 0.5–1 g q6–8h to a max of 100 mg/kg for severe infections. Endocarditis/septicemia: 1–1.5 g q6h. Pneumococcal pneumonia: 0.5 g q12h. Preoperative: 1 g 30–60 min before surgery. During surgery: 0.5–1 g. Postoperative: 0.5–1 g q6–8h × 24 h and up to 5 d.

Cefepime hydrochloride [Maxipime] is a fourth-generation cephalosporin with broader spectrum activity than other cephalosporins.

Drug Interactions: none noted.

Side Effects Similar to penicillin

Dosage: IM, IV: 500 mg–2 g q12h.

Cefixime [Suprax], a third-generation cephalosporin, is used to treat uncomplicated urinary tract infections, otitis media, pharyngitis, and tonsillitis caused by susceptible bacteria.

Drug Interactions: none noted.

Side Effects

Nervous System: bowel—diarrhea/flatulence, dizziness, dyspepsia, headache, nausea/vomiting.

Endocrine System: (Pregnancy Category B) fever.

Immune System: genital pruritus, skin reactions.

Dosage: PO 200 mg bid. Tablets or powder to be made into a suspension containing 100 mg/5 mL.

Cefonicid sodium [Monocid], a second-generation cephalosporin, is used to treat moderate to severe infections.

Off Label: Uncomplicated gonorrhea.

Drug Interactions: Decreased renal elimination with probenecid.

Incompatibilities

Solution/Additive and Y-site: aminoglycosides.

Side Effects

Nervous System: bowel—diarrhea, burning sensation, myalgia, nausea/vomiting, pain—injection site.

Endocrine System: (Pregnancy Category B) fever.

Immune System: anaphylaxis,* enterocolitis—pseudomembranous*, flu-like syndrome, neutropenia, skin—allergic reactions, phlebitis (with IV), superinfections.

Dosage: IM, IV 0.5–2 g/d divided or daily. Surgical prophylaxis: 1 g 60 min before surgery. May give × 2 days if needed.

Cefoperazone sodium [Cefobid], a third-generation cephalosporin, is used to treat infections of skin and skin structures: urinary tract, respiratory tract; peritonitis and other intraabdominal infections; pelvic inflammatory disease, endometritis, and other female genital tract infections; septicemia.

Off Label: Children < 12 y.

Drug Interactions: Disulfiram-like reaction with alcohol. Decreased renal elimination with probenecid.

Incompatibilities

Solution/Additive: aminoglycosides, doxapram.

Y-site: aminoglycosides, labetalol, meperidine, perphenazine.

Side Effects

Nervous System: bloating, bowel—diarrhea, cramps—abdominal, pain—IM site.

Endocrine System: (Pregnancy Category B) BUN/alkaline phosphatase/serum creatinine—elevated, oliguria.

Immune System: AST/ALT—elevated, colitis—pseudomembranous,* eosinophilia, abnormal PT/PTT—hypoprothrombinemia, skin—allergic reactions, superinfections.

Dosage: IM, IV 2–4 g q12h to a maximum of 16 g/d.

* Life-threatening side effect.

Cefotaxime sodium [Claforan], a third-generation cephalosporin, is used to treat serious infections of lower respiratory tract, skin and skin structures, bones and joints, CNS, and GU tract infections. It is also used to treat septicemia and intraabdominal infections, as well as for perioperative prophylaxis.

Off Label: To treat disseminated gonococcal infections. Drug of choice for gonococcal ophthalmia.

Drug Interactions: Decreased renal elimination with probenecid.

Incompatibilities

Solution/Additive: aminoglycosides, aminophylline, sodium bicarbonate.

Y-site: aminoglycosides, aminophylline, doxapram, sodium bicarbonate.

Side Effects

Nervous System: bowel—diarrhea, nausea/vomiting, pain—abdominal.

Endocrine System: (Pregnancy Category B) anorexia, fever, night sweats.

Immune System: AST/ALT—elevated, colitis—pseudomembranous,* LDH/bilirubin/alkaline phosphatase—elevated, skin—allergic reactions. IV site: phlebitis/thrombophlebitis.

Dosage: Moderate to severe infections: IM, IV 1–2 g q6–8h, up to 2 g q4h to maximum of 12 g/d. Surgical prophylaxis: IM, IV 1 g 30–90 min before surgery.

Cefotetan disodium [Cefotan] is a cephamycin similar to cephalosporins and with typical uses.

Drug Interactions: Disulfiram-like reaction with alcohol. Decreased renal elimination with probenecid.

Incompatibilities

Solution/Additive: aminoglycosides, doxapram, heparin, promethazine, tetracyclines.

Y-site: aminoglycosides, promethazine.

Side Effects

Nervous System: bowel—diarrhea, disulfiram-like reaction, nausea/vomiting, pain—abdominal, injection site.

Endocrine System: (Pregnancy Category B) chills, fever.

Immune System: colitis, prolonged bleeding time/PTT, skin—allergic reactions.

Dosage: IM, IV 1–2 g q12h. Surgical prophylaxis: IM, IV 1–2 g 30–60 min before surgery.

Cefoxitin [Mefoxin], a second-generation cephalosporin, is used to treat infections of the lower respiratory tract, urinary tract, skin and skin structures, and bones and joints, as well as intraabdominal endocardio, gynecologic infections, septicemia, and uncomplicated gonorrhea. It is also used for perioperative prophylaxis in prosthetic arthroplasty and cardiovascular surgery. It is specific for mixed aerobic–anaerobic infections.

Drug Interactions: Decreased renal elimination with probenecid.

Incompatibilities

Solution/Additive and Y-site: aminoglycosides.

Side Effects

Nervous System: bowel—diarrhea, pain—IM site.

Endocrine System: (Pregnancy Category B) fever.

Immune System: colitis—pseudomembranous,* nephrotoxicity/interstitial nephritis,* skin—allergic reactions/exfoliative dermatitis, thrombophlebitis—IV site.

Dosage: IM, IV 1–2 g q6–8h to maximum of 12 g/d. Surgical prophylaxis: IM, IV 2 g 30–60 min before surgery; then 2 g q6h for 24 h. For uncomplicated gonorrhea: IM, IV 2g with PO 1 g probenecid.

Cefpodoxime [Vantin], a third-generation cephalosporin, is used to treat gonorrhea, otitis media, lower and upper respiratory infections, and urinary tract infections.

Off Label: Skin and soft tissue infections.

Drug Interactions: Decreased absorption with antacids, ranitidine.

Drug–Food Interactions: Food may increase the absorption.

Side Effects

Nervous System: asthenia, bowel—diarrhea/flatulence, cough, dizziness, fatigue, insomnia, itching—eye, nausea/vomiting, pain—abdominal, psyche—anxiety/nightmares, malaise.

Endocrine System: (Pregnancy Category B) anorexia, fever, flushing.

Immune System: colitis—pseudomembranous,* epistaxis, superinfections.

Dosage: Respiratory tract, skin, soft tissue: PO 200 mg q12h for 10 d. UTI: PO 100 mg q12h. Gonorrhea: PO 200 mg in 1 dose.

Cefprozil [Cefzil], a second-generation cephalosporin, is used to treat upper and lower respiratory tract infections, otitis media, and skin infections.

Drug Interactions: Decreased renal elimination with probenecid.

---

* Life-threatening side effect.

Side Effects

Nervous System: headache, nause/vomiting, pain—abdominal.

Endocrine System: (Pregnancy Category B) none noted.

Immune System: allergic responses, superinfections.

Dosage: PO 250–500 mg q12–24h for 10–14 d.

Ceftazidime [Ceptaz, Fortaz, Tazicef, Tazidime], a third-generation cephalosporin, is used to treat infections of lower respiratory tract, skin and skin structures, urinary tract, and bones and joints. It is also used to treat septicemia, gynecologic, intraabdominal, and CNS infections.

Off Label: Surgical prophylaxis.

Drug Interactions: Increased renal elimination with probenecid.

Incompatibilities

Solution/Additive: aminoglycosides.

Y-site: aminoglycosides, fluconazole.

Side Effects

Nervous System: bowel—diarrhea, nausea/vomiting, metallic taste, pain—abdominal.

Endocrine System: (Pregnancy Category B) fever.

Immune System: colitis—pseudomembranous,* fungal infections, skin—allergic reactions, superinfections.

Dosage: IM, IV 1–2 g q8–12h. Up to 2g q6h.

Ceftizoxime sodium [Cefizox] is a third-generation cephalosporin.

Drug Interactions: Increased renal elimination with probenecid.

Incompatibilities

Solution/Additive and Y-site: aminoglycosides.

Side Effects

Nervous System: bowel—diarrhea, nausea/vomiting, paresthesia.

Endocrine System: (Pregnancy Category B) fever.

Immune System: cellulitis, colitis—pseudomembranous,* phlebitis, skin—allergic reactions.

Dosage: IM, IV 1–2 g q8–12h. Up to 2 g q4h.

Ceftriaxone sodium [Rocephin] is a third-generation cephalosporin.

Drug Interactions: Increased renal elimination with probenecid. Disulfiram-like reaction with alcohol.

Incompatibilities

Solution/Additive: aminoglycosides, clindamycin.

Y-site: aminoglycosides.

Side Effects

Nervous System: cramps, diarrhea, pain—IM site

Endocrine System: (Pregnancy Category B) chills, fever.

Immune System: biliary sludge, fungal infections, skin—allergic reactions.

Dosage: IM, IV 1–2 g q12–24h to maximum of 4 g/d. Meningitis: IM, IV 2 g q12h. Surgical prophylaxis: IM, IV 1 g 30–120 min before surgery. Uncomplicated gonorrhea: IM 250 mg in 1 dose.

Cefuroxime axetil [Ceftin], Cefuroxime sodium [Kefurox, Zinacef] are second-generation cephalosporins.

Drug Interactions: Decreased renal elimination with probenecid.

Incompatibilities

Solution/Additive: aminoglycosides, doxapram, sodium bicarbonate.

Y-site: aminoglycosides, sodium bicarbonate.

Side Effects

Nervous System: bowel—diarrhea, nausea/vomiting, IV site—burning/pain.

Endocrine System: (Pregnancy Category B) BUN/serum creatinine—increased, creatinine clearance—decreased.

Immune System: anemia, colitis, superinfections, thrombophlebitis—IV site.

Dosage: PO 250–500 mg q12h. IM, IV 750 mg–1.5 g q6–8h. Meningitis: IM, IV 3 g q8h. Surgical prophylaxis: IM, IV 1.5 g 30–60 min before surgery; then 750 mg q8h for 24 h.

Cephalexin [Keflex, others] is a broad-spectrum first-generation cephalosporin.

Drug Interactions: Decreased renal elimination with probenecid.

Side Effects

Nervous System: bowel—diarrhea, dizziness, fatigue, headache, nausea/vomiting.

Endocrine System: (Pregnancy Category B) anorexia.

Immune System: anaphylaxis,* angioedema,* rash, superinfections.

* Life-threatening side effect.

Dosage: PO 250–500 mg q6h. Integumentary infection: PO 500 mg q12h.

<u>Cephalothin sodium [Keflin, Seffin]</u> is a first-generation cephalosporin prototype.

Drug Interactions: Decreased renal elimination with probenecid.

Incompatibilities

Solution/Additive: aminoglycosides, aminophylline, bleomycin, calcium chloride, calcium gluceptate, calcium gluconate, cimetidine, colistimethate, cytarabine, diphenhydramine, dopamine, erythromycin, methylprednisolone, metoclopramide, penicillin G, phenobarbital, polymyxin B, tetracyclines.

Y-site: aminoglycosides, cytarabine, erythromycin, metoclopramide, polymyxin B, tetracyclines.

Side Effects

Nervous System: bowel—diarrhea/flatulence, cramps, dizziness, fatigue, headache, malaise, nausea/vomiting, vertigo.

Endocrine System: (Pregnancy Category B) anorexia, fever.

Immune System: agranulocytosis,* anaphylaxis,* enterocolitis—pseudomembranous,* skin—allergic reactions, thrombophlebitis—IV site.

Dosage: IM, IV 250 mg–2 g q4–6h up to 2 g q4h to maximum of 12 g/d. Surgical prophylaxis: IM, IV 1–2 g 30–60 min before surgery; then q6h for 24 h.

<u>Cephapirin sodium [Cefadyl]</u> is a first-generation broad-spectrum antibiotic.

Drug Interactions: Decreased renal elimination with probenecid.

Incompatibilities

Solution/Additive: aminoglycosides, aminophylline, ascorbic acid, epinephrine, mannitol, norepinephrine, phenytoin, tetracyclines, thiopental.

Y-site: aminoglycosides, phenytoin, tetracyclines, thiopental.

Side Effects

Nervous System: bowel—diarrhea, cramps—abdominal, nausea/vomiting.

Endocrine System: (Pregnancy Category B) fever.

Immune System: anaphylaxis,* eosinophilia, serum sickness-like symptoms, skin—allergic reactions.

---

* Life-threatening side effect.

Dosage: IM, IV 500 mg–1 g q4–6h to maximum of 12 g/d.

<u>Cephradine [Anspor]</u> is a first-generation broad-spectrum antibiotic.

Drug Interactions: Decreased renal elimination with probenecid.

Incompatibilities

Solution/Additive and Y-site: aminoglycosides, other antibiotics, TPN solutions.

Side Effects

Nervous System: bowel—diarrhea, chest tightness, dizziness, heartburn, pain—abdominal/IV site/joint, paresthesias.

Endocrine System: (Pregnancy Category B) none noted.

Immune System: skin—allergic reactions, superinfections, thrombophlebitis—IV site, induration/tissue sloughing—IM site.

Dosage: IM, IV 500 mg–1 g q4–6h up to 12 g/d. Perioperative prophylaxis: IM, IV. 1–2 g 30–60 min before surgery; 1–2 g during surgery; then 1–2 g q6h × 24 h.

LINCOSAMIDES

Lincosamides came from the soil of Lincoln, Nebraska, and are useful in anaerobic infections.

<u>Clindamycin salts [Cleocin, others]</u>, refined from lincomycin, has fewer adverse effects than lincomysin.

Off Label: Toxoplasmosis, in combination with pyrimethamine in AIDS patients.

Drug Interactions: Enhanced neuromuscular blocking with neuromuscular blocking agents. Decreased effect with chloramphenicol, erythromycin.

Incompatibilities

Solution/Additive: ceftriaxone, fluconazole, ranitidine, tobramycin.

Side Effects

Nervous System: bloating, cardiac arrest* (with rapid IV), flatulence, hypotension—post IM, myalgia, nausea/vomiting, pain—abdominal/IM site, taste changes.

Endocrine System: (Pregnancy Category B) fever.

Immune System: agranuloytosis,* colitis—pseudomembranous*, eosinophilia, jaundice, leukopenia, liver function tests—abnormal, skin—allergic reactions, sterile abscess, superinfections, thrombocytopenia.

Dosage: PO 150–450 mg q6h. IM, IV 300–900 mg q6–8h to maximum of 2700 mg/d. Acne vulgaris: Topical to affected areas bid.

Lincomycin hydrochloride [Lincocin] is used for patients with penicillin allergy. It is bacteriostatic or bactericidal depending on dosage and organism sensitivity.

Drug Interactions: Decreased absorption with kaolin pectin. Enhanced neuromuscular blockade with neuromuscular blockers.

Incompatibilities

Solution/Additive: ampicillin, carbenicillin, methicillin, penicillin G, phenytoin.

Side Effects

Nervous System: bowel—diarrhea, cardiopulmonary arrest,* cramps—abdominal, dizziness, headache, hypotension, nausea/vomiting, syncope, taste changes.

Endocrine System: (Pregnancy Category B) anorexia.

Immune System: agranulocytosis,* angioedema,* aplastic anemia,* colitis—pseudomembranous*, acute enterocolitis, glossitis, leukopenia, neutropenia, skin—allergic reactions, thrombocytopenia.

Dosage: PO 500 mg q6–8h to maximum of 8 g/d. IM 600 mg q12–24h. IV 600 mg–1 g q8–12h.

MACROLIDES

The macrolides, in addition to their antimicrobial activity, also "inhibit activation and chemotaxis of neutrophils" (Kelly & Kamada in Dipiro 1997). Because they may cause liver toxicity, they are of limited usefulness. In addition, they may increase theophylline levels to the point of seizures.

Azithromycin [Zithromax] is a macrolide antibiotic for treatment of mild to moderate infections caused by pyogenic streptococci.

Off Label: Bronchitis, *Helicobacter* gastritis and *Mycobacterium avium-intracellulare* complex infections.

Drug Interactions: Decreased peak level with antacids.

Drug–Food Interactions: Decreased absorption with food by 50%.

Side Effects

Nervous System: bowel—diarrhea, dizziness, headache, nausea/vomiting, pain—abdominal.

Endocrine System: (Pregnancy Category B) none noted.

Immune System: hepatotoxicity, liver function tests—slightly elevated.

Dosage: PO 500 mg on day 1. Then 250 mg q24h for 4 more days. IV 500 mg qd × 2 d minimum. Sexually transmitted disease: PO 2 g in a single dose.

Clarithromycin [Biaxin] is a semisynthetic macrolide antibiotic. It is used to treat aerobic and anaerobic gram-positive and gram-negative organisms.

Drug Interactions: Increased theophylline levels by 20%. Possible toxicity of carbamazepine, digoxin, ergotamine, triazolam, warfarin.

Side Effects

Nervous System: abdominal discomfort, bowel—diarrhea, dyspepsia, headache, nausea, abnormal taste.

Endocrine System: (Pregnancy Category C) none noted.

Immune System: eosinophilia, skin—allergic reactions.

Dosage: PO 250–500 mg bid for 10–14 d. Mycobacterial infections: PO 500 mg q12h. *H. pylori* infections: PO 500 mg tid.

Dirithromycin [Dynabac] is an erythromycin analog more active against gram-positive organisms than gram-negative organisms.

Drug Interactions: Increased theophylline levels possible.

Side Effects

Nervous System: asthenia, bowel—diarrhea/flatulence, cough, dizziness, dyspepsia, dyspnea, headache, nausea/vomiting, pain—abdominal/chest.

Endocrine System: (Pregnancy Category C) GGT—elevated.

Immune System: ALT/AST—elevated, asthmatic symptoms, pharyngitis, rhinitis, skin—allergic reactions.

Dosage: PO 500 mg qd.

Erythromycin and Salts

These bacteriostatic macrolides inhibit protein synthesis and have a spectrum similar to the penicillins.

Erythromycin [E-Mycin, others], erythromycin estolate [Ilosone], erythromycin stearate [Eramycin, others], is used to treat chlamydia, *Hemophilus influenzae, Neisseria gonorrhoeae,* and pneumococcal pneumonia. It is an alternative antibiotic to penicillin.

Drug Interactions: Increased serum levels/toxicities of carbamazepine, cyclosporin, digoxin, theophylline, triazolam, warfarin. Increased peripheral vasospasm possible with ergotamine.

---

* Life-threatening side effect.

Side Effects

Nervous System: bowel—diarrhea, cramps—abdominal, hearing loss—reversible, heartburn, nausea/vomiting, tinnitus, vertigo.

Endocrine System: (Pregnancy Category B) anorexia, fever.

Immune System: anaphylaxis,* cholestatic hepatitis syndrome, eosinophilia, skin—allergic reactions.

Dosage: PO 250–500 mg q6h or 333 mg q8h. *C. trachomatis:* PO 500 mg qid or 666 mg q8h.

Erythromycin ethylsuccinate [E.E.S., others] has the same uses as erythromycin.

Drug Interactions: Increased serum levels of carbamazepine, cyclosporin, digoxin, theophylline, triazolam, warfarin possible. Ergotamine may induce ischemia and peripheral vasospasm.

Side Effects

Nervous System: bowel—diarrhea, cramps—abdominal, nausea/vomiting.

Endocrine System: (Pregnancy Category B) anorexia.

Immune System: ototoxicity, skin—allergic reactions, stomatitis, superinfections.

Dosage: PO 400 mg q6h to maximum of 4 g/d.

Erythromycin glucepate [Ilotycin Glucepate] is used when oral administration is not possible.

Drug Interactions: Possible increase of serum levels or toxicity of carbamazepine, cyclosporin, digoxin, theophylline, triazolam, warfarin. Possible ischemia and peripheral vasospasm with ergotamine.

Incompatibilities

Solution/Additive: amikacin, aminophylline, ampicillin, cephalothin, colistimethate, heparin, metaraminol, metoclopramide, pentobarbital, secobarbital, streptomycin, tetracyclines, vitamin B complex with C.

Y-site: aminophylline, heparin, tetracyclines.

Side Effects

Nervous System: bowel—diarrhea, cramps—abdominal, nausea/vomiting, pain—post injection.

Endocrine System: (Pregnancy Category B) none noted.

Immune System: anaphylaxis,* liver function test variations, superinfections.

Dosage: IV 250 mg–1 g q6h to maximum of 4 g/d.

---

* Life-threatening side effect.

Troleandomycin [Tao] so resembles erythromycin (though less active) that it is seldom used unless the infection is not susceptible to other antibiotics.

Drug Interactions: Increased levels and toxicity of carbamazepine, cyclosporins, theophylline possible. Cholestatic jaundice possible with oral contraceptives. Possible increased prothrombin time with warfarin. Possible ischemia and peripheral vasospasm with ergotamine.

Side Effects

Nervous System: bowel—abdominal cramps/diarrhea, nausea/vomiting.

Endocrine System: (Pregnancy Category B) none noted.

Immune System: anaphylaxis,* cholestatic jaundice, skin rash, superinfections, urticaria.

Dosage: PO 250–500 mg q6h.

TETRACYCLINES

Ironically, the Pfizer Company looked at almost 1000 soil samples from around the world without success, only to find the source of tetracycline in the soil under their noses at their own Indiana plant. Tetracyclines are bacteriostatic, blocking bacterial protein synthesis of RNA, and are effective against chlamydia, rickettsia, brucellosis, cholera, typhus relapsing fever, and chronic lung infections, and in long-term acne therapy. They can prevent traveler's diarrhea. Tetracyclines are broad-spectrum against gram-negative and gram-positive bacteria, protozoa, spirochetes, rickettsia, mycoplasmas, conjunctivitis (trachoma), granuloma inguinale, and chancroid (venereal infections). Their sclerosing effect in chest instillation decreases pericardial and pleural effusions of malignancies. Tetracyclines act synergistically with the sulfonamides to increase their potency against brain abscess. Tetracyclines have a deadly potential in combination with the anesthetic methoxyflurane. The newer generation of tetracyclines is excreted through bile and reabsorbed. The older forms are excreted mainly through the kidneys. They should be taken on an empty stomach. Tetracyclines reduce the effect of penicillin, birth control pills, and digoxin. They can permanently stain small children's teeth. Note that the generic names of the tetracyclines end in "cycline."

Doxycycline hyclate [Vibramycin, others] has similar uses to those of tetracycline.

Off Label: Acute PID and leptospirosis. Prophylaxis for rape victims, suppression and chemoprophylaxis of chloroquine-resistant *Plasmodium falciparum* malaria, traveler's diarrhea. Intrapleural malignant pleural effusions.

Drug Interactions: Possible decreased absorption with antacids, iron preparations, calcium, magnesium kaolin-pectin, sodium bicarbonate, zinc. Antagonized effects of doxycycline and desmopressin. Increased digoxin absorption and toxicity. Increased risk of renal failure with methoxyflurane.

Side Effects

Nervous System: bowel—diarrhea, nausea/vomiting, vision—color interference.

Endocrine System: (Pregnancy Category D) anorexia.

Immune System: enterocolitis, photosensitivity, skin—allergic reaction, superinfections, thrombophlebitis (with IV use).

Dosage: PO, IV 100 mg q12h on day 1; then 100 mg/d as single dose to maximum of 100 mg q12h. Gonorrhea: PO 200 mg stat; follow with 100 mg hs; then 100 mg bid for 3 d. Primary and secondary syphilis: PO 300 mg/d in divided doses for at least 10 d. Travelers' diarrhea: PO 100 mg/d during risk (up to 2 wk) beginning day 1 of travel.

Tetracycline hydrochloride [Achromycin, others] is used to treat amebiases, chlamydial, mycoplasmal, rickettsial, spirochetal, uncommon infections.

Off Label: Actinomycosis, acute exacerbations of chronic bronchitis, Lyme disease, pericardial effusion, acute PID, sexually transmitted epididymoorchitis. With quinine for multidrug-resistant strains of *P. falciparum* malaria. Antiinfective prophylaxis for rape victims. Recurrent cystic thyroid nodules. Melioidosis. Fluorescence test for malignancy.

Drug Interactions: Decreased absorption with antacids, calcium, magnesium. Increased hypoprothrombinemia with anticoagulants. Decreased absorption with kaolin and pectin. Possible fatal nephrotoxicity with methoxyflurane.

Drug–Food Interactions: Dairy products and iron supplements decrease absorption.

Side Effects

Nervous System: bowel—diarrhea, discomfort—abdominal, dyspepsia, dysphagia, headache, heartburn, hypertension—intracranial, nausea/vomiting, pain—retrosternal, shock*—irreversible.

Endocrine System: (Pregnancy Category D) acidosis, azotemia, BUN/serum creatinine—increased, hyperphosphatemia, dry mouth, serum cholesterol—decreased. With outdated drug: aminoaciduria, glycosuria, polydypsia, polyuria, proteinuria acidosis.

Immune System: anaphylaxis,* drug fever, phototoxicity, serum sickness, skin—allergic reactions.

Dosage: PO 250–500 mg bid–qid to maximum of 1–2 g/d. IM 250 mg qd or 300 mg/d in 2–3 divided doses.

Acne: PO 500–1000 mg/d in 4 divided doses. Topical: bid to cleansed areas.

QUINOLONES

This group's names are, with one exception, recognizable by the ending "oxacin." They are broad spectrum and inhibit DNA-gyrase, preventing bacterial DNA replication and blocking transcription, recombination, repair, and transposition in many gram-negative and gram-positive bacteria. They are not effective against many strains of streptococci.

Cinoxacin [Cinobac] is used for initial and recurrent UTIs.

Drug Interactions: Decreased renal elimination with probenecid.

Side Effects

Nervous System: arthropathy, bowel—constipation/diarrhea, cramps—abdominal, dizziness, gums—sore, insomnia, itching—rectal, nausea/vomiting, photophobia, psyche—agitation/anxiety, taste—metallic, tinnitus, vision—blurred.

Endocrine System: (Pregnancy Category B) anorexia.

Immune System: skin—allergic reactions, swelling—extremities.

Dosage: PO 1 g/d in 2–4 divided doses.

Ciprofloxacin hydrochloride [Cipro] is used for bone and joint, lower respiratory, and urinary tract infections in adults. Absorption is decreased by antacids containing magnesium or aluminum. Caution is needed in patients on theophylline because the combination raises theophylline blood levels. Caution is also required in patients with a history of seizures.

Drug Interactions: Possible increase of theophylline levels 15–30%. Decreased absorption with antacids, sucralfate, iron. Possible increased PT with warfarin.

Incompatibilities

Solution/Additive: aminophylline, clindamycin, dexamethasone, furosemide, heparin, hydrocortisone, magnesium sulfate, methylprednisolone, mezlocillin, phenytoin, sodium bicarbonate, theophylline.

Y-site: aminophylline, clindamycin, furosemide, heparin, phenytoin, sodium bicarbonate, theophylline.

Side Effects

Nervous System: bowel—diarrhea/gas, cramps, fatigue, headache, insomnia/somnolence, malaise, nausea/vomiting, psyche—confusion/depression/restlessness, seizures* (caution with rapid IV), vertigo, vision—

---

*Life-threatening side effect.

blurred. Ophthalmic: foreign body sensation, itching.† IV site: burning, pain.

Endocrine System: (Pregnancy Category X) alkaline phosphatase/BUN/lactic dehydrogenase/serum creatinine—elevated, fever.

Immune System: SGOT/SGPT/WBC/neutrophils/hematocrit/eosinophilia—decreased, erythema at infusion site, phlebitis, pruritus, rash, tendon rupture. Ophthalmic: crystalline precipitate on superficial portion of cornea/lid margin/conjunctival hyperemia/crusting/scales.

Dosage: UTI: PO 250 mg q12h. IV 200 mg q12h, infused over 1 h. Difficult infections: PO 500–750 mg q12h. IV 200–400 mg q12h, infused over 1 h. Corneal ulcers: 2 gtt q15min for 6 h; then 2 gtt q30min for next 18 h; then 2 gtt q1h for 24 h; then 2 gtt q4h for 14 d.† Conjunctivitis 1–2 gtt in conjunctival sac q2h while awake for 2 d; then 1–2 gtt q4h while awake for 5 d.† Acute sinusitis: PO 500 mg bid × 10d.

Levofloxacin [Levaquin] is a fluoroquinolone used to treat acute maxillary sinusitis caused by *Streptococcus hemophilus influenzae* or *Moraxella catarrhalis* and other URIs caused by *Staphylococcus aureus, S. pneumoniae, H. influenzae, M. catarrhalis.* It is also used to treat community acquired pneumonia due to *S. aureus, S. pneumoniae, H. influenzae, H. oarainfluenzae, Klebsiella pneumoniae, M. catarrhalis, Chlamydia pneumoniae, Legionella pneumonophila,* or *Mycoplasma pneumoniae.* It is also used for mild to moderate infections of the integumentum due to *S. aureus* or *Streptococcus pyogenes,* and mild to moderate complicated UTI due to *E. faecalis, E. cloacae, E. coli, K. pneumoniae, P. mirabilis,* or *P. aeruginosa,* and moderate pyelonephritis due to *E. coli.*

Drug Interactions: Decreased levels of oral levofloxacin with antacids containing magnesium or aluminum, sucralfate, metal cations such as iron, and multivitamin preparations with zinc; these agents should be taken either 2 h before or after oral levofloxacin administration. Increased levels of theophylline with oral levofloxacin. Increased risk of CNS stimulation or seizures with concomitant NSAIDs administration.

Side Effects

Nervous System: bowel—constipation/diarrhea/flatulence, dizziness, dyspepsia, fatigue, headache, malaise, nausea/vomiting, pain—abdominal, psyche—anxiety/insomnia/nervousness/sleep disorders, taste perversion, tremor.

Endocrine System: (Pregnancy Category C) anorexia, edema, sweating.

Immune System: leukorrhea, pruritus, rash, urticaria, vaginitis.

Dosage: PO, 500 mg q24h × 10 d. IV 500 mg infused over 60 min q24h × 7–14 d. UTI, pyelonephritis PO 250 mg q24h × 10 d. IV 250 mg infused over 60 min q24h × 10d.

Caution: Avoid rapid infusion. All IV dosages are reduced with renal insufficiency.

Nalidixic acid [Neg Gram], a synthetic quinolone, is used to treat urinary tract infections caused by susceptible gram-negative bacteria.

Off Label: GI tract infections caused by susceptible strains of *Shigella sonnei.* Prophylaxis of bacteriuria and for bladder irrigation for low-grade cystitis. Nalidixic acid has many of the side effects of the quinolones, but may be used in children older than 3 mo.

Drug Interactions: Decreased absorption with antacids possible. Increased effects of warfarin.

Side Effects

Nervous System: arthralgia, bowel—diarrhea/abdominal pain, dizziness, drowsiness, headache, malaise, myalgia, nausea/vomiting, psyche—confusion/depression/excitement/insomnia, seizures,* syncope, vertigo, weakness

Endocrine System: (Pregnancy B) chills, cholestasis, eosinophilia, fever.

Immune System: anaphylaxis,* angioedema,* AST—transient increase, hemolytic anemia (especially with G6PD deficiency), hypersensitivity, peripheral neuritis, photosensitivity, pneumonitis, pruritus, rash, urticaria

Dosage: UTI PO acute therapy 4 g per day in 4 doses for 1–2 weeks. For chronic therapy: 500 mg qid.

Ofloxacin [Floxin, Ocuflox] is used to treat *Chlamydia trachomatis* infections, uncomplicated gonorrhea, prostatitis, respiratory tract infections, skin and skin structure infections, urinary tract infections by susceptible bacteria, and superficial ocular infections.

Off Label: ENT infections, *Helicobacter pylori* infections, salmonella gastroenteritis.

Drug Interactions: Decreased absorption with magnesium- or aluminum-containing antacids and other cations, eg, calcium, iron, zinc.

Side Effects

Nervous System: bladder—dysuria, bowel—diarrhea, burning, dizziness, dysmenorrhea, GI discomfort, headache, insomnia, nausea/vomiting, pain, psyche—hallucinations.

---

† Eye related.

* Life-threatening side effect.

Endocrine System: (Pregnancy Category C) none noted.

Immune System: menorrhagia, pruritus, rash, vaginal discharge, vaginitis.

Dosage: Uncomplicated gonorrhea: PO 400 mg for 1 dose. UTI, respiratory tract, integumentary infections: PO 200–400 mg q12h for 7–10 d. IV 400 mg q12h for 7 d. Prostatitis: PO 300 mg bid for 6 wk. IV 300 mg q12h for 10 d; then PO for 6 wk. Superficial ocular infections: 1–2 gtt q2–4h on first 2 d; then qid up to 5 more days. Ophthalmic: Instill 1–2 gtt q2–4h for first 2 d; then qid for up to 5 additional days.[†]

Sparfloxacin [Zagam] is an aminodifluorquinilone that treats infections of a wide range of gram-negative and gram-positive infections by inhibiting bacterial DNA gyrase.

Drug Interactions: Decreased absorption with aluminum and magnesium antacids or sucralfate formulations and with zinc or iron salts.

Side Effects

Nervous System: arrhythmias—bradycardia/QT interval prolonged, bowel—diarrhea/flatulence, insomnia, nausea/vomiting, pain—abdominal.

Endocrine System: (Pregnancy Category C) concentrated urine.

Immune System: colitis—pseudomembranous,* photosensitivity.*

Dosage: PO 400 mg loading dose on day 1; 200 mg qd for 10 days.

MISCELLANEOUS ANTIMICROBIAL AGENTS

The following antimicrobials do not easily fit into categories.

Atovaquone [Mepron] is used to treat the protozoan diseases caused by Pneumocystis carinii and Plasmodium in patients intolerant of cotrimoxazole.

Off Label: Cerebral toxoplasmosis.

Drug Interactions: Three- to fourfold increased oral absorption with food, especially fatty food.

Side Effects

Nervous System: bowel—diarrhea, cough, dizziness, dyspepsia, headache, hypotension, insomnia, nausea/vomiting, pain—abdominal.

Endocrine System: (Pregnancy Category C) anorexia, fever, hypoglycemia, hyponatremia.

Immune System: anemia, neutropenia, sinusitis, skin—allergic reactions, thrush.

Dosage: PO 750 mg (5 mL) suspension bid for 21 d.

Chloramphenicol and salts [Chloromycetin, others], discovered in the soil of Caracas, Venezuela, is able to cross the BBB, making it useful in treating brain abscess. It is used only in severe infections resistant to other antibiotics. Chloramphenicol is also useful for treating typhoid, meningitis, epiglottitis, rickettsia, lymphogranuloma, and psittacosis. This is no trivial drug, and can cause bone marrow suppression and aplastic anemia. CBC must be monitored closely (qod).

Drug Interactions: Decreased metabolism and prolonged activity of chlorpropamide, dicumarol, phenytoin, tolbutamide possible. Decreased levels with phenobarbital. Delayed response to folic acid, iron preparations, vitamin B_{12}.

Incompatibilities

Solutions/Additives: chlorpromazine, glycopyrrolate, metoclopramide, polymyxin B, prochlorperazine, promethazine, tetracyclines, vancomycin.

Side Effects

Nervous System: bowel—diarrhea, dyspnea, nausea/vomiting, paresthesias—digital, psyche—confusion/delirium/depression, taste—unpleasant, visual disturbances.

Endocrine System: (Pregnancy Category C) fever, increased plasma iron.

Immune System: anaphylaxis,* angioedema,* agranulocytosis,* anemia—hypoplastic,* bone marrow depression,* enterocolitis, glossitis, gray syndrome, Hb—reduction, hypoprothrombinemia, leukemia,* leukopenia, neuritis—optic/peripheral, optic nerve atrophy, paroxysmal nocturnal hemoglobinuria, reticulocytosis, skin—allergic reactions, stomatitis, superinfections, thrombocytopenia.

Dosage: PO, IV 50 mg/kg/d in 4 divided doses. Ophthalmic solution: Topical: 1–2 gtts q3–6h or small strip of ophthalmic ointment in lower conjunctival sac q3–6h[†] or 2–3 gtt of otic solution in ear tid. Meningitis: IV 75–100 mg/kg/d divided q6h.

Demeclocycline [Declomycin] is a broad-spectrum tetracycline. It is absorbed more readily and excreted more slowly, with a longer duration of effective blood levels allowing longer intervals between doses. It can inhibit protein synthesis, increase tissue breakdown, and damage kidneys with the increased waste products of tissue breakdown.

[†] Eye related.
* Life-threatening side effect.

Off Label: Used to treat chronic SIADH by inhibiting antidiuretic hormone (ADH).

Drug Interactions: Decreased absorption with antacids, calcium, iron, kaolin-pectin, magnesium, sodium bicarbonate, zinc. Increased digoxin absorption. Increased risk of renal failure with methoxyflurane. Effects of desmopressin, cephalosphorins, and demeclocycline antagonized.

Food–Drug Interactions: Absorption decreased with dairy products and food.

Side Effects

Nervous System: bowel—diarrhea, nausea/vomiting, pain/cramps—abdominal.

Endocrine System: (Pregnancy Category D) anorexia, azotemia, diabetes insipidus.

Immune System: anaphylaxis,* esophageal—irritation or ulceration, pericarditis,* photosensitivity, skin—allergic reactions.

Dosage: PO 150 mg q6h or 300 mg q12h to maximum of 2.4 g/d. Gonorrhea: PO 600 mg; then 300 mg q12h for 4 d. Excessive ADH secretion: PO 600–1200 mg/d in 3–4 divided doses.

Metronidazole [Flagyl, MetroGel, others] is used to treat asymptomatic/symptomatic trichomoniasis, acute intestinal amebiasis, and amebic liver abscess; it is used for preoperative prophylaxis in colorectal surgery, elective hysterectomy or vaginal repair, and emergency appendectomy. IV route is used to treat serious infections by susceptible anaerobic bacteria in intraabdominal infections, skin infections, gynecologic infections, septicemia, and for both pre- and postoperative prophylaxis.

Topical: Bacterial vaginosis, rosacea.

Off Label: pseudomembranous colitis, Crohn's disease.

Drug Interactions: Increased hypoprothrombinemia with oral anticoagulants. Disulfiram-like reaction possible with alcohol. Acute psychosis with disulfiram. Increased metabolism with phenobarbital. Increased lithium levels. Transient neutropenia with fluorouracil, azathioprine.

Incompatibilities

Solution/Additive: aztreonam, dopamine, TPN.

Side Effects

Nervous System: arrhythmias—ECG changes, ataxia, bladder—dysuria/incontinence, bowel—constipation, cramps—abdominal, drowsiness, dyspepsia, fatigue, headache, insomnia, nausea/vomiting, fleeting pain—

joint, paresthesia, psyche—confusion/irritability/restlessness, sensory disturbances, sexual function—decreased libido/dyspareunia, taste changes, vertigo, weakness.

Endocrine System: (Pregnancy Category B) anorexia, fever, flushing, dry mouth, polyuria, vaginal/vulvar dryness.

Immune System: nasal congestion, cystitis, proctitis.

Dosage: Trichomoniasis, giardiasis, *Gardnerella:* PO 2 g once or 250 mg tid, 375 mg bid, or 500 mg bid for 7 d. Vaginal: qd or bid for 5 d. Amebiasis: PO 500–750 mg tid. Anaerobic infections: PO 7.5 mg/kg q6h to maximum of 4 g/d. IV 15 mg/kg loading dose; then 7.5 mg/kg q6h to maximum of 4 g/d. Pseudomembranous colitis: PO 200-500 mg tid. IV 250–500 mg tid or qid. Bacterial vaginosis: PO [Flagyl ER] 750 mg qd × 7 d.

Pentamidine isethionate [NebuPent, Pentam 300] is an antiprotozoal used to treat *P. carinii* pneumonia.

Off Label: African trypanosomiasis and visceral leishmaniasis.

Drug Interactions: Increased risk of nephrotoxicity with aminoglycosides, amphotericin B, cyclosporin, vancomycin.

Side Effects

Nervous System: arrhythmias—various ventricular tachycardia,* brochospasm,* cough, dizziness, hypotension*—swift/severe, nausea/vomiting, neuralgia, pain—chest, psyche—confusion/hallucinations, shortness of breath, taste—unpleasant.

Endocrine System: (Pregnancy Category C) anorexia, hyperkalemia, hypoglycemia,* acute renal failure, sweating. IV: facial flush.

Immune System: anemia, laryngitis, leukopenia, pneumothorax,* Stevens–Johnson syndrome,* thrombocytopenia.

Dosage: *Pneumocystis carinii* pneumonia: IM, IV 4 mg/kg qd for 14–21 d. Infuse IV over 60 min. Prophylaxis of *P. carinii* pneumonia: inhaled 300 mg per nebulizer q4wk.

Vancomycin hydrochloride [Vancocin, others] is a parenteral antibiotic that treats bacterial infections that are nonsensitive or resistant to other antimicrobial drugs.

Drug Interactions: Increased toxicity of ototoxic and nephrotoxic drugs including aminoglycosides, amphotericin B, colistin, polymyxin B.

Incompatibilities

Solution/Additive: aminophylline, barbiturates, chloramphenicol, chlorothiazide, dexamethasone, heparin, methicillin, sodium bicarbonate, warfarin.

---

* Life-threatening side effect.

Y-site: heparin.

Side Effects

Nervous System: hearing loss, nausea, severe pain, shock.*

Endocrine System: (Pregnancy Category C) fever, uremia.*

Immune System: anaphylaxis,* eosinophilia, leukopenia—transient, nephrotoxicity,* rash, thrombophlebitis—injection site.

Dosage: IV 500 mg q6h or 1 g q12h. Infuse slowly (60–90 min). *Clostridium difficile* colitis: 125–500 mg q6h.

A Single-Dose Antibiotic

The practice of some patients to stop taking their prescribed course of antibiotics once they feel better and saving the remainder to take the next time they feel ill has helped some bacteria to become resistant to those antibiotics. A one-dose antibiotic provides patient convenience and prevents the practices that lead to antibiotic resistance.

Fosfomycin tromethamine [Monurol] is used to treat uncomplicated urinary tract infections caused by *Enterococcus faecalis* and *E. coli.*

Drug Interactions: Metoclopramide lowers serum levels and renal excretion, as do other drugs that increase GI motility.

Side Effects

Nervous System: asthenia, bowel—diarrhea/dyspepsia, dizziness, headache, nausea/vomiting.

Endocrine System: (Pregnancy Category B) anorexia, fever.

Immune System: flu syndrome, pruritus.

Dosage: PO 3 g single-dose sachet. Dissolve in ½ cup of cold water. Administer immediately.

ANTISEPTICS

The antiseptics make the environment inhospitable to microbes and inhibit their growth and reproduction.

Methenamine hippurate [Hiprex, Urex], methenamine mandelate [Mandelamine, Mandameth] becomes formaldehyde in acid urine, making the environment uninhabitable for bacteria.

Drug Interactions: Forms an insoluble precipitate with sulfamethoxazole in acid urine. Hydrolysis to formal-

dehyde may be prevented by acetazolamide, sodium bicarbonate.

Side Effects

Nervous System: bladder—dysuria/frequency, bowel—diarrhea, cramps—abdominal, nausea/vomiting, pain—abdominal.

Endocrine System: (Pregnancy Category C) albuminuria, anorexia, crystalluria.

Immune System: bladder irritation, hematuria.

Dosage: 1 g bid.

Methylene blue [Urolene Blue], though sometimes used to treat UTIs, is also an antidote for cyanide poisoning, a diagnostic agent, an indicator dye, and also used to treat oxalate phosphate lithiasis.

Off Label: Cutaneous viral infections. Diagnosis of gastroesophageal reflux in pediatrics.

Drug Interactions: none noted.

Side Effects

Nervous System: arrhythmias, bowel—diarrhea, nausea/vomiting, pain—abdominal/precordial.

Endocrine System: (Pregnancy Category C) profuse sweating.

Immune System: anemia—with continued use, hemolysis, methemoglobinemia.

Dosage: PO 65–130 mg bid or tid pc. Cyanide poisoning: IV 1–2 mg/kg 1% solution injected slowly over several minutes.

SULFONAMIDES

Gerhard Domagk won the Nobel Prize in medicine in 1939 for discovering sulfonamides, but Hitler would not let him accept the award. Perhaps more valuable to Domagk, however, was that sulfa saved his daughter from septicemia after she pricked herself with a needle (Sneader 1985). The sulfonamides differ from antibiotics made from microbes. Derived from industrial compounds used to dye wool, the sulfonamides act as antimetabolites to deprive bacteria of essential nutrients, starving them by inhibiting an enzyme that makes folic acid usable in the production of thymine, part of bacterial DNA. They cannot be used in purulent wounds, however, where bacteria can get all the DNA building blocks they need from pus. Rapidly excreted by the kidneys, they are useful in most UTIs except glomerulonephritis. Their pH makes them perfect for treating eye infections. They are also useful in treating lymphogranuloma venereum. They may decrease birth control pill effectiveness, sometimes indicated by breakthrough bleeding.

---

* Life-threatening side effect.

<u>Dapsone [DDS]</u> has value in treating *Mycobacterium leprae, Mycobacterium tuberculosis, Pneumocystis carinii,* and *Plasmodium.*

Drug Interactions: Decreased absorption and enterohepatic circulation with activated charcoal. Increased risk of adverse hematologic reactions with pyrimethamine, trimethoprim. Decreased levels 7- to 10-fold with rifampin.

Side Effects

Nervous System: headache, insomnia, malaise, nausea/vomiting, pain—abdominal, paresthesias, psyche—nervousness, tinnitus, vertigo, vision—blurred, weakness.

Endocrine System: (Pregnancy Category C) anorexia, fever, male infertility.

Immune System: agranulocytosis,* ALT/AST—increased, anemia, aplastic anemia,* toxic epidermal necrolysis* Heinz body formation, hemolysis, hepatic necrosis, infectious mononucleosis–like syndrome, jaundice, LDH/bilirubin—increased, LE, lymphadenopathy, methemoglobinemia with cyanosis, rhinitis, skin—allergic reactions, sulfone syndrome.

Dosage: Dermatitis herpetiformis: PO 50 mg/d; increase to 300 mg/d if needed to maximum of 500 mg/d. Lepromatous/borderline lepromatous leprosy: PO 100 mg/d ≥ 10 y. Tuberculoid/indeterminate-type leprosy: PO 100 mg/d with 6 mo of rifampin 600 mg/d ≥ 3 y. Prophylaxis for close contacts of multibacillary leprosy: PO 50 mg/d.

<u>Nitrofurantoin [Furadantin, Macrodantin, Macrobid, others]</u> starves bacteria by interfering with their use of carbohydrates. It can cross the BBB.

Drug Interactions: Decreased absorption with antacids. Antagonized antimicrobial effects with nalidixic acid and other quinolones.

Side Effects

Nervous System: arthralgia, bowel—diarrhea, drowsiness, headache, nausea/vomiting, possibly irreversible neuropathy—peripheral, pain—abdominal, vertigo, vision—nystagmus.

Endocrine System: (Pregnancy Category B) anorexia, cholestatic jaundice, crystalluria, dark yellow or brown urine.

Immune System: agranulocytosis,* anaphylaxis,* anemia—hemolytic or megaloblastic, asthma—in asthmatic patients, eosinophilia, exfoliative dermatitis,* allergic pneumonitis, interstitial pneumonitis or fibrosis,* hepatic necrosis,* pulmonary sensitivity reactions, skin—allergic reactions, superinfections—GU.

---

* Life-threatening side effect.

Dosage: Pyelonephritis, cystitis: PO 50–100 mg qid or Macrobid 100 mg bid. Chronic suppressive therapy: PO 50–100 mg hs.

<u>Nitrofurazone [Furacin]</u> has no antifungal activity. It is bacteriocidal against most organisms on skin surfaces.

Drug Interactions: none noted.

Side Effects

Nervous System: none noted.

Endocrine System: (Pregnancy Category C) none noted.

Immune System: allergic dermatitis, superinfections.

Dosage: Topical: applied directly to dressings or to lesion qd or q4–5d for second-degree burn with minimum exudation.

<u>Silver sulfadiazine [Silvadene]</u> is a combination whose action is unlike either compound alone in its bacteriocidal ability. It has the same toxicity as other sulfonamides.

Drug Interactions: The silver inactivates proteolytic enzymes.

Side Effects

Nervous System: burning, itching, pain.

Endocrine System: (Pregnancy Category C) none noted.

Immune System: reversible leukopenia, rash, sulfonamide toxicity.

Dosage: Apply 1% cream 1⁄16-in. thickness with a sterile glove to debrided, cleansed wound qd or bid. The patient may require analgesia before treatment.

<u>Sulfamethoxazole [Gantanol]</u> is an intermediate-acting sulfonamide. It is used to treat susceptible infections such as acute, recurrent, or chronic urinary tract infections, and lymphogranuloma venereum.

Drug Interactions: none noted.

Side Effects

Nervous System: arthralgia, ataxia, auditory—hearing loss/tinnitus, bowel—diarrhea, convulsions,* headache, malaise, nausea/vomiting, neuropathy, pain—abdominal, psyche—depression/drowsiness/insomnia/acute psychosis.

Endocrine System: (Pregnancy Category B) anuria, chills, crystalluria, fever, goiter, hematuria, hypoglycemia.

Immune System: acute hemolytic anemia (especially with G6PD deficiency), agranulocytosis,* allergic myocarditis, anaphylaxis,* aplastic anemia,* eosinophilia, exfoliative dermatitis, hypoprothrombinemia, infection by nonsusceptible organisms, jaundice, LE phenomenon, leuko-penia, pancreatitis, photosensitivity, pruritus, rash, Stevens-Johnson syndrome,* stomatitis, thrombocytopenia, vascular lesions.

Dosage: For mild to moderate infections: PO 2 g loading dose; then 1 g q8–12h.

Sulfisoxazole [Gantrisin] is a short-acting sulfonamide used to treat gram-positive and gram-negative organisms. It is bacteriostatic through interference with folic acid biosynthesis in bacteria.

Drug Interactions: Sulfa effect possibly antagonized by PABA-containing local anesthetics. Hypoprothrombinemia potentiated with anticoagulants. Possible increase of sulfonylurea-induced hypoglycemia.

Side Effects

Nervous System: arthralgia, ataxia, auditory—hearing loss/tinnitus, bowel—diarrhea, convulsions,* headache, malaise, nausea/vomiting, neuropathy, pain—abdominal, psyche—depression/drowsiness/insomnia/acute psychosis.

Endocrine System: (Pregnancy Category B; D if near term) anuria, chills, crystalluria, fever, goiter, hematuria, hypoglycemia. (Kernicterus in newborns.)

Immune System: acute hemolytic anemia (especially with G6PD deficiency), agranulocytosis,* allergic myocarditis, anaphylaxis,* aplastic anemia,* eosinophilia, exfoliative dermatitis, hypoprothrombinemia, infection by nonsusceptible organisms, jaundice, LE phenomenon, leukopenia, pancreatitis, photosensitivity, pruritus, rash, Stevens–Johnson syndrome,* stomatitis, thrombocytopenia, vascular lesions.

Dosage: PO start with 2 g. Then 1 g q8–12h.

Trimethoprim [Proloprim, others] is an antiinfective and folic acid antagonist with slow bacterial action to treat initial stages of acute UTIs.

Off Label: To treat and prevent chronic and recurrent UTI and traveler's diarrhea.

Drug Interactions: May inhibit phenytoin metabolism.

Side Effects

Nervous System: epigastric discomfort, nausea/vomiting, taste changes.

Endocrine System: (Pregnancy Category C) fever, BUN/serum transaminases—increase.

Immune System: exfoliative dermatitis,* glossitis, leukopenia, megaloblastic anemia, methemoglobinemia,

neutropenia, photosensitivity, skin—allergic reactions, thrombocytopenia.

Dosage: UTI 100 mg bid or 200 mg qd. Traveler's diarrhea: PO 200 mg bid.

Trimethoprim and sulfamethoxazole (TMP-SMZ) [Bactrim, Septra, others] is used to treat initial episodes of acute, uncomplicated UTIs.

Off Label: Treatment and prevention of chronic and recurrent UTIs. Used in conjunction with dapsone in initial episode of *Pneumocystis carinii*.

Drug Interactions: May inhibit phenytoin metabolism. Increased effect of sulfonylureas and anticoagulants. Decreased effect of cyclosporins.

Side Effects

Nervous System: arthralgia, bowel—diarrhea, myalgia, nausea/vomiting, pain—abdominal, weakness.

Endocrine System: (Pregnancy Category C) anorexia, anuria, crystalluria, oliguria, renal failure.

Immune System: agranulocytosis,* anemia—aplastic*/megaloblastic, enterocolitis—pseudomembranous,* hepatitis, hypoprothrombinemia, allergic myocarditis,* photosensitivity, stomatitis, thrombocytopenia, toxic epidermal necrolysis.*

Dosage: PO 160 mg TMP/800 mg SMZ (1 DS tab) q12h. IV 8–10 mg/kg/d TMP (IV dosage is based on TMP) divided q6–12h infused over 60–90 min. *Pneumocystis carinii* pneumonia: IV 20 mg/kg/d TMP divided q6h infused over 60–90 min. Prophylaxis for *Pneumocystis carinii* pneumonia: PO 160 mg TMP/800 mg SMZ q24h.

Trimetrexate [Neotrexin], an orphan drug, is an antimetabolite, immunosuppressant, and antineoplastic that has found use in treating *Pneumocystis carinii* pneumonia.

Off Label: Advanced non-small-cell lung cancer, metastatic cancer of the head and neck, metastatic colorectal adenocarcinoma, pancreatic carcinoma.

Drug Interactions: Increased levels and toxicity possible with cimetidine, erythromycin, azole antifungals. Decreased levels possible with rifampin. Increased hematologic toxicity with zidovudine.

Incompatibilities

Solution/Additive and Y-site: chloride-containing solutions, foscarnet.

Side Effects

Nervous System: nausea/vomiting.

Endocrine System: (Pregnancy Category D) serum creatinine—slight transient elevations.

---

* Life-threatening side effect.

Immune System: granulocytopenia, liver function—slight transient elevations, myelosuppression,* thrombocytopenia, rash.

Dosage: *Pneumocystis carinii* pneumonia PO 60 mg/m²/d. The IV solution may be given PO to AIDS patient with PCP. IV 45 mg/m² as infusion over 60–90 min concurrent with leucovorin 20 mg/m² q6h (IV or PO). 21 days of trimetrexate and 24 days of leucovorin.

MYCOBACTERIAL INFECTIONS AND DRUGS TO TREAT THEM

Mycobacterium tuberculosis and *Mycobacterium avium* are closely related. TB has been a part of human history for thousands of years; *M. avium* had been relatively benign until the AIDS epidemic. In AIDS patients, *M. avium* infects the lungs, liver, intestines, spleen, blood, and lymph nodes. Mycobacteria take their time. They can lie dormant until conditions turn favorable. They send no toxins to signal their presence. Sulfonamides such as trimethoprim and dapsone, in addition to antitubercular antibiotics such as streptomycin, amikacin, ethambutol, rifampin, and other antibiotics (ciprofloxacin, imipenem, and clofazimine), are showing some success in the treatment of *M. avium* when used in combination.

Tuberculosis was once the most common killer in the temperate climates. Large sanitariums were built just to house and treat TB patients. Now tuberculosis is treated with little or no hospitalization. Public health nurses follow up on patients as they take these medications at home over months. Always an occupational hazard for street sweepers exposed to the dried sputum of people who spit on streets, in recent years TB cases have increased proportionate to the increased numbers of immigrants coming from areas where TB is still common. Add these factors to the mounting TB infections in AIDS patients. Tuberculosis can affect not only lungs, but bones, kidneys, adrenals, meninges, and the GI tract. Treatment takes months to years and requires the patient's cooperation.

Aminosalicylic acid [P.A.S.] prevents folic acid synthesis in a manner similar to the sulfonamides and is used in conjunction with streptomycin or isoniazid or both to treat TB.

Off Label: Lipid lowering.

Drug Interactions: Increased hypoprothrombinemic effects of oral anticoagulants. Increased risk of crystalluria with ammonium chloride, ascorbic acid. Decreased intestinal absorption of cyanocobalamine, folic acid. Decreased absorption of digoxin possible. Inhibited absorption possible with antihistamines. Increased or decreased phenytoin levels. Decreased elimination with probenecid, sulfinpyrazone. Increased toxicity possible with salicylates.

---

* Life-threatening side effect.

Side Effects

Nervous System: diarrhea, dyspepsia, malaise, nausea/vomiting, pain—joint.

Endocrine System: (Pregnancy Category C) anorexia, chills, fever, goiter (with long treatment).

Immune System: agranulocytosis,* anemia—hemolytic, eosinophilia, acute hepatitis, leukopenia, lymphocytosis, skin—allergic reactions, thrombocytopenia.

Dosage: For TB: PO 10–12 g/d divided bid or tid.

Capreomycin [Capastat Sulfate] is used in conjunction with other antitubercular drugs when the disease is resistant to first-line drugs of isoniazid and rifampin cannot be tolerated.

Drug Interactions: Increased risk of nephrotoxicity, ototoxicity with aminoglycosides, amphotericin B, cisplatin, colistin, polymixin B, vancomycin.

Side Effects

Nervous System: hearing loss, neuromuscular blockage—large doses, pain—IM site, respiratory depression/arrest,* weakness.

Endocrine System: (Pregnancy Category C) electrolyte imbalances.

Immune System: eosinophilia, eighth cranial nerve damage, hepatic dysfunction, leukocytosis, leukopenia, nephrotoxicity,* skin—allergic reactions, sterile abscess—IM site, tubular necrosis.*

Dosage: For TB: IM 20 mg/kg/d for 60–120 d; then 1 g 2–3 ×/wk for 6–12 mo or longer.

Cycloserine [Seromycin], produced from *Streptomyces orchidaceus* or *S. garyphalus,* inhibits bacterial cell wall synthesis by blocking incorporation of D-alanine into the wall. It is used in conjunction with other tuberculostatics as a secondary drug.

Off Label: Sjögren's syndrome and ulcerative colitis and to prevent rejection of heart–lung and pancreatic transplants.

Drug Interactions: Increased levels possible with aminoglycosides, danazol, diltiazem, doxycycline, erythromycin, ketoconazole, methylprednisolone, metoclopramide, nicardipine, NSAIDs, prednisolone, verapamil. Decreased levels possible with carbamazepine, isoniazid, octreotide, phenobarbital, phenytoin, rifampin. Increased risk of nephrotoxicity with acyclovir, aminoglycosides, amphotericin B, cimetidine, cotrimoxazole, erythromycin, ketoconazole, melphalan, ranitidine, trimethoprim. Possible hyperkalemia with potassium-sparing diuretics, ACE inhibitors.

Side Effects

Nervous System: arrhythmias, convulsions,* drowsiness, dysarthria, dyskinesia, headache, hyperreflexia, neuropathy—peripheral, paresis, paresthesias, photophobia, psyche—anxiety/confusion/depression/hyperirritability/psychosis, tics, vision—disturbances/pain.

Endocrine System: (Pregnancy Category C) vitamin B_{12}/folic acid deficiency.

Immune System: anemia—megaloblastic/sideroblastic, dermatitis, photosensitivity.

Dosage: TB: 250 mg q12h for 2 wk; may increase to 500 mg q12h to maximum of 1 g/d. (Vitamin B_6/pyridoxine 100 mg tid may prevent neuropathy.) UTI: PO 250 mg q12h for 2 wk.

Ethambutol hydrochloride [Myambutol] is used in conjunction with other antituberculosis drugs.

Off Label: Atypical mycobacterial infections.

Drug Interactions: none noted.

Side Effects

Nervous System: dizziness, headache, nausea/vomiting, pain—abdomen/joint, paresthesias, photophobia, psyche—confusion/hallucinations, vision—changes/pain.

Endocrine System: (Pregnancy Category B) anorexia.

Immune System: anaphylaxis,* ocular toxicity, anterior optic neuritis, retinal hemorrhage/edema, retrobulbar optic neuritis.

Dosage: PO 15 mg/kg q24h. Retreatment: start with 25 mg/kg/d for 60 d; then decrease to 15 mg/kg/d.

Ethionamide [Trecator-SC] is derived from isonicotinic acid and possibly inhibits bacterial peptide synthesis in *M. tuberculosis, M. avium,* and *M. leprae.* To avoid GI side effects the patient should take the drug with food.

Off Label: Atypical mycobacterial infections and tuberculosis meningitis.

Drug Interactions: Increased neurotoxic effects possible with cycloserine, isoniazid.

Side Effects

Nervous System: ataxia, bowel—diarrhea, dizziness, drowsiness, epigastric distress, headache, hypotension—postural, nausea/vomiting, paresthesias, psyche—depression/hallucinations/restlessness, seizures,* sexual function—impotence, taste—metallic.

---

* Life-threatening side effect.

Endocrine System: (Pregnancy Category D) anorexia, hypothyroidism, sialorrhea.

Immune System: ALT/AST—elevated, hepatitis, jaundice, menorrhagia.

Dosage: PO 0.5–1 g/d divided q8–12h.

Isoniazid [INH] is more potent than streptomycin, the classic TB antibiotic. It inhibits cell growth and kills cells.

Off Label: Atypical mycobacterial infections, tuberculosis meningitis, action tremor in multiple sclerosis.

Drug Interactions: Increased CNS toxicity with cycloserine, ethionamide. Increased phenytoin levels possible. Decreased GI absorption with aluminum-containing antacids. Possible coordination difficulties/psychotic reactions with disulfiram.

Drug–food Interactions: Decreased rate/extent of absorption with food. Take 1 h before meals.

Side Effects

Nervous System: bladder—urinary retention (male), bowel—constipation, dizziness, dyspnea, headache, nausea/vomiting, neuropathy—peripheral, paresthesias, psyche—hallucinations, tinnitus, weakness.

Endocrine System: (Pregnancy Category C) acetonuria, chills, fever, electrolyte imbalances, glycosuria, gynecomastia, metabolic acidosis, pellagra, proteinuria, vitamin B_{12}/pyridoxine—decreased.

Immune System: agranulocytosis,* aplastic anemia,* AST/ALT—elevated, bilirubin—elevated, eosinophilia, hepatitis/jaundice, methemoglobinemia, rheumatic and LE-like syndromes, skin—allergic reactions, thrombocytopenia

Dosage: For TB: PO, IM 5 mg/kg to maximum of 300 mg/d. Prophylaxis: PO 300 mg/d.

Purified protein derivative PPD [Aplisol, Tubersol] is the tuberculin skin test given to identify subclinical or active TB. A positive reaction does not mean infection, but does indicate prior exposure to the organism and T lymphocyte production.

Dosage: Intradermal, using a TB syringe: 0.1 mL of test solution. Read in 48 h. Induration (swelling, not redness) greater than 5–9 mm indicates TB antibodies and requires further screening with chest X-ray and sputum smear culture.

Pyrazinamide [Tebrazid] is a nicotinamide analog used in combination with other antituberculosis drugs.

Drug Interactions: none noted.

Side Effects

Nervous System: arthralgia, bladder—dysuria, headache, nausea/vomiting

Endocrine System: (Pregnancy Category C) none noted.

Immune System: anemia—hemolytic, fatal hemoptysis,* liver function tests—abnormal, lymphadenopathy, peptic ulcer aggravation, plasma prothrombin—decreased, skin—allergic reactions, splenomegaly.

Dosage: PO 15–35 mg/kg/d divided tid or qid to a maximum of 2 g.

<u>Rifampin [Rifadin]</u>, developed by the French and named after a gangster movie, is used in tandem with other antituberculosis drugs.

Off Label: Chemoprophylaxis for *H. influenzae* type B infection. Used to treat leprosy alone or in combination with dapsone and other antiinfectives. Used to treat susceptible gram-negative and gram-positive infections not responding to other antiinfectives. Used to treat Legionnaire's disease in combination with erythromycin or tetracycline.

Drug Interactions: Increased risk of hepatotoxicity with alcohol, isoniazid. Decreased levels with *p*-aminosalicylic acid. Decreases levels of barbiturates, benzodiazepines, clofibrate, oral contraceptives, corticosteroids, dapsone, digitoxin, fluconazole with potential for therapeutic failure, ketoconazole, methadone, metoprolol, progestins, propanolol, quinidine, sulfonylureas, warfarin.

Side Effects

Nervous System: ataxia, bowel—cramps/diarrhea/flatulence, drowsiness, fatigue, hearing loss—transient, nausea/vomiting, numbness—generalized, psyche—inability to concentrate/confusion, vision—disturbances.

Endocrine System: (Pregnancy Category C) anorexia, fever, menstrual disorders.

Immune System: anemia–hemolytic, colitis—pseudomembranous,* eosinophilia, flu-like syndrome, hematuria, hemoglobinuria, hemoptysis, hepatorenal syndrome* (with intermittent therapy), liver function tests—transient elevation, acute real failure, * skin—allergic reactions. With overdose: GI symptoms, liver enlargement/tenderness, jaundice, brown-red or orange skin/sweat/saliva/tears/feces, unconsciousness.

Dosage: TB: PO/IV 600 mg qd with other anti-TB agents. Meningococcal carriers PO 600 mg bid for 2 consecutive d.

---

* Life-threatening side effect.

▶ ANTIFUNGALS

Fungi, a kingdom of life more complex than viruses or bacteria, but neither plant nor animal, thrive on death. Without fungi the earth would be littered with dead plants and animals. Fungi cover the entire body, eating dead tissue (keratin) from skin, hair, and nails and waiting for us to die in order to consume what is left. Bacteria and the immune system hold fungi in check, but when one is weakened, burned, or pregnant, the fungi have the advantage.

During long-term antibiotic therapy or after radiation, fungi can overwhelm the host. Fungal infections can also arise from contact with spores in public showers, by use of other people's brushes and personal items, or by breathing in infested dust from soils and bird droppings. Some fungi found in decaying organic matter in soil cause histoplasmosis, coccidioidomycosis, and blastomycosis. Histoplasmosis can result from contact with birds and bats and can affect the respiratory tract, liver, and spleen among other organs. Ringworm and athlete's foot are mold infections (tinea). *Candida albicans* infection (called thrush when it infects the mouth and monilia or candidiasis when the vagina is infected) poses a serious threat to burn patients, people on total parenteral alimentation (TPA), patients getting prosthetic heart valves, and the immunosuppressed, for example, AIDS and chemotherapy patients.

Antifungal treatment usually takes weeks, as new uninfected skin grows out and infected layers are shed. Fungal cell membranes are more like human cell membranes, rather than bacterial cell membranes, and thus antibiotics do not work on them.

<u>Amphotericin B [Fungizone], amphotericin B lipid complex [ABELCET]</u> binds to ergosterol, a cholesterol-like substance in fungal cell walls. It is used as IV treatment for systemic fungal infections: aspergillosis, blastomycosis, coccidioidomycosis, cryptococcosis, disseminated candidiasis, histoplasmosis, paracoccidioidomycosis, sporotrichosis, and others.

Off Label: Candiduria, fungal endocarditis, meningitis, septicemia, fungal UTI, paracoccidioidomycosis, and amebic meningoencephalitis.

Drug Interactions: Increased nephrotoxicity possible with aminoglycosides, capreomycin, carboplatin, cisplatin, colistin, cyclosporin, furosemide, mechlorethamine, vancomycin. Hypokalemia possible with corticosteroids; hypokalemia increases digitalis toxicity risk with digitalis glycosides.

Incompatibilities

Solution/Additive: calcium chloride, calcium gluconate, cimetidine, edetate calcium disodium, metaraminol, methyldopa, polymyxin, potassium chloride, ranitidine, saline solutions, TPN solutions, verapamil.

Y-site: aminoglycosides, clindamycin, cotrimoxazole, diphenhydramine, dobutamine, dopamine, fluconazole, heparin, lidocaine, penicillins, phenothiazines, procaine, tetracycline, vitamins.

Side Effects

Nervous System: arthralgia, bowel—diarrhea, burning sensation, cramps—epigastric, dyspnea, headache, hearing loss, nausea/vomiting, pain—muscle, sedation, tinnitus, vertigo, weakness.

Endocrine System: (Pregnancy Category B) anorexia, fever, hypokalemia, hypomagnesemia, dry skin, urine—low specific gravity, weight loss.

Immune System: allergy—rash, anaphylaxis,* anemia, erythema, lesion exacerbation, nephrotoxicity,* pruritus, superinfections, thrombocytopenia, thrombophlebitis (at IV site), urticaria.

Dosage: Most indications: IV initial dose to follow test dose.§ IV 250 μg/kg/d infused over 4–6 h in a single dose. Adjusted daily in increments of 250 μg/kg/d or faster if tolerated to maximum of 1.0 mg/kg/d or 1.5 mg/ kg/d qod. Not to exceed daily total dose of 1.5 mg/g. Candiduria bladder irrigation: Continuous bladder irrigation per 3-way closed drainage catheter system at 1 L/24 h: 5–50 mg/L sterile water. [ABELCET] IV 5 mg/kg/d at 2.5 mg/kg/h.

Butenafine [Mentax] is a cream used to treat interdigital tinea pedia.

Drug Interactions: none noted.

Side Effects

Nervous System: burning, itching, stinging.

Endocrine System: (Pregnancy Category B) none noted.

Immune System: dermatitis, erythema, irritation, worsened infection.

Dosage: Topical application to affected area qd for 4 wk.

Ciclopirox olamine [Loprox] inhibits transport of amino acids within fungal cell to interfere with DNA, protein, and RNA synthesis. It is used to treat tinea cruris and tinea corporis caused by *Trichophyton rubrum*, *Trichophyton mentagrophytes*, *Epidermophyton floccosum*, and *Microsporum canis*, and tinea versicolor caused by *Candida albicans*.

Drug Interactions: None noted.

---

* Life-threatening side effect.
§ Test dose: IV 1 mg in 20 mL of D5W over 10–30 min to avoid anaphylactic risk.

Side Effects

Nervous System: burning.

Endocrine System: (Pregnancy Category B) none noted.

Immune System: condition—worsening, irritation, pruritus.

Dosage: Topical: To affected area and surrounding skin bid.

Clotrimazole [Gyne-Lotrimin, Lotrimin, Mycelex] increases fungal cell membrane permeability, resulting in leakage of intracellular contents and loss of ability to replicate. It is used to treat skin infections.

Off Label: Trichomoniasis.

Drug Interactions: none noted.

Side Effects

Nervous System: nausea/vomiting. Topical: stinging. Vaginal: bloating, mild burning, cramps—lower abdominal, itching, pain/soreness with intercourse, mild urinary frequency.

Endocrine System: (Pregnancy Category Topical—B, Oral—C) none noted.

Immune System: Topical: edema, erythema, desquamation, liver function tests—abnormal, pruritus, skin fissures, urticaria, vesication. Vaginal: cystitis, urethritis.

Dosage: Topical: Small amount applied to affected areas AM and PM. Intravaginal: Insert 1 applicatorful or one 100 mg vaginal tablet into vagina at hs for 7 d; or one 500 mg vaginal tablet hs for one dose. Thrush: PO 1 troche 5 times/d q3h for 14 d.

Econazole nitrate [Spectazole] also acts on the fungal membrane and is used to treat tinea and moniliasis.

Off Label: Erythrasma; in conjunction with corticosteroids, for bacterial or fungal dermatoses associated with inflammation.

Drug Interactions: none noted.

Side Effects

Nervous System: burning/stinging sensation.

Endocrine System: (Pregnancy Category C) none noted.

Immune System: erythema, pruritus.

Dosage: Topical: 1% cream to infected areas bid. Tinea versicolor: qd is sufficient.

Fluconazole [Diflucan] interferes with ergosterol in the fungal cell membrane. It is used to treat cryptococcal meningitis, oropharyngeal and systemic candidiasis, and vaginal candidiasis.

Drug Interactions: Increased PT with warfarin. Increased phenytoin, cyclosporine levels. Hypoglycemic reactions with sulfonylureas. Decreased levels with rifampin, cimetidine.

Incompatibilities

Solution/Additive: piperacillin.

Y-site: amphotericin B, ceftazidime.

Side Effects

Nervous System: bowel—diarrhea, headache, nausea/vomiting, pain—abdominal.

Endocrine System: (Pregnancy Category C) none noted.

Immune System: AST—increase in cryptococcal and AIDS patients, rash.

Dosage: Oropharyngeal, esophageal candidiasis: PO, IV 200 mg day 1; then 100 mg qd for 2 wk (oropharyngeal) or 3 wk (esophageal). Systemic candidiasis: PO, IV 400 mg on day 1; then 200 mg qd for 4 wk. Vaginal candidiasis: PO 150 mg for 1 dose. Cryptococcal meningitis: PO, IV 400 mg on day 1; then 200 mg qd for 10–12 wk.

Flucytosine [Ancobon, others] is used alone or in combination with amphotericin B for serious systemic infections by cryptococcus and candida.

Off Label: Chromomycosis.

Drug Interactions: Synergy with amphotericin B may decrease flucytosine renal clearance and increase toxicity.

Side Effects

Nervous System: bloating, bowel—diarrhea, headache, nausea/vomiting, psyche—confusion/hallucinations, sedation, vertigo.

Endocrine System: (Pregnancy Category C) serum alkaline phosphatase/BUN/serum creatinine—elevated.

Immune System: agranulocytosis,* anemia, AST/ALT—elevated, bone marrow hypoplasia, eosinophilia, enterocolitis, hepatitis, hepatomegaly, leukopenia, thrombocytopenia.

Dosage: PO 50–150 mg/kg/d divided q6h.

Griseofulvin [Fulvicin-U/F, Grifulvin V, Grisactin], griseofulvin ultramicrosize [Fulvicin P/G, Grisactin Ultra, Gris-PEG] acts on mitotic spindles to disrupt cell division of fungi. It is used to treat fungal infections of hair, nails, and skin. A second appropriate topical agent may be required.

Off Label: Angina pectoris, gout, Raynaud's disease.

Drug Interactions: Flushing, tachycardia possible with alcohol. Decreased effect possible with barbiturates. Decreased hypoprothrombinemic effects of oral anticoagulants possible. Increased estrogen metabolism possible, manifested by breakthrough bleeding and decreased oral contraceptive effectiveness.

Side Effects

Nervous System: bowel—diarrhea/flatulence, fatigue, headache—severe, heartburn, insomnia, nausea/vomiting, psyche—confusion/psychotic symptoms, taste—acuity decrease/unpleasant, vertigo.

Endocrine System: (Pregnancy Category C) anorexia, estrogen-like effects in children, proteinuria, dry mouth, thirst.

Immune System: angioedema*—severe, punctate basophilia, fixed drug eruption, granulocytopenia, hepatotoxicity, leukopenia, monocytosis, mouth—furred tongue/thrush, nephrotoxicity,* neutropenia, photosensitivity, pruritus, serum sickness syndromes, urticaria.

Dosage: Tinea corporis, tinea cruris: PO 500 mg microsize or 330–375 mg ultramicrosize qd in single or divided doses. Tinea pedis, tinea unguium: PO 0.75–1 g microsize or 660–750 mg ultramicrosize qd in single or divided doses. Decrease microsize doses to 500 mg/d after response is noted.

Haloprogin [Halotex] is a fungicidal or fungistatic iodinated phenolic ether that helps heal superficial infections of *Candida, Epidermophyton, Malassezia, Microsporum,* and *Trichophyton.*

Drug Interactions: none noted.

Side Effects

Nervous System: burning sensation.

Endocrine System: (Pregnancy Category B) none noted.

Immune System: irritation, lesion exacerbation, maceration increase, pruritus, sensitization.

Dosage: Topical: 1% cream or solution to affected area bid for 2–3 wk.

Itraconazole [Sporanox] is used to treat systemic fungal infections caused by aspergillosis, blastomycosis, histoplasmosis, onychomycosis.

Off Label: Superficial candida, pityriasis versicolor, systemic and vaginal candidiasis.

Drug Interactions: Hypoglycemia possible with sulfonylureas. Decreased levels with carbamazepine, H$_2$-antagonists, phenytoin, rifampin. Increased cyclosporin, digoxin levels possible. May increase cisapride levels, causing dan-

---

* Life-threatening side effect.

gerous arrhythmias. Enhanced anticoagulant effects of warfarin possible.

Side Effects

Nervous System: bowel—diarrhea/flatulence, dizziness, drowsiness, dyspepsia, fatigue, headache, nausea/vomiting, pain—abdominal, psyche—euphoria, sexual function—libido decrease/impotence, somnolence. With high doses: hypertension.

Endocrine System: (Pregnancy Category C) anorexia, hypertriglyceridemia, gynecomastia. With high doses: hypokalemia, adrenal insufficiency.

Immune System: gastritis, pruritus, serum transaminases/alkaline phosphatase/bilirubin—elevated, rash.

Dosage: Pulmonary and extrapulmonary blastomycosis, nonmeningeal histoplasmosis: PO 200 mg qd; may increase to maximum of 200 mg bid if no improvement; continue for 3 mo. Life-threatening infections: Start with 200 mg tid for 3 d; then 200–400 mg/d. Oropharyngeal candidiasis: PO 200 mg qd × 1–2 wk. Esophageal candidiasis: PO 100 mg qd to a maximum 200 mg/d × 3 wk minimum. Vaginal candidiasis: PO 200 mg qd for 3 d. Onychomycosis: PO 200 mg qd for 3 mo.

Ketoconazole [Nizoral] is used to treat blastomycosis, candidiasis, chromomycosis, coccidioidomycosis ("San Joaquin Valley fever"), histoplasmosis, paracoccidioidomycosis.

Topical: Tinea corporis and tinea cruris.

Off Label

Oral: Cushing's syndrome associated with adrenal or pituitary adenoma, dysfunctional hirsutism, onychomycosis, precocious puberty, vaginal candidiasis; swish-and-swallow liquid form as prophylaxis for immunocompromised patients.

Topical: cutaneous candidiasis, psoriasis, tinea manum, tinea pedis, seborrheic dermatitis.

Drug Interactions: Photosensitivity with alcohol. Decreased absorption with antacids, anticholinergics, H₂-blockers. Increased drug metabolism with isoniazid, rifampin. Decreased levels of ketoconazole and phenytoin. Increased levels, toxicity of cyclosporine possible. Increased hypoprothrombinemia of warfarin possible. Increased levels of and arrhythmias with cisapride, astemizole possible.

Side Effects

Nervous System: bowel—constipation/diarrhea, nausea/vomiting, pain—breast/epigastric/abdominal, sexual function—loss of libido/impotence, stinging.

Endocrine System: (Pregnancy Category C) ACTH-induced corticosteroid serum levels, anorexia, gyneco-mastia—males, hair loss, hypoadrenalism*—acute, hyponatremia—rare, renal hypofunction, serum cholesterol/triglycerides—transient decreases, lowered serum testosterone/oligospermia.

Immune System: anaphylaxis,* angioedema,* erythema, hepatic necrosis,* pruritus, rash, urticaria, uterine bleeding.

Dosage: PO 200–400 mg qd. Topical: Apply 1–2 ×/d to affected and surrounding area. Dandruff: shampoo 2 ×/wk for 4 wk; lather and then massage scalp for 1 min, rinse and repeat, leaving shampoo on scalp for 3 min; rinse thoroughly.

Miconazole [Monistat IV], miconazole nitrate [Monistat, Micatin, others] is used to treat tinea corporis, tinea cruris, tinea pedis, tinea versicolor. It is given parenterally for severe systemic infections and intrathecally for meningitis. Bladder irrigation is used for bladder infections.

Drug Interactions: Decreased antifungal activity of amphotericin B and miconazole. Increased PT with warfarin possible. Severe hypoglycemia possible with sulfonylureas.

Side Effects

Nervous System: arrhythmias/tachycardia, bowel—diarrhea, cramps—pelvic, drowsiness, headache, itching, nausea/vomiting, vulvovaginal burning.

Endocrine System: (Pregnancy Category B) fever, flushing, hyperlipidemia, hyponatremia—transient.

Immune System: anaphylaxis,* hematocrit decrease, hives, phlebitis, pruritus, rash, thrombocytopenia.

Dosage: Intravaginal: 1 applicatorful of cream or one 100-mg suppository hs for 7 d, or one 200-mg suppository hs for 3 d. IV (slow to avoid arrhythmias): 200–3600 mg/d in 3 divided doses or 20 mg intrathecally q3–7d. Bladder installation: 200 mg of diluted solution bid to qid or continuous infusion.

Nystatin [Mycostatin, Nilstat, others] is used to treat a broad spectrum of fungal infections. It is nontoxic and nonsensitizing.

Drug Interactions: none noted.

Side Effects

Nervous System: bowel—diarrhea, nausea/vomiting

Endocrine System: (Pregnancy Category C) none noted.

Immune System: none noted.

Dosage: Candida: PO 500,000–1,000,000 U tid. 1–4 troches 4–5 ×/d. Suspension 400,000–600,000 U qid. Vaginal: 1–2 tabs qd for 2 wk.

---

* Life-threatening side effect.

<u>Terbinafine cream [Lamisil]</u> is fungicidal. It is used to treat tinea corporis, tinea cruris, and interdigital tinea pedis caused by *Epidermophyton floccosum*, *Trichophyton mentagrophytes*, or *Trichophyton rubrum*.

Drug Interactions: none noted.

Side Effects

Nervous System: bowel—diarrhea, dyspepsia, lethargy, malaise, pain—abdominal, taste disturbance.

Endocrine System: (Pregnancy Category C) none noted.

Immune System: rash.

Dosage: Onychomycosis of nails: PO 250 mg qd for 6 wk (fingernails) or 12 wk (toenails). Topical for tinea corporis/cruris or cutaneous candidiasis: qd or bid for 1–7 wk.

▶ DRUGS FOR PARASITE INFESTATIONS

Viruses, bacteria, and molds are not the only life forms seeking humans out as food. Protozoa, spirochetes, worms, and insects also infest and infect humans. Some of the same drugs used to treat bacterial infections are also effective against the parasites.

▶ ANTIMALARIALS

Because humans travel all over the world so easily now, nurses may treat patients for diseases they picked up far away—diseases such as malaria. The name *malaria* comes from the Italian words for "bad air," which was once thought to be the cause of the disease. The female *Anopheles* mosquito, the vector, carries the plasmodium infection. The plasmodium offspring, called merozoites, develop in the liver. Liver cells rupture and the merozoites are released into the blood, where they enter the RBCs. The RBCs then rupture, releasing gametocytes, and the cycle goes around again. When the RBCs rupture, in cycles of 36–72 hours, the body responds with chills and fever. Drugs for malaria treat the acute attack or prevent the disease.

<u>Chloroquine hydrochloride [Aralen Hydrochloride]</u>, <u>chloroquine phosphate [Aralen Phosphate]</u> serves as malaria prophylaxis and is used to treat the acute stage. It is also used to treat giardiasis and amebiasis outside of the GI tract.

Off Label: An antiinflammatory in the treatment of rheumatoid arthritis and discoid and systemic LE, porphyria cutanea tarda, solar urticaria, polymorphous light eruptions.

Drug Interactions: Decreased absorption with aluminum- or magnesium-containing antacids and laxatives. Give 4 h before or after antacids. May interfere with rabies vaccine response.

Side Effects

Nervous System: arrhythmias—ECG changes, bowel—diarrhea, cramps—abdominal, fatigue, headache, hypotension, myalgia, nausea/vomiting, paresthesias, psyche—confusion/irritability/nightmares, reduced reflexes, vertigo, vision changes—accommodation/blurred/photophobia/scotomas, weakness.

Endocrine System: (Pregnancy Category C) anorexia, fever, slight weight loss.

Immune System: alopecia, anemia—hemolytic (with G6PD deficiency), corneal edema/opacity/deposits, hair bleaching/freckles, lymphedema—upper limbs, ototoxicity, pruritus.

Dosage: Malaria prophylaxis: PO 5 mg/kg/wk to maximum of 300 mg for 2 wk prior to entering a malaria zone and 4–6 wk after leaving. Acute stage: Load with PO 600 mg; then 300 mg at 6, 24, 48 h. IM 200 mg q6h to maximum of 800 mg/24 h. Amebicide: PO 600 mg qd for 2 d; then 300 mg for 2–3 wk. Rheumatoid arthritis/SLE: PO 150 mg qd at evening meal.

<u>Hydroxychloroquine sulfate [Plaquenil Sulfate]</u> is derived from and acts like chloroquine by preventing DNA replication to prevent malaria or treat acute episodes.

Off Label: Porphyria.

Drug Interactions: Decreased absorption with aluminum- or magnesium-containing antacids and laxatives. Give 4 h before or after antacids. May interfere with rabies vaccine response.

Side Effects

Nervous System: bowel—diarrhea, cramps—abdominal, fatigue, headache, nausea/vomiting, psyche—anxiety/mood changes, vertigo.

Endocrine System: (Pregnancy Category C) anorexia, weight loss.

Immune System: agranulocytosis,* aplastic anemia,* hair—bleaching or loss, hemolysis (in G6PD deficiency), itching, rash, retinopathy, thrombocytopenia.

Dosage: Malaria prophylaxis: PO 310 mg base qwk on same day 2 wk before entering malaria zone and for 4–6 wk after leaving the zone. Acute malaria: PO 620 mg base; then 310 mg base at 6, 18, and 24 h. LE: PO 310 mg

---

* Life-threatening side effect.

base 1–2/d. RA: PO 400–600 mg/d until response. Then decrease to lowest maintenance levels.

<u>Mefloquine hydrochloride [Lariam]</u> is effective against all types of malaria, including chloroquine-resistant malaria.

Drug Interactions: Prolonged cardiac conduction possible with beta blockers, calcium channel blockers, and possibly digoxin. Decreased levels with quinine possible. Increased risk of seizures due to possible decreased levels of valproic acid.

Side Effects

Nervous System: arrhythmias—bradycardia, dizziness, headache, itching, nausea/vomiting, psyche—confusion/nightmares/psychosis, syncope, vision—disturbances.

Endocrine System (Pregnancy Category C): none noted.

Immune System: rash.

Dosage: Malaria: PO 1250 mg (5 tabs) in 1 dose with a minimum of 8 oz of water. Malaria prophylaxis: PO 250 mg qwk for 4 wk. Start 1 wk before entering malarial zone; then 250 mg qwk for duration of exposure and 250 mg qwk for 4 wk after leaving zone.

<u>Primaquine phosphate</u> prevents initial and recurrent malarial attacks by interfering with plasmodial metabolism in its mitochondria, and also by interrupting erythrocytic parasite development. Primaquine cannot be used to treat the acute attack, but it destroys the parasites outside the RBCs.

Drug Interactions: Increased toxicity of both primaquine and quinacrine.

Side Effects

Nervous System: arrhythmias, cramps—abdominal, epigastric distress, headache, psyche—confusion/depression, vision disturbance—accommodation, vomiting.

Endocrine System: (Pregnancy Category C) none noted.

Immune System: agranulocytopenia, agranulocytosis,* anemia, granulocytopenia*/acute hemolytic anemia (with G6PD deficiency), leukocytosis, leukopenia, methemoglobinemia, pruritus.

Dosage: Prophylaxis: PO 15 mg qd for 14 d upon leaving the malaria zone. Relapse prevention: same dosage in addition to chloroquine or hydroxychloroquine on first 3 d of acute attack.

<u>Pyrimethamine [Daraprim]</u> is a folic acid antagonist or antimetabolite that selectively inhibits dihydrofolate re-

ductase in malarial plasmodia and *Toxoplasma gondii.* Working in different stages of folic acid synthesis, pyrimethamine is used in combination with sulfonamides, which are also antimetabolites, and with quinine for chloroquine-resistant. *P. falciparum.*

Drug Interactions: Decreased effectiveness against toxoplasmosis with folic acid, *p*-aminobenzoic acid (PABA).

Side Effects

Nervous System: (large doses) bowel—diarrhea, cramps—abdominal, vomiting. Acute toxicity: convulsions,* respiratory failure.*

Endocrine System: (Pregnancy Category C) with large doses: anorexia, folic acid deficiency.

Immune System: With large doses: atrophic glossitis, pancytopenia, rashes, thrombocytopenia.

Dosage: Malaria prophylaxis: PO 25 mg qwk. Toxoplasmosis: Start with PO 50–75 mg qd with a sulfonamide for 1–3 wk; then decrease both drugs by half and continue for 4–5 wk longer.

<u>Quinacrine [Atabrine]</u> can be used to treat malaria, but it has generally been replaced by more effective antimalarials. Quinacrine is also used to treat dwarf tapeworms, giardiasis, and cestodiasis. As a sclerosing agent intrapleurally, quinacrine can prevent recurrence of pneumothorax. Quinacrine inhibits RNA transcription and DNA replication, blocking protein synthesis in parasites.

Drug Interactions: Disulfiram-like reaction possible with alcohol. Increased toxicity with primaquine.

Side Effects

Nervous System: bowel—diarrhea, convulsions,* cramping, dizziness, GI upset, headache, nausea/vomiting, psyche—agitation/confusion/irritability/nightmares/toxic psychosis, vertigo, visual disturbances.

Endocrine System: (Pregnancy Category C) anorexia, fever.

Immune System: aplastic anemia,* dermatitis, corneal edema/deposits, exfoliative dermatitis,* hepatitis.

Dosage: Malaria suppression: PO 100 mg qd for 1–3 mo. Dwarf tapeworm: PO 300 mg quinacrine on empty stomach in 3 portions every 20 min; follow in 1.5 h with a sodium sulfate purge. Tapeworm: Before treatment, bland diet preceding day and fast after dinner; saline enema before treatment and 1–2 h after; on day of treatment, 200 g q10min for 4 doses and 600 mg sodium bicarbonate with each dose. Giardiasis: PO 100 mg tid for 5–7 d.

---

* Life-threatening side effect.

Quinine sulfate [Quinamm] is derived from from the bark of the cinchona tree. It is the classic, or prototypical, antimalarial, used alone or with pyrimethamine plus a sulfonamide. Quinine affects plasmodial DNA and enzymes, decreasing oxygen uptake and carbohydrate metabolism. Another use is the treatment of nocturnal leg cramps that accompany arteriosclerosis, arthritis, diabetes, thrombophlebitis, and varicose veins. This second use is the result of quinine's effect on intracellular calcium, extending the refractory period and decreasing the motor end-plate excitability.

Drug Interactions: Increased vagolytic effects with anticholinergics and possible antagonized cardiac effects. Increased digoxin levels possible. Decreased effect with anticonvulsants, barbiturates, rifampin due to increased quinine metabolism. Decreased renal elimination and increased toxicity with carbonic anhydrase inhibitors, frequent antacids, sodium bicarbonate. Increased hypothrombinemia of warfarin possible.

Side Effects

Nervous System: angina, bowel—diarrhea, dizziness, dyspnea, gastric distress, headache, hearing impairment, nausea/vomiting, psyche—apprehension/confusion/delirium/excitement, syncope, tinnitus, vertigo, vision impairment. Toxicity: cardiovascular collapse,* coma,* death.*

Endocrine System: (Pregnancy Category X) fever.

Immune System: hemolytic anemia, agranulocytosis,* hypoprothrombinemia, leukopenia, pruritus, thrombocytopenia. Toxicity: blackwater fever,* death.*

Dosage: Acute malaria: PO 650 mg q8h for 3 d. Malaria prophylaxis: PO 325 mg bid for 6 wk. For information on leg cramps please refer to Chapter 4.

▶ DRUGS FOR OTHER PARASITIC CONDITIONS

Just as antimalarial drugs can treat parasites other than plasmodia, there are drugs for treating these other parasites too. The following are among them.

Emetine hydrochloride is an amebicide that acts in the intestinal wall and the liver to block parasitic cell protein synthesis.

Drug Interactions: none noted.

Side Effects

Nervous System: Toxicity: arrhythmias—tachycardia and others, bowel—diarrhea, cramps—abdominal, dizziness,

dyspnea, epigastric burning/pain, faintness, headache, hypotension, muscle—ache/pain/tenderness, nausea/vomiting, pain—precordial, stiffness, tremors. Injection/lesion sites: pain/tenderness.

Endocrine System: (Pregnancy Category X) none noted.

Immune System: With large doses: abscess, cellulitis, acute lesions in GI tract/heart*/kidney/liver/skeletal muscle, necrosis, pericarditis, skin—allergic reactions.

Dosage: Amebic dysentery: IM, deep SC 1 mg/kg bid to maximum of 65 mg/kg/d for no more than 10 d. Hepatic amebiasis or abscess: Same, but do not repeat in less than 6 wk.

Paromomycin [Humatin] is produced from *Streptomyces rimosus* and resembles kanamycin and neomycin. Paromomycin is both bactericidal and amebicidal, especially inside the GI tract, where it can also help eradicate tapeworms. Because it kills intestinal flora, paromomycin is used to kill nitrogen-forming bacteria during hepatic coma. This drug was also discussed under *Aminoglycosides* earlier in this chapter.

Pentamidine isethionate [Pentam 300] is used to treat *P. carinii* pneumonia, a usually rare sporozoan pneumonia, now commonly seen with AIDS.

Off Label: African trypanosomiasis and visceral leishmaniasis, the drug interferes with RNA and DNA production. It is a toxic drug and can damage the kidneys, cause blood dyscrasias, and lower blood pressure, blood sugar, and blood calcium. For side effects and dosage, see *Miscellaneous Antimicrobial Agents* earlier in this chapter.

INSECT PARASITES

Throughout history, humans have carried crawling vermin on their bodies—once the norm rather than an exception; human hosts simply endured the itching and misery. During the Middle Ages and Renaissance, fancy ladies carried vermin-eating pets such as ermine on gold chains to eat scurrying insects on their bodies. The chains were meant to keep the pet from finding someone with more vermin to eat. In this day and age, scabies and lice are found where people cannot or will not keep their bodies clean. Occasionally health professionals may, in the course of their work, be exposed to these parasites. Children may contact them in school. Scabies leave characteristic trails under the skin where they have burrowed. Lice leave tiny nits on the hair. Eradication includes thorough cleaning of clothes, bedding, rugs, furniture, brushes, and combs.

Lindane [Gamabenzene, Kwell, Scabene] kills parasites and their ova to treat head lice, body lice, and scabies.

---

* Life-threatening side effect.

Drug Interactions: none noted.

Side Effects

Nervous System: CNS stimulation, convulsions* (usually with product misuse), dizziness, restlessness, tremors. Inhalation: headache, nausea/vomiting.

Endocrine System: (Pregnancy Category B) none noted.

Immune System: eczematous eruptions. Inhalation: ENT irritation

Dosage: Topical. Scabies: Warm, not hot, shower and apply; rinse off after 24 h. Lice: Rub into area, leave on for 5 min, and shampoo out. Avoid facial contact. Do not repeat in <1 wk.

Note: A hot shower prior to application may contribute to systemic absorption of the insecticide. When absorbed, lindane concentrates in fatty tissue, even that of the brain. GABA drugs are used to treat overdose. (See Chapter 6 on GABA drugs.) Insects die as the result of neuronal destabilization.

Malathion (See Chapter 3 for cholinergic pesticides and antidote.)

---

* Life-threatening side effect.

Chapter Highlights

- Plagues will always be a threat.

- Infections by bacteria, fungi, and viruses, as well as infestations of parasites, remain a constant threat to human life, killing millions of people every year.

- The antimicrobials and antiparasite drugs aid the body's immune system in defending against those forms of life that threaten our own.

- Such drugs must always be used carefully and according to directions to lessen the chance of drug resistance developing in the infecting organism.

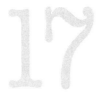

Drugs to Treat Cancer: Antineoplastics

drug list

- aldesleukin [Proleukin]
- altretamine [Hexalen]
- amifostine [Ethyol]
- aminoglutethimide [Cytadren]
- anastrazole [Arimidex]
- asparaginase [Colaspase Elspar]
- bacillus Calmette-Guérin (BCG) vaccine [Tice, TheraCys]
- bicalutamide [Casodex]
- bleomycin sulfate [Blenoxane]
- busulfan [Myleran]
- carboplatin [Paraplatin]
- carmustine [BiCNU]
- chlorambucil [Leukeran]
- cisplatin [Platinol]
- cladribine [Leustatin]
- cyclophosmamide [Cytoxan]
- cytarabine [Cytosar-U, others]
- dacarbazine [DTIC, DTIC-Dome, Imidazole Carboxamide]
- dactinomycin [Actinomycin-D, Cosmegen]
- daunorubicin hydrochloride [Cerubidine]
- dexrazoxane [Zinecard]
- docetaxel [Taxotere]
- doxorubicin hydrochloride [Adriamycin]
- epoetin alfa (human recombinant erythropoietin) [Epogen, Procrit]
- estramustine phosphate sodium [Emcyt]
- etoposide [VePesid, others]
- floxuridine [FUDR]
- fludarabine phosphate [Flurada]
- fluorouracil (FU) [Adrucil, others]
- flutamide [Eulexine]
- gemcitabine [Gemzar]
- goserelin acetate [Zoladex]

drug list

- hexamethylmelamine [Hexalen]
- idarubicin hydrochloride [Idamycin]
- ifosfamide [Ifex]
- interferon alfa: alfa-2A [Roferon-A], alfa-2B [Intron A]
- irinotecan [Camptosar]
- leucovorin calcium [Calcium Folinate, others]
- leuprolide acetate [Lupron, Lupron Depot]
- lomustine [CeeNU]
- mechlorethamine hydrochloride [Mustargen]
- megestrol acetate [Megace, Pallace]
- melphalan [L-PAM, L-Sarcolysin, others]
- mercaptopurine [Purinethol]
- mesna [Mesnex]
- methotrexate [Mexate, MTX, others]
- mitomycin [Mutamycin]
- mitoxantrone hydrochloride [Novantrone]
- nilutamide [Nilandron]
- paclitaxel [Taxol]
- pentostatin [Nipent]
- plicamycin [Mithracin, Mithramycin]
- procarbazine hydrochloride [Matulane]
- sargramostin [Leukine, Prokine]
- streptozocin [Zanosar]
- tamoxifen citrate [Nolvadex]
- thioguanine (TG)
- thiotepa [Thioplex, TSPA]
- topotecan [Vumon]
- tretinoin [Retin-A, Vesanoid, others]
- vinblastine sulfate [Velban]
- vincristine sulfate [Oncovin]
- vinorelbine tartrate [Navelbine]

▶ THE NATURE OF CANCERS

A cancer begins when one daughter cell mutates in response to an agent, perhaps viral, bacterial, chemical, or radiation, which causes a genetic change. Succeeding generations keep acquiring mutations until at last, a descendent cell acquires the final mutation needed to cross the line into malignancy. Losing its distinctive shape and ability to suppress the cell cycle or respond to external signals to stop dividing, the cell spins out of control. Multiplying wildly, the new formation of mutant cells compresses and damages healthy tissue, and malignant cells metastasize by slipping into the bloodstream to colonize faraway sites (Cavenee, 1995).

The name *cancer* comes from the pincer-like protrusions from the primary tumors that looked to early researchers like crab claws. Cancers can arise in solid tissue, lymph glands, and bone and spread to the rest of the body. For example, the two kinds of leukemia—lymphogenous, which begins in the lymph glands, and myelogenous, which begins in the bone—eventually invade the spleen and liver. Finally, leukemic cells will be produced in many other parts of the body in vast numbers that weaken and pain the bone.

Malignant tumors require postsurgical follow-up therapy, because, "the knife is never enough . . . if one cancerous cell gets away the cancer can metastasize" (Rosenberg, 1992). Traditionally, cancer treatment has been to directly attack and kill malignant cells with radiation and chemicals. While radiation can be pinpointed at cancerous sites, the drugs used have been aimed broadly to kill cancerous cells that may have traveled far from the original site. Some of these drugs are extremely toxic and kill, not only malignant cells, but also healthy cells. When these drugs destroy blood-forming cells in the bone, they compromise the immune system, leaving the patient vulnerable to infection and even other types of cancer. In addition, they may cause genetic mutations in healthy cells too, which can also cause cancer.

Some antineoplastic drugs are cell-cycle specific and are given when the cancer cells are in vulnerable phases of development. Because the cells in a tumor are in different phases simultaneously, drugs are often given in combination to enhance the chances of killing cells at various phases of development. Ironically, the cell-killing toxic drugs may become ineffective when cancerous growths, in order to survive, develop resistance by pumping the drugs back out of the cells.

Hormones of the endocrine system can be involved in triggering certain cancers and also in cancer treatment. When tumors of the reproductive system are hormone dependent, one modality of treatment is to block sex hormone receptors. The cytotoxic effect of corticosteroids is utilized in treating blood cell cancers: lymphocytic leukemia, lymphoma, multiple myeloma, and plasma cell cancer. Corticosteroids offer palliation of other cancers and cancer therapy effects such as drug reactions, bone marrow graft-vs-host reactions, hypercalcemia, and pain resulting from nerve compression or edema (Balmer, 1996).

Some of the drugs to treat cancer have been used for decades and may simply offer more hope than cure, but medicine is learning the language of the immune system. Harnessing of the immune system messenger molecules, vaccines, and drugs to prevent angiogenesis offer promising avenues to treat and prevent cancer.

▶ CLASSIFICATION OF ANTINEOPLASTIC DRUGS

Antineoplastic drugs fall into seven groups, in addition to chemoprotectants: alkylating agents, which include nitrosourteas, antimetabolites, cytokines, DNA intercalating drugs, hormonal drugs and antagonists, mitotic inhibitors, and miscellaneous drugs. Many of these drugs are given in cycles to interrupt specific stages of cell de-

velopment and halt cell multiplication. A great number of these drugs are toxic; the side effects are those of chemical poisoning. They can also cause cancer and must be handled with care. Drugs of the nervous system are used to treat the nausea and vomiting and discomfort of chemotherapy.

ALKYLATING AGENTS

Alkylating agents were derived from the toxic mustard gas used in World War I after doctors noticed that mustard gas made the lymph nodes shrink. These agents cross-link or tangle DNA and stop the malignant cells' replication. They are not cell-cycle specific, but are most effective in rapidly dividing cells.

<u>Altretamine, hexamethylmelamine [Hexalen]</u> is used to treat ovarian cancer.

Drug Interactions: During week 1 of treatment, incapacitating dizziness and syncope with concomitant administration of altretamine and tricyclic antidepressants, monoamine oxidase inhibitors, or selegiline possible.

Side Effects

Nervous System: ataxia, hyporeflexia, muscle weakness, nausea/vomiting, numbness—peripheral, Parkinson-like tremors.

Endocrine System: (Pregnancy Category D) slight increase in serum creatinine.

Immune System: alopecia, eczema, leukopenia, thrombocytopenia.

Dosage: PO 260 mg/m^2/d qid pc and hs for 14 or 21 consecutive d in a 28-d cycle.

<u>Busulfan [Myleran]</u> is cell-cycle nonspecific. Because it damages myeloid cells more than lymphoid cells, it is the drug of choice for controlling primary thrombocythemia and thrombocytosis in polycythemia vera and myelofibrosis; it is palliative for chronic myelogenous leukemia.

Drug Interactions: Increased uric acid levels possible with probenecid, sulfinpyrazone.

Side Effects

Nervous System: bowel—diarrhea, dizziness, hypotension, muscle weakness, nausea/vomiting.

Endocrine System: (Pregnancy Category D) Addison-like syndrome, breast enlargement, sterility, weight loss.

Immune System: cataracts, false-positive cytology, hair loss, infections, myelosuppression,* pigmentation, pulmonary fibrosis,* renal failure.*

---

* Life-threatening side effect.

Dosage: PO 4–8 mg qd divided. Maintenance: 1–4 mg qd

Carboplatin [Paraplatin] is a combination of carboplatin, a platinum compound, and mannitol. This drug, like cisplatin, is cell-cycle nonspecific. Carboplatin cross-links DNA and is a palliative treatment for ovarian carcinoma that recurs after prior chemotherapy. No pretreatment or posttreatment forced hydration or diuresis is necessary.

Drug Interactions: Increased risk of ototoxicity, nephrotoxicity possible with aminoglycosides. May decrease phenytoin levels.

Incompatibilities

Solution/Additive: dextrose solutions.

Side Effects

Nervous System: bowel—constipation/diarrhea, dysgeusia, hypogeusia, nausea/vomiting, neuropathy—peripheral, tinnitus.

Endocrine System: (Pregnancy Category D) anorexia, mild electrolyte imbalances.

Immune System: alopecia, anemia,* hypersensitivity reactions, leukopenia,* liver enzymes—elevated, nephrotoxicity, neutropenia,* rash, thrombocytopenia.

Dosage: Ovarian cancer: IV 360 mg/m² on day 1 q 4 wk. The infusion is run more than 15 min. Head/neck/small-cell lung cancer: IV 300–400 mg/m² q4wk.

Chlorambucil [Leukeran] is a nitrogen mustard derivative and probably the least toxic and slowest acting of its group. Cell-cycle nonspecific, it can be used alone or in combination with other antineoplastics for treating chronic lymphocytic leukemia, lymphomas, Hodgkin's, and carcinomas of breast, ovaries, and testes. Uses for non-neoplastic conditions include rheumatoid arthritis complicated by vasculitis, autoimmune hemolytic anemia connected with cold agglutinins, lupus glomerulonephritis, idiopathic nephrotic syndrome, and macroglobulinemia.

Drug Interactions: Hyperuricemia possible with allopurinol, colchicine.

Side Effects

Nervous System: nausea/vomiting—infrequent, neuropathy—peripheral, pulmonary complications, seizures* (with high doses).

Endocrine System: (Pregnancy Category D) hyperuricemia, sterility.

Immune System: alopecia, anemia, bone marrow depression,* hepatotoxicity,* leukopenia, papilledema, rashes, thrombocytopenia.

---

* Life-threatening side effect.

Dosage: PO. Start with 0.1–0.2 mg/kg/day for 3–6 wk. Decrease dosage if WBC drops. Usual dose: 4–10 mg/d.

Cisplatin [Platinol] is composed of a platinum atom circled by two chloride atoms and two ammonia molecules in the cis position. DNA on malignant cell surfaces makes the surface more negative. Lymphocytes have positive charges on their surfaces, and are thus repelled. Cisplatin (platinum) not only cross-links DNA, but removes surface DNA from tumor cells, increasing malignant cell vulnerability to attack by the immune system. As an alkylating, non-cell-specific agent, cisplatin cross-links DNA in rapidly multiplying cells; in combination with vinblastine and bleomycin for metastatic testicular tumors; or with doxorubicin for metastatic ovarian tumors in addition to surgery and radiation. Cisplatin is also used to treat carcinomas of the head, neck, endometrium, and bladder. To decrease the chances of damage to hearing or kidney function, the patient must be kept well hydrated beginning 8–12 h before treatment with 1–2 L of IV fluids. A Foley catheter is inserted to spare the patient frequent voidings that disrupt rest. Output must be maintained at over 100 mL/h with a specific gravity of less than 1.030 for up to 24 h after treatment is completed.

Drug Interactions: Increased nephrotoxicity and acute renal failure with aminoglycosides, amphotericin B, vancomycin, other nephrotoxic drugs. Try to separate by at least 1–2 wk. Increased risk of ototoxicity with aminoglycosides, furosemide.

Incompatibilities

Solution/Additive: 5% dextrose, sodium bicarbonate, metoclopramide.

Side Effects

Nervous System: arrhythmias, bowel—constipation/diarrhea, headache, hearing loss, movement—uncoordinated, nausea/vomiting—severe, neuropathies—worsened with exercise/may be irreversible, taste loss, vertigo, vision changes, tinnitus.

Endocrine System: (Pregnancy Category D) anorexia, SIADH—elevated, hypocalcemia, hypomagnesemia, hyperuricemia, xerostomia.

Immune System: anaphylaxis,* AST—elevated, hemolytic anemia, hemolysis, leukopenia, myelosuppression, nephrotoxicity—dose-related/cumulative, stomatitis, thrombocytopenia.

Dosage: IV. Metastatic testicular tumor: cisplatin 20 mg/m² days 1–5 q3–4wk in combination with bleomycin 30 U/wk on day 2 for 12 wk and vinblastine 0.15–0.2 mg/kg on days 1 and 2 q3wk for a total of 8 doses.

Metastatic ovarian tumor: cisplatin 50 mg/m² day 1 q3wk plus doxorubicin 50 mg/m² day 1 q3wk in sequence. As a single agent: 100 mg/m² q3–4wk. The drug is diluted in 2 L dextrose in 1/2 or 1/3 normal saline containing 37.5 g of the osmotic diuretic mannitol (to prevent renal toxicity) and infused over 6–8 h.

Cyclophosphamide [Cytoxan] is cell-cycle nonspecific, blocking DNA, RNA, and protein synthesis probably through cross-linking DNA strands. Cyclophosphamide suppresses immunity and triggers antidiuretic hormone (ADH) release. It is used alone or in combination to treat malignant lymphoma, multiple myeloma, leukemia, and malignant lung neoplasms. It is also used for advanced neuroblastoma, ovarian adenocarcinoma, and breast carcinoma. Nonneoplastic uses include the treatment of mycosis fungoides, severe rheumatoid arthritis, multiple sclerosis, systemic lupus erythematosus, Wegener's granulomatosis, and nephrotic syndrome and the prevention of homotransplantation rejection. Immunosuppression and leukopenia can be fatal in as soon as 2–8 d after the first dose and as late as 1 mo after a series. Even purulent wounds may not appear to be infected because WBCs fall to a level too few to create pus. Careful intake and output (I&O) is required and fluids must be pushed to prevent kidney damage. Water intoxication may occur, manifested by confusion, headache, lethargy, tremors, and seizures. Hematuria may occur briefly or last for months and require blood replacement.

Drug Interactions: Prolonged neuromuscular blocking activity with succinylcholine. Increased cardiac toxicity with doxorubicin possible.

Side Effects

Nervous System: bowel—diarrhea, dizziness, fatigue, nausea/vomiting.

Endocrine System: (Pregnancy Category C) facial flushing, hyperkalemia—severe, hyperuricemia, hyponatremia, sweating, SIADH, water intoxication, weight—loss/gain.

Immune System: alopecia, anaphylaxis,* anemia, bladder fibrosis, sterile hemorrhagic/nonhemorrhagic cystitis,* drug fever, emboli—pulmonary,* edema—pulmonary, poor healing, hematuria, hepatotoxicity, leukopenia,* acute myeloid leukemia,* mucositis, nails—ridging/pigmentation, neoplasms, nephrotoxicity, neutropenia, pneumonitis, interstitial pulmonary fibrosis,* skin—pigmentation/allergy, thrombophlebitis.

Dosage: PO. Start with 1–5 mg/kg/d. Maintenance: q7–10d. IV. Start with 40–50 mg/kg divided doses for 2–5 d to maximum of 100 mg/kg. Maintenance: 10–15 mg/kg q7–10d or 3–5 mg/kg twice a week.

Dacarbazine [DTIC, DTIC-Dome, Imadazole Carboxamide] is a cell-cycle nonspecific triazine with alkylating characteristics; it acts as an antimetabolite during purine synthesis. It has minimal immunosuppressive activity and is more apt to cause severe nausea and vomiting than most of the alkylating agents. It can be used alone or in combination with other antineoplastics for the treatment of refractory Hodgkin's disease, metastatic malignant melanoma, neuroblastoma, and sarcomas. Dacarbazine is also a nitrosourea, making it lipophilic and able to readily cross the BBB.

Off Label: Malignant glucagonoma and soft tissue metastatic sarcoma. Hemorrhage is possible from platelet decrease.

Incompatibilities

Solution/Additive: heparin.

Side Effects

Nervous System: facial paresthesia, headache, malaise, myalgia, nausea/vomiting, pain—injected vein, psyche—confusion, seizures,* vision—blurred.

Endocrine System: (Pregnancy Category C) anorexia, facial flushing.

Immune System: alopecia, anaphylaxis,* anemia—mild, erythematosus, flu-like syndrome, hemorrhage,* hepatotoxicity, leukopenia*—severe, rashes, thrombocytopenia—severe.*

Dosage: IV 2–4.5 mg/kg/d for 10 d q4wk, or 250 mg/m²/d for 5d. Repeat at 3-wk intervals. Hodgkin's: IV 150 mg/m²/d for 5 d with other drugs q4 wk or 375 mg/m² on day 1 with other drugs and repeat q15d.

Ifosfamide [Ifex] is related to the nitrogen mustards. Its alkylated metabolites cross-link DNA and RNA strands and inhibit protein synthesis:

Drug Interactions: Increased hepatic conversion to an active metabolite with hepatic enzyme inducers (barbiturates, phenytoin, chloral hydrate). Corticosteroids may inhibit conversion to active metabolites.

Side Effects

Nervous System: bowel—diarrhea, coma,* cranial nerve dysfunction, nausea/vomiting, psyche—confusion/hallucinations, seizures,* somnolence.

Endocrine System: (Pregnancy Category D) anorexia, metabolic acidosis.

Immune System: alopecia, hemorrhagic cystitis,* hepatic dysfunction, nephrotoxicity,* neutropenia,* skin—necrosis/extravasation, thrombocytopenia.*

---

* Life-threatening side effect.

Dosage: IV 1.2 g/m²/d over at least 30 min for 5 consecutive days. Repeat q3wk or after recovery from hematologic toxicity.

Mechlorethamine hydrochloride [Mustargen] is a cell-cycle nonspecific mustard gas analog that interferes with DNA, RNA, and protein synthesis. It is myelosuppressive and weakly immunosuppressive with vesicant activity. It can be used alone or in combination with other antineoplastic agents for palliative treatment of Hodgkin's, lymphosarcoma, mycosis fungoides, polycythemia vera, chronic lymphocytic and myelocytic leukemia, and bronchial carcinoma. When drug is administered into a cavity, the patient must be repositioned every 5–10 min for 1 h to bring the drug into contact with all of the cavity. Extra fluid may be removed by paracentesis after 24–36 h.

Drug Interactions: May raise serum uric acid levels thus decreasing effectiveness of anti-gout drugs.

Side Effects

Nervous System: coma,* diarrhea, drowsiness, headache, lightheadedness, nausea/vomiting, neuropathy—peripheral, psyche—cerebral deterioration, tinnitus, vertigo, weakness.

Endocrine System: (Pregnancy Category D) amenorrhea, anorexia, azoospermia, hyperuricemia.

Immune System: agranulocytosis,* alopecia, anemia, chromosomal abnormalities, herpes zoster, hyperheparinemia, hypersensitivity reactions, leukopenia, lymphocytopenia, pruritus, thrombocytopenia. Extravasation site: pain, inflammation, sloughing, thrombosis, thrombophlebitis.

Dosage: IV 0.4 mg/kg or 10 mg/m² for a single course of treatment or in divided doses q3–6wk based on blood counts. Advanced Hodgkin's: IV 6 mg/m² on day 1 and 8 of a 28-d cycle.

Melphalan [L-PAM, L-Sarcolysin, others] is a nitrogen mustard similar to mechlorethamine with its myelosuppressive and immunosuppressive activity, but without vesicant properties. It is palliative for multiple myeloma, but may be used for Hodgkin's and breast and ovary carcinomas.

Drug Interactions: Increased risk of nephrotoxicity with cyclosporin.

Incompatibilities

Y-site: amphotericin B, chlorpromazine.

Side Effects

Nervous System: nausea/vomiting

---

* Life-threatening side effect.

Endocrine System: (Pregnancy Category D) uremia.

Immune System: agranulocytosis,* alopecia, anemia, angioedema,* acute nonlymphatic leukemia, leukopenia, pulmonary fibrosis, stomatitis, thrombocytopenia.

Dosage: Multiple myeloma: PO 6 mg qd for 2–3 wk. Stop for 4–5 wk. Maintenance: 2 mg qd once WBC and platelets start to rise. IV 16 mg/m² over 15 min q2wk for 4 doses. Epithelial ovarian carcinoma: PO 0.2 mg/kg/d for 5 d. Repeat q4–5wk based on hematology.

Mitomycin [Mutamycin], an antitumor antibiotic, is cell-cycle specific (G and S). As an alkylating agent, it cross-links DNA and is sometimes effective in tumors resistant to older alkylating drugs. It is used to treat cancers of head, neck, breasts, lungs, prostate, GI tract, and pancreas as well as superficial bladder cancer.

Incompatibilities

Solution/Additive: dextrose-containing solutions.

Side Effects

Nervous System: bowel—diarrhea, acute bronchospasm,* cough—nonproductive, dyspnea, edema, fatigue, headache, nausea/vomiting, pain, paresthesias.

Endocrine System: (Pregnancy Category D) anorexia.

Immune System: alopecia, anemia, bone marrow toxicity* (4–6 wk after treatment starts), hematemesis, hemolytic uremic syndrome,* hemoptysis, nail bed—purple discoloration, pneumonia, pneumonitis—interstitial,* renal toxicity, thrombophlebitis. Injection site: cellulitis/desquamation/induration/necrosis.

Dosage: IV 20 mg/m² q6–8wk. Additional doses based on hematologic response.

NITROSOUREAS

The nitrosoureas are also alkylating agents, but they are lipophilic and thus able to readily cross the BBB to treat tumors of the CNS.

Carmustine [BiCNU] alkylates DNA and RNA and inhibits several enzymatic processes. It is used to treat CNS tumors, Hodgkin's disease, other lymphomas, and multiple myeloma resistant to other drugs. It is also used in combination with other drugs for stomach cancer.

Drug Interactions: Increased neutropenia and thrombocytopenia possible with cimetidine.

Side Effects

Nervous System: ataxia, dizziness, nausea/vomiting.

Endocrine System: (Pregnancy Category D) none noted.

Immune System: MI,* myelosuppression,* pulmonary infiltration*/fibrosis, retinal hemorrhage, stomatitis, thrombocytopenia. Injection site: pain/flushing/hyperpigmentation.

Dosage: IV 150–200 mg/m² q6wk in 1 dose or over 2 d. Mycosis fungoides: Topical: 0.05–0.4% solution or ointment qd or bid for 6–8 wk.

<u>Lomustine [CeeNU]</u> is a lipid-soluble alkylating nitrosourea with activity similar to that of carmustine. Being lipid-soluble, it passes through the BBB more readily for palliative treatment of primary and metastatic brain tumors. Lomustine is also used to treat Hodgkin's disease as well as carcinomas of the GI tract, lungs, and kidneys.

Drug Interactions: None noted.

Side Effects

Nervous System: ataxia, disorientation, itching, lethargy, nausea/vomiting.

Endocrine System: (Pregnancy Category D) anorexia.

Immune System: alopecia, anemia, leukopenia*—cumulative, liver function tests—transient elevations, nephrotoxicity, pulmonary toxicity (rare), rash, thrombocytopenia*—cumulative.

Dosage: PO 130 mg/m² in one dose. Repeat in 6 wk. Then give according to WBCs over 4000 mm³ and platelet counts over 100,000 mm³.

<u>Procarbazine hydrochloride [Matulane]</u> is cell-cycle specific (S phase). It disrupts DNA in a manner similar to alkylators and radiation and also interferes with transfer RNA synthesis. It is sometimes given in combination with mechlorethamine, prednisone, and vincristine. It is used to treat Hodgkin's disease and some solid tumors. It has MAO action with tyramine foods, crosses the BBB, and can raise BP to crisis.

Drug Interactions: Increased CNS depression with alcohol, phenothiazines, other CNS depressants. Hypertensive crisis, hyperpyrexia possible with tricyclic antidepressants, ephedrine, MAOIs, phenylpropanolamine, sympathomimetics.

Food–Drug Interactions: hypertensive crisis possible with tyramine-containing foods.

Side Effects

Nervous System: arrhythmias—tachycardia, arthralgia, ataxia, bowel—diarrhea/constipation, coma,* cough, dizziness, dysphagia, edema—rare, fatigue, footdrop, headache, hearing changes—rare, hypotension, insomnia, lethargy, myalgia, nausea/vomiting, neuropathies,

paresthesias, psyche—apprehension/confusion/depression/hallucinations/nervousness/nightmares/acute psychosis, reflexes—decreased, seizures,* tremors.

Endocrine System: (Pregnancy Category D) anorexia, chills, fever, flushing, gynecomastia, dry mouth, spermatogenesis—decreased, sweating, testes—atrophy.

Immune System: alopecia, anemia, ascites, bleeding, bone marrow suppression,* dermatitis, hemolysis, herpes, hoarseness, hyperpigmentation, infections, jaundice, photosensitivity, pleural effusion, pruritus, rash, retinal hemorrhage—rare.

Dosage: Adjunct for Hodgkin's: PO 2–4 mg/kg qd or qd divided for 1 wk. Increase to 4–6 mg/kg/d to reach maximum response, unless contraindicated by blood count.

<u>Streptozocin [Zanosar]</u> is cell-cycle nonspecific, but more effective in the G₂-M phase. It blocks DNA synthesis. It is used for pancreatic islet cell cancers (in drug combination), for colorectal cancer (in combination), and also for Hodgkin's disease. It concentrates in pancreas beta cells, blocks glucogenesis, decreases insulin production, causes liver and kidney toxicity, and is a vesicant. CBC, BUN, serum creatinine, and electrolytes must be monitored during treatment.

Drug Interactions: Increased hematologic toxicity with myelosuppressive agents. Increased risk of nephrotoxicity with nephrotoxic agents including aminoglycosides, amphotericin B, cisplatin, vancomycin. Reduced cytotoxic effect on pancreatic beta cells with phenytoin.

Side Effects

Nervous System: bowel—diarrhea, nausea/vomiting, psyche—confusion/depression.

Endocrine System: (Pregnancy Category D) acetonuria, alkaline phosphatase—transient increase, aminoaciduria, anuria,* azotemia,* glucose tolerance abnormalities, glucosuria, glycosuria without hyperglycemia, hyperchloremia,* hypoalbuminemia, hypocalcemia, hypokalemia, hypophosphatemia,* insulin shock*—rare, proteinuria,* proximal renal tubular reabsorption defects, urine—alkaline pH.

Immune System: ALT/AST—increased, anemia, duodenal ulcer—rare, myelosuppression, nephrotoxicity.* IV site: necrosis after extravasation.

Dosage: IV 500 mg/m² for 5 d q6wk or 1000 mg/m²/wk for 2 wk. Then increase to 1.5 g/m²/wk. Infuse dose over 15 min–6 h.

<u>Thiotepa [Thioplex, TSPA]</u> is cell-cycle nonspecific. It cross-links DNA by selective reaction with phosphate groups. It

---

* Life-threatening side effect.

is used with other drugs for breast, superficial bladder, and ovarian cancer, cancerous meningitis, and malignant pleural or peritoneal effusions.

Drug Interactions: none noted.

Off Label: Prevention of pterygium recurrences after postoperative beta-irradiation; leukemia, malignant meningeal neoplasms.

Side Effects

Nervous System: headache, nausea/vomiting, throat—tight sensation. Intravesical: pain.

Endocrine System: (Pregnancy Category D) amenorrhea, anorexia, fever, hyperuricemia, spermatogenesis-impaired.

Immune System: anemia,* hives, intestinal mucosa ulceration, leukopenia,* pancytopenia,* pruritus, rash, response-slowed in heavily irradiated site, thrombocytopenia.* Injection site: pain/weeping. Intravesical: hematuria, hemorrhagic chemical cystitis, vesical irritability.

Dosage: IV 0.3–0.4 mg/kg q1–4wk. Intracavitary: 0.6–0.8 mg/kg qwk. In bladder: 60 mg in 30–60 mL distilled water, retain for 2 h weekly for 4 wk. Intratumor: Start with 0.6–0.8 mg/kg; maintenance: 0.07–0.08 mg/kg q1–4 wk.

ANTIMETABOLITES

The antimetabolites are also known as folate antagonists. Essentially, these agents starve cancer cells by blocking an enzyme that reduces folate vitamins to the active forms needed to synthesize thymidylate and purine to create the DNA needed for cell replication.

Cladribine [Leustatin] inhibits DNA synthesis and repair in dividing and quiescent lymphocytes and monocytes.

Incompatibilities: Do not mix with other diluents/drugs.

Side Effects

Nervous System: bowel—diarrhea, dizziness, headache, nausea.

Endocrine System: (Pregnancy Category D) fever, serum creatinine—elevated.

Immune System: anemia, myelosuppression,* thrombocytopenia.

Dosage: Hairy cell leukemia: IV 0.09 mg/kg/d by 7-d continuous infusion. Chronic lymphocytic leukemia: IV 0.1 mg/kg/d continuous infusion, or 0.028–0.14 mg/kg/d as 2-h bolus infusion for 5 consecutive days.

---

* Life-threatening side effect.

Cytarabine [Cytosar-U, others] is cell-cycle specific (S) and converts into a triphosphate nucleotide that inhibits DNA synthesis. The 60–80% remission rate in acute non-lymphocytic leukemia is a treatment breakthrough. It is potentially carcinogenic and mutagenic, as are many of the antineoplastics. Cytarabine is combined with daunorubicin and/or thioguanine, and is a second drug of choice for acute lymphocytic leukemia. It is also effective for lymphoblastic lymphoma. High-dosage cytarabine plus daunorubicin is used for the last phase of chronic myelogenous leukemia. Remission requires extreme myelosuppression.

Drug Interactions: GI toxicity may decrease digoxin absorption. Decreased aminoglycoside activity against *Klebsiella pneumoniae.*

Incompatibilities

Solution/Additive: cephalothin, fluorouracil, gentamicin, heparin, insulin, nafcillin, oxacillin, penicillin G.

Side Effects

Nervous System: bladder—retention, bowel—diarrhea, headache, lethargy, nausea/vomiting, neuropathy—brachial plexus/peripheral, pain—injection site, photophobia, psyche—confusion/personality changes, somnolence, vertigo.

Endocrine System: (Pregnancy Category D) anorexia, fever, renal dysfunction, weight loss.

Immune System: anemia, bleeding, bulla formation, cellulitis, conjunctivitis, desquamation, erythema, esophagitis, freckles, hemorrhage,* hepatotoxicity, inflammation/ulceration—anal/oral, jaundice, leukopenia, megaloblastosis, myelosuppression, neurotoxicity,* pericarditis,* rash, skin ulcers, sore throat, stomatitis, thrombocytopenia. Injection site: thrombophlebitis.

Dosage: Leukemias: IV 200 mg/m² by continuous infusion over 24 h. SC 1 m/kg 1–2 ×/wk. Intrathecal: 5–75 mg once q4d or once/d for 4 d.

Floxuridine [FUDR] a pyrimidine antagonist, is cell-cycle specific. The body catabolizes it into fluorouracil.

Drug Interactions: none noted.

Side Effects

Nervous System: angina, bowel—diarrhea, cramps, hemiplegia, hiccups, nausea/vomiting, psyche—depression, seizures,* vertigo.

Endocrine System: (Pregnancy Category D) anorexia, fever, renal insufficiency, dry skin.

Immune System: alopecia, dermatitis, esophagopharyngitis, low immunity, leukopenia, myocardial ischemia, photosensitivity, pruritic ulcerations, rash.

Dosage: Intraarterial 0.1–0.6 mg/kg by continuous infusion.

Fludarabine phosphate [Fludara], a vidarabine analog, causes DNA chain interruption and is effective in treating chronic lymphocytic leukemia, low-grade non-Hodgkin's lymphoma, and also mycosis fungoides.

Drug Interactions: none noted.

Side Effects

Nervous System: bowel—diarrhea, coma,* cough, dyspnea, myalgia, nausea/vomiting, vision—blindness.

Endocrine System: (Pregnancy Category D) chills, fever.

Immune System: anemia, infection, myelosuppression, rash.

Dosage: 25 mg/m²/d for 5 d. Give over 30 min in 100–125 mL of D5W or NS. Refrigerate the drug before reconstitution and use within 8 h after reconstitution.

Fluorouracil (FU) [Adrucil, others] is cell-cycle specific (S) and interferes with DNA and RNA synthesis. It is used in breast and metastatic breast cancers, prostatic cancers resistant to normal treatment, GI and pancreatic cancers, and sometimes head and neck cancers.

Incompatibilities

Solution/Additive: cytarabine, diazepam, doxorubicin, droperidol.

Y-site: droperidol.

Side Effects

Nervous System: angina, bowel—diarrhea, acute cerebellar syndrome, malaise, nausea/vomiting, psyche—euphoria, optic disturbances.

Endocrine System: (Pregnancy Category D) alkaline phosphatase/serum transaminase/lactic dehydrogenase—elevated, fever.

Immune System: epistaxis, GI tract inflammations, leukopenia,* ulcers, hair loss, myocardial ischemia, rashes, serum bilirubin—elevated. Topical: burning, dermatitis, pruritus, suppuration, swelling, toxic granulation.

Dosage: IV. Start with 12 mg/kg qd for 4 d. If there is no toxicity, 6 mg/kg on days 6, 8, 10, and 12. Maintain on same course every 30 d. Multiple actinic or solar keratoses, superficial basal cell carcinoma, and (unlabeled) condylomata acuminata: Topical bid to lesions. DC when inflammation reaches erosion, necrosis, and ulceration. Healing may take up to 2 mo.

* Life-threatening side effect.

Gemcitabine [Gemzar], an analog of cytarabine, inhibits ribonucleotide reductase and reduces the normal pool of deoxycytidine triphosphate, thus inhibiting DNA synthesis. Survival rates are minimal in breast, pancreatic, and non-small-cell lung cancers.

Drug Interactions: none noted.

Side Effects

Nervous System: arthralgia, bowel—diarrhea, fatigue, headache, nausea/vomiting.

Endocrine System: (Pregnancy Category D) chills, fever.

Immune System: anemia, bleeding, liver transaminases—elevated, rashes, thrombocytopenia.

Dosage: IV 1 g/m²/wk infused over 30 min for 7 consecutive weeks. Rest for 1 wk. Then once per week for 3 wks with 1 wk rest thereafter.

Mercaptopurine [Purinethol] is cell-cycle specific (S). It inhibits DNA and RNA synthesis and suppresses humoral and cellular immune response. It is used for maintenance in acute nonlymphocytic and lymphocytic leukemia, with other drugs for chronic myelogenous leukemia (blast phase), and suppression of the immune response in bowel inflammation disease.

Drug Interactions: Increased toxicity with allopurinol possible. May potentiate or antagonize anticoagulant effects of warfarin.

Side Effects

Nervous System: bowel—diarrhea, nausea/vomiting.

Endocrine System: (Pregnancy Category D) anorexia, hyperuricemia, oliguria, renal dysfunction.

Immune System: anemia, bleeding, bone marrow hypoplasia, eosinophilia, GI tract—inflammation/ulceration, hepatic necrosis,* leukopenia,* liver function—impaired, pancytopenia, thrombocytopenia.*

Dosage: PO 2.5 mg/kg/d for 4 wk. Increase to 5 mg/kg/d if no therapeutic response. Maintenance: 1.25–2.5 mg/kg qd.

Methotrexate [Mexate, MTX, others] is a cell-cycle specific (S) that blocks the use of folic acid for DNA synthesis. Methotrexate administration is followed with leucovorin to replenish the depleted folate needed by the patient ("leucovorin rescue"). It is used to treat osteogenic sarcoma and lymphomatous and carcinomatous meningitis. It is used PO for maintenance for acute lymphocytic leukemia, and intrathecally to prevent CNS recurrence in combination with other drugs for non-Hodgkin's lymphoma, choriocarcinoma, and solid tumors of breast, ovary, testicles, prostate, bladder, lung, neck, and head.

Methotrexate is also used for advanced mycosis fungoides and psoriatic arthritis.

Drug Interactions: Increased risk of hepatotoxicity with alcohol. Increased levels and toxicity possible with chloramphenicol, NSAIDs, PABA, penicillin, phenylbutazone, phenytoin, salicylates, sulfonamides, sulfonylureas, tetracyclines. Altered response possible with folic acid.

Incompatibilities

Solution/Additive: bleomycin, droperidol, heparin, metoclopramide, prednisolone, ranitidine.

Y-site: droperidol, ranitidine.

Side Effects

Nervous System: aphasia, ataxia, bowel—diarrhea, coma,* convulsions* (after intrathecal), sudden death,* dizziness, drowsiness, headache, hemiparesis, nausea/vomiting, tremors, vision—blurred.

Endocrine System: (Pregnancy Category D) abortion, chills, fetal defects, fever, infertility, menstrual dysfunction, metabolic changes precipitating diabetes, osteoporosis.

Immune System: alopecia, anemia, aplastic bone marrow,* hepatic cirrhosis,* hepatotoxicity,* hypogammaglobulinemia, inflammation—oral cavity structures, leukopenia, myelosuppression,* nephropathy, photosensitivity, pneumonitis,* pulmonary fibrosis,* rashes, resistance to infection—decreased, septicemia, telangiectasis, systemic toxicity (after intrathecal/intraarterial), thrombocytopenia. Intraarterial catheter site: thrombophlebitis.

Dosage: Leukemia: IM/IV induction: 3.3 mg/m²/d. PO, IM, IV maintenance 20–30 mg/m² twice weekly. Lymphoma: PO 12–25 mg/d × 4–8 d with 7–10 d rest intervals. Psoriasis PO 2.5–5 mg q12h for 3 doses each wk up to 25–30 mg/wk. IM, IV 10–25 mg/wk. Rheumatoid arthritis PO 2.5–5 mg q12h × 3 doses qwk or 7.5 mg qwk. Trophoblastic neoplasm PO 15–30 mg/d × 3–5 courses q12wk. IM, IV as with PO.

Drug respites are necessary. Also see *leucovorin calcium* for rescue later in this chapter.

Pentostatin [Nipent] inhibits adenosine deaminase, resulting in a buildup of deoxyadenosine and several phosphorylated derivatives, depleting cellular ATP and inhibiting DNA synthesis in lymphatic tumor cells. It is cell-cycle specific for the G_1 phase.

Drug Interactions: Skin rashes possible with allopurinol. Enhanced effects with vidarabine. Fatal pulmonary toxicity with fludarabine phosphate. Acute pulmonary edema/hypotension carmustine, etoposide, high-dose cyclophosphamide.

Side Effects

Nervous System: coma,* fatigue, lethargy, nausea/vomiting.

Endocrine System: (Pregnancy Category D) none noted.

Immune System: lymphocytopenia, frequent severe systemic infection, nephrotoxicity.*

Dosage: Hairy cell leukemia: IV bolus ≥ 3–5 min 4 mg/m² qowk.

Thioguanine (TG) is cell-cycle specific (S), disrupting DNA by replacing guanine and inhibiting RNA synthesis. It is used with other drugs for acute nonlymphocytic leukemia, and with still others for lymphocytic leukemia. Thioguanine is used as a palliative for chronic myelogenous leukemia.

Drug Interactions: none noted.

Side Effects

Nervous System: ataxia—rare, bowel—diarrhea, nausea/vomiting.

Endocrine System: (Pregnancy Category X) anorexia, hyperuricemia.

Immune System: anemia, possibly fatal hepatic vein occlusion,* jaundice, leukopenia,* rash, stomatitis, thrombocytopenia.*

Dosage: PO 2 mg/kg qd for 4 wk. May increase to 3 mg/kg/d if no response.

CYTOKINES

The immune system communicates with messenger molecules called cytokines. The interferons, a type of cytokine, are protein molecules that regulate the immune response and have antiviral and antiproliferative activity. Interferons can potentiate the macrophages. Recombinant DNA technology makes commercial production of these molecules possible. In addition to their promise in the treatment of cancer, interferons are being used to treat multiple sclerosis.

Aldesleukin [Proleukin], produced by activated T lymphocytes, binds to T-cell receptors to induce proliferative response and differentiation into lymphokine-activated killer (LAK) cells in the blood and tumor-infiltrating lymphocytes (TIL-cells) in specific tumors.

Drug Interactions: May affect CNS function with psychotropic drugs. May increase myelotoxicity with cytotoxic

---

* Life-threatening side effect.

chemotherapy. May increase nephrotoxicity with aminoglycosides, indomethacin. May increase cardiotoxicity with doxorubicin. May increase hepatotoxicity with methotrexate, asparaginase. Antitumor effectiveness may be decreased with glucocorticoids.

Side Effects

Nervous System: bowel—diarrhea, cardiovascular collapse,* coma,* edema, hypotension, nausea/vomiting, pulmonary insufficiency, psyche—psychosis.

Endocrine System: (Pregnancy Category D) serum creatinine/transaminases—increased, chills, fever, oliguria.

Immune System: anemia, increased bilirubin, capillary leak syndrome, cardiovascular toxicity,* edema—pulmonary/interstitial, eosinophilia, MI,* nasal congestion, rash, thrombocytopenia.

Dosage: Metastatic renal cell carcinoma: IV 600,000 IU/kg over 15 min q8h for 14 doses. Repeat after 9 d to a total of 28 doses.

Bacillus Calmette-Guérin (BCG) vaccine [Tice, TheraCys] is

an attenuated strain of the bacillus Calmette-Guérin strain of *Mycobacterium bovis* used to immunize against tuberculosis. Used intravesically in bladder cancer in situ, it may cause a local, chronic inflammatory response, which draws macrophages and leukocytes to the site to destroy superficial tumor cells.

Off Label: Malignant melanoma.

Drug Interactions: Antagonized or inhibited vaccine-mediated immune response with concurrent antimycobacterial therapy (aminosalicylic acid, capreomycin, cycloserine, ethambutol, ethionamide, isoniazid, pyrazinamide, rifabutin, rifampin, streptomycin). Live vaccines may interfere with immune response to BCG. Possible sensitivity to tuberculin with previous vaccination or other exposure to BCG. Possible booster effect after repeat tuberculin testing if individual has had prior BCG vaccination.

Side Effects

Nervous System: bladder—spasms/decreased flow and capacity/dysuria/incontinence/nocturia/clot retention, bowel—constipation/diarrhea, dizziness, headache, malaise, pain—abdominal/penal, weakness.

Endocrine System: (Pregnancy Category C) anorexia, fever.

Immune System: abscess, allergy, anaphylaxis,* anemia, hemorrhagic cystitis, DIC,* eosinophilia, leukopenia, lymphadenitis, pulmonary infection, thrombocytopenia.

Dosage: Intravesical. TheraCys: 3 vials (27 mg each, or 81 mg total) of BCG reconstituted with accompanying diluent, diluted in 50 mL of sterile, preservative-free 0.9% NaCl and instilled into bladder slowly by gravity flow via urethral catheter; suspension is retained for 2 h, after which time the patient voids. Treatments are begun 7–14 d after biopsies or transurethral resections, and are administered once a week for total of 6 wk. Then one treatment at 3, 6, 12, 18, and 24 mo. Tice: 1 vial per intravesical instillation; usually repeated weekly for 6 wk followed by monthly instillation for 6–12 months.

Interferon alfa: Alfa-2A [Roferon-A], alfa-2B [Intron A]

are cytokines that bind to specific membrane receptors and are taken up intracellularly to affect diverse functions, for example, increased activity of natural killer (NK) lymphocytes and phagocytic macrophages.

Drug Interactions: none noted.

Side Effects

Nervous System: arthralgia, headache, hypertension, malaise, myalgia, nausea, tachycardia. Very high doses: confusion, dizziness, somnolence.

Endocrine System: (Pregnancy Category D) anorexia, chills, fever.

Immune System: AST/LDH/alkaline phosphatase—slight elevation, flu-like syndrome, leukopenia, thrombocytopenia.

Dosage: Alfa-2a for hairy cell leukemia: SC, IM 3 million U/d × 16–24 wk. AIDS-related Kaposi's sarcoma: SC, IM 36 million U/d × 10–12 wk. Then may reduce to 3 × per wk. Genital and anal warts: intralesional 1 million U per lesion 3 × per wk on alternate days × 3 wk. Chronic viral hepatitis: SC, IM 1–3 million U/d × 1 wk. Then 3 × per wk × 48–52 wk. Alfa-2b for hairy cell leukemia: IM, SC million U/m² 3 × per wk. Kaposi's sarcoma: IM, SC 30 million U/m² 3 × per wk. Condylomata acuminata: IM, SC 1 million U/m² 3 × per wk. Chronic hepatitis B or C: SC 3 million U 3 × per wk × 18–24 wk.

DNA INTERCALATING DRUGS

Intercalating agents interfere with DNA synthesis by binding to the strands and causing a break in DNA and preventing its repair. Many intercalating drugs are anthracene derivatives with broad-spectrum anticancer activity. They are extremely toxic and cause severe nausea and vomiting, mucositis, alopecia, and myelosuppression. They can cause both acute and chronic cardiac damage. Acute toxicity causes arrhythmias, including PVCs. Chronic toxicity results in sarcoplasmic reticulum damage and the inability of the cardiac muscle to bind

---

* Life-threatening side effect.

with the calcium necessary to contract muscle cells. Pericarditis and congestive heart failure can prove fatal. The drugs also carry the risk of extravasation. Drug resistance may occur when cancerous cells are able to pump out the drug.

Dactinomycin [Actinomycin-D, Cosmegen] is cell-cycle specific (G and S). It binds to guanine in DNA and interferes with DNA-dependent polymerase. It is used to treat testicular cancer and choriocarcinoma resistant to methotrexate, childhood tumors, soft tissue sarcomas, and Kaposi's sarcoma. Dactinomycin is a vesicant.

Drug Interactions: Elevates uric acid levels requiring dose adjustment of anti-gout agents. Increased effects of both dactinomycin and other myelosuppressants. Increased effects of both radiation and dactinomycin. May reactivate erythema from previous radiation therapy. Decreased antihemorrhagic effects of vitamin K, leading to prolonged clotting time and potential hemorrhage.

Side Effects

Nervous System: bowel—diarrhea, dysphagia, fatigue, lethargy, malaise, myalgia, nausea/vomiting.

Endocrine System: (Pregnancy Category C) anorexia, fever, gonadal suppression, hyperuricemia, hypocalcemia.

Immune System: acne, agranulocytosis,* alopecia, anemia, aplastic anemia,* cheilitis, glossitis, hepatitis, leukopenia,* pancytopenia, proctitis, reticulopenia, skin reactions—often over previously irradiated areas, stomatitis, thrombocytopenia,* ulceration—GI. Extravasation site: contractures/necrosis/sloughing.

Dosage: IV 500 μg/d for 5 d. May repeat at 2- to 4-wk intervals as tolerated. Isolation perfusion: IV 50 μg/kg for lower extremity or pelvis. Use 35 μg/kg for upper extremity.

Daunorubicin hydrochloride [Cerubidine] is cell-cycle specific (S). It binds with DNA and interferes with RNA synthesis. Daunorubicin is used to treat acute lymphocytic leukemia (with vincristine and prednisone) and, with cytarabine, acute myelogenous leukemia, lymphoma, childhood tumors, and leukemia.

Drug Interactions: none noted.

Incompatibilities

Solution/Additive: dexamethasone, heparin.

Side Effects

Nervous System: arrhythmias, bowel—diarrhea, CHF,* edema—peripheral, acute nausea/vomiting.

Endocrine System: (Pregnancy Category D) anorexia, fever, gonadal suppression, hyperuricemia.

Immune System: alopecia, anemia, bone marrow depression,* cellulitis—severe, leukopenia, mucositis, stomatitis, thrombocytopenia. IV site extravasation: necrosis.

Dosage: IV 30–60 mg/m² qd for 3–5 d q3–4wk. With cytarabine: IV 30–45 mg/m² for 3 d; then subsequent 2-d courses with cytarabine 100 mg/m² qd for 7 d.

Doxorubicin hydrochloride [Adriamycin] is cell-cycle specific (S) and interferes with DNA replication and RNA synthesis; effective for acute leukemia, lymphoma, Hodgkin's, soft tissue sarcomas, and also breast, ovarian, lung, thyroid, stomach, and bladder cancers. The side effects are similar to those of daunorubicin.

Drug Interactions: Decreased effect with barbiturates. Prolonged half life with streptozocin, may require reduced dosage of doxorubicin.

Incompatibilities

Solution/Additive: aminophylline, cephalothin, dexamethasone, diazepam, fluorouracil, furosemide, hydrocortisone, heparin, vinblastine.

Y-site: furosemide, heparin.

Side Effects

Nervous System: arrhythmias–ventricular arrhythmias,* CHF, acute left ventricular failure, diarrhea, drowsiness, hyper-/hypotension, lethargy, nausea/vomiting.

Endocrine System: (Pregnancy Category D) anorexia, chills, fever, hyperuricemia. With too rapid IV infusion: facial flushing

Immune System: alopecia, anaphylaxis,* anemia, angioedema,* erythema, hyperpigmentation—buccal mucosa/nail beds/tongue, lacrimation, leukopenia,* lymphangitis, myelosuppression—severe, phlebosclerosis, pruritus, rash, skin reaction (with prior radiation), thrombocytopenia, urticaria. Red flare around injection site. Extravasation: severe cellulitis, tissue necrosis, vesication.

Dosage: IV 60–75 mg/m² q21d or 30 mg/m² for 3 d. Repeat q4wk to maximum cumulative dose of 500–550 mg/m².

Idarubicin hydrochloride [Idamycin] is a daunorubicin derivative with greater potency and perhaps less cardiotoxicity than other anthracyclines.

Drug Interactions: None noted.

Incompatibilities

Solution/Additive and Y-site: acyclovir, alkaline solutions, ampicillin/sulbactam, cefazolin, ceftazidime, clindamycin, dexamethasone, etoposide, furosemide, gentamicin, heparin, hydrocortisone, imipenem/cilastatin, meperidine, methotrexate, mezlocillin, sargramostim, sodium bicarbonate, vancomycin, vincristine.

Side Effects

Nervous System: atrial fibrillation, bowel—diarrhea, CHF,* nausea/vomiting, pain—chest/abdominal.

Endocrine System: (Pregnancy Category D) none noted.

Immune System: alopecia, anemia,* hepatotoxicity, leukopenia,* MI,* mucositis, nephrotoxicity, rash, thrombocytopenia.

Dosage: Acute myelogenous leukemia (AML): IV 12 mg/m² qd for 3 d. Inject slowly over 10–15 min.

Mitoxantrone hydrochloride [Novantrone] blocks DNA/RNA transcription; it is not cell-cycle specific. It is used as combination therapy with other agents to treat acute nonlymphocytic leukemia and alone to treat ovarian cancer and lymphoma. It discolors sclera, skin, urine.

Off Label: Breast cancer, refractory lymphomas.

Drug Interactions: May impair vaccine immune responses. Increased risk of infection with yellow fever vaccine possible.

Side Effects

Nervous System: arrhythmias—tachycardia/left ventricle (decreased function), bowel—diarrhea, CHF,* nausea/vomiting.

Endocrine System: (Pregnancy Category D) edema.

Immune System: alopecia, hepatotoxicity,* leukopenia,* MI* (cumulative doses of > 80–100 mg/m²), thrombocytopenia.*

Dosage: Induction therapy: IV 12 mg/m² on days 1–3. If needed, repeat induction. Dilute with at least 50 mL 0.9% NaCl or D5W. Introduce over 30–60 min into a freely running IV infusion. Consolidation therapy: IV 12 mg/m² on days 1 and 2. Do not exceed 80–120 mg/m² lifetime exposure.

Plicamycin [Mithracin, Mithramycin] is cell-cycle specific, probably disrupting DNA synthesis. It blocks bone reabsorption at the osteoblast level. Plicamycin is used in treating testicular cancer or other unresponsive malignancies.

Drug Interactions: Increased hypercalcemia with vitamin D.

Side Effects

Nervous System: bowel—diarrhea, dizziness, drowsiness, headache, nausea/vomiting, psyche—depression/irritability, weakness.

Endocrine System: (Pregnancy Category C) anorexia, facial flushing, fever, hypocalcemia, hypokalemia, hypophosphatemia, renal function tests—abnormal.

Immune System: abnormal liver function tests, bleeding/coagulation disorders* (dose related), hemoptysis, intestinal hemorrhage, leukopenia, phlebitis, rash, thrombocytopenia.

Dosage: IV 25–30 μg/kg qd for 8–10 d or until toxicity requires discontinuation to maximum of 30 μg/kg/d for 10 d.

HORMONAL DRUGS AND ANTAGONISTS

The corticosteroids have cytotoxic capabilities, and the sex hormones can block hormone-dependent tumor cell receptors. These are probably the least toxic of all anticancer agents, and the corticosteroids alleviate some of the side effects of other drugs and some effects of the cancers. Their affinity for sodium does, however, cause edema. The nonsteroids may be used to block hormonal production or influence in hormone-dependent cancers.

Aminoglutethimide [Cytadren] is not cell-cycle specific. It blocks steroid synthesis by preventing enzyme change of cholesterol to pregnenolone (precursors of cortisol and aldosterone) and blocks the nonadrenal enzyme change of androgens to estrogens. Aminoglutethimide is used for advanced estrogen receptor–positive breast tumors and when the patient has relapsed after first responding to tamoxifen. It is also used for Cushing's disease resulting from adrenal or adrenocortical tumors or growths. In response to the drop in corticosteroids the pituitary releases ACTH. To counter possible ACTH release, hydrocortisone is given with aminoglutethimide. *Note:* Aminoglutethimide is used after tamoxifen and progestin.

Drug Interactions: Decreased effect with dexamethasone. Decreased anticoagulant response to warfarin.

Side Effects

Nervous System: arrhythmias—tachycardia, clumsiness, dizziness, drowsiness, headache, hypotension, lethargy, nausea/vomiting, vision—uncontrolled eye movements (dose related).

Endocrine System: (Pregnancy Category D) anorexia, masculinization.

Immune System: blood disorders (rare)—agranulocytosis*/anemia/Coombs negative/leukopenia/neutrope-

---

* Life-threatening side effect.

nia/pancytopenia*/thrombocytopenia, hepatotoxicity, pruritus, rash.

Dosage: Breast cancer: PO 250 mg bid and hydrocortisone 60 mg hs, 20 mg AM and 20 mg at 2 PM qd for 2 wk; then 250 mg qid and hydrocortisone 20 mg hs, 10 mg in AM, and 10 mg at 2 PM thereafter. Cushing's Disease: PO 250 mg q6h; may increase 250 mg/d q1–2 wk if needed to maximum of 2 g/d.

Anastrazole [Arimidex] See *aminoglutethimide.*

Dosage: PO 1 mg qd.

Bicalutamide [Casodex] is a nonsteroidal agent with an affinity for androgen receptors in prostatic carcinoma, blocking the androgen-dependent tumor. It is used in the treatment of advanced prostate cancer in conjunction with luteinizing hormone–releasing hormone (LHRH) analog.

Drug Interactions: Increased effects of oral anticoagulants possible.

Side Effects

Nervous System: bladder—incontinence/dysuria/frequency/nocturia/retention/urgency, bowel—constipation/diarrhea, CHF, cramps—legs, dizziness, dyspepsia, edema—peripheral, headache, hypertension, myalgia, myasthenia, nausea/vomiting, neuropathy, pain—abdominal/bone/chest, paresthesia, psyche—anxiety/confusion/insomnia/nervousness, sexual function—impotence/decreased libido.

Endocrine System: (Pregnancy Category X) anorexia, edema—peripheral, gynecomastia, gout, hot flashes, hyperglycemia, dry mouth, sweating, weight—loss/gain.

Immune System: alopecia, anemia, arthritis, flu syndrome, hematuria, infection, liver function tests—increased levels, melena, pathologic bone fractures, pruritus, UTI.

Dosage: PO 50 mg qd.

Flutamide [Eulexin] blocks both testosterone and dihydrotestosterone in target tissue.

Drug Interactions: none noted.

Side Effects

Nervous System: bowel—diarrhea, drowsiness, edema, encephalopathy, nausea/vomiting, psyche—anxiety/confusion/depression/nervousness, sexual function—impotence/libido loss.

Endocrine System: (Pregnancy Category D) anorexia, edema, galactorrhea, gynecomastia, hot flashes.

Immune System: anemia, hepatic necrosis, hepatitis, jaundice, leukopenia, rash, SGOT/SGPT/bilirubin—may increase, thrombocytopenia.

Dosage: PO 250 mg q8h.

Estramustine phosphate sodium [Emcyt] is a combination of two standard therapies: a hormone and an alkylating agent.

Drug–Food Interactions: Decreased absorption possible with dairy products, calcium supplements.

Side Effects

Nervous System: bowel—diarrhea/flatulence, burning sensation—throat, CHF, cramps—leg, dyspnea, edema—peripheral, headache, insomnia, lethargy, nausea/vomiting, psyche—anxiety/lability, sexual function—impotence.

Endocrine System: (Pregnancy Category X) anorexia, breast tenderness, edema—peripheral, flushing, glucose tolerance—decreased, gynecomastia, hypercalcemia, dry skin, thirst.

Immune System: bone marrow depression* (rare), bruising, CVA,* pulmonary emboli,* GI bleeding, hair thinning, liver function tests—abnormal, leukopenia, MI,* rash, thrombocytopenia, thrombophlebitis.

Dosage: PO 14 mg/kg/d in 3–4 divided doses.

Nilutamide [Nilandron] is a nonsteroidal antiandrogen used to treat metastatic prostatic cancer by blocking androgen receptors.

Drug Interactions: Possible delayed elimination of phenytoin, theophylline, and vitamin K antagonists.

Side Effects

Nervous System: bladder—nocturia, bowel—constipation, dizziness, dyspnea, dyspepsia, headache, hyperesthesia, hypertension, nausea/vomiting, pain—abdominal/back/bone/chest, psyche—depression/insomnia, sexual function—impotence/decreased libido, vision—abnormal/chromatopsia/impaired adaptation to dark.

Endocrine System: (Pregnancy Category C) anorexia, edema—peripheral, fever, hot flushes, gynecomastia, body hair loss, dry skin, sweating, testicular atrophy.

Immune System: ALT/AST—increased, anemia, flu syndrome, hematuria, pneumonia, rash, URI, UTI.

Dosage: PO 50-mg tabs. Start with 6 tabs qd for 30 d. Follow with 150 mg qd thereafter.

Gonadotropin-releasing Hormone Analogs
Releasing hormones from the hypothalamus cause the pituitary to secrete the hormones that stimulate the go-

---
* Life-threatening side effect.

nads to produce sex hormones. By blocking the releasing hormones, sex-hormone tumors are deprived of the hormones they require to sustain them.

<u>Goserelin acetate [Zoladex]</u> inhibits pituitary gonadotropin release to treat cancers of breast or prostate.

Drug Interactions: None noted.

Side Effects

Nervous System: headache, nausea/vomiting, pain—bone.

Endocrine System: (Pregnancy Category X) breast—swelling/tenderness, hot flashes, sexual function—impotence/decreased libido, vaginal—dryness/spotting/breakthrough bleeding.

Immune System: tumor flare.

Dosage: SC 3.6 mg q28d. Depot: 10.8 q12 wk.

<u>Leuprolide acetate [Lupron, Lupron Depot],</u> a synthetic analog of porcine or bovine gonadotropin-releasing hormone (GnRH), is used to block and desensitize pituitary GnRH receptors and ultimately suppress gonadotropin secretion and steroidogenesis, resulting in prostatic and testicular atrophy. It may inhibit hormone-dependent tumors.

Drug Interactions: none noted.

Side Effects

Nervous System: asthenia, arrhythmias, bowel—constipation/diarrhea, dizziness, dysuria, edema—peripheral, headache, myalgia, nausea/vomiting, pain—bone/flank, paresthesia, sexual function—impotence/decreased libido, taste—sour.

Endocrine System: (Pregnancy Category X) amenorrhea, anorexia, breast tenderness, edema—peripheral, fever, hot flashes, gynecomastia, hypoglycemia, vaginal bleeding, thyroid enlargement.

Immune System: flare—disease/pulmonary fibrosis, Hct/Hb—decrease, hematuria, GI bleeding, MI,* pleural rub, rash, swelling-face. Injection site: irritation.

Dosage: Palliation of prostate cancer: SC 1 mg/d; IM 7.5 mg/mo of Depot. Endometriosis, anemia: IM 3.75 mg q mo.

<u>Megestrol acetate [Megace, Pallace].</u> The antineoplastic activity of this drug is not well understood, but possibly it has a pituitary-mediated antiluteinizing action. It is palliative for advanced carcinoma of the breast or endometrium.

---

* Life-threatening side effect.

Drug Interactions: None noted.

Side Effects

Nervous System: breast tenderness, headaches, nausea/vomiting, psyche—depression.

Endocrine System: (Pregnancy Category X) amenorrhea, breakthrough bleeding and spotting, cervical and breast secretions, edema, fever, hirsutism, changes in menstrual bleeding, weight fluctuations.

Immune System: allergic reactions, alopecia, thrombi.

Dosage: Breast cancer: PO 40 mg qid. Endometrial cancer: PO 40–320 mg/d in divided doses.

<u>Tamoxifen citrate [Nolvadex]</u> competes with estrogen for its receptors. It decreases the number of unoccupied estrogen receptors, thus decreasing hormone response. It is used to treat advanced estrogen receptor–positive and stage II breast cancer, advanced prostate cancer, renal cell cancer, and, occasionally, melanoma.

Drug Interactions: Enhanced clotting effects of warfarin possible.

Side Effects

Nervous System: shortness of breath, distaste, dizziness, headache, lightheadedness, nausea/vomiting, pain—bone, sleepiness, vision changes.

Endocrine System: (Pregnancy Category C) anorexia, hot flashes, hypercalcemia, menstrual changes, milk production/leaking, dry skin, weight gain.

Immune System: hair loss, leukopenia, photosensitivity, pruritus vulvae, rash, thrombosis,* vaginal—discharge/bleeding.

Dosage: PO 10—20 mg bid. Stimulate ovulation: PO 5–40 mg bid for 4 d.

MITOTIC INHIBITORS

During the metaphase of mitosis or cell division, the microtubular spines of the dividing cell's two asters begin to form the mitotic spindle. Mitotic inhibitors interfere with this step in cell replication.

<u>Docetaxel [Taxotere]</u> is a semisynthetic derivative of the taxoid family extracted from the needles of the yew tree, *Taxus baccata.* It binds to microtubule tubulin sites and causes clumps to form and halt cell division in metaphase in refractory breast and non-small-cell lung cancers.

Drug Interactions: Modified metabolism with concomitant administration of compounds that induce, inhibit, or are metabolized by cytochrome P450 3B4, eg, cyclosporine, erythromycin, ketoconazole, troleandomycin.

Side Effects

Nervous System: chest tightness, dyspnea, edema, nausea/vomiting, pain—low back, paresthesia, peripheral nerve numbness.

Endocrine System: (Pregnancy Category C) edema, facial flushing.

Immune System: alopecia, anemia, edema—pulmonary, neutropenia, rash, thrombocytopenia.

Dosage: IV 60–100 mg/m² infused over 1 h q21d. Premedicate with dexamethasone 8 mg bid for 5 d starting 1 d prior to decrease fluid retention.

Etoposide [VePesid, others] is cell-cycle specific (G2). It poisons spindles and breaks single-stranded DNA. It is used with other drugs for small-cell anaplastic lung cancer, sarcomas, and solid tumors in breast and lung. It is used as a fall back in combination for testicular germ cell tumors, large cell lymphoma, and Hodgkin's disease.

Drug Interactions: none noted.

Side Effects

Nervous System: arrhythmias—tachycardia, bowel—constipation/diarrhea, bronchospasm,* cramps—abdominal, dyspepsia, dyspnea, hypotension, nausea/vomiting, neuropathy—peripheral, pain—body/chest/throat, paresthesias, psyche—confusion, somnolence, weariness.

Endocrine System: (Pregnancy Category D) anorexia, chills, fever, sweating.

Immune System: alopecia, anaphylaxis, anemia, edema—pulmonary, pleural effusion, leukopenia, severe myelosuppression.* IV site extravasation: necrosis, pain, thrombophlebitis.

Dosage: IV 50–100 mg/m² for 5 d q3–4wk for 3–4 courses, or 100 mg/m² on days 1, 3, and 5, q3–4wk for 3–4 courses. PO: Double the IV dose rounded to the nearest 50 mg. Small-cell lung carcinoma: IV 35 mg/m²/d for 4 d to 50 mg/m²/d for 5 d q3–4wk. PO: Double the IV dose rounded to the nearest 50 mg.

Irinotecan [Camptosar] breaks single strands in DNA in the treatment of advanced colorectal cancer when fluorouracil fails.

Drug Interactions: Increased risk of severe myelosuppression after previous pelvic or abdominal irradiation. Dexamethasone increases risk of lymphocytopenia. Increased chance of akathisia with prochlorperazine. Increased risk of dehydration, secondary to vomiting/diarrhea.

Side Effects

Nervous System: bowel—diarrhea, nausea/vomiting

Endocrine System: (Pregnancy Category D) none noted.

Immune System: leukopenia, myelosuppression.

Dosage: IV. Start with 125 mg/m² in 500 mL of D5W over 90 min weekly for 4 wk. Rest × 2 wk. If no toxicity, subsequent doses may be repeated q6wk.

Paclitaxel [Taxol] is derived from the bark of pacific yew tree *Taxus brevifolia*. It binds to tubulin proteins to cause abnormal microtubule polymerization and cell cycle arrest in metaphase.

Drug Interactions: Increased myelosuppression if cisplatin precedes paclitaxel.

Incompatibilities

Solution/Additive: PVC bags and infusion sets should be avoided due to leaching of DEHP (plasticizer). Do not mix with other medications.

Side Effects

Nervous System: arrhythmias—bradycardia, arthralgia, bronchospasm,* chest pain, hypotension, myalgia, numbness, nausea/vomiting, paresthesias.

Endocrine System: (Pregnancy Category D) flushing.

Immune System: alopecia, anaphylaxis,* cardiotoxicity, neutropenia, urticaria.

Dosage: Ovarian cancer: IV 135 mg/m² 24 h infusion q22d. Breast cancer: IV 175 mg/m² over 3 h q3wk. Kaposi's sarcoma: IV 135 mg/m² infused over 3 h q3wk or 100 mg/m² infused over 3 h q2wk. Solid tumors, malignant melanoma: IV 250 mg/m² over 24 h q3wk.

Note: To reduce hypersensitivity reactions premedicate with dexamethasone PO or IV 20 mg 14 and 7 h prior to taxol infusion; diphenhydramine IV 50 mg 30 min prior to taxol; and cimetidine IV 300 mg or ranitidine IV 50 mg 30 min prior to taxol.

Topotecan [Vumon] is cell-cycle specific (S and G₂ phase) with actions similar to those of etoposide. It is used to treat lymphoma or acute leukemia. It is carcinogenic.

Drug Interactions: Prolonged duration of neutropenia with filgrastim. Increased morbidity/mortality in concomitant use with other neoplastics. Increased myelosuppression with cisplatin.

Side Effects

Nervous System: bowel—diarrhea, dyspnea, headache, hypotension, nausea/vomiting, paresthesia.

Endocrine System: (Pregnancy Category D) none noted.

Immune System: alopecia, anaphylaxis,* myelosuppression. IV site: phlebitis.

---

* Life-threatening side effect.

Dosage: IV 1.5 mg/m² qd × 5 d of a 21-d course for 4 courses.

Vinca Alkaloids

The vinca alkaloids are mitotic inhibitors derived from the periwinkle or vinca plant. They bind to the tubulin protein that forms the microtubules of the spindles, and thus poison the spindles during mitosis.

Vinblastine sulfate [Velban] is cell-cycle specific (M). It stops the metaphase by crystallizing microtubular and spindle proteins. It is used instead of vincristine in Hodgkin's disease and in combination with other drugs for testicular cancer. It is also used alone for renal cancer, choriocarcinoma, breast cancer, and advanced Hodgkin's disease. It is a vesicant.

Drug Interactions: none noted.

Incompatibilities

Solution/Additive: furosemide, heparin.

Y-site: furosemide.

Side Effects

Nervous System: bladder—retention, bowel—constipation/diarrhea, bronchospasm,* convulsions,* ileus, nausea/vomiting, pain—abdominal/muscular/parotid/tumor site, paresthesias—extremities/tongue, psyche—depression, deep tendon reflex—loss, weakness.

Endocrine System: (Pregnancy Category D) anorexia, aspermia, fever, hyperuricemia, weight loss.

Immune System: alopecia, anemia, bleeding—old peptic ulcer/rectal, enterocolitis—hemorrhagic,* leukopenia,* pharyngitis, photosensitivity, Raynaud's, stomatitis, vesiculation. Injection site: cellulitis, phlebitis, sloughing after extravasation.

Dosage: IV 3.7 mg/m² over 1 min qwk. Increase qwk to maximum of 18.5 mg/m² if tolerated.

Vincristine sulfate [Oncovin] is cell-cycle specific (M). It stops metaphase by crystallizing microtubule and spindle proteins in treating Hodgkin's and non-Hodgkin's lymphoma and childhood tumors. It is combined with other drugs for acute lymphocytic leukemia, but is not useful in solid tumors. It is also used for thrombocytopenic purpura (a condition that often goes with SLE). It has more toxicity than the other vinca alkaloids, though most are dose-related and reversible.

Drug Interaction: none noted.

Incompatibilities

Y-site: furosemide.

* Life-threatening side effect.

Side Effects

Nervous System: ataxia, athetosis, bladder—dysuria/polyuria/retention, bowel—constipation (severe)/diarrhea, bronchospasm,* convulsion* (with hypertension), cramps—abdominal, dysphagia, foot/hand drop, headache, hyper-/hypotension, malaise, nausea/vomiting, pain—neuritic, paralytic ileus, paresthesias, psyche—depression, sensory loss, vision—cortical blindness (transient)/diplopia/photophobia/ptosis, deep tendon reflexes loss, weakness—larynx/extrinsic eye muscles.

Endocrine System: (Pregnancy Category D) anorexia, fever, hyperkalemia, hyperuricemia, weight loss.

Immune System: alopecia, hepatotoxicity,* optic atrophy with blindness, parotitis, pharyngitis, rash, SIADH, stomatitis, uric acid nephropathy, urticaria. IV site: cellulitis/phlebitis after extravasation.

Dosage: IV 1.4 mg/m²/wk to a max of 2 mg/m².

Vinorelbine tartrate [Navelbine], a semisynthetic vinca alkaloid, inhibits polymerization of tubules into microtubules, disrupting mitotic spindle formation.

Drug Interactions: Increased granulocytopenia with cisplatin. Increased risk of acute pulmonary reactions with mitomycin.

Incompatibilities

Solution/Additive: acyclovir, aminophylline/theophylline, amphotericin B, ampicillin, cefoperazone, ceforanide, cefotetan, ceftriaxone, fluorouracil, furosemide, ganciclovir, methylprednisolone, mitomycin, piperacillin, sodium bicarbonate, thiotepa, trimethoprim–sulfamethoxazole.

Y-site: acyclovir, aminophylline/theophylline, amphotericin B, cefoperazone, ceforanide, cefotetan, ceftriaxone, fluorouracil, furosemide, ganciclovir, methylprednisolone, mitomycin, piperacillin, sodium bicarbonate, thiotepa, trimethoprim–sulfamethoxazole.

Side Effects

Nervous System: asthenia, bowel—constipation/diarrhea, fatigue, myalgia, nausea/vomiting, pain—injection site/jaw, paralytic ileus, paresthesia, peripheral neuropathy, deep tendon reflex decrease, weakness.

Endocrine System: (Pregnancy Category D) none noted.

Immune System: alopecia, anemia, granulocytopenia,* hepatotoxicity, mucositis, neutropenia,* stomatitis, thrombocytopenia, thrombophlebitis.

Dosage: Non-small-cell lung or breast cancer: IV 30 mg/m²/wk.

MISCELLANEOUS AGENTS

These drugs do not easily fit into any category.

Asparaginase [Colaspase Elspar] is cell-cycle specific. It interferes with DNA/RNA synthesis during the post-mitotic G_1 phase of cell division and disrupts protein synthesis in malignant cells deficient in asparagine synthetase. Extremely toxic, it is used in the acute stages of lymphocytic leukemia and lymphoblastic lymphoma, but not in long term-therapy of solid tumors.

Drug Interactions: Decreased hypoglycemic effects of insulin/sulfonylureas. Increased toxicity possible if given with or immediately before corticosteroids, vincristine. Antitumor effect of methotrexate blocked if asparaginase is given with or immediately before it.

Side Effects

Nervous System: bowel—diarrhea, cramps—abdominal, dizziness, drowsiness, dyspnea, fatigue, nausea/vomiting (severe), pain—flank, Parkinson-like syndrome, psyche—agitation/confusion/depression/hallucinations.

Endocrine System: (Pregnancy Category C) anorexia, azotemia, chills, fever, glycosuria, hyperglycemia, fatal hyperthermia,* hyperuricemia, hypoalbuminemia, hypocalcemia, proteinuria, sweating, weight loss.

Immune System: anaphylaxis,* clotting factors V, VII, VIII, IX—decreased, fibrinogen/platelets—decreased, leukopenia, liver function test—abnormalities, rashes.

Dosage: IV 200 IU/kg qd for 28 d. Inject over at least 30 min into running IV.

Bleomycin sulfate [Blenoxane] is an antitumor antibiotic made from the fungus *Streptomyces*. It is cell-cycle specific (G_2 and M phases); it targets DNA and prevents thymidine attachment to the DNA chain. It is used to treat Hodgkin's (with doxorubicin, vinblastine, and dacarbazine); lymphoma (with cyclophosphamide, vincristine, doxorubicin, and prednisone); and testicular, head, neck, esophageal, skin, and cervical cancers.

Drug Interactions: Increased bone marrow toxicity with other neoplastic agents. Decreased effects of digoxin, phenytoin.

Incompatibilities

Solution/Additive: aminophylline, ascorbic acid, carbenicillin, cephalosporins, diazepam, hydrocortisone, methotrexate, mitomycin, nafcillin, penicillin G, terbutaline.

---

* Life-threatening side effect.

Side Effects

Nervous System: bowel—diarrhea, headache, nausea/vomiting, pain—tumor site, psyche—confusion.

Endocrine System: (Pregnancy Category D) anorexia, weight loss.

Immune System: anaphylaxis.*

Dosage: Lymphoma: SC, IM, IV 10–20 U/m² 1–2 ×/wk after a 1–2 U test dose. Carcinoma/sarcoma and Hodgkin's: SC, IM, IV 10–20 U/m² or 0.25–0.5 U/kg 1–2×/wk to a total dose of 300–400 U. Hodgkin's maintenance: IM, IV 1 U/d or 5 U/wk.

Tretinoin [Retin-A, Vesanoid, others] a combination of retinoic acid and vitamin A acid used to treat acne vulgaris and flat warts and for remission-induction treatment of acute promyelocytic leukemia.

Drug Interactions: Increased inflammation and peeling possible with topical acne medications. Stinging possible with topical products containing alcohol or menthol.

Side Effects

Nervous System: nausea/vomiting

Endocrine System: (Pregnancy: Category B) none noted.

Immune System: blistering, erythema, temporary hyper-/hypopigmentation, local inflammation, scaling.

Dosage: Acute promyelocytic leukemia: PO 45 mg/m²/d. Acne: Topical: Apply q hs.

▶ CHEMOPROTECTANTS

Chemoprotectants help decrease some of the toxic effects of cancer chemotherapy.

Amifostine [Ethyol] is a thiophosphate compound. It is metabolized by membrane-bound alkaline phosphatase to the reduced thiol metabolite to help bind electrophilic metabolites from DNA-binding antineoplastics or ionizing radiation. It is also used as a prophylactic to block cisplatin-induced nephrotoxicity and neurotoxicity without altering antitumor efficacy in patients with advanced ovarian cancer.

Drug Interactions: May potentiate hypotension with antihypertensive drugs.

Side Effects

Nervous System: hypotension, nausea/vomiting, sneezing, somnolence, taste—metallic.

Endocrine System: (Pregnancy Category C) flushing, sensation of cold hands.

Immune System: none noted.

Dosage: IV 910 mg/m² qd in NS over 15 min, 30 min prior to cisplatin, but never with the cisplatin.

Dexrazoxane [Zinecard] intracellularly converts to an iron chelating agent, interfering with iron-mediated free radical generation believed partly responsible for one form of cardiomyopathy. It is used in conjunction with doxorubicin in treating women with metastatic breast cancer who have received a cumulative doxorubicin dose of 300 mg/m².

Drug Interactions: none noted.

Side Effects

Nervous System: none noted.

Endocrine System: (Pregnancy Category C) None noted.

Immune System: granulocytopenia,* leukopenia,* thrombocytopenia.* (It is not clear if these side effects are the result of the dexrazoxane or of the antineoplastics.)

Dosage: IV 10 parts dexrazoxane to 1 part doxorubicin or 500 mg/m² for q 50 mg/m² of doxorubicin q3wk. Administration by slow IV push or rapid IV infusion in 0.9% NaCl or D5W within 6 h of reconstitution. Start doxorubicin within 30 min of beginning dexrazoxane.

Leucovorin calcium [Calcium Folinate, others] is a reduced form of calcium readily available to the cell. An essential cell growth factor given during antineoplastic therapy to protect cells from the action of folic acid antagonists.

Drug Interactions: none noted.

Incompatibilities

Solution/Additive and Y-site: droperidol.

Side Effects

Nervous System: nausea/vomiting, wheezing.

Endocrine System: (Pregnancy Category C) none noted.

Immune System: pruritus, rash, thrombocytosis, urticaria.

Dosage: Megaloblastic anemia: IM, IV no more than 1 mg/d. Leucovorin rescue for methotrexate toxicity: PO, IM, IV 10 mg/m², followed by 10 mg/m² q6h for 72 h. Further doses based on serum methotrexate. Leucovorin rescue for other folate antagonist toxicity: PO, IM, IV 5–15 mg/d. Adjunct in treatment of pneumocystosis or toxoplasmosis: PO, IM, IV 3–6 mg tid.

---

* Life-threatening side effect.

Mesna [Mesnex] reacts in the kidney with urotoxic ifosfamide metabolites to detoxify them and decrease hematuria.

Drug Interactions: Not compatible with cisplatin.

Incompatibilities

Solution/Additive: cisplatin.

Side Effects

Nervous System: nausea/vomiting, taste—foul.

Endocrine System: (Pregnancy Category B) soft stools.

Immune System: none noted.

Dosage: IV dose = 20% of ifosfamide dose and is given at time of ifosfamide administration and 4 and 8 h after ifosfamide administration.

▶ HEMATOPOIETIC GROWTH FACTOR

When therapeutic interventions suppress blood cell production, the patient is vulnerable to hemorrhage and infection. Hematopoietic growth factor spurs cell replacement. Also, patients with chronic renal insufficiency, as well as those with anemias induced by malignancies and AIDS, may need stimulation of RBC production.

Epoetin alfa (human recombinant erythropoietin) [Epogen, Procrit] stimulates bone marrow production of RBCs.

Drug Interactions: none noted.

Side Effects

Nervous System: arthralgias, bowel—diarrhea, headache, hypertension, nausea, pain—bone, seizures.*

Endocrine System: (Pregnancy Category C) iron deficiency, sweating.

Immune System: clotting of AV fistula, thrombocytosis.

Dosage: SC, IV 3–500 U/kg/dose 3 ×/wk. Start with 50–100 U/kg/dose until target Hct range of 30–33% is reached. To maximum of 36%. Rapid increase (over 4 points in a 2-wk period) increases risk of serious adverse reactions. If after 8 wk Hct has not increased 5–6 points, increase dose; then reduce dose after target range is reached or the Hct increases by over 4 points in a 2-wk period. Dose usually increased or decreased by 25 µg/kg increments.

Sargramostim [Leukine, Prokine], a recombinant human granulocyte–macrophage colony stimulating factor (GM-CSF) from yeast, stimulates proliferation and differentiation of hematopoietic progenitor cells in the granulocyte–macrophage pathways.

Drug Interactions: May increase myeloproliferative effects with corticosteroids and lithium.

Incompatibilities

Solution/Additive: haloperidol, hydrocortisone, hydroxyzine.

Y-site: acyclovir, amphotericin B, cefonicid, cefoperazone, chlorpromazine, idarubicin, lorazepam, mitomycin, morphine, nalbuphine, ondansetron, vancomycin.

Side Effects

Nervous System: arrhythmias—abnormal ST segment depression/supraventricular arrhythmias/tachycardia, bowel—diarrhea, arthralgia, edema, fatigue, headache, hypotension, lethargy, malaise, myalgia, nausea/vomiting, pain—bone.

Endocrine System: (Pregnancy Category C) anorexia, fever, hyperuricemia, weight gain.

Immune System: anemia, pericardial effusion,* pericarditis, pleural effusion, pruritus, rash, thrombocytopenia.

First Dose Reaction

Nervous System: arrhythmias—tachycardia, dyspnea, hypotension, nausea/vomiting, pain—leg, rigors, spasms—leg.

---

* Life-threatening side effect.

Endocrine System: (Pregnancy Category C) fever, flushing, sweating.

Immune System: none noted.

Dosage: Autologous bone marrow transplant: IV 250 $\mu g/m^2/d$ infused over 2 h for 21 d. Begin 2–4 h after bone marrow transfusion and not less than 24 h after last dose of chemotherapy or 12 h after last radiation therapy. Neutropenia: SC 3–15 $\mu g/kg/d$.

Chapter Highlights

- Cancer is the result of mutations accumulated over generations of cell replications that begin after one daughter cell acquires the incipient mutation.

- The original anticancer drugs affect the cancer cell nucleus to damage the genetic material in order to halt cell replication.

- Some cancers may become refractory to toxic antineoplastics and even pump them back out of the malignant cells.

- The nurse must use caution in the handling and administration of the toxic carcinogenic drugs.

- Corticosteroids have cell-killing properties and are used in conjunction with other antineoplastics.

- Hormone-dependent cancers are treated with hormone-blocking agents.

- Newer approaches to treating cancer are using the immune system's ability to protect and defend the body.

18 Drugs to Increase or Suppress Immunity

Medical science has learned how to manipulate the immune system to initiate the immune response to many viral and bacterial diseases that decimated whole populations in recurrent epidemics and pandemics that were so severe they changed the course of history. Witness the destruction of indigenous peoples by diseases brought to the western hemisphere by Europeans. Immunizations have now prevented unnecessary pain, suffering, and death. On the other hand, the ability to suppress the immune response has made organ transplant possible. Has the immune system been tamed and domesticated? Not really—not yet. The search continues for vaccines for AIDS and some cancers. But even if there were a vaccine for every disease, new ones would develop. Plagues will probably always be one viral or bacterial mutation away.

The use of vaccination to prevent infectious disease dates back to 1796, when the English physician Edward Jenner tested a hunch that cowpox protected against smallpox infection by vaccinating a boy, considered expendable as a subhuman member of the underclass, with a preparation of live cowpox. The boy survived the vaccination. Aggressive programs of vaccination to prevent smallpox have eradicated that viral plague from the planet some 200 years after Jenner's experiment. In 1881, Louis Pasteur infected chickens with aged cholera culture and found that the aged cultures seemed not to infect the chickens, so he infected them with fresh cultures, which also failed to sicken them. He realized that the weak, aged cultures had somehow made the chickens immune to the fresh cholera culture.

Following Pasteur's lead, modern vaccines are made from weakened (attenuated) or killed infectious organisms, which stimulate the immune system to create antibodies to mark the foreign proteins of the vaccine and protect against future infection. Routine immunization of infants and children against once-common diseases like mumps, measles, pertussis, and polio has decreased childhood morbidity and mortality. However, the protein preparations used may pose a small risk of allergic reaction, and immunization cannot be fully guaranteed in all cases. In addition, on rare occasions, the preparation may actually cause the disease. The nurse should always have an allergy kit with epinephrine on hand and a doctor's order to use it when giving inoculations. The nervous system, endocrine system, and immune system (Master Systems) responses to inoculation include the following:

Nervous System: fatigue, malaise, myalgia, and pain at injection site.

Endocrine System: (Pregnancy Category C) fever. With the possible exception of rubella, vaccination during pregnancy is not contraindicated.

Immune System: allergy, anaphylaxis, the actual disease—rare, encephalopathy (within 7 d after vaccination)

▶ ROUTINE IMMUNIZATIONS FOR CHILDHOOD DISEASES

Routine immunization for childhood diseases has cut infant mortality from preventable infectious diseases and improved life expectancy rates. Prior to the discovery of vaccines, it was not unusual for a family to lose one or more infants and children to diseases now rarely seen, such as diphtheria. Though some parents fear that such immunizations may cause serious side effects, the nurse may assure the parents that the side effects are extremely rare, but that the unprevented disease may cost the child unnecessary suffering, possible physical sequelae, and even death.

Hepatitis B vaccine recombinant [Engerix-B, Recombivax HB] contains inactivated and purified hepatitis B surface antigen (HBsAg) derived from human plasma, but no human plasma is used in its production. A gene splicing technique is used. The vaccine protects against hepatitis B viral infection, which is associated with liver cancer. Even adults should be vaccinated.

Dosage: IM Recombivax: 1 mL at 0, 1, and 6 mo. Engerix B: 1 mL at 0, 1, and 6 mo or 0, 1, 2, and 12 mo.

Mumps vaccine [Mumpsvax] protects against mumps, an acute viral infection characterized by swollen parotid glands. It is most often acquired between the ages of 5 and 15, but adults can be infected, and severely.

Dosage: SC 0.5 mL at 12 mo, with a booster before the child enters school.

Pertussis vaccine protects against whooping cough, a gram-negative coccobacillus infection of the respiratory tract, characterized by paroxysmal coughing that ends in a loud, "whooping" inspiration. It is usually contracted by infants and children less than age 4 y.

Dosage: See *combinations*.

Sabin vaccine [Orimune] protects against poliovirus. Poliovirus is caused by one or more of three RNA viruses. The vaccine is trivalent.

Dosage: PO 0.5 mL in 4 doses at 2 mo, 4 mo, and 18 mo, then after 4–6 y (before the child enters school).

Rubella vaccine [Meruvax II] protects against German measles, a viral, droplet-spread infection causing URI and a fine red maculopapular rash.

Dosage: SC 0.5 mL at 12 mo, with a booster before the child enters school.

Rubeola vaccine [Attenuvax] protects against rubeola, a paramyxovirus contagion also called measles, spread by droplets from the nose, mouth, and throat and causing URI and a spreading maculopapular rash.

Dosage: SC 0.5 mL at 12 mo, with a booster before the child enters school, usually in combination with mumps and rubella.

Note: Mumps, measles, and rubella vaccines (MMR) are given at 12 mo and at 4–6 y or before the child enters school.

Varicella vaccine [Varivax]

Dosage: SC 0.5 mL; 2 doses 4–8 wk apart. Children: one dose.

▶ COMBINATIONS

Diphtheria, pertussis, and tetanus toxoid vaccine (DPT) protects against all three diseases.

Dosage: IM 0.5 mL for 3 doses q4–6wk. Give at 2 mo, 4 mo, 6 mo. Boosters at 15 mo and 4–6 y.

Diphtheria and tetanus toxoids (DT) protects against the two diseases.

Dosage: IM 0.5 mL in 2 doses 4 wk apart. Boosters in 1 y and at school enrollment age.

▶ VACCINATIONS FOR HIGH-RISK SITUATIONS

Cholera vaccine protects against cholera, a diarrheal infectious disease.

Dosage: Over 10 y: SC, IM 0.5 mL. Repeat in 4 wk and then q6mo as needed. (6 mo–4 y: 0.2 mL, 5–10 y: 0.3 mL.)

Hemophilus B polysaccharide vaccine is for a disease usually of preschool children. Although not a routine immunization, it is recommended for all children 2 mo–6 y, especially those in day-care facilities.

Dosage: SC 0.5 mL. Option 1: 2 mo, 4 mo, 6 mo, with a booster at 15 mo. Option 2: 2 mo, 4 mo, and 12 mo.

Hepatitis A vaccine provides active immunization for people 2 y of age or older. Primary immunization should be completed at least 2 wk before expected exposure to hepatitis A. It is recommended for travelers to areas where the disease is endemic and for persons engaging in high-risk sexual activity, residents of a community experiencing hepatitis A outbreak, users of illicit injectable drugs, certain institutional workers (eg, caretakers for the developmentally challenged), employees of child day-care centers, laboratory workers who handle live hepatitis A virus, and handlers of primate animals that may be harboring hepatitis A. For those requiring both immediate and long-term protection, hepatitis A vaccine may be administered concomitantly with immune globulin.

Dosage: IM 1 mL 2 doses given 1 mo apart. Booster 6–12 mo after primary course. (24–18 y: 0.5 mL.)

Influenza vaccine is formulated each year to anticipate the viruses most likely to cause an epidemic. Scientists go yearly to the farms and markets of Asia, looking for viral variations that signal a new flu strain. These flu viruses appear to originate in Asia and then spread around the globe. Consider some of their names: Asian flu, Shanghai flu, Hong Kong flu . . .

Dosage: SC 0.5 mL every year.

Meningitis vaccine is from *N. meningitides* groups A and C or A, C, Y, and W-135. Children under 2 y should receive only group A.

Dosage: SC 0.5 mL.

Plague vaccine protects against plague.

Dosage: IM 1.0 mL; then 0.2 mL in 1–3 mo; third dose after 3–6 mo.

Pneumococcal vaccine [Pneumovax 23, Pnu-imune 23], a polyvalent, is for adults with chronic debilitating disease to protect them from 23 pneumococcal strains.

Dosage: SC, IM 0.5 mL in 1 dose.

Rabies vaccine protects against rabies either before or after exposure.

Dosage: IM 1.0 mL. Repeat in 1 wk and 4 wk after initial dose. Boosters q2y. Postexposure prophylaxis: IM 1 mL. Repeat 3, 7, 14, and 28 d later. In addition, rabies immune globulin is given with first dose for passive immunity.

Tetanus toxoid is used to prevent a neuromuscular dysfunction caused by the exotoxin of *Clostridium tetani*.

Dosage: IM 0.5 mL. Repeat in 4–8 wk, and in again in 6–12 mo.

Tuberculin skin test reveals antibody formation and thus exposure to TB, but not infection.

Dosage: Intradermal, using a TB syringe. 0.1 mL of test solution to raise a weal. Read after 48 h.

Tuberculosis vaccine protects against TB.

Dosage: Intradermal using multiple puncture. 0.1 mL.

Typhoid vaccine [Vivotif Berna] is recommended for persons traveling to areas where typhoid is endemic.

Dosage: SC 0.5 mL. Repeat in 4 wk. Booster SC 0.5 mL or intradermal 0.1 mL q3y. PO 1 capsule on 4 alternate days, 1 h ac with cold to lukewarm water. (<10 y: 0.25 mL q3 y)

Yellow Fever vaccine [YF-Vax] is recommended for persons traveling to areas where yellow fever is endemic.

Dosage: SC 0.5 mL. Booster q10y.

▶ ANTITOXINS AND IMMUNE SERUMS

Though vaccines prevent some contagious diseases by purposely introducing specific antigens into the body to stimulate the creation of antibodies, antitoxins and immune serums provide passive immunity when the patient has been exposed to potentially virulent and deadly microbes without being vaccinated first, or when there is no vaccine for the disease. Passive immunity agents include antitoxins, the antibodies developed by

other species, and immune serums, the antibodies or globulins that are harvested from pooled human plasma. Antitoxins require a sensitivity test first to rule out potentially serious immune response to the donor animal's proteins. Serums are less likely to cause allergic response.

ANTITOXINS

Botulism antitoxin is for the severe food poisoning caused by the toxins of *Clostridium botulinus*. The antitoxin is available from the Centers for Disease Control and Prevention in Atlanta, Georgia, (404-639-3670; www.cdc.gov).

Dosage: Test first for sensitivity. Then give IV one 10-mL vial intravenously and 1 vial IM. If symptoms worsen after 4 h, give another vial IV. Then 1 more vial after 12–24 h.

Diphtheria antitoxin is given in conjunction with the appropriate antibiotic, eg, erythromycin, penicillin, or tetracycline, to further protect the patient.

Dosage: Prophylactically: IM 5000–10,000 U. As part of the treatment: IV 20,000–120,000 U.

Rabies antirabies serum is given in addition to rabies vaccine when the patient has suffered deep multiple bites, especially near the brain and spinal cord.

Dosage: IM 55 U/kg, with half of the dose injected around the bites.

Tetanus antitoxin is used in the event no tetanus immune globulin, human, is available.

Dosage: SC, IM 1500–5000 U within 24 h or 10,000–20,000 U within 48 h of the injury. Treatment of tetanus: IM, IV (divide dosage and use both routes) 50,000–100,000 U.

IMMUNE SERUMS

Gamma-globulin, immune globulin intramuscular, immune serum globulin [Gammar], immune globulin intravenous [Gamimune N, Iveegam, others] are made from plasma pooled from many donors. They contain immunoglobulin G (IgG), which, in turn, contains concentrated antibodies to such diseases as bacterial infections, hepatitis, rubella, and rubeola. Gamma globulin provides passive immunity to either prevent the disease or decrease its severity in relatively healthy individuals as well as in those compromised by immunoglobulin deficiency or severe infection or burns.

Dosage: Hepatitis A exposure: IM 0.02–0.04 mL/kg as soon as possible. For prolonged exposure give 0.05–0.06 mL/kg once q4–6mo. Hepatitis B exposure: IM

0.02–0.06 mL/kg as soon as possible after exposure if HBIG is not available. Rubella: Only the susceptible pregnant woman needs the vaccine to protect the fetus in the first trimester: IM 20 mL. Rubeola: IM 0.25 mL/kg within a week of exposure. Varicella-zoster Exposure: IM 0.6–1.2 mL/kg as soon as possible. Immunoglobulin deficiency: IM 1.2 mL/kg followed by 0.6 mL/kg q2–4wk. IV: Gammagard or others: 100 mg/kg/mo. Idiopathic thrombocytopenic Purpura: IV 400 mg/kg for 5 consecutive d or 1 g/kg qod for up to 3 doses.

Hepatitis B immune globulin [H-Big, Hep-B-Gammagee, Hyper Hep].

Dosage: IM 0.06 mL/kg as soon as possible, preferably within 24 h. Repeat in 1 mo.

Lymphocyte immune globulin [At-gam] contains antibodies that attack the recipient's own cell-mediated and humoral immunity, destroying T lymphocytes and other immune factors in organ transplant patients to prevent transplant rejection.

Dosage: IV 10–30 mg/kg/d.

Rabies immune globulin [Hyperab] is given in conjunction with rabies vaccine after exposure.

Dosage: IM 20 U/kg with half the dose injected around the bite(s) or broken skin.

Tetanus immune globulin [Hyper-Tet] is given in addition to tetanus toxoid upon exposure.

Dosage: Prophylaxis: IM 250 U. Treatment: IM 3000–6000 U.

▶ IMMUNITY DURING PREGNANCY

During pregnancy the woman's immune response to foreign proteins in the blood and tissue of the gestating embryo/fetus is suppressed by the products of conception. Understanding the process promises to unlock some mysteries of the immune system. The closer the embryo's genetic endowment is to the mother's, the less vigorous the embryo's suppressing action, leading to a greater chance of spontaneous abortion, perhaps decreasing the chances for congenital defects being passed on.

THE Rh FACTOR

Rh-positive blood from an embryo/fetus stirs a vigorous immune response by the Rh-negative mother's immune system. This occurs either when the pregnancy is aborted

or at birth when blood from each makes contact. Subsequent Rh-positive pregnancies are threatened when the mother's immune system develops antibodies against the Rh factor.

Rho(D) immune globulin [Gamulin Rh, HypRho-D, Rho GAM] is given to impart a passive immunity for the Rh factor to the mother, thus preventing the development of antibodies that would reject future Rh-positive pregnancies.

Dosage: IM 1 vial at ≤ 28 wk and within 72 hours of exposure. Obstetrics: 1 vial for every 15 mL fetal packed red cells. Transfusion accident: 1 vial for every 15 mL of Rh-positive packed red cell volume.

▶ DRUGS TO SUPPRESS THE IMMUNE RESPONSE

The immune response is meant to help us survive against a sea of infectious diseases, but sometimes the response is unwelcome. Drugs to suppress the immune response have been invaluable in making organ transplant possible. Without such drugs the immune system would reject the foreign tissue. In addition, in the quest to treat allergy, drugs are being developed that suppress the immune response that causes asthma.

Azathioprine [Imuran] inhibits DNA, RNA, and normal protein synthesis in rapidly growing cells and suppresses T-cell effects before transplant rejection.

Side Effects

Nervous System: arthralgia, bowel—diarrhea, dysarthria, nausea/vomiting.

Endocrine System: (Pregnancy Category C) anorexia, biliary stasis, alkaline phosphatase—elevated, steatorrhea.

Immune System: agranulocytosis,* alopecia, anemia, AST/ALT/bilirubin—increased, bone marrow depression,* carcinogenisis, esophagitis, hepatitis/toxic hepatitis, infections, leukopenia, rash, teratogenisis, thrombocytopenia.

Dosage: Renal transplantation: PO 3–5 mg/kg/d; may be able to reduce to 1–3 mg/kg/d. IV 3–5 mg/kg/d; may be able to reduce to 1–3 mg/kg/d. Rheumatoid arthritis: PO 1 mg/kg/d; may increase by 0.5 mg/kg/d at 4- to 6-wk intervals if needed to maximum of 2.5 mg/kg/d.

Cyclosporin [Sandimmune], discovered in the mud of a Norwegian forest, calls off the attack of the WBCs that

---

* Life-threatening side effect.

would destroy a transplanted organ without killing the WBCs. This drug in combination with corticosteroids makes organ transplant feasible.

Side Effects

Nervous System: ataxia, bladder—frequency/retention, bowel—constipation/diarrhea, convulsions,* cramps—legs, discomfort—abdominal, headache, hearing—loss/tinnitus, hyperesthesia, hypertension, insomnia, lethargy, nausea/vomiting, night sweats, pain—chest, paraparesis, paresthesias, psyche—anxiety/flat affect/amnesia/confusion/depression/visual hallucinations, tremor, weakness.

Endocrine System: (Pregnancy Category C) anorexia, chills, edema, fever, flushing, gynecomastia, hirsutism, hyperglycemia, hyperkalemia, hypermagnesemia, hyperuricemia, oliguria, oily skin, serum bicarbonate—decreased, weight loss.

Immune System: acne, anemia, gastritis, gingival hyperplasia, infections, leukopenia, lymphoma, MI*—rare, nephrotoxicity, sinusitis, sore throat, thrombocytopenia.

Dosage: PO 14–18 mg/kg 4–12 h preoperatively. Maintenance: 5–10 mg/kg qd. IV 5–6 mg/kg 4–12 h preoperatively. Continue until PO is feasible. RA: PO 2.5 mg/kg/d in 2 doses; gradual increase q4wk to max of 4 mg/kg/d. Severe psoriasis: PO 1.25 mg/kg bid. If needed after 4 wk increase 0.5 mg/kg/d q2wk to a max of 4 mg/kg/d.

Muromonab-CD3 [Orthoclone OKT3], a murine monoclonal antibody, targets the T3 (CD3) molecule in the antigen recognition site of the T cell, causing removal of CD3-positive T cells from circulation. The product is used to prevent renal inflammation and destruction in kidney transplant and should be given as soon as signs of rejection are noted. **Caution:** Only a physician may administer. Have crash cart available.

Side Effects

Nervous System: arrhythmias—tachycardia, bowel—diarrhea, dyspnea, malaise, nausea/vomiting, pain—chest, tremors, wheezing.

Endocrine System: (Pregnancy Category C) chills, fever.

Immune System: pulmonary edema*—severe, susceptibility to infection by molds, bacteria, and viruses such as cryptococcus, cytomegalovirus, gram-negative bacteria, herpes simplex, *Pneumocystis carinii, Serratia.*

Dosage: IV bolus in under 1 min. 5 mg qd for 10–14 d.

---

* Life-threatening side effects.

▶ LEUKOTRIENE INHIBITORS

Leukotrienes are messenger molecules in the immune system—fatty acids that mediate inflammation as they bind to smooth muscle cells in the airway.

Cromolyn sodium [Disodium Cromoglycate, DSCG Intal, Gastrocrom, Nasalcrom] stabilizes mast cells and is used in conjunction with glucocorticoids so that the steroids can be reduced or discontinued (Fig. 18–1). Like the glucocorticoids, this drug is not for the treatment of the acute asthma attack. Rather, it helps to prevent attacks, especially exercise- or antigen-induced attacks. Cromolyn sodium inhibits the release of leukotrienes and histamine from mast cells. But histamine is not the culprit in asthma. The slow-reacting substance of anaphylaxis from sensitized pulmonary mast cells is implicated in asthma. Cromolyn sodium is used for IgE-mediated or extrinsic asthma caused by exposure to specific allergens, eg, dander, dust, and pollens. Cromolyn may interfere with calcium transport across cell membranes.

Drug Interactions: none noted.

Side Effects

Nervous System: arrhythmias—palpitations/PVCs/tachycardia, arthralgia, bladder—dysuria/frequency, bronchospasm,* convulsions,* cough, dizziness, dyspnea, fatigue, headache, legs—stiff/weak, lethargy, lightheadedness (pc), migraine, myalgia, nausea/vomiting, pain—chest, psyche—anxiety/behavior change/depression/hallucinations/insomnia/nervousness/psychosis, slightly bitter after-taste, tinnitus.

Endocrine System: (Pregnancy Category B) edema, flushing.

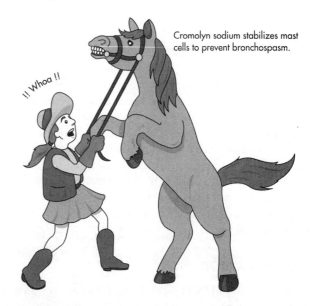

Cromolyn sodium stabilizes mast cells to prevent bronchospasm.

!! Whoa !!

Figure 18-1. Cromolyn sodium preventing a "broncho" spasm.

Immune System: anaphylaxis,* angioedema,* contact dermatitis, peripheral eosinophilia, erythema, esophagitis, eyes—itchy/puffy, hepatic function tests—abnormal, LE syndrome, nasal congestion/stinging/burning, swollen parotids, peripheral neuritis, photosensitivity, pruritus, purpura, rash, throat/trachea irritation, urticaria.

Dosage: PO 100 mg-capsule qid 30 min ac and hs. Open the capsule and dissolve in ½ glass of hot water. Add ½ glass of cold water while stirring. Do not use juices. Inhalation per metered inhaler or capsule: 1 spray qid. Nasal solution: 1 spray in each nostril 3–6 ×/d at regular intervals. Prevent further eye inflammation: Ophthalmic 4% solution 1–2 gtt (1.6 mg/gtt) per eye 4–6 ×/d.[†]

<u>Glatiramer acetate for injection [Copaxone]</u> modifies the immune processes in the treatment of multiple sclerosis. Its use comes from the fact that it reduces the incidence and severity of experimental allergic encephalomyelitis (EAE)—a condition induced in several animal species through immunization against CNS-derived material containing myelin and often used as an experimental animal model of MS.

Drug Interactions: none noted.

Side Effects

Nervous System: arrhythmias—tachycardia, arthralgia, bladder—urgency, bowel—diarrhea, dyspnea, edema—peripheral, foot drop, gastrointestinal disorder, hypertonia, laryngismus, migraine, pain—back/chest/ear/neck, palpitations, psyche—agitation/anxiety/confusion/nervousness, speech disorder, syncope, tremor, vertigo, vision—disorders/nystagmus.

Endocrine System: (Pregnancy Category B) anorexia, chills, dysmenorrhea, edema, fever, flushing, sweating, weight gain.

Immune System: bacterial infection, bronchitis, cyst, ecchymosis, edema—facial, erythema, flu syndrome, herpes simplex, gastroenteritis, infection, lymphadenopathy, pruritus, rash, rhinitis, skin nodules, urticaria, vaginal moniliasis. Injection site: erythema/hemorrhage/induration/inflammation/mass/pain/pruritus/urticaria/welt.

Dosage: SC 20 mg qd for relapsing-remitting MS.

<u>Zafirlukast [Accolate]</u> is the first in a new line of drugs called leukotriene inhibitors, which prevent leukotrienes from mobilizing immune cells in response to allergens. Zafirlukast competes for the receptor sites of leukotriene D_4 and E_4, part of the chemical cascade of slow-reacting substance of anaphylaxis (SRSA). SRSA is associated with the inflammation process in asthma that accounts for airway edema, smooth muscle constriction, and altered cellular activity.

Drug Interactions: Increased PT of warfarin. Decreased levels with erythromycin. Decreased plasma levels with theophylline.

Side Effects

Nervous System: asthenia, diarrhea, dizziness, dyspepsia, myalgia, nausea/vomiting, pain—abdominal/back.

Endocrine System: (Pregnancy Category B) fever.

Immune System: ALT—elevation, URI—increased in patients over 55.

Dosage: PO 20 mg tab AM and hs 1 h ac or 2 h pc.

 Chapter Highlights

- Immunizations have prevented countless instances of infection, suffering, and death by providing passive immunity or stimulating active immunity.

- Immunosuppressants have saved the lives of people requiring organ transplant.

- Inroads have been made on countering the slow-reacting substance of anaphylaxis, which causes the allergic response of asthma.

- Learning to harness the power of the immune system offers the potential to gain an advantage over the infectious and allergic agents that surround us.

[†] Eye related.

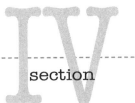

section IV

The Gastrointestinal Tract and Drugs

This section contains only one chapter. It describes a part of us that is also not a part of us. It is not nervous system or endocrine system or immune system. The alimentary canal is a paradox. It is us, but it is also not us. A river truly runs through us. The nervous system controls its flow with muscular waves of peristalsis that force its contents along. The endocrine system seeks nutrients from the canal. The immune systems patrols the lining of the lumen, killing swarms of pathogens that are vying for the same nutrients in this watery mass and enter the bloodstream to the liver, which is also heavily guarded. Drugs that work in the lumen can help kill pathogens directly, aid breakdown of food, influence water content and bulk, and coat or irritate the lining. But aside from the vitamins, medical agents that work in the canal tend to act locally and not enter the body. To better understand how the alimentary canal works, here is the story of a hamburger (Max Burgher) making its way through the canal (Fig. IV–1).

THE STORY OF MAX

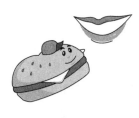

Max Burgher enters the alimentary canal,

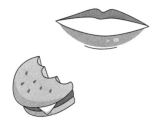

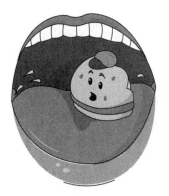

little jets in the salivary glands spray Max with amylase to break down his starch. Teeth tear at him and grind him smaller and smaller until . . . he is swallowed and, after a six-second fall, he finds himself in bits and pieces in a great bag filled with hydrochloric acid, secreted in response to histamine from gastric parietal cells. Max is held here while he is kneaded into a slimy mass more appropriately called "Max Chyme."

Figure IV–1. The travels of Max Burgher (*continued*).

281

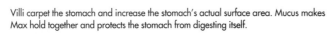

Villi carpet the stomach and increase the stomach's actual surface area. Mucus makes Max hold together and protects the stomach from digesting itself.

Max's proteins are broken down by pepsin, which hydrochloride (HCl) makes from pepsinogen. Gastric lipase goes to work on Max's emulsified fats. Rennin waits to break down milk products.

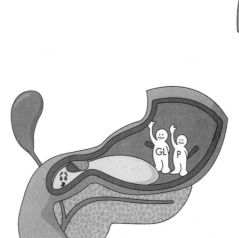

Max Chyme doesn't know which way is up. Rings of muscle squeeze him into little Max Chymes or boluses—slowly swirled by long ribbons of muscle, swayed to and fro by the local muscles. The villi carpet fans the mixed-up Max even more. To add to all this motion, peristalsis, caused by more muscle rings, keeps Max Boluses moving ever onward into the . . .

DUODENUM . . .

Because Max started out as a solid, he will move more slowly than if he had been a liquid. And because of his high caloric content, his exit from the stomach will be slowed.

Special cells lining the duodenum and jejunum produce and secrete secretin to stimulate pancreatic secretions to neutralize the acid Max Bolus has picked up in the stomach. This watery solution contains much sodium and some potassium, calcium, and magnesium. It's a little like offering Max Bolus a TUMS. At the same time the gallbladder contracts and squeezes bile onto Max Bolus.

Bile contains sodium bicarbonate, chloride, bile acids, electrolytes in solution, lecithin, cholesterol, pigment, some protein, and whatever the liver has metabolized in the way of detoxified drugs, etc.

Cholecystokinin in the duodenum is what stimulates the gallbladder to contract. Its twin, pancreozymin, plus secretin stimulate the pancreas.

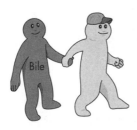

Bile will travel with Max Bolus through the intestine, helping to emulsify fat. Biliary acids will dissolve cholesterol and free any fatty acids and fat-soluble vitamins.

Most of the bile is reabsorbed and goes back to the liver to start over.

Some of it is attacked by bacteria.

Only about 5% of the secreted bile will make the great escape from the end of the alimentary canal.

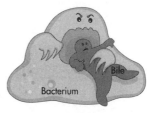

MEANWHILE. . . .

Back at the pancreas, enzymes are released to break down raw or cooked starch and glycogen (amylolytic enzyme). Lipolytic enzymes work on the fats bile doesn't coat. (The pancreas also releases three enzymes—trypsin, chymotrypsin, and catboxypeptidase—to break down protein.)

The starches become sugars. Proteins are broken down into their smaller parts.

Figure IV-1 (continued). The travels of Max Burgher (*continued*).

AT LAST . . . ABSORPTION . . .

"Max Sugars," "Max Proteins," and "Max Fats" leave the intestine by different paths. Some pass through the mucosa into the portal blood. Some move from greater to lesser concentration . . . that's osmosis.

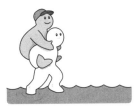

Some are carried or ferried, and still others are engulfed and drawn into the portal blood system.

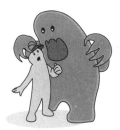

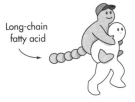

Long-chain fatty acid

To lymph

Protein carrier

Most fats are carried by proteins into the lymph circulation. The lymphatic circulation ultimately empties into the general blood circulation.

By the time Max Bolus has traveled the 20-plus feet of the small intestine, the sugars, fats, and proteins have found the exits to blood and lymph circulation. The portal system carries blood from the gut to the liver for further processing and detoxification—sanitizing.

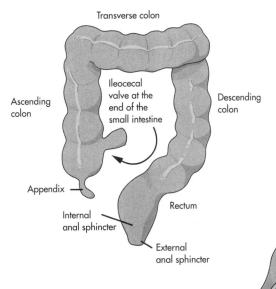

Transverse colon

Ascending colon

Ileocecal valve at the end of the small intestine

Descending colon

Appendix

Internal anal sphincter

Rectum

External anal sphincter

In the colon, most of the water that held all the digesting fluids that poured on Max Burgher is reabsorbed. (More or less twice the water that Max Burger once had.)

Of course, sodium (Na) and H_2O have an intimate relationship and Na is absorbed here with the H_2O. Other minerals exit here too.

Bacteria create vitamin K and some of the B vitamins. The vitamins are absorbed from the colon. The bacteria also create hydrogen sulfide and methane gases.

As Max Feces prepares to leave, he is a jumble of fiber, bacteria, water, and protein sloughed from the walls of the alimentary canal.

THE END

Figure IV-1 (continued). The travels of Max Burgher.

Drugs That Work
in the Intestinal Lumen

- activated charcoal, liquid antidote [Actidose, Charcoaid, others]
- antacids [Gelusil, Maalox, others]
- bisacodyl [Dulcolax]
- bismuth subsalicylate [Pepto-Bismol]
- cascara sagrada [Cas-Evac]
- cholestyramine resin [Questran, others]
- colestipol [Colestid]
- docusate calcium [Surfak, others]
- docusate sodium [Colace, Doxinate, others]
- folate sodium [Volvite Sodium]
- glycerin [Glycerol, Glyrol]
- ivermectin [Stromectol]
- lactulose [Cephulac, Chronulac]
- magnesium citrate solution [Citrate of Magnesium, Citroma, Citro-Nesia]
- magnesium hydroxide [Milk of Magnesia (MOM)]
- mebendazole [Vermox]
- mineral oil [Fleet Mineral Oil, Petrogalar, Fleet Mineral Oil Enema]
- pancrelipase [Cotazym, Pancrease, others]
- piperazine citrate [Antepar]
- polyethylene glycolelectrolyte solution [GoLYTELY]
- psyllium hydrophilic mucilloid [Metamucil, others]
- pteroylglutamic acid [Folacin, others]
- pyrantel pamoate [Antiminth]
- senna pod preparation [Black-Draught, Gentlax B, Senexon, Senokot, Senolax]
- sodium phosphate, sodium biphosphate [Fleet Phosphosoda, Fleet Enema]
- sucralfate [Carafate]
- thiabendazole [Mintezol]
- vitamin A
- vitamin B_1 (thiamine hydrochloride)
- vitamin B_2 (riboflavin)
- vitamin B_3 (niacin) [Niac, Nicobid, others]

- vitamin B$_6$ (pyridoxine)
- vitamin B$_9$ (folic acid)
- vitamin B$_{12}$ (cyanocobalamin)
- vitamin B$_{12A}$ (hydroxocobalamin)
- vitamin C (ascorbic acid) [Ascorbicap, others]
- vitamin E (tocopherol) [Aquasol E, others]

▶ PANCREATIC ENZYMES

Pancreatic enzymes replace missing or insufficient naturally occurring enzymes that break down raw or cooked starch, glycogen, and fat. Some such enzymes can be purchased over the counter, whereas others require prescriptions.

Pancrelipase [Cotazym, Pancrease, others] is made from pork and replaces missing enzyme in malabsorption syndrome due to cystic fibrosis or other conditions of exocrine pancreatic insufficiency.

Drug Interactions: Decreased absorption of iron possible.

Side Effects

Nervous System: High doses: diarrhea/nausea/vomiting.

Endocrine System: (Pregnancy Category C) High doses: hyperuricosuria.

Immune System: none noted.

Dosage: PO. Capsules or tabs 1–3 ac or with food to maximum of 8, or 1–2 packets of powder 1–2 h ac, with meals or 1 h pc, with an extra dose with food between meals.

▶ ANTACIDS

These weakly basic inorganic salts neutralize gastric acid, thereby inhibiting pepsin's action. The aluminum salts bind phosphate and bile salts. They give relief for heartburn and indigestion in peptic ulcer disease (PUD) and gastroesophageal reflux disease (GERD).

Antacids [Gelusil, Maalox, others] are usually combinations of aluminum hydroxide plus magnesium hydroxide. Though they act in the lumen of the digestive tract, their cations do get absorbed to a degree. They may decrease absorption of other drugs.

Drug Interactions: Aluminum hydroxide preparations decrease absorption of chloroquine, cimetidine, ciprofloxacin, digoxin, isoniazid, iron salts, NSAIDs, norfloxacin, ofloxacin, phenytoin, phenothiazines, quinidine, tetracycline, thyroxine. Systemic alkalosis possible with sodium polystyrene sulphonate. Magnesium hydroxide preparation decreases absorption of chlordiazepoxide, dicumarol, digoxin, isoniazid, quinolones, tetracyclines.

Side Effects

Nervous System: bowel—constipation/diarrhea.

Endocrine System: (Pregnancy Category C) alkalosis, hypercalcemia, hypermagnesemia, hypophosphatemia, nephrolithiasis.

Immune System: nosocomial pneumonia.

Dosage: GERD: PO 10–30 mL prn or 1 and 3 h pc and hs. PUD: PO 100–160 mEq of acid-neutralizing capacity per dose 1 and 3 h pc and hs for 4–8 wk or until healed.

Note: *Sometimes simethicone is added to these preparations to decrease gas in the GI tract.*

▶ LOCALIZED ULCER TREATMENT

A combination of sulfated sucrose and aluminum hydroxide is used to treat ulcers by combining with the surface of the ulcer and forming a cover to protect the ulcer from further damage by gastric acids, pepsin, and bile salts.

Sucralfate [Carafate] is used to treat gastric ulcers.

Drug Interactions: Decreased absorption possible of digoxin, phenytoin, quinolones, tetracycline.

Side Effects

Nervous System: constipation, diarrhea, nausea.

Endocrine System: (Pregnancy Category B) dry mouth.

Immune System: none noted.

Dosage: PO 1 g 1 h ac and hs. Maintenance: 1 g bid. If antacids are also used, administer them 1/2 h before or after the sucralfate.

▶ BILE AND CHOLESTEROL BINDERS

Bile and cholesterol binders adhere to fatty substances in the gut to prevent their absorption and to reduce circulating cholesterol. Forming an insoluble mass, they are excreted in the feces.

Psyllium hydrophilic mucilloid [Metamucil, others] is thought to bind with dietary cholesterol, preventing absorption. It also creates bulk to stimulate peristalsis and elimination.

Drug Interactions: Decreased absorption of antibiotics, digoxin, nitrofurantoin, salicylates, warfarin.

Side Effects

Nervous System: Excessive use: cramps—abdominal, diarrhea, nausea/vomiting. In dry form: abdominal cramps, GI tract strictures.

Endocrine System: (Pregnancy Category C) none noted.

Immune System: Excessive use: eosinophilia.

Dosage: 1–2 rounded tsp or 1 packet daily to tid in fluid.

Cholestyramine resin [Questran, others] acts in the gut to bind bile acids and thus decrease fat absorption. It helps eliminate lindane, a chlorinated hydrocarbon that causes CNS excitation.

Drug Interactions: Decreased absorption of oral anticoagulants, digoxin, iron salts, penicillins, phenobarbital, tetracyclines, thiazide diuretics, thyroid hormones, fat-soluble vitamins.

Side Effects

Nervous System: belching, bowel—bloating/constipation/diarrhea/flatulence/impaction, heartburn, nausea/vomiting, pain—abdominal, uveitis, sexual function—increased libido.

Endocrine System: (Pregnancy Category C) acidosis—hyperchloremic, anorexia, deficiencies—calcium/iron/vitamins A, D, K, folate levels—decreased in erythrocytes, steatorrhea, weight loss.

Immune System: hemorrhoids, hypoprothrombinemia, irritation—perianal/skin/tongue, rash.

Dosage: PO 4 g/d ac or with meals and hs to maximum of 24 g/d. Hyperlipoproteinemia: PO 4–8 g bid to qid ac and hs. Pruritus: PO 4 g bid to qid and hs.

Note: When given for lindane poisoning, do not make the patient vomit.

Colestipol [Colestid] has an action similar to that of cholestyramine.

Drug Interactions: Decreased absorption of oral anticoagulants, digoxin, iron salts, penicillins, phenobarbital, tetracyclines, thiazide diuretics, thyroid hormones, fat-soluble vitamins.

Side Effects

Nervous System belching, bowel—constipation/diarrhea/flatulence/distention, nausea/vomiting, pain—joint/muscle, shortness of breath.

Endocrine System: (Pregnancy Category C) serum chloride and phosphorus—transient increases, serum sodium and potassium—decreased.

Immune System: arthritis, dermatitis, liver enzymes—transient increases, urticaria.

Dosage: PO 15–30 g/d in 120–180 mL of water bid–qid in divided doses. Digitalis toxicity: 10 g followed by 5 g q6–8 h as needed.

▶ ANTIBIOTICS

As noted in Chapter 16, some antibiotics actually do microbe-to-microbe combat in the lumen of the gut, killing the flora and cleaning the gut in preparation for diagnostic procedures or surgery. See Chapter 16 for drugs and dosages.

Bismuth subsalicylate [Pepto-Bismol], a venerable agent, is not an antibiotic; however, it seems to have direct antimicrobial action in treating traveler's diarrhea caused by *E. coli* and *V. cholerae*. It also has an antisecretory effect in the stomach.

Off Label: *H. pylori.*

Drug Interactions: Decreased absorption or effect of tetracyclines, quinolones possible. Increased toxicity of aspirin, hypoglycemics, warfarin.

Side Effects

Nervous System: bowel—impaction, ear—hearing loss/tinnitus, headache, muscle spasms/weakness, psyche—anxiety/confusion/mental depression, slurred speech. High doses: bismuth toxicity: encephalopathy, seizures.*

*Life-threatening side effect.

High doses: subsalicylate toxicity: arrhythmias—tachycardia, cardiovascular collapse,* coma,* death,* hyperpnea, nausea/vomiting, psyche—confusion, respiratory failure,* seizures* (in severe overdose), tinnitus.

Endocrine System: (Pregnancy Category C; D in third trimester) stools—gray/black, tongue discoloration. High doses: subsalicylate toxicity: hyperpyrexia, metabolic acidosis, respiratory alkalosis.

Immune System: High doses: bismuth toxicity: methemoglobinemia. High doses: subsalicylate toxicity: edema—cerebral/pulmonary.

Dosage: Diarrhea: PO 30 mL or 2 tab q30–60min prn up to 8 doses/d. Traveler's diarrhea: PO 2–4 tab or 15–30 mL qid for 3 wk.

▶ LAXATIVES

Laxatives are used to clean out the bowel before diagnostic examinations or before surgery in the abdomen. They are also used to relieve constipation (dehydrated stool). Laxatives are of vital use in preventing constipation, which causes straining at stool and poses a potential hazard for patients with cardiovascular conditions. Such straining can cause a Valsalva maneuver, or forced exhalation against a closed airway. During the straining, thoracic and venous pressures rise. Venous return to the heart decreases. Blood pressure drops. Pulse rises. Upon relaxation of the maneuver, blood rushing into the heart can overload it and cause cardiac arrest. Straining can also cause cerebral circulation problems. Possibly the simplest way to prevent ordinary constipation is to drink adequate amounts of water and eat a high fiber diet. To prevent cardiac or cerebrovascular complications, keep the mouth open during a bowel movement.

ANTHRAQUINONE CATHARTICS

Irritant or stimulant cathartics (anthraquinones) irritate the mucous membranes and draw water into the bowel. The fecal mass moves too fast for the bowel to reabsorb water.

Cascara sagrada [Cas-Evac] is used for temporary relief of constipation and to prevent straining at stool.

Note: *"Black and white" is the name given to the combination of cascara sagrada and milk of magnesia.*

Drug Interactions: none noted.

---

* Life-threatening side effect.

Side Effects

Nervous Systems: Large doses: gripping, nausea, abnormally loose stools. Chronic use: rebound constipation.

Endocrine System: (Pregnancy Category C) anorexia, impaired glucose tolerance, hypocalcemia, hypokalemia, urine discoloration. Chronic use: black stools.

Immune System: none noted.

Dosage: PO 325-mg tab or 1 mL fluid extract at hs. 5 mL aromatic fluid extract at hs.

Senna pod preparation [Black-Draught, Gentlax B, Senexon, Senokot, Senolax] is similar to but more potent than cascara sagrada. It stimulates peristalsis to treat acute constipation and for preoperative and preradiographic bowel evacuation.

Side Effects

Nervous System: bowel—cramps/flatulence, nausea. Prolonged use: watery diarrhea.

Endocrine System: (Pregnancy Category C) Prolonged use: electrolyte and water loss, weight loss.

Immune System: Prolonged use: reversible melanotic segmentation of colonic mucosa.

Dosage: PO 1 level tsp qd or bid. Syrup 2–3 tsp qd or bid. Tab 1–2 qd or bid.

Note: *Use only half the dose for gynecologic, obstetric, and geriatric patients.*

DIPHENYLMETHANE CATHARTICS

These cathartics increase fluid in the bowel and stimulate peristalsis.

Bisacodyl [Dulcolax] stimulates peristalsis to treat acute constipation and for preoperative and preradiographic bowel evacuation. Bisacodyl also increases intestinal fluid volume through increased epithelial permeability.

Drug Interactions: Early dissolution of enteric-coated tablets with antacids.

Side Effects

Nervous System: mild cramping, diarrhea, nausea.

Endocrine System: (Pregnancy Category C) fluid and electrolyte imbalances.

Immune System: none noted.

Dosage: PO 10–15 mg. Rectal suppository 10 mg.

Glycerin [Glycerol, Glyrol] is used to treat constipation by absorbing water from tissues to create greater fecal mass.

Off Label: Reduces mortality due to strokes in the elderly. Glycerin's main use is in the treatment of constipation, but in the oral form it also reduces the pressure of narrow-angle glaucoma; the topical ophthalmic preparation reduces corneal edema.

Drug Interactions: none noted.

Side Effects

Nervous System: arrhythmias, bowel—diarrhea/abdominal cramps/rectal discomfort, dizziness, headache, nausea/vomiting, psyche—disorientation.

Endocrine System: (Pregnancy Category C) dehydration, glycosuria, hyperglycemia, hyperosmolar nonketotic coma.*

Immune System: hyperemia.

Dosage: Constipation: Rectal 3 g suppository or 5–15 mL of enema high into rectum and retain for 15 min.

SALINE AND MAGNESIUM CATHARTICS

Saline cathartics retain water in the intestinal lumen, distending the bowel, which increases peristalsis and speeds the passage of the fecal mass.

Lactulose [Cephulac, Chronulac], a lactose derivative with a laxative action, causes increased acidity of colon contents and thus decreases blood ammonia levels created by intestinal flora.

Drug Interactions: Laxatives may distort signs of therapeutic action of lactulose.

Side Effects

Nervous System: abdomen—cramps/distention/pain/belching, borborygmi, diarrhea, flatulence. Excessive dose: hydrogen gas accumulation, nausea/vomiting.

Endocrine System: (Pregnancy Category C) Excessive dose: hypernatremia.

Immune System: none noted.

Dosage: Chronic constipation: PO 30–60 mL/d prn. Prevention and treatment of portal-systemic encephalopathy: PO 30–45 mL tid–qid. Severe portal-systemic encephalopathy: 30–45 mL q1–2h, reducing dosage when stools reach 2–3/d. Rectal 300 mL diluted in 700 mL water per rectal balloon catheter and retain for 30–60 min. May repeat in 4–6 h if necessary or until patient can take PO.

Magnesium citrate solution [Citrate of Magnesia, Citroma, Citro-Nesia] is a bowel cleanser used prior to some surgical and diagnostic procedures. It is also used after treatment with antiparasitic drugs to help eliminate parasites. It causes osmotic retention of fluid to increase fecal mass, distend the colon, and stimulate peristalsis.

Drug Interactions: none noted.

Side Effects

Nervous System: abdominal cramps, nausea.

Endocrine System: (Pregnancy Category B) fluid and electrolyte imbalances. Prolonged use: hypermagnesemia.

Immune System: none noted.

Dosage: PO 240 mL hs.

Magnesium hydroxide [Milk of Magnesia (MOM)] draws water from the bowel to increase fecal mass, distend the colon, and stimulate peristalsis for short-term treatment of constipation. In low doses, it has antacid activity. It is also used to treat mineral acids and arsenic poisoning and to neutralize the oral acidity.

Drug Interactions: Decreased absorption of chlordiazepoxide, dicumarol, digoxin, isoniazid, quinolones, tetracycline.

Side Effects

Nervous System: Excessive use: abdominal cramps, diarrhea, nausea/vomiting. Hypermagnesemia: arrhythmias—bradycardia/complete heart block*/other ECG abnormalities,* coma,* respiratory depression,* hyporeflexia, hypotension, lethargy, nausea/vomiting, psyche—depression, weakness.

Endocrine System: (Pregnancy Category B) Excessive use: alkalinization of urine, dehydration. Prolonged use: electrolyte imbalance.

Immune System: none noted.

Dosage: PO 15–60 mL hs. Follow with 1 glass of water for laxative effect.

Polyethylene glycolelectrolyte solution [GoLYTELY] is used to clean the bowel before gastrointestinal examination per osmotic activity with no net absorption or excretion of ions or water.

Drug Interactions: May flush oral medications from the bowel when administered within 1 h of polyethylene glycoelectrolyte solution.

Side Effects

Nervous System: bloating, cramps—abdominal, feeling of fullness, nausea/vomiting.

---

* Life-threatening side effect.

Endocrine System: (Pregnancy Category C) none noted.

Immune System: anal irritation, anaphylaxis/dermatitis/rhinorrhea/urticaria—rare.

Dosage: PO 240 mL q10min until 4 L is consumed. Per NG tube at 20–30 mL/min (1.2–1.8 L/ph).

Sodium Phosphate, Sodium Biphosphate [Fleet Phospho-soda, Fleet Enema] relieves occasional constipation. It is also used for bowel cleansing prior to surgery or x-ray or endoscopic examination.

Drug Interactions: None noted.

Side Effects

Nervous System: none noted.

Endocrine System: (Pregnancy Category C) serum sodium/potassium—elevated, serum calcium/potassium—decreased, possible hypocalcemia, hyperphosphatemia, hypernatremia, acidosis.

Immune System: none noted.

Dosage: PO 20 mL in 8 oz of water. Enema form 60–120 mL.

BULK-FORMING LAXATIVES

Bulk-forming laxatives swell up with water. The enlarged fecal mass stimulates peristalsis and defecation.

Psyllium [Metamucil, others] See *psyllium hydrophin mucilloid* as bile and cholesterol binder earlier in this chapter.

SURFACTANT LAXATIVES

Surfactant laxatives (stool softeners) decrease surface tension of the fecal mass so that water penetrates. As a detergent, they soften the stool by mixing fat and water in the stool.

Docusate calcium [Surfak, others], docusate sodium [Colace, Doxinate, others] lowers the surface tension of stool, permitting water and fats to penetrate and soften fecal mass for easier passage. Helps prevent straining during stool.

Drug Interactions: Increased systemic absorption of mineral oil.

Side Effects

Nervous System: bowel—mild abdominal cramps/diarrhea, nausea, bitter taste.

Endocrine System: (Pregnancy Category C) none noted.

Immune System: rash. Liquid preparation: throat irritation.

Dosage: PO 50–500 mg qd. PR 50–100 mg added to enema fluid.

Mineral oil [Fleet Mineral Oil, Petrogalar, Fleet Mineral Oil Enema] softens and lubricates hard stools to ease their passage. Indicated for relief of fecal impaction or when straining must be avoided. Removes barium sulphate residues after barium GI series or outlining the left atrium.

Note: Sometimes an elderly patient may use mineral oil as a "salad dressing" to prevent or relieve constipation. He or she must be made aware that mineral oil may coat the vegetables and reduce absorption of vitamins from them.

Side Effects: None noted in any system.

Dosage: PO 15–30 mL hs. Enema 90–120 mL.

▶ ANTHELMINTICS—WORMING DRUGS

The following drugs directly kill worms in the intestine. (Also see Chapter 16.)

Ivermectin [Stromectol] is an anthelmintic used to treat intestinal infestations of the nematodes *Strongyloides stercoralis* and *Onchocerca volvulus*. Ivermectin increases invertebrate chloride ion channels in nerve and muscle cells, resulting in paralysis and death of the parasite.

Side Effects

Nervous System: arrhythmias—tachycardia, bowel—constipation/diarrhea/distension, dizziness, fatigue, myalgia, nausea/vomiting, pain—abdominal, psyche—somnolence, tremor, vertigo.

Endocrine System: (Pregnancy Category C) anorexia, fever.

Immune System: facial edema, pruritus, rash, urticaria.

Dosage: Strongyloides: PO 200 µg/kg in 1 dose. Onchocerciasis: 150 mcg/kg in 1 dose.

Mebendazole [Vermox] blocks worms' glucose uptake and starves them. It is used to treat infestations of *Ancylostoma duodenale* (common hookworm), *Ascaris lumbricoides* (roundworm), *Enterobius vermicularis* (pinworm), *Necator americanus* (American hookworm), *Trichuris trichiura* (whipworm).

Off Label: Beef, dwarf, and pork tapeworm and threadworm infections. Only 10% of the drug enters the host system.

Drug Interactions: none noted.

Side Effects

Nervous System: bowel—diarrhea, dizziness, pain—abdominal.

Endocrine System: (Pregnancy Category C) fever.

Immune System: possible tissue necrosis in cysts.

Dosage: PO 100 mg AM and hs for 3 d. If necessary, repeat in 3 wk. Pinworms may only require a single 100-mg dose.

Piperazine citrate [Antepar] is used to eliminate round-worms and pinworms. An exception to killing worms directly, it increases peristalsis to expel the live worms from the intestine. With low toxicity, its side effects usually result only for high dosage.

Drug Interactions: Exaggerated extrapyramidal effects and seizures possible with phenothiazines.

Side Effects

Nervous System: arthralgia, ataxia, bronchospasm,* choreiform movements, convulsions,* cramps—abdominal, productive cough, EEG abnormalities, diarrhea, nausea/vomiting, paresthesia, psyche—emotional detachment/memory defects, tremors, vertigo, vision—blurred/defects in accomodation/nystagmus/paralytic strabismus, weakness.

Endocrine System: (Pregnancy Category B) fever.

Immune System: anemia*—hemolytic, cataracts, erythema multiform, photosensitivity, urticaria.

Dosage: Pinworms: PO 65 mg/kg qd for 7–8 d to maximum of 2.5 g. Roundworms: PO 3.5 g/kg qd for 2 d.

Pyrantel pamoate [Antiminth] paralyzes roundworms, hook-worms, and pinworms. The side effects are dose related.

Drug Interactions: May be antagonistic with piperazine.

Side Effects

Nervous System: bowel—diarrhea, abdominal distension, dizziness, drowsiness, insomnia, nausea/vomiting, tenesmus.

Endocrine System: (Pregnancy Category C) anorexia.

Immune System: AST—transient elevation, rash.

Dosage: Pinworms, roundworms: PO 11 mg/kg for 1 d to maximum of 1 g. Hookworms: same dosage for 3 d.

Thiabendazole [Mintezol] suppresses egg and larva production for pinworms, threadworms, and sometimes hookworms, roundworms, and whipworms by inhibiting helminth-specific enzymes.

Drug Interactions: none noted.

Side Effects

Nervous System: arrhythmias—bradycardia, bowel—diarrhea, dizziness, drowsiness, enuresis, gastric distress, headache, hypotension, nausea/vomiting.

Endocrine System: (Pregnancy Category C) anorexia, cholestasis, crystalluria, hyperglycemia, malodor of urine.

Immune System: allergy, AST—transient rise, hematuria, leukopenia—transient, nephrotoxicity, perianal rash, pruritus.

Dosage: Weight <70 kg: PO 25 mg/kg bid pc for 2 d. Weight > 70 kg: 1.5 g bid (maximum 3 g/d × 2 d).

▶ DRUGS TO TREAT POISON INGESTION

The antidote activated charcoal is not absorbed from the gut, but rather acts externally to the surface of the bowel to adsorb toxins from the mucosa.

Activated charcoal, liquid antidote [Actidose, Charcoaid, others] increases drug diffusion rate from plasma into GI tract for adsorption from the bowel mucosa. It is used in the treatment of overdose of most drugs and chemicals. Repetitive doses are termed gastric dialysis and used in uremia to adsorb waste products from the GI tract. It also adsorbs intestinal gases in treatment of distension, dyspepsia, flatulence and is used as a topical deodorant for foul-smelling ulcers and wounds.

Drug Interactions: Decreased absorption of oral medications possible; administer at least 2 h apart.

Side Effects

Nervous System: With rapid ingestion: vomiting.

Endocrine System: (Pregnancy Category C) none noted.

Immune System: none noted.

Dosage: PO. Start with 30–100 g (1 g/kg or 5–10 times the weight of poison ingested) in 6–8 oz of water. Repeated administration (gastric dialysis) 20–40 g q6h for 1–2 d.

Note: *Not for use in the following ingestions: cyanide, caustic alkalis, ethanol, iron, methanol, mineral acids, and organic solvents.*

▶ NUTRIENTS FROM THE RIVER: VITAMINS

Vitamins maintain vital body functions. They come to us from the plants, animals, and fluids that we ingest into the river that flows through us. We absorb vitamins and minerals from what we eat. The late astronomer Carl Sagan said that, "We are made from the stuff of stars." In essence the food we eat comes from the sun's light, which is captured in plant leaves by photosynthesis. We get our power from the sun. The cells in the mucosa of the alimentary canal absorb that converted energy and the vitamins we need. This section explains what the

---

* Life-threatening side effect.

vitamins do. The minerals are covered in other chapters in the context of their actions.

Misnamed "vital amines," vitamins are not amines, but they are vital to survival. Vitamins A, D, and K have been described earlier in the text. Vitamin A is essential to the development of healthy cells. Vitamin D is essential to maintaining calcium levels, and vitamin K decreases clotting functions.

<u>Vitamin A</u> comes from animal sources, though plants containing orange pigments or carotene are called provitamin A. Vitamin A becomes retinal and acts on the retina to enhance night vision. It also maintains the integrity of cells in the epithelium and mucous membranes. Hypervitaminosis occurs at plasma levels over 1200 IU/dL.

Side Effects

Nervous System: headache, intracranial hypertension/increased intracranial pressure, psyche—irritability, vision—miosis/nystagmus. Hypervitaminosis A syndrome: abdominal discomfort, migratory arthralgia, lethargy, malaise, sweating.

Endocrine System: (Pregnancy Category A; X if > RDA) exophthalmos, papilledema. Hypervitaminosis A syndrome: retarded or slow growth, hypercalcemia, hypomenorrhea, polydipsia/polyuria.

Immune System: Hypervitaminosis A syndrome: alopecia, anemia—hypoplastic, gingivitis, hepatosplenomegaly, leukopenia, nails—brittle, sedimentation rate/PT—elevated, skin—desquamation/drying/cracking/lip fissures/pigmentation increase, subperiosteal thickening—radius/tibia/occiput. IV: anaphylaxis,* death.*

Dosage: PO (male) 1000 mcg, (female): 800 mcg.

<u>Vitamin B$_1$ (thiamine hydrochloride)</u> is needed to prevent beriberi.

Side Effects

Nervous System: cardiovascular collapse,* cyanosis, GI hemorrhage, nausea, pulmonary edema, restlessness, throat tightness, weakness. Rapid IV: slight fall in BP.

Endocrine System: (Pregnancy Category A) sweating, sense of warmth.

Immune System: anaphylaxis,* angioedema,*

Dosage: Dietary supplement: PO 5–30 mg/d. Deficiency: IM/IV 50–100 mg tid. Beriberi: IM, IV 10–500 mg tid × 2 wk.

<u>Vitamin B$_2$ (riboflavin)</u>, an apparently safe flavoprotein enzymes component, works with proteins as catalysts in cellular respiratory reactions for energy. (Pregnancy Category A; C if > RDA)

Dosage: Dietary supplement: PO 5–10 mg/d. Dietary deficiency: PO 5–30 mg/d in divided doses.

<u>Vitamin B$_3$ (niacin) [Niac, Nicobid, others]</u> converts protein, carbohydrate, and fat into energy. It has a direct action on vascular smooth muscles and inhibits hepatic synthesis of VLVD, cholesterol, and triglyceride, and, indirectly, LDL.

For Side Effects, see Chapter 8.

Dosage: Deficiency: PO 10–20 mg/d. SC, IM, slow IV 25–100 mg 2–5 ×/d. Pellagra: PO 300–500 mg/d in divided doses. Hyperlipidemia: PO 1.5–3g/d in divided doses. May increase up to 6g/d as needed.

<u>Vitamin B$_6$ (pyridoxine)</u> becomes pyridoxal, a coenzyme in protein, fat, and carbohydrate metabolism. It is also a part of enzyme reactions to transform amino acids and to convert tryptophan to niacin and serotonin. The nervous system uses it in energy transformation. It may stimulate heme production.

Side Effects

Nervous System: Possible with large parenteral doses: paresthesias/seizures*/ somnolence. Injection site: burning/stinging pain.

Endocrine System: (Pregnancy Category A; C if >RDA) large parenteral doses: flushing/sense of warmth, low folic acid levels.

Immune System: none reported.

Dosage: Dietary deficiency: PO, IM, IV 2.5–10 mg/d for 3 wk; then may reduce to 2.5–5 mg/d. Pyridoxine deficiency syndrome: PO,IM, IV. Start with up to 600 mg/d. Maintenance: up to 50 mg/d. Isoniazid-induced deficiency: PO, IM, IV 100–200 mg/d for 3 wk; then 25–100 mg/d.

<u>Vitamin B$_9$ (folic acid), pteroylglutamic acid [Folacin, others], folate sodium [Volvite Sodium]</u> is apparently nontoxic and essential to production of RBCs, WBCs, and platelets. (Pregnancy Category A)

Dosage: PO, IM, IV ≤1 mg/d. Maintenance: PO, IM, IV ≤ 0.4 mg/d.

<u>Vitamin B$_{12}$ (cyanocobalamin)</u> has many functions, including myelin synthesis, protein and carbohydrate metabolism, normal growth, cell reproduction, RBC maturation, and nucleoprotein synthesis.

Side Effects

Nervous System: bowel—mild transient diarrhea, CHF, itching, sensation of body swelling.

Endocrine System: (Pregnancy Category A; C if parenteral) flushing, hypokalemia.

---

* Life-threatening side effect.

Immune System: anaphylaxis,* sudden death,* edema—pulmonary, severe optic nerve atrophy in Leber's disease, peripheral vascular thrombosis. Existing polycythemia vera may be revealed when B$_{12}$ deficiency is remedied.

Dosage: B$_{12}$ deficiency: IM, deep SC 30 µg/d for 5–10 d; then 100–200 µg/mo. Pernicious anemia: IM, deep SC 100–1000 µg/d for 2–3 wk; then 100–1000 µg/d for 2–3 wk; then 100–1000 µg q2–4 wk. Diagnosis of megaloblastic anemia: IM, deep SC 1 µg/d for 10 d while on a low-folate and low-vitamin B$_{12}$ diet. Schilling Test: IM, deep SC 1000 µg × 1 dose. Dietary supplement: PO 1–25 µg/d.

Vitamin B$_{12A}$ (hydroxocobalamin) is similar to cyanocobalamin, but with slower absorption from injection site and possible increased liver uptake.

Dosage: Deficiency: IM 30 µg/d for 5–10 d; then 100–200 µg/mo or 1000 mcg qod until remission; then 1000 µg/mo.

Vitamin C (ascorbic acid) [Ascorbicap, others] supports wound healing, synthesis and maintenance of collagen and intercellular ground substance of body tissue cells, blood vessels, bones, cartilage, skin, tendons, and teeth. It is essential to the production of catecholamines during stress and to the immune system's protective responses.

Side Effects

Nervous System: bladder—dysuria, bowel—diarrhea, cramps—abdominal, headache, insomnia, nausea/vomiting. Injection site: soreness. Rapid IV: dizziness, faintness.

Endocrine System: (Pregnancy Category C) crystalluria, hyperoxaluria, hyperuricemia.

Immune System: heartburn, sickle cell crisis, urethritis. With G6PD deficiency: acute hemolytic anemia.

---

* Life-threatening side effect.

Dosage: PO, IM, IV, SC 150–500 mg in 1–2 doses. Prophylactic: PO, IM, IV, SC 45–60 mg/d. Urine acidifier: PO, IM, IV, SC 4–12 g/d in divided doses.

Vitamin E (tocopherol) [Aquasol E, others] is an antioxidant that protects cells against damage by free radicals. Vitamin E aids digestion and metabolism of polyunsaturated fats, maintains cell membrane integrity, decreases platelet aggregation, helps utilize vitamin A, and promotes muscle health.

Side Effects

Nervous System: bowel—cramps/diarrhea, fatigue, headache, nausea, vision—blurred, weakness—skeletal muscle.

Endocrine System: (Pregnancy Category A) creatinuria, gonadal dysfunction, serum creatine kinase/cholesterol/triglycerides—increased, serum thyroxine/triiodothyronine—decreased, urinary androgens/estrogens—increased

Immune System: sterile abscess, contact dermatitis, thrombophlebitis.

Dosage: Deficiency: PO, IM 60–75 IU/d. Prevention of deficiency: PO 12–15 IU/d.

 ## Chapter Highlights

- The alimentary canal is a descriptive term for the river that runs through us.
- Mucosal cells absorb the fluids, vitamins, and fuels we need to sustain us.
- Worming agents kill the parasites that compete for food in the canal, but parasites are not the only life in the canal.
- The three Master Systems have equal responsibilities for the canal.
- The nervous system propels the contents of this foreign space.
- The endocrine system oversees nutrition.
- The immune system patrols the mucosal tissue to destroy invaders.

section V

Critical Thinking

The nurse is entrusted with enormous responsibility when ordering and administering drugs, and observing the effects. Each procedure requires care and concentration and critical thinking. As students, nurses are taught the proper procedures for drug administration which include the *Five Rights:*

1. The Right Time.
2. The Right Drug.
3. The Right Route.
4. The Right Dose.
5. The Right Patient.

With practice these procedures become as easy as riding a bicycle. However, they must never be unconscious motions. At each of the 5 steps the nurse must consciously think and answer the question embedded in the word "right." In addition, the nurse must never be timid about questioning a drug order that seems improper. The nurse has that right.

The patient has rights too. The patient has a right to know the name of the drug and its effect and possible side effects. The nurse needs to be sure that the patient understands what is happening to his body. In this era of shorter hospital stays patients are often discharged home with medications they or a family member will have to administer. The nurse must make sure the patient and, or caregiver know exactly what to do. Dr. Ruth Grendell, one of the authors of this section, tells the story of a patient who was taught how to give injections of his medications by injecting an orange. The man thought that he was to inject the medication into the orange and then eat the orange. Even patients need to know the right route.

There are other "rights" involved in drug administration. As the observer, the nurse must always be alert to the patient's response to the drug and ask herself if the patient is having the right or expected response to the drug. Following proper procedures of drug administration may become second nature for the nurse, but each patient presents the nurse with unique challenges. The nurse must be aware of the expected therapeutic outcomes and ever alert for the unexpected. Always the observer, the nurse is also the teacher, and thus must always be learning about the drugs administered.

In short, by following the Five Rights of Drug Administration the nurse has five chances to practice critical thinking skills. The critical thinking continues after drug administration, extending into observation and assessment of therapeutic outcomes or unwanted drug effects. The nurse is not alone in these daunting responsibilities. Pharmacists are an essential part of the health team and dispense knowledge as well as drugs. The nurse should never hesitate to seek needed information from the pharmacist.

To help the reader develop necessary critical thinking skills this section contains a number of patient vignettes and a discussion of pharmacokinetics. Dr. Ruth Grendell, who has taught pharmacology to student nurses for many years, has developed the vignettes to inform and test the reader's critical thinking skills. Dawn Metresin, a practicing pharmacist, has responded to the vignettes with her expertise and describes what happens to a drug molecule after administration. In "The Nurse Takes Action", the reader will get to see some common disease conditions, the drugs to treat them, and the important nursing interventions involved. In "Over the Counter," the reader will get the pharmacist's point of view.

The nurse must always observe the Five Rights of Drug Administration, and, in addition, never stop learning about drugs and using careful assessment skills in order to provide safety and the optimal therapeutic outcome for the patient. The patient has the right to expect only the best critical thinking skills from the nurse.

20 Over the Counter: The Pharmacist Speaks

Dawn L. Metrisin

When a person swallows a pill or receives a parenteral medication, the action is not totally determined by the drug's chemical composition. "Drugs do not create functions but modify existing functions within the body" (Clark, Queener, & Karb, 1997, p. 4). Picture a drug broken into tiny "medicine molecules" that could be followed all over the body. Throughout this chapter you will follow the "molecule" and visualize the actions taking place. The "molecules" can interact not only with the body but also other "molecules" present as well.

Adverse drug reactions, drug toxicity, or drug interactions may result from any one or a combination of things. In addition, the person's age, weight, gender, and physical and mental status can influence outcomes. Pharmacists play a significant role in preventing or minimizing problems by monitoring an individual's drug profile and serving as a patient educator and/or a resource. Whether involving a combination of over-the-counter and prescription medications or use of multiple drugs, the incidence of drug interactions is increasing. Many new drugs approved by the Federal Drug Administration (FDA) are entering the market every month, thus increasing the potential for new or unknown drug interactions.

Nurses must also be knowledgeable in clinical pharmacology and must implement strategies to avoid or alleviate problems for individuals. Knowledge of the basic types of drug interactions facilitates recognition of biologic reactions according to drug families. Drugs classified within the same master system may produce similar side effects both within that system and across the interconnecting systems.

▶ MASTER SYSTEM DRUG EFFECTS

Many nervous system medications have a profound effect on drug interactions. Interactions in this system may result in loss of seizure control, cardiac arrhythmias, or exacerbation of hypertension. Drugs classified within the endocrine system are influenced by the negative feedback system, which regulates the various circulating hormone levels. Thus the introduction of a drug to treat one hormone disorder may affect other endocrine gland functions. Many of the immune system drug interactions are due to the use of multiple drugs to combat inflammatory and infectious diseases and may result in blood dyscrasias, allergic responses, or superinfections (ulcers, stomatitis, gingivitis).

This chapter will identify the various classifications of drug interactions within a specific system and across the master systems and in the alimentary canal, describe the physiologic consequences of these reactions, and profile specific patient populations susceptible to drug reactions. Drug interactions and precautions related to the case studies in Chapter 21 will also be discussed.

▶ DRUG INTERACTIONS

Two primary processes are involved when drugs enter the body. *Pharmacokinetic* actions include the four subprocesses of *absorption, distribution, metabolism, and excretion* (ADME). Many pharmacokinetic drug interactions are assessed using plasma or serum drug levels and by monitoring the clinical status of the patient. Although these interactions are important, the potential for danger is more limited than from pharmacodynamic interactions.

Pharmacodynamic actions include a drug's effect at the physiologic or cellular level. Pharacodynamic interactions are common and the clinical relevance is significant. Examples include *synergistic,* or enhanced, effect of two concurrently administered drugs, and *antagonis-*

tic, or opposing, effects of two competing drugs. Drug interactions can be beneficial or have adverse effects on physiologic and psychological functions. (See Tables 21–1 through 21–9 on drug interaction.)

▶ PHARMACOKINETIC DRUG PROCESSES AND INTERACTIONS

ABSORPTION

Approximately 80% of all drugs are taken orally. The mouth is the first stop and the first contact a pill has with the master systems. This is of course a brief stop, and the pill continues down into the stomach. Upon arrival in the stomach, enzymes, acids, and bacteria break this pill down into the absorbable "medicine molecules." The bioavailability of the "medicine molecule" can be defined as how ready this "molecule" is for body action. Bioavailability of a drug is affected by several factors. For example, the drug form, route of administration, gastrointestinal motility, presence of food or other drug, the level of liver function, and degree of blood flow to the liver are just a few factors the "medicine molecule" encounters when it first enters the body.

Absorption of an oral drug is the movement from the gastrointestinal tract to the body tissues (1) via diffusion across membranes, (2) with help of a carrier enzyme or protein, or (3) by pinocytosis, an engulfment by the cell membrane. This initial contact is also the first area for potential drug interactions. Oral drugs, which must be in solution for absorption to take place, are most often absorbed in the slightly acidic stomach environment. Factors influencing absorption include the acid–base environment, motility, presence of other drugs or foods (especially hot and fatty foods), amount of resident bacteria in the gastrointestinal tract, and drug–drug interactions. The presence of pain or stress can also cause significant pharmacokinetic changes. Lipid-soluble and non-ionized drugs are absorbed more quickly than water-soluble and ionized drugs, because the cell membranes also have a high lipid content. Some drugs bypass the systemic circulation and enter the liver via the portal vein directly from the intestine (Kee & Hayes, 1997).

Acid–Base Environment

The pK_a value of any substance stipulates the pH level at which the substance will ionize (form ions) or be non-ionized (have no positive or negative charge). In the highly acidic or low pH environment of the gastric secretions, an acidic drug like aspirin becomes inert or nonactive and can then readily diffuse across the gastric membrane and be rapidly absorbed. However, acidic drugs can be very irritating to the gastric mucosa. The addition of an antacid (eg, Tums) raises the gastric pH

and results in ionization of the aspirin, thus delaying absorption but also the drug's clinical effect. Drug manufacturers frequently advertise that the addition of protective or enteric coatings to anti-inflammatory, acidic medications (eg, Ecotrin) will avoid the common side effect of gastric irritation. The enteric coatings are also beneficial for drugs that might be destroyed by gastric secretions and, thus, allow absorption to take place in the intestine.

The addition of histamine$_2$ blocking agents such as cimetidine (Tagamet) and famotidine (Pepcid) that reduce gastric acid production can also simulate the higher pH intestinal environment and cause premature dissolving of acidic drugs, thus creating more gastric irritation. The problem can be alleviated by staggering the dose intervals by at least 2 hours between the two different medications, and possibly diminish the need for additional doses of the histamine$_2$ blocking agents.

Bacteria

Bacteria normally present in the intestine are destroyed by some antibiotics. However, the absorption of some medications (eg, oral contraceptives) is dependent upon the presence of the bacteria. Therefore, a decrease in serum levels of an oral contraceptive can result in either an unexpected outcome of uterine bleeding or a pregnancy.

Motility

Any GI disturbance such as vomiting and diarrhea affects absorption of a drug. When a person takes a drug that alters the normal movement in the gastrointestinal tract, other serum drug levels are affected. For example, when metoclopramide [Reglan], which increases GI motility, is given concurrently with digoxin, a cardiac glycoside that is absorbed in the stomach, the result is a lower therapeutic serum digoxin level and possible added cardiovascular problems.

Drug–Drug Interactions

Sometimes our "molecule" is not alone. Occasionally the molecule has to share the stomach and intestinal environment. The "molecules" are trying to catch the next "bus" (carrier) to the next "town" (tissues), but keep getting pushed back from the door by other "molecules." A drug–drug interaction is one of the most frequent and easily preventable absorption problems. Insoluble complexes are formed when there is a chemical binding of one drug to another drug, and absorption is canceled. A classic example of this type of interaction is the combination of tetracycline (an antibiotic) and iron. Iron and tetracycline chelate or bind together and are not absorbed. Administering these drugs at wider spaced intervals prevents this drug interaction.

Parenteral Drug Absorption

The administration of drugs by the several parenteral routes bypasses absorption via the GI tract. Intravenous medications are absorbed directly into the bloodstream and are the preferred route for maintaining continuous drug concentrations. In this case our "molecule" is already available for action into the system. This "molecule" is prepackaged and ready for work in the body. Intravenous absorption "molecules" must already be pH balanced the same as the bloodstream and be a small enough size to fit into the smallest of veins. Glucose and regular insulin [Humulin R, Novolin R] are just a few "molecules" of this caliber.

Intramuscular medications are best absorbed from muscles with a good blood supply. Rate of absorption can be increased by applying heat or massage to the site. The rate can also be slowed by the application of ice packs or by the addition of a vasoconstricting medication such as epinephrine. Big "molecular molecules" such as anabolic steroids and vaccines cannot be handled by direct venous contact, so these "molecules" enter the body intramuscularly.

Absorption of subcutaneous medications is primarily through the capillaries. This route is often used when slow systemic absorption is desired. "Molecules" such as NPH insulin [Humulin N and Novolin N] and sumatriptan HCl [Imitrex injection] start their journey underneath the subcutaneous fat layers of the skin.

Just like humans, each "molecule" is different, and some molecules require other forms of entry into the body. Eventually the "molecule" reaches the bloodstream, but it may arrive there in a different form. Systemic absorption of transdermal and topical medications is through the skin. Other drugs are absorbed by mucous membranes and by inhalation. The numerous capillaries of the rectal mucosa promote both local and systemic absorption of suppositories and fluids. Drugs can also be injected into the spinal column (intrathecal) and even into body cavities or joints when direct access to these areas is needed.

DRUG DISTRIBUTION

Body Fluid Composition

Approximately 60% of the adult body is composed of water. The total body water content is determined by age, gender, and weight ratio of body muscle and fat. Males have a higher amount of total body water because they have a lower percentage of body fat content than do females. Younger adults have higher concentrations of body water than elderly persons, whereas newborns and infants have an even higher water concentration than adults. In fact, newborns have such a high content of body water that drug dosages must be drastically decreased.

Body water is distributed into the intracellular, extracellular, and intravascular areas of the body. Any drug deposited in the extracellular fluid will not be active in the body, almost as if our "molecule" is lost. The distribution of drugs is affected by any alteration in body fluid composition. Drug distribution is primarily a result of the "molecule's" affinity for a hydrophilic (water-loving) or hydrophobic (water-hating) tissues. After metabolism by liver enzymes, most drugs are deposited into the hydrophilic, water-soluble regions of the body.

Two issues of concern involving drug distribution for the elderly are the amount of body fat concentration and plasma proteins. Body fat increases and water content decreases during the aging process. Water-soluble drugs affected by this change include digoxin, alcohol, and lithium (a psychotropic drug), which are all classified as nervous system drugs. As a result, dosages of these medications must be adjusted to a person's lean body weight. Fat-soluble drugs, on the other hand, are also often found in the nervous system drug classification. Examples include Elavil, Tofranil, Prozac (antidepressants); Xanax, Ativan, Valium, popular benzodiazepines (used as antidepressants and anxiolytics); and phenobarbital, a barbiturate (used in antiseizure therapy and for mild sedation). Since most of the nervous system medications are widely prescribed for adults, caution is warranted if the individual has high body fat content because toxic drug concentrations in these tissues can ensue.

Plasma Proteins

Other influencing factors on drug distribution include blood flow and a drug's protein-binding ability. Our medicine "molecule" carries a key that fits into the receptor site on plasma proteins for distribution to the target tissues. The receptor site is the keyhole for the "molecule," but the molecule is stuck there. The key fits, but not enough to cause any action for the body tissues. When a drug binds with the protein, it is pharmacologically inactive. After all protein receptor sites are saturated, the remaining amount of drug is free to circulate and, eventually, bind with tissue receptor sites where drug action takes place. This is where the "molecule" "key" fits and opens the "door" to tissue activity. Diffusion into tissues is facilitated by a high concentration of free drug. As the amount of free drug is diminished, more protein-bound drug is released into the circulation to maintain a balance of free drug available to target tissues. The protein-bound drug can serve as a reservoir for an extended period of time and prevent harmful effects from higher concentrations of free drug.

Our "molecule's" "key" is not the only one around. Two drugs can have affinity for the same protein receptor site. Concurrent administration of these competing drugs displaces one of the drugs, resulting in circulation of the unbound or free drug, and thereby promoting a bond at the tissue receptor sites. An example is the coadministration of phenytoin [Dilantin], an antiseizure agent, and warfarin [Coumadin], an anticoagulant, which are both highly protein-bound by blood carrier proteins, especially by albumin. The result could be a loss of seizure control or severe bleeding.

Albumin and globulin are two of the most important plasma proteins. Lowered protein levels, especially albumin, create a compensatory increase in circulating drugs. The elderly patient gradually experiences a loss of plasma proteins. Other disorders contributing to protein loss include malnutrition, cirrhosis of the liver, and kidney failure. Loss of protein binding sites can lead to an excess of free drug and can, eventually, lead to drug toxicity and be life threatening. Decreased doses of medications are frequently prescribed for individuals with these conditions. Drug distribution is also hindered within body glands, tumors, abscess areas, and exudates. Some drugs accumulate in tissues such as fat, bone, liver, eyes, and muscles.

METABOLISM/BIOTRANSFORMATION

Metabolism is one of the many intricate and delicate processes involving all three master systems. The major site of drug metabolism is the liver, although the white blood cells, lungs, skin, kidneys and bacteria in the GI tract are involved to a minor extent. Our medicine "molecule" rides a "roller coaster" through the body and eventually comes to a stop. Some drugs enter the body through the GI tract in a biologically inactive form, are not extensively metabolized, and are eliminated in the urine unchanged. Other inactive drug forms are activated by liver enzymes. An example is the drug cyclophosphamide, which is used in cancer therapy (Clark, Queener, & Karb, 1997). Metabolism can be compared to a factory assembly line in which drugs are transported by the blood to the liver from the stomach or intestines. Through a complex process, the liver determines whether the drug is useful to the body or if it should be eliminated. This process is referred to as the *first-pass effect*. The drug metabolites are either sent on their way for distribution throughout the body or are excreted. Some drugs that are already active are metabolized into inactive forms for excretion. (Most drugs are fat-soluble and must be converted into water-soluble substances prior to excretion.) These important processes are repeated during subsequent passes through the liver to prevent indefinite circulation and prolonged drug effects. Many of the liver enzymes are non-drug specific and are capable of metabolizing many different drugs. The liver can also synthesize more enzymes to metabolize a drug that is given repeatedly. The use of alternate routes for drug administration may avoid the first-pass effect, for example, drugs that are absorbed directly across the mucous membranes for rapid entry into the systemic circulation (Clark, Queener, & Karb, 1997).

The *half-life* ($t_{1/2}$) of a drug refers to the time required for one-half of a drug concentration to be eliminated from the body and is affected by both metabolism by the liver and excretion processes. The half-life is prolonged in persons with decreased liver or kidney function, thus contributing to an accumulation of the drug. A drug may go through several half-lives before a major portion of the drug is eliminated. Continued doses of a drug can also contribute to accumulation and adverse side effects. Four to eight hours is considered to be a short half-life and 24 hours or longer to be a long half-life (Kee & Hayes, 1997). Drugs with a shorter half-life must be given more frequently to achieve and maintain a therapeutic effect.

Any alteration in the drug metabolism process contributes to a potential drug interaction. Causes in alteration include cirrhosis or liver failure that results in diminished production of the liver metabolizing enzymes. In these conditions, drugs are poorly metabolized. Consequently, lower doses of drugs are prescribed and often spaced over longer time intervals. Drugs not requiring metabolism by the liver can also be used.

Interactive Effects of Drugs and Liver Enzymes

Enzyme Induction: Drugs can either induce or inhibit liver enzyme activity. Enzyme induction occurs when a drug stimulates production of excess cytochrome P-450, the chemical term for liver enzymes. As a result, an increase in hepatic enzymes also increases the metabolism of drugs taken concurrently. A decrease in therapeutic activity reduces a clinical response for up to 2 weeks following the addition of an enzyme-stimulating drug. Drug serum levels should be monitored for individuals taking these drugs to determine the need for adjusting drug doses or scheduling, or for a change to a non-interacting medication. For example, cigarette smoking induces liver enzyme activity, and therefore a smoker would require higher doses of Theo-Dur (theophylline) to achieve the intended bronchodilating effects for clinical control of asthma.

Enzyme Inhibition: Inhibition of enzyme production rapidly occurs in the body when two drugs compete for the same binding site on the metabolizing enzyme. If such an interaction occurs, a change in homeostasis can develop as quickly as 24 hours following the addition of the competing drug or change in the dosing schedule compared to the 2-week response seen with induced enzyme production.

EXCRETION/ELIMINATION

If drugs were not excreted, they would continue to circulate throughout the body indefinitely. It is at this point our medicine "molecule" has finished the journey and has begun the process of leaving the body. The "molecule" cannot just leave; it must be prepared in a way that it can exit the body safely. The primary source of excretion, or elimination, is through the renal system. Alternate routes include the bile, feces, lungs, saliva, sweat, and breast milk. Free, unbound, water-soluble, and unchanged drugs are filtered by the renal nephrons. The kidneys are also capable of forming substances to biotransform drugs in preparation for excretion from the body. Protein-bound drugs remain in the body until they are released into the general circulation from the protein receptor site (Kee & Hayes, 1997).

Renal excretion is through active tubular secretion and passive tubular reabsorption. Active tubular secretion uses anionic or cationic protein carriers for a more rapid drug elimination than the passive processes. Active excretion of the antibiotic penicillin G is very rapid compared to the slower passive elimination process for the antibiotic tetracycline.

Passive reabsorption involves diffusion of substances across the tubular membranes. Passive reabsorption is dependent upon a specific urine pH, which can vary from 4.5 to 8. An acidic pH ionizes weak basic drugs and facilitates excretion; acidic drugs remain nonionized and are then reabsorbed by passive diffusion. Alkaline urine promotes excretion of weak acid drugs such as aspirin, whereas acid urine promotes excretion of weak basic drugs such as bicarbonate. For example, concurrent administration of Dyazide (a thiazide diuretic) and lithium (a psychotherapeutic drug) causes decreased clearance of lithium and contributes to lithium toxicity. In addition, adverse and toxic effects can result when an unmetabolized drug reaches the kidney and cannot be excreted. Some drugs, including aminoglycoside antibiotics, are nephrotoxic and therefore inhibit their own excretion (Clark, Queener, & Karb, 1997).

► ALIMENTARY CANAL FUNCTIONS

The alimentary canal plays a primary role in many of the pharmacokinetic processes. Oral drugs can be given in tablet, capsule, or liquid form. A major portion of the solid forms can include buffers or fillers, lubricants, binders to prevent disintegration, or compounds to facilitate disintegration in the proper environment. Solid drug forms must be broken down or dissolved for absorption in the GI tract. Drugs from different manufacturers may contain varying amounts of these added compounds, which can alter the dissolution process. Older drugs may dry out on the shelf and take longer to disintegrate in the GI tract.

The presence of food delays absorption of drugs and some drugs should be given on an empty stomach.

Other drugs, such as griseofulvin, an antifungal agent, should be taken with fatty foods. Gastric emptying time varies from individual to individual and can vary with the time of day, thus affecting the time that a drug is exposed to the acidic gastric contents. Infants, children, and the elderly have less stomach acid than young-to-middle-aged adults, leading to less degradation of drugs and more rapid absorption. The presence of other drugs in the GI tract can also enhance or inhibit absorption.

The pH of GI contents changes throughout the GI tract. Changes in motility caused by vomiting and diarrhea also drastically affect absorption and distribution of drugs. Absorption is also dependent upon the amount of available surface area and the presence or absence of digestive enzymes. (See Chapter 21 for additional information on drug action within the Master Systems and for the discussion on alimentary canal processes.)

► PHARMACODYNAMIC INTERACTIONS

SYNERGISM

Synergism is a phenomenon whereby the combination of two drugs produces more of a response than their individual effects (1 + 1 = 3). For example, the administration of Percocet, a narcotic analgesic, and Benadryl, an antihistamine, increases the central nervous system (CNS) effect of drowsiness produced by both drugs. Some drugs can combine with several different receptor sites.

ANTAGONISM

Antagonism occurs when an interaction between two drugs results in the effect of either or both drugs being decreased. Coumadin (warfarin) is commonly used as an anticoagulant as prophylaxis for persons who are susceptible to cardiovascular accidents (CVAs) by decreasing the likelihood for clots to form in small veins. However, co-administration of Coumadin and vitamin K, the antidote to Coumadin, will cancel action of one or both drugs.

Nurses and other health care providers should be aware of all medications that individuals take, whether nonprescription, herbals, or prescription drugs. Many of the drug interactive problems experienced by patients could be the result of synergistic action of two similar-acting drugs rather than a side effect of a specific drug. An accurate drug history and skillful assessment are essential throughout the drug regimen, as well as documentation and reporting patient responses to the physician. Rather than adding a drug to counteract a side effect of drowsiness from two sedating drugs, the physician may alter the dose schedule or prescribe alternate drugs. If there is any doubt regarding possible drug interactions or therapeutic plasma (serum) levels, and therapeutic index, or safety level, it is wise to consult with a pharmacist or obtain information from a drug reference or manual. (Please refer to Table 21–1.)

EXAMPLES OF NERVOUS SYSTEM DRUG INTERACTIONS

Many of the drugs classified within the nervous system category were chosen as examples in the previous discussion on pharmacokinetic and pharmacodynamic drug interactions. Additional selected examples are included here.

Digitalis (digoxin), a cardiac drug, is one of the most highly interactive drugs in the nervous system. Digoxin's absorption can be slowed by the use of antacids. Its half-life can be decreased and therapeutic serum levels lowered by phenytoin [Dilantin] and phenobarbital [Luminal], which are both used in anticonvulsant therapy. Digoxin's serum levels can be elevated through enzyme inhibitors such as cimetidine, an anti-ulcer agent, and isoniazid, an antiinfective prescribed as tuberculosis therapy. In addition, the competition for albumin receptor sites between quinidine [Quinaglute], an antiarrhythmic agent, and verapamil [Calan or Calan SR], a calcium channel blocker and digoxin results in displacement of digoxin into free circulation, thus increasing serum levels. Hyperkalemia also increases digoxin levels. Any of these can result in digoxin toxicity.

Cimetidine [Tagamet] an anti-ulcer agent prescribed for allergy therapy, interacts with many other medications. Cimetidine now is also available as an OTC drug and is a popular choice due to its minimal drowsiness side effect. A potent inhibitor of liver enzyme production, cimetidine will frequently increase levels of any drug metabolized extensively by the liver including (1) warfarin [Coumadin], an anticoagulant; (2) theophylline [Theo-Dur], a bronchodilator; (3) calcium channel blockers [ie, Calan], prescribed as antihypertensives; (4) benzodiazepine [ie, Diazepam], an anticonvulsant and anxiolytic; and (5) tricyclic antidepressants [ie, Elavil].

EXAMPLES OF ENDOCRINE SYSTEM DRUG INTERACTIONS

The endocrine system intertwines hormones in the brain, primarily through the hypothalamus and the pituitary gland, and other major organs in the body. Some endocrine drugs, like prednisone, secreted by the adrenal gland, constantly maintain homeostasis or balance. The steroids and thyroid hormones are secreted or prevented from entering the bloodstream by the hypothalamus after it receives information on blood levels of circulating hormones from feedback loops. These messenger hormones aid in controlling the amounts of hormone secreted by the target glands in what is commonly referred to as the

negative feedback system. Lower circulating hormone levels trigger releasing hormones from the hypothalamus that induce the pituitary gland to send the specific stimulating hormone to the corresponding gland. The target glands respond by secreting additional hormone into the circulating blood. Any alteration in this feedback system will change blood concentration of targeted endocrine hormones.

An example is the current protocol for the use of oral contraceptive agents. To achieve the primary goal of preventing pregnancy and to minimize the many potential side effects, the lowest dose strength is prescribed. However, the consequence at this dose level is a very narrow therapeutic range in plasma levels. Breakthrough bleeding or pregnancy can result from any alteration of the absorption or metabolism processes.

Plasma concentrations of oral contraceptives can also be adversely affected by some antibiotics, phenytoin [Dilantin] and carbamazepine [Tegretol], or anticonvulsants. Antibiotics affect the absorption process and phenytoin and carbamazepine interfere with metabolism.

Insulin, a fragile protein peptide, is not absorbed at all through the intestinal tract owing to the destructive effects of the gastric acid pH. Therefore, insulin is given subcutaneously; *but only regular insulin* can be given intravenously, as well. Most drug interactions with insulin involve the pharmocokinetic processes of absorption and distribution of insulin from the subcutaneous layers of the skin, which depend upon blood flow and/or fat distribution. Local massaging of the skin and exercise enhance absorption. Common injection sites include the upper arm, thigh, or abdominal area.

Drug interactions resulting in hypoglycemia or hyperglycemia states related to oral antidiabetic or hypoglycemic agents can occur during the metabolism process. The combination of beta blockers, such as propranalol [Inderal], alcohol, and anabolic steroids with the oral antidiabetic agents can result in hypoglycemia. Corticosteroids, furosemide [Lasix], phenytoin [Dilantin], and lithium combined with the oral antidiabetics can exacerbate hyperglycemia.

EXAMPLES OF IMMUNE SYSTEM DRUG INTERACTIONS

Drug interactions in the immune system primarily involve combinations of anticoagulants, antibiotics, antiviral agents, and other antiinfective drugs. Many treatment regimens for infections involve either multiple antibiotics or medications to relieve the common symptoms of an illness, such as sneezing, nasal discharge, watery eyes, cough, or pain. Antihistamines, decongestants and cough syrups, and aspirin or Tylenol are among the medications for the treatment of viral or bacterial infections. Caregivers should interview the patient to determine what OTC or prescriptive medications the patient may be taking. The addition of nasal decongestants can induce a serious hypertensive crisis for a person taking MAO (monamine-oxidase) inhibitor drugs (antidepressants).

The addition of aspirin may cause increased bleeding for persons who are taking warfarin [Coumadin], which has a very narrow therapeutic plasma range. Any slight change in plasma levels creates either bleeding or clotting. Any drug affecting the metabolism enzymes in the liver will undoubtedly alter warfarin plasma levels.

Theophylline [Theo-Dur], an important asthma medication, also has a very narrow therapeutic plasma level. Caution must be observed if the patient is currently taking an enzyme-inducing or -inhibiting drug. Low theophylline levels can exacerbate asthma symptoms, whereas excess levels can result in hypotension, brain damage, seizures, and even death.

▶ PATIENT PROFILES

Determining which patient populations are susceptible to drug interactions can be a challenge. Any individual who has preexisting decreased liver or kidney function has the most potential for drug interactions. These individuals metabolize drugs slowly, if at all, and require adjustment to a lower dose or a prolonged interval between doses. For example, rather than taking a medication four times a day, the dose could be lowered to once or twice a day. Some medications could be administered on alternate days.

Alcoholics and cigarette smokers also present unique challenges. Chronic alcohol abuse and cigarette smoking induce production of liver enzymes. Cigarette smokers often have asthma and take theophylline; they may require more than a 40% higher dose than nonsmokers (Hendeles & Weinberger, 1983; Kee & Hayes, 1997).

Children and the elderly have different metabolism rates than young and middle-aged adults. Neonates and infants have less plasma protein and higher percentages of body water. Phenytoin [Dilantin], an anticonvulsant agent, and other highly protein-bound drugs are given in much smaller doses to these populations because of the decreased availability of plasma proteins. Theophylline distributes rapidly into the aqueous portions of the body. A neonate, with approximately 75% body water content, will require larger doses of theophylline (Clark, Queener & Karb, 1997).

Polypharmacy, or multiple drug therapy, in the elderly is a primary concern. It is common for an elderly person to have five, ten, or more medications in the prescription file. Polypharmacy is compounded when these individuals have their prescriptions filled at different pharmacies because of cost differences, convenience of location, and so on. This practice should be discouraged because pharmacies are not computer-linked to each other for determining what drugs are in the individual's file.

Decreased metabolism and excretion rates in the elderly also contribute to altered and increased responses to medications. Excretion of cimetidine [Tagamet], digoxin, and the cephalosporin antibiotics is often delayed. Kidney function tests such as creatinine clearance (Cl_{cr}) to determine glomerular filtration rate (GFR) should be performed to determine whether adjustment to lower doses is needed.

Persons with seizure disorders, diabetes, hypertension, congestive heart failure, or chronic infectious diseases such as AIDS also require multiple drug therapy. It is imperative, especially for patients with seizures, that adequate administration and careful monitoring be done. Many of the antiseizure drugs inhibit and induce enzyme production at the same time, thus presenting a complicated clinical picture. Any change or discontinuation of therapy needs to be addressed.

▶ CONCLUSION

It is extremely important to remember the significance of drug interactions. Any of the pathways that the drug may take in the body is a potential site for drug interactions. Whether in the GI tract, the bloodstream, liver, or kidney, any drug may act differently in the presence of another drug. An interaction may be as minor as the chemical binding in the stomach or as major as the displacement of a drug from plasma proteins via a competing drug or drugs.

Throughout this chapter, we have discussed the origins of drug interactions and the consequences of those interactions on the three Master Systems. All three systems are affected and no one drug is taken without the potential for drug interactions.

However, modern drug manufacturers continue their attempts to create the "perfect" drug—one that is virtually drug-interaction free. Many drugs classified in the nervous system, such as the cardiovascular agents and antiseizure agents, have been improved to prevent variable human responses. The many improvements made in antibiotics, immune system medications, have made it virtually impossible to have absorption or metabolism problems. Insulin, an endocrine system drug, has been improved, and now human insulin, which is more compatible than other animal insulins, has been developed and is more rapidly absorbed.

Quality health care will be provided as health care givers continue to monitor and prevent possible drug interactions. Knowledge of the numerous drug interactions and interventions to alleviate them will be the keys to future patient-client satisfaction and good health. (See pharmacist's discussion related to case study drug interactions that are presented in Chapter 21.)

21

The Nurse Takes Action

Ruth N. Grendell

The focus of this chapter is the nursing roles in drug therapy, which include drug administration and patient/client education. A thorough understanding of the patterns of communication among body cells and the influence of drugs on cell function is essential in preparing nurses to fulfill these roles. The use of the nursing process and the holistic framework provided by the interactive networking of the three Master Systems form general guidelines for the nurse's action. To illustrate the various nursing actions, a surgical case study will be interpreted throughout the following discussion.

▶ ASSESSMENT PART ONE— THE NURSE COLLECTS DATA

First, let's talk about some of the major information that the nurse needs to know about a *person* receiving drug therapy. Mary Thompson, a 45-year-old woman admitted to your medical/surgical unit, is scheduled for an exploratory laparotomy with a possible colon resection the next morning. The physician's written orders include several diagnostic tests, a bowel prep, and preoperative medications. Your assignment is to admit Mrs. Thompson and to prepare her both psychologically and physiologically for the surgical procedure. Nursing assessment is essential to establish a baseline for your plan of care. Mrs. Thompson can supply you with her history background, your physical assessment will provide objective data, and further information that you need can be obtained from other sources, for instance, the client's record and diagnostic testing reports.

Important facts about the person are:

- Age, gender, weight, height, vital signs.
- Allergies, nature of the current health problem as well as all previous problems.

- Reasons for current medications (including over-the-counter drugs and vitamins).
- Her knowledge about her drugs, attitude toward drugs, reactions, and compliance.
- Genetic/ethnic/cultural background (potential factors in response to medications).
- General health habits/risk factors, including diet, smoking, alcohol use, exercise.
- Fear/anxiety level related to surgery and outcome.

Other questions to include are:

- Has she previously been hospitalized? For what reasons? When?
- Has she had previous surgery? If so, when? Were there complications?
- Is she sexually active and when was her last menstrual period? (Some girls under 12 and women over 50 are sexually active and do become pregnant, which does pose a potential complication to the surgical outcome.)
- Does she have family or support persons who will be available to assist her?

(In some cases, you may want to include questions on recreational drug use, recent travels, and immunizations.)

QUESTIONS ABOUT CLIENT'S MEDICATIONS

Next, you will need to obtain information about the client's *medications*. You may need to refer to a drug text to answer these questions. Edwards (1997) indicated that almost all drugs interact adversely with at least one other drug!

- What is the purpose of the drug? How does it "speak" to the body cells? (What Master System is used to classify this drug? How does it affect other systems?)

- Will the addition of a new drug change effectiveness of other drugs, or vice versa?
- Does the drug cause changes in mental status, vital signs, elimination, homeostasis?
- Does the drug alter electrolyte action potential? Change diagnostic tests? Cause blood dyscrasias?
- How does mode of drug administration affect person's response to drug?

NURSE'S RESPONSIBILITIES RELATED TO DRUG ADMINISTRATION

You will also need to know what your responsibilities are related to:

- Adhering to the "five rights" of drug administration—Right time, Right drug, Right dose Right route, and Right patient.
- Special measures required before administering the drug (ie, taking the pulse, blood pressure; checking blood drug levels).
- Potential for drug dependence/tolerance.
- Potential hazardous or adverse reactions.
- Effects the drug may have for an elderly person; for a very young person; or for the pregnant woman, including contraindications and/or dosage.
- Providing adequate information about the drugs in the teaching plan.

DRUGS AND THE ELDERLY

This group of individuals comprise a large portion of the patient population and present a special challenge to the health care provider. Even the well elderly have physiologic changes that affect metabolism and elimination of drugs, thus placing them at risk for adverse side effects. Risks increase for elders with one or more chronic diseases that require multiple drugs. See the box describing the various risk factors associated with the aging process and response to drug therapy.

OTHER FACTORS THAT AFFECT DRUG THERAPY

Assessment of a person's attitude toward drug use is also important in devising a plan of care. Many people associate taking medicine with getting well and, thus, adhere to the drug regimen. However, a person's perception and expectations regarding outcomes of drug therapy can be influenced by culture or family beliefs. Some people rely on traditional home remedies, which may interfere with the prescribed therapy. Others may view medications as unnecessary or damaging and refuse to take them.

Gender can affect a person's response to drugs. Men may metabolize certain drugs more quickly than women. Certain ethnic groups may also respond differently to drugs. For example, the response of African-Americans to adrenergic beta-blocker agents commonly used to control hypertension is less than the response of Caucasians; Chinese people seem to be more sensitive to these drugs than either of the other two groups (Clark, Queener, & Karb, 1997). In addition, some ethnic groups are deficient in specific enzymes that can alter response to drugs.

▶ ASSESSMENT PART TWO— THE NURSE ANALYZES DATA

Your next step is to *analyze* all the described information to make appropriate nursing diagnoses and to state the desired client outcomes related to drug therapy. Organizing data into clusters or patterns aids in the analysis. For example, grouping all data pertaining to anxiety, or all data pertaining to risks for infection or fluid and electrolyte imbalance, will structure your plan of action. These preliminary steps are crucial in building the foundation for the remaining phases of the nursing process—nursing diagnoses, effective outcomes, planning, implementation, and evaluation. Four important concepts to remember are:

- Drug effects depend on the specific drug, the dosage, and the individual patient.
- Drugs mimic the way cells talk to each other.
- Drugs are created to modify existing functions within the body—NOT to create new functions.
- No drug has a single action, and all drugs have potential for causing a response from more than one system.

NURSING DIAGNOSES/CLIENT OUTCOMES

Every nursing diagnosis should have at least one *measurable* client outcome, or response/behavior, that can be achieved within a defined time frame. When anticipated outcomes are shared with the client and family (or support persons), these persons can actively participate in care and making decisions. Measurable outcome statements should be specific and realistic and incorporate the person's desire and capabilities to meet the expected outcome. For example: "The client will administer own insulin correctly without coaching within three days." The time period for process outcomes, for example, "Patient will maintain a patent airway," would be ongoing until a particular problem is resolved. Process outcomes are monitored by the nurse and documented to assure that interventions are directed toward meeting the individual's need.

Integrating your knowledge of normal and abnormal physiologic functions with information on drug actions will assist you in selecting appropriate diagnoses and the plan of care. Identifying the client's strengths and use of wellness diagnoses, for instance, health-seeking behaviors, also aid in establishing attainable goals. Examples of wellness diagnosis statements are: (1) Making appropriate changes in lifestyle or attitude, (2) Adapting to illness, (3) Acquiring/learning new information and/or skills (Stolte, 1997). North American Nursing Diagnosis Association (NANDA) approved nursing diagnoses will be used in the following discussions.

Nursing diagnoses and outcomes for Mary Thompson, your perioperative patient, could include:

- N.D. (Neurologic System) Anxiety related to the surgical experience and management of postoperative discomfort.
  Outcomes: Relief of anxiety, increased knowledge of surgical proceedings and assurance of adequate postoperative analgesia. (Timelines can be added for measurement purposes.)
- N.D. (Endocrine System) Risk for fluid and electrolyte imbalance related to NPO status.
  Outcome: Fluid and electrolyte balance will be maintained. (Add timeframe.)
- N.D. (Immune System) Potential for infection related to surgical procedure.
  Outcomes: Patient will remain free of infection as evidenced by absence of fever and other vital signs within normal limits, and normal lab values, eg, white blood count. (Add timeframe.)

Nursing diagnoses and their related outcomes serve as guides for planning and implementing interventions in collaboration with the client (and, frequently, with other health care team members). Selected interventions related to *medication therapy* for the above diagnoses would include: (1) Provide time to discuss Mrs. Thompson's concerns; discuss postoperative pain control; provide adequate postoperative analgesia. (2) Provide fluids as appropriate; maintain accurate fluid intake–output record; give supplemental electrolytes (if ordered), monitor person's response to prescribed electrolyte therapy. (3) Assess vital signs, assess surgical wound for signs of infection, maintain aseptic technique, and administer antibiotics as ordered.

Common nursing diagnoses related to drug therapy are:

- Noncompliance R/T side effects of medication or forgetfulness, denial, etc.
- Noncompliance R/T overuse or underuse.
- Knowledge deficit R/T directions or purpose of drug or its importance.
- Risk for injury R/T adverse side effects of medication.

The nurse can incorporate these diagnoses into the teaching plan.

Expected client outcomes related to *all* drug therapy include the following. The client will:

- Describe purpose and importance of medication therapy; comply with prescribed regimen; *not* adjust dosage schedule or amount without permission; *not* over or under use drug, or share drug with others.
- Demonstrate how to manage side effects, take measures to avoid side effects, report any adverse effects of drug(s) and possible reactions related to other drugs and foods.
- Consult with health care provider/pharmacist before using OTC drug, eg, cold medicines.

Risk Factors of Aging Process and Response to Drug Therapy

DRUG-RELATED PROBLEM	CONTRIBUTING FACTOR
Altered response to drug (delay in absorption, distribution, metabolism, excretion of drug).	Natural "slowing physiologic changes" due to aging process.
Potential for additive and synergistic drug effects.	Polypharmacy regimen commonly used to manage more than one health problem.
Self-medication with over-the-counter drugs/interactions with prescribed drugs.	Individuals do not understand potential for interactions.
Poor nutrition/limited exercise/altered serum drug levels.	Fatigue, limited income, physical disabilities, anorexia, dental and digestive problems.
Misdiagnosis of adverse effects of drugs/diminished quality of life.	Drug side effects can mimic aging behaviors or caregivers' stereotypical perception of elder behavior.
Noncompliance—denial of problem resulting in threat to health. (An especially high incidence in this age population.)	Over/underuse of drugs due to: impaired memory, serious side effects of drugs, knowledge deficit of purpose of drug, delay in communicating with health care provider.

- Inform all health care providers (including dentist) about health problems, allergies, medications, including use of OTC drugs, herbal remedies, vitamins, or alcohol.
- Practice safety precautions related to drug therapy that would be detrimental to self or others (avoid any dangerous or hazardous activity if dizzy or unsteady).

A defined time period may be added to meet measurement criteria.

PLANNING—SETTING THE PRIORITIES

This phase sets the stage for nursing interventions. The nursing diagnoses are ranked in order of their importance, and strategies are designed to meet short- and long-term outcome goals. An individualized plan is developed using all factual data about the person, the specific health problem, and the resources available. Appropriate interventions are those that are acceptable to the client and that meet nursing and agency standards. A written plan serves as a communication tool to assure continuity of care for the client's present and future needs.

Mrs. Thompson's major concerns prior to surgery are her anxiety over the surgical outcome and how her postoperative pain will be managed. (She probably hasn't even thought about the possibility of infection or fluid and electrolyte imbalances.) Your first priority, then, would be to relieve anxiety for Mrs. Thompson and her family by describing basic procedures, explaining the potential sequence of events, and assuring them that she will have adequate postoperative analgesia and continuity of care. An assessment of their coping strategies will also assist in developing strategies for including their involvement in the plan of care. Your plan would include instructions on when to report her pain for appropriate medication management, how to facilitate analgesia through relaxation, and the rationale for precautions taken following administration of medication.

The second priority nursing diagnosis is the potential for infection. Your plan of prevention includes instructing Mrs. Thompson and her family on the importance of (1) deep breathing and coughing techniques to minimize postoperative lung congestion, (2) maintaining a clean surgical site, (3) maintaining adequate nutrition and fluid balance, and (4) providing a rationale for completing the antibiotic schedule as prescribed. The nurse would also encourage mobility and exercise, monitor for systemic and localized signs and symptoms of infection, and promote adequate nutritional and fluid intake. The third diagnosis, fluid and electrolyte imbalances, is of particular importance during surgery and in the postoperative period. The nurse assumes primary responsibilities for maintaining the intravenous solution containing electrolytes at the appro-

priate rate, monitoring the client's responses, and reporting any deviations from the expected values (McCloskey & Bulechek, 1996). Mrs. Thompson is encouraged to drink fluids and eat nutritious foods when able. All three diagnoses are interrelated and their outcomes are affected by each other. Anxiety and pain affect the ability to cope and participate in self-care, alter the healing process, and may influence the individual's responses to medication. Inadequate fluids and electrolytes alter pharmacokinetics and can increase the person's susceptibility to infection. Infection robs the person of needed energy, can increase risk for adverse drug reactions, and prolongs convalescence.

IMPLEMENTING—THERAPEUTIC NURSING INTERVENTIONS

Certain interventions are standard for all persons receiving drug therapy. Some medications may require specific procedures prior to administration, for instance, assessment of vital signs, serum drug levels, compatibility of drugs being taken, and time schedule. Today's emphasis on patient-focused care requires active participation by the client, as well as family and support persons, in managing drug therapy. Teaching individuals about their drug regimen and how to monitor drug effects are major components of that process. Some of these standard interventions are to:

- Determine factors that preclude the client from taking medication as ordered and behavior modification toward a healthy lifestyle. (Client's readiness and willingness to learn are important factors, as well as the influence of culture and beliefs on an individual's attitude.)
- Evaluate client's (and/or family/caregiver's) ability to administer medication.
- Consult with other health care team members regarding teaching materials related to diet, exercise, additional lifestyle changes, medication management. (The pharmacist may assist in planning dosage schedule that will have minimal impact on a person's lifestyle; stating what major safety precautions to take; strategies to take when dose is missed; interactions with OTC drugs, herbs, and foods; dangers of sharing drugs and abrupt withdrawal of drug.)
- Enlist help from other health care providers for innovative teaching methods for persons with sensory disabilities, comprehension difficulties, etc.
- Instruct client and family about medications; provide written and visual materials to aid learning and as reinforcement; demonstrate use and care of devices used for administering medication; instruct what procedures to take prior to administering medication (monitoring pulse, glucose level, etc) as appropriate.
- Stipulate preventive measures for storage of drug to avoid accidental use by child (or others) and the actions to take if an accident occurs.

Client's Questions to Guide Medication Teaching Plan

- Why do I need (name of medication)?
- What effect does my health problem (disease) have on my life?
- What is the usual treatment for this problem?
- How does (name of medication) differ from the other medicines used for this problem?
- How quickly will I benefit from (name of medication)? What happens if (name of medication) doesn't do what it is supposed to do?
- How do I take (name of medication)?
- What are the common side effects? How long do they last? Will they interfere with my lifestyle, my work, etc?
- Are there any serious side effects? Could that happen to me? What are the symptoms?
- What does my doctor/health care provider need to know about me to decrease my risks of serious side effects from (name of medication)?
- Can I take other medications when I'm taking (name of medication)? What about OTC drugs, vitamins, foods, herbal remedies?
- [For female clients] What if I become pregnant while taking (name of medication)?
- Are there any other risks (eg, smoking, alcohol) that I should know about?
- Where do I get more information about (name of medication)?

Standard Nursing Instructions on Medication Safety

- Provide essential information related to purpose of medication, dosage schedule, what to do when dose is missed, potential common drug side effects, precautions to take, what symptoms to report to physician/health care provider.

Note: Clients may be ordering several months' supply through the mail and may not read or understand written instructions if they are provided. Also, clients may not have easy access to the health care provider.

- Inform clients that altering dose amount without notifying the health care provider may be harmful. Reinforce written instructions. (Determine if client can read and understand instructions.) Answer questions as needed.

Standard Nursing Instructions on Medication Safety (continued)

- Provide sufficient information about health problem/disease for client to realize its impact on life, need for drug therapy, and importance of making appropriate decisions.
- Inform of possible incidence of serious side effects, the individual's particular risks, symptoms, strategies to take, and what to report to doctor/health care provider immediately. Encourage clients with allergies and chronic illnesses to inform <u>all</u> health care providers and to wear identification tag detailing health problems/medications.
- Caution client to avoid taking OTC drugs, vitamins, home remedies, or other drugs without consulting with physician/health care provider.
- Clients taking multiple drugs should maintain a current list, keep it with them, and provide all health care providers with update.
- Provide rationale for not stopping medications abruptly. Reinforce instructions to take all of prescription, if directed to do so.
- Instruct client not to share drugs with others. Inform on proper storage of drugs and caution to keep drugs out of children's reach. Use childproof caps if children are in home. Do not refer to medicine as candy. Instruct client not to mix different medications in same container. Teach proper disposal of unused drugs.
- Demonstrate how to administer drugs, eg, instillation of eye/ear drops. Obtain feedback to assure that client understand directions.
- Collaborate with interdisciplinary health team members in designing appropriate medication management. Suggest strategies that will assist client in adherence to drug regimen. Encourage client's active participation in self-care.
- Provide name(s) of resource persons for further information.

- Provide name(s) of resource persons to answer questions and concerns regarding medication and self-care, costs, medication alert devices.
- Inform how to renew prescription, proper disposal of expired drugs.
- Evaluate client's learning/understanding.

See the box depicting a client's questions that guide an individualized medication teaching plan and the boxes that describe standard nursing interventions related to drug administration and instruction.

EVALUATION—THE NURSE DETERMINES OUTCOME ACHIEVEMENT

The expected outcomes can be used as indicators of goal achievement and effectiveness of the plan, or demonstrate deviations. Evaluation is ongoing throughout the nursing process and dictates any modifications or continuance of the plan. The nursing process is cyclic in nature, requiring reexamination of each step or phase.

► CONCLUSION

A holistic approach is crucial to the success in administration of drugs, monitoring client responses, maintaining drug therapy, and evaluating client outcomes (Kee & Hayes, 1997). The systematic format of the nursing process provides an effective method to support successful results from the prescribed therapy. The current managed care environment requires the client to become a more active member of the health care team. The most appropriate decisions are made by informed individuals. One of the greatest gifts nurses can give to their clients is empowerment through knowledge. This requires the nurse to have a thorough understanding of physiologic functions and pathophysiologic effects and to be able to differentiate normal from abnormal symptoms and reactions. An understanding of psychosocial variables and individual responses is also necessary.

A case study approach is used in this chapter to illustrate these various factors. Several additional case studies have been designed to assist the student in the application of critical-thinking skills in all phases of the nursing process. The student is invited to use these vignettes and concepts presented in the chapter as springboards in planning and implementing individualized and effective drug therapy plans.

The "Pharmacist's Response" is a feature that is used to provide information on drug actions and actual and/or potential drug interactions related to the the case study vignettes from the perspective of a pharmacist. Additional general information is supplied regarding interactions of these medications and other drugs within the nervous system and among the other Master Systems.

The critical thinking questions are used to encourage the reader to research information that will assist in planning, implementing, and evaluating care to be provided for these individuals.

► NURSING ACTION CASE STUDIES

The following case studies related to medication therapy are designed to illustrate the language and patterns of communication among the three Master Systems. Multiple drugs are included in each case study to reflect actual clinical practice. Examples include drugs that affect action potential, agents that mimic or block parasympathetic and sympathetic nervous system actions, and drugs that primarily influence functions within the endocrine and immune systems. Yet each drug designed for a specific effect has impact on the total person. Questions related to the nurse's role in drug therapy are placed within the framework of the nursing process to stimulate critical thinking.

 # Case Study 1 Vignette

Mr. Jackson, an African-American, age 67, has been diagnosed with hypertension, with a systolic range of 160–179 and diastolic range of 100–109. For the last several weeks, he has also experienced chest pains upon exertion. Prior to these symptoms, he had episodes of shortness of breath accompanied by generalized weakness and dizziness when he climbed a flight of stairs or walked up an incline, forcing him to stop and rest. Sometimes he could feel a rapid pulse beat "pounding" in his ears. Yesterday, the pain occurred shortly after eating a steak dinner "with all the trimmings" at a restaurant in celebration of his son's 40th birthday. The viselike pain was more intense than usual and radiated to his jaw and shoulders. "I thought I was having a heart attack and was going to die," he said, "just like my father did when he was only 60."

Mr. Jackson admitted that he has seldom sought medical help. His last checkup was more than a year ago. At that time, his blood pressure was moderately elevated (155/98), pulse rate was 88–92, and his serum cholesterol was 244 mg/dL (normal is < 240 mg/dL). He had noticed some swelling of his legs at the end of the day. His doctor prescribed metoprolol tartrate [Lopressor], a cardioselective beta$_1$ blocker agent, and hydrochlorothiazide (HCTZ) (for mild diuresis); however, he did not keep a return appointment scheduled for 2 months later. The doctor also recommended a low-salt, reduced-calorie diet and moderate exercise, but Mr. Jackson has not adhered to this regimen. He did not like the side effects of the drugs or the restriction of his favorite foods, and exercise was "too much bother." In fact, he has gained a few pounds since his retirement, and he now weighs 170 lb. His height is 5 ft 9½ in. He has limited cigarette smoking to one-half pack a day for the past year.

For purposes of this discussion, Mr. Jackson was placed on nifedepine [Procardia] sustained-release tablets and sublingual nitroglycerin tablets to take as needed for chest pain.

 The Pharmacist's Response

Mr. Jackson, age 67. Diagnosed with cardiovascular problems and hypertension. Medications include nifedepine [Procardia]—calcium-channel blocker, and nitroglycerine—sustained-release and sublingual—a vasodilator agent

Actions

Drugs classified as calcium-channel blockers, such as Procardia XL and Cardizem, are some of the most frequently used drugs prescribed for hypertension and angina. The effects on the nervous system are shown through action on the cells of the heart itself and the vasculature.

Mr. Jackson has a multitude of health factors that affect many drug actions. First, he has been noncompliant with the earlier drug regimen. It is difficult to treat someone who does not want to take responsibility for his own care. Therefore, the choice of treatment for these individuals is by the simplest and easiest methods, which includes once-a-day dosage of one medication that produces the desired action with minimal side effects. Procardia XL is an excellent choice, for these reasons. Also, several major biologic functions are altered by his disease processes, his age (67), and his ethnicity. Alterations in the cardiovascular system and the aging process can particularly affect metabolism and excretion of drugs, and African-Americans do not respond to some antihypertensive drugs as well as Caucasians.

The only potential problem to effective drug action with either Procardia XL or nitroglycerin would be absorption. Ab-

sorption problems are virtually eliminated when nitroglycerin is given sublingually. If Mr. Jackson swallows the Procardia XL pill whole without chewing the tablet, the medication is released slowly all day long and the potential problem with drug absorption is minimized.

 Critical Thinking Questions

1. Using the history information cited in the vignette, list key factors related to the neurologic system that have contributed to the progression of Mr. Jackson's health problems.

2. Why are calcium channel blockers, eg, nifedipine, effective in relieving angina pain and hypertension?

3. What would you include in the teaching plan for Mr. Jackson related to nifedipine? What specific instructions would you include for the sustained-release form?

4. Identify at least four outcomes you would expect to see as the result of Mr. Jackson's adherence to the plan of care (for nifedipine). Include at least one beneficial outcome in each of the three Master Systems.

5. What information would you give to Mr. Jackson regarding the use of sublingual nitroglycerin to relieve an attack of angina? As a prophylactic measure?

6. What are two common <u>adverse</u> side effects of nitroglycerin?

7. What measures can Mr. Jackson take to minimize these effects?

TABLE 21-1   Interactions of Calcium-Channel Blocking Agents With Other Nervous System Agents

Calcium-Channel Blocker	Nervous System Drug	Interaction	Intervention
Nifedipine [Procardia]	Quinidine (Duraquin)—antiarrhythmic	Increases quinidine clearance	Stagger dosage schedule or reduce dosage
Verapamil [Calan SR]	Quinidine	Decreases quinidine clearance—hypotension	Stagger dosage schedule
Nifedipine & verapamil	Carbamazepine [Tegretol] antiseizure drug	Increase levels of antiseizure drug	Change to another calcium-channel blocker, stagger dosage, or reduce dosage of Tegretol
Nifedipine & verapamil	Cimetidine & ranitidine (especially) H₂ antagonists—antigastric ulcer therapy	Increase bioavailability of calcium-channel blockers	Reduce dosage of calcium drugs or change to less interacting H₂ antagonists, ie, nizatidine [Axid] or famotidine [Pepcid]
Nifedipine & verapamil	Fentanyl [Sublimaze]—analgesic	Severe hypotension	Schedule analgesic & calcium-channel blockers at wider intervals

TABLE 21-2   Interaction of Calcium Channel Blocking Agents With Immune System Drugs

Calcium-Channel Blockers	Immune System Drugs	Interaction	Intervention
Felodipine [Plendil]	Erythromycin—a potent enzyme inhibitor	Felodipine levels greatly increased	
All	Warfarin [Coumadin]—anticoagulant	Warfarin levels increased	Closely monitor prothrombin time to determine dose adjustments
All	Cyclosporin [Sandimmune, Neoral]—prevent organ transplant rejection (patient may be on hypertensives also)	Increased levels of cyclosporin	May be advantageous Combination of drugs can achieve desired effect at a lower cost

 ## Case Study 2 Vignette

Your next client is Ken Anderson, age 40, who is an accountant. He has been an insulin-dependent diabetic since age 12. He has now been diagnosed with secondary open-angle glaucoma. He has recently noticed recurrent blurring of vision with gradual loss of peripheral vision, difficulty adjusting to darkened conditions, and seeing colored rings around lights. He also has experienced an increase in pain and redness of his eyes, particularly at the end of the day. He said that his mother also had glaucoma.

The usual daily medication therapy for glaucoma includes: (1) topical miotics (direct-acting cholinergic) to constrict the pupil and increase outflow of aqueous humor, eg, pilocarpine or (2) topical beta-adrenergic antagonists, eg, timolol [Timoptic] to suppress production of aqueous humor; (3) an oral carbonic anhydrase inhibitor, eg, acetazolamide [Diamox] may be added for its diuretic action and suppression of aqueous humor production. The effectiveness of beta-adrenergic antagonists in most types of glaucoma and their fewer systemic effects make them the current drug category of choice. A combination of drugs is often prescribed.

 ## Critical Thinking Questions

1. What is the sequence and schedule for administering the eye medications when more than one medication is ordered?

2. What information would you give Mr. Anderson to allay his fears about the systemic effects of timolol and pilocarpine on his diabetes management?

3. Are there any specific instructions you should give him about his adjustment to dim light or when he is in bright sunlight?

 ## Case Study 2 Vignette (Continued)

Several months later, Mr. Anderson experienced a flare-up of his seasonal allergy symptoms. A co-worker recommended that he try some of his astemizole [Hismanal] because it had worked so well on his own symptoms. Mr. Anderson declined because of the previous instructions regarding OTC drugs, and also because of his concern about its effect on his diabetes control. You commend him on this action and state that the reference books indicate that Hismanal is to be used cautiously for persons with increased intraocular pressure (IOP).

Following a thorough history and examination, the physician prescribes a low dose of Hismanal, and advises Mr. Anderson to return for IOP check within 1 week.

 ### The Pharmacist's Response

Mr. Ken Anderson, age 40. Diagnosed with glaucoma and insulin dependency. Medications include pilocarpine/timolol—adrenergic beta-blocking agents and astemizole [Hismanal]—an antihistamine agent.

Actions

Most insulin-dependent diabetics have impaired circulation and are susceptible to glaucoma and other related diseases. Most persons do not think that absorption of drugs through the eye reaches systemic circulation—but it does. In fact, systemic absorption from the eye is quite extensive. However, ophthalmic medications are in small concentrations and given in minute doses, and systemic effects are not as profound as when the medication is given in tablet or pill form. Pilocarpine does not have many drug–drug interactions; however, timolol (beta-adrenergic blocker and astemizole [Hismanal], an antihystamine, do. Most precautions related to use of pilocarpine are due to the disease of glaucoma itself. Some OTC medications might exacerbate glaucoma, as mentioned in the vignette.

Beta-blockers are nervous system medications used orally and ocularly. When beta-blockers are given orally, significant drug interactions can occur for persons with diabetes. Beta-blockers can inhibit beta$_1$ cells in the heart and beta$_2$ cells throughout the body. Oral administration of drugs that act on beta$_1$ cells are preferred for diabetic clients because there is less potential for hypoglycemia. However, it is necessary to prescribe a beta$_2$ action drug for its ocular effects for Mr. Anderson. The lowest possible dose would be prudent, and its effect on glucose control would be minor.

In the immune system, astemizole [Hismanal] and is a potent antihistamine with the potential for serious drug interaction effects. Such medications have a "black-box warning" in package inserts. Serious cardiovascular conditions may ensue following therapy. An individual may experience a prolongation of the QT interval of the cardiac cycle and ventricular arrhythmias. Persons with liver disorders are also strongly discouraged from taking these antihistamines for the same reasons. Most of the adverse events occur when an individual takes interacting medications or has liver dysfunction.

 Critical Thinking Questions

1. What would you include in a patient/family teaching plan related to administration of Hismanal and potential side effects in the nervous, endocrine, and immune systems?

2. Since Mr. Anderson is so concerned about a drug's effect on his diabetic control, what information would you give him to lessen his concern?

3. What symptoms would indicate adverse side effects related to his glaucoma?

TABLE 21-3 Drug Interactions Related to Timolol and Hismanal

Drug	Interaction	Result/Treatment
Timolol (beta-blocker)	Synergistic—added effects with other nervous systemic beta-blockers	Increases levels of quinidine and verapamil, resulting in bradycardia
Hismanal	Increased Hismanal levels by enzyme inhibition from macrolide antibiotics (erythromycin, clarithromycin) and azole antifungals (fluconazole, itraconazole)	Treatment: Withdraw use of antihistamine or use loratidine [Claritin], which is a noninteracting, nonsedating antihistamine, until other drug therapy is over

 # Case Study 3 Vignette

Mrs. Nancy Pringle, age 65, was brought to the emergency department by ambulance after being awakened early in the morning by severe dyspnea accompanied by an episode of incessant coughing and production of thick, viscous sputum. Her husband said she felt as if she was suffocating and he noticed that her skin was quite gray; her hands were cold and clammy. Her breathing sounded very "noisy and wet." She appeared extremely anxious, almost in a state of panic. When he took her pulse, it was very fast and weak. She became very confused. This attack was worse than any other, and he knew immediate help was necessary. The swelling in her feet and legs had increased during the past month, she had gained 4 lb, and she experienced labored breathing with the slightest exertion. She was constantly fatigued "even though she has taken all her medicines."

Mr. Pringle said that she had been a semi-invalid since her heart attack 4 months ago. He admitted that they usually rely on frozen dinners, canned foods, and takeout meals.

Their daughter and grandchildren's weekly visits are short, "because my wife tires easily when they're around." Mr. Pringle works as an auto mechanic and Mrs. Pringle is home alone except on Thursdays, when the housekeeper is there. He expressed his great concern about the outcome of his wife's present condition. Mrs. Pringle has been on a daily maintenance dose of verapamil (calcium channel blocker/antiarrhythmic), hydrochlorothiazide [HydroDiuril] (a diuretic), and a potassium supplement.

Following the initial workup, Mrs. Pringle was admitted to the CCU with the diagnosis of pulmonary edema. (Her reported symptoms are typical.) Medical management included the administration of *oxygen* to relieve hypoxia and dyspnea; *morphine* to relieve anxiety and pain; intravenous furosemide [Lasix] for rapid removal of fluids; and digoxin to assist the impaired cardiac function. (Two additional drugs, naloxone hydrochloride [Narcan], an antagonist to morphine, and aminophylline may also be ordered to relax the bronchioles and to facilitate gas exchange.)

★ The Pharmacist's Response

Mrs. Nancy Pringle, age 65. Diagnosed with pulmonary edema old MI, and congestive heart failure. Medications include digitalis (digoxin), a cardiotonic, and aminophylline (theophylline), a bronchodilator.

Congestive heart failure (CHF) is a disease for which multiple drug therapies are used. Medications to control CHF affect potassium and fluid levels. Many times, the patient requires multiple drugs as a result of adding only one additional drug. This problem cannot be avoided, because the patient could not survive without any one of the medications.

The major problem in treating Mrs. Pringle is that she takes many drugs and thereby increases her risks for drug interactions. A treatment goal for Mrs. Pringle would be to use the lowest possible drug doses and as few drugs as possible, and still control CHF symptoms. (Refer to critical thinking questions at end of case vignette for further research on Mrs. Pringle's many other drugs and their potential interactions.)

Actions

Aminophylline is a form of theophylline salt that is 79% plain theophylline. Theophylline drug interactions will be used for this discussion. It is well documented that theophylline is highly metabolized by the liver and requires specific blood levels for effective therapy. Theophylline has a very narrow therapeutic serum level and any alteration in theophylline levels can be dangerous. A standard practice is to closely monitor patient responses and serum levels until a steady state is reached.

Caregivers for Mrs. Pringle must consider that she is elderly and assure that she does not smoke before taking aminophylline. The elderly do not normally have efficient metabolizing capabilities as younger people do. Also, smokers have

elevated enzyme metabolism of theophylline, thus frequently requiring higher drug doses than nonsmokers.

Theophylline is one of thee medications that interact with many drugs in each of the master systems. All of the following drugs increase theophylline serum levels. Erythromycin and quinolone antibiotics [Cipro, Noroxin] in the immune system must be used sparingly with theophylline. Verapamil [Calan SR] and propranolol [Inderal], nervous system agents, must be used cautiously for persons with Mrs. Pringle's health problems. Oral contraceptives, endocrine system drugs, can also increase theophylline serum levels. Usually if the patient needs to be on both interacting medications, and there is no alternative, physicians will monitor the patient and adjust the interacting drugs accordingly. This will minimize the possible effects of drug interaction on the prescribed therapy.

Digoxin toxicity is a common phenomenon. Owing to the narrow therapeutic serum range, patients receiving digoxin must be closely monitored until a steady serum level is reached. Many drugs given concurrently with digoxin interact unfavorably. Many of the interactions can be avoided by close monitoring.

Clinicians must find a digoxin dose that helps Mrs. Pringle's heart to beat more strongly and decrease potential for interactions with the furosemide [Lasix] diuretic prescription. Frequently these medications are used together despite the interaction side effect. This is a situation in which the treatment outcome must outweigh the potential risk of drug interaction. The goals are for Mrs. Pringle to breathe more easily and for a halt in the progression of her disease.

Critical Thinking Questions

1. What are the hallmark indicators of morphine toxicity to include in your assessment following administration of morphine analgesia?

2. What safety precautions would you incorporate into your plan of care for a client receiving narcotic analgesia? What instructions would you provide to the client?

3. How does naloxone [Narcan] reverse narcotic action? Why is it necessary to closely monitor the individual for a period of time following administration of Narcan even though it produces a rapid response?

4. When planning the schedule for administering bid doses of Lasix, what times in the day would you use? What is your rationale?

5. The risk for digitalis toxicity is great owing to the combined effects of digoxin and furosemide [Lasix]

(and similar diuretics). Describe the common symptoms of digitalis toxicity.

6. What is the most common electrolyte imbalance resulting from the digoxin/furosemide combined actions? What are the adverse side effects related to this electrolyte imbalance?

7. How does digoxin improve cardiac function? Describe the assessment parameters and rationale

for withholding a prescribed dose of a digitalis preparation.

8. When aminophylline is given to relax the bronchioles and facilitate gas exchange, what potential effect would it have on the beta$_1$ receptors of the heart?

TABLE 21-4 Digoxin Drug Interactions

Interacting Drugs	Interaction	Interventions
Nervous system drugs— quinidine, verapamil, amiodarone, propafenone	Reduce renal clearance of digoxin—resulting in toxicity	Reduce dose approximately 50% and closely monitor for signs of digoxin toxicity
Metoclopramide	Reduces bioavailability of digoxin by stimulating GI movement	Use either elixir or capsules of digoxin to increase bioavailability
Endocrine system drugs— sprinolactone, ACE inhibitors (captopril, lisinopril, etc)	Reduce renal clearance of digoxin	Reduce digoxin dose by 50% and monitor serum levels and individual responses
Immune system drugs—tetracycline & erythromycin	These antiinfectives can contribute to hypokalemia which subsequently can lead to digitalis toxicity.	If possible, change antibiotic therapy or reduce dose of digoxin
Alimentary canal—Questran and antacids	Greatly hinder absorption or inactivate drug by binding with it	Stagger doses between digoxin and interacting drugs by at least 1–2 hours

Case Study 4 Vignette

Mary Noble, age 77, has experienced many of the cardinal symptoms of Alzheimer's disease (AD) over the past 3 years. Her husband, Carl, died 5 years ago, and she lived alone until she moved in with her married daughter, Susan, and her family last year. During the family conference, Susan and her husband, Charles, learn that the incidence of Alzheimer's disease (also referred to as degenerative or senile dementia) is commonly associated with age; however, it can occur in younger adults (40–50), particularly when there is a familial relationship. Symptoms have a gradual onset and can run a course of 3–20 years until the person's death. Neuropathologic and biochemical changes result in progressive memory loss, personality changes, failure to recognize familiar persons and objects, inability for abstract thinking, restlessness, wandering, becoming lost, and self-care deficits.

Mary is diagnosed with moderate-level symptoms. Susan quit her secretarial position to care for her mother because of safety issues. Mary has become combative at times and appears very depressed. Sometimes, she wanders during the night; at other times few symptoms are evident. The physician has decided on a trial use of tacrine [Cognex], which

is classified as a cholinergic (parasympathomimetic) drug. It also inhibits the reuptake of norepinephrine, serotonin, and dopamine.

Critical Thinking Questions

1. Describe the symptoms you would usually expect to see as a result of parasympathomimetic drug action. What is the rationale for prescribing tacrine for Mary?

2. How does the presence of food affect the absorption rate of tacrine? When are the best times of the day to administer tacrine?

3. What instructions would you give to Susan about potential adverse effects related to initiation of tacrine therapy? What are the potential delayed adverse effects?

4. What indicators would you use to evaluate the effectiveness of tacrine therapy? When would you expect to see improvement in Mary's behavior? What information would you provide to Susan and her family regarding expectations of tacrine therapy?

 # Case Study 4 Vignette (Continued)

Several months later, Mary still experiences insomnia and becomes easily agitated and confused, especially later in the day (sundowner syndrome). The family has considered institutionalization, but are willing to try one more option. Mary's physician adds haloperidol decanoate [Haldol] to her drug regimen. The treatment plan to help control these symptoms begins with low doses of haloperidol twice daily followed by gradual dosage increases if there is no adverse response

★ The Pharmacist's Response

Mrs. Mary Noble, age 77. Diagnosed with Alzheimer's disease. Medications include tacrine [Cognex] and haloperidol [Haldol], an antipsychotic agent.

Memory loss is a significant problem in maintaining drug therapy for people with Alzheimer's disease. These individuals frequently must rely on others to remind them to take their medication correctly and for optimal therapy. When this obstacle is overcome, the risk for other drug interactions is decreased.

Action

Tacrine [Cognex] is metabolized by the cytochrome P-450 hepatic enzyme system. Since Mrs. Noble does not have asthma or gastric ulcers, there will not be a concern for interactions with other common drugs metabolized by these enzymes, such as cimetidine and theophylline.

Haloperidol [Haldol] can be classified as a butyrophenone antipsychotic. The blocking action on dopamine is important in the treatment of Alzheimer's disease. However, since this medication is an active nervous system medication, many drug interactions are either synergistic or antagonistic toward the effects of Haldol on the body.

Fortunately, Mary Noble has no other medical problems. Adding Haldol does not interact with the tacrine and actually can help her condition to become more stable. She is heavily relying on nervous system medications to function, so additional nervous system medications should be used cautiously to avoid synergistic effects.

Haloperidol drug interactions occur primarily with other nervous system drugs. Meperidine [Demerol] and alcohol cause synergistic CNS effects. Lithium and Prozac use can lead to severe extrapyramidal symptoms (EPS). Concurrent use of Haldol with anorexants, anticholinergics, barbiturates, or carbamazepine may result in decreased serum levels, especially with the anticholinergic drugs. Serum levels may be increased by haloperidol for phenytoin, propranolol, and tricyclic antidepressants.

 ## Critical Thinking Questions

1. Describe the extrapyramidal reactions that may occur from the use of haloperidol [Haldol]. How would these reactions be controlled? Why would Haldol be contraindicated for a person with Parkinson's disease?

2. A potentially hazardous side effect is neuroleptic malignant syndrome (NMS). What symptoms/ reactions to haloperidol would you assess to indicate the presence of this condition?

3. State the potential side effects of haloperidol on the endocrine and immune systems.

4. Because of its long half-life, how quickly will you expect to see haloperidol's therapeutic effects?

TABLE 21-5 Tacrine Drug Interactions

Interacting Drug	Interaction	Intervention
Nervous system drug—cimetadine	Causes increase in tacrine serum levels via enzyme inhibition	Reduce tacrine dose or switch to less interacting agent (nizatidine, famotidine)
Nervous system drugs—anticholinergics— Cogentin, Donnatal, Pro-Banthine, Atrovent—even Benadryl	Antagonistic action; tacrine, a cholinesterase inhibitor, increases acetylcholine levels— opposite action to interacting drugs	Drugs are not compatible Concurrent use contraindicated
Nervous system drug—theophylline	Decreased renal clearance of theophylline resulting in increased serum levels of theophylline	Closely monitor and reduce theophylline dose according to diagnostic results

Case Study 5 Vignette

Mrs. Kathleen Adams, age 72, was diagnosed with Parkinson's disease 4 years ago. (Parkinson's disease usually develops in people over the age of 60. Mrs. Adams exhibits the three cardinal hallmarks of tremor, rigidity, and bradykinesia, or slow movements.) Her first notable symptom was a tremor, or a "pill-rolling" movement of her right thumb and fingers when at rest that usually slows or stops with voluntary movement. There has been a recent increase in the tremor in her right arm and a "clumsiness" in fine motor skills. She has the typical shuffling gait with absence of arm movement, and she falls frequently. At times, she "freezes" in place (akinesia, or lack of movement). Other behaviors are the typical stooped posture, the "masklike" facial expression, and drooling of saliva. She is frequently constipated. Her husband, John, has noticed her increased memory loss, confusion, and agitation. She cannot care for herself independently. He is her primary caregiver and is very concerned about his ability to continue in this role. Both Kathleen and John are very depressed. (Intellectual ability often remains intact; however, some individuals have symptoms similar to those of Alzhiemer's disease.)

Mrs. Adams has taken carbidopa-levodopa [Sinemet] for 2 years, but its effectiveness has decreased. She has been admitted to the hospital for monitoring the addition of selegiline [Eldepryl], a parasympatholytic agent, developed as adjunctive therapy when response to carbidopa-levodopa has deteriorated.

 ## The Pharmacist's Response

Mrs. Kathleen Adams, age 72. Diagnosed with Parkinson's disease. Medications: selegiline [Eldepryl].

Actions

Diet is an important consideration for patients taking selegiline [Eldepryl]. Selegiline, a monoamine oxidase inhibitor (MAOI), specifically acts upon the MAO-B enzyme. Nardil and Parnate are well-known as MAO-A inhibitors. Addition of aged cheeses, red wine, or other tyramine-containing foods can

cause a severe hypertensive crisis. The irony in this therapy is that Eldepryl is three to four times more bioavailable when taken with food. Patient education about the dangers and necessity to avoid these foods is very important. Since Mrs. Adams may also rely on other people to achieve optimum therapy results, caregivers should be aware that the diet has a very important role in drug interactions.

Mrs. Adams is also depressed. Antidepressants must be chosen with caution due to potentially serious drug interactions.

 ## Critical Thinking Questions

1. What are the potential neurologic side effects related to selegiline?

2. When selegiline is used as adjunctive therapy, how will the dose of carbidopa-levodopa [Sinemet] be adjusted?

3. How does the addition of carbidopa increase the effectiveness of levodopa? What instructions would you give to Mr. and Mrs. Adams on the effects of abrupt withdrawal of carbidopa-levodopa?

4. What teaching would you provide them to manage orthostatic hypotensive effects of selegiline [Eldepryl]?

5. Describe the "on–off" phenomenon that can occur after prolonged therapy with levodopa. What are the symptoms of dyskinesia?

6. Prepare an instructional plan to assist Mrs. Adams in the management of constipation that may be a drug side effect.

 # Case Study 6 Vignette

The primary reason for Nancy Garretson's visit to the outpatient clinic is for assessment of a recent episode of palpitations. The blood pressure reading was 178/98. Nancy, age 56, takes estradiol [Estrace] 1 mg daily five times a week pre-

scribed after her total hysterectomy 15 years ago. She is an executive secretary in a large insurance firm. She believes her recent divorce has been a major cause of her rise in blood pressure. She has occasional migraine headaches, but rates her overall health as good. The palpitation incident worries her, because both of her parents had cardiac and hypertensive problems.

Nancy, who is 5 ft, 3 in. tall, is somewhat overweight at 150 lbs. Several weight-reduction attempts have resulted in poor long-term effects. She frequently skips lunch and admits to overeating at dinnertime. Her work is quite demanding and she frequently works extra days, thus leaving little free time for recreational activities. However, she likes to walk and occasionally swims at the condominium pool.

Following the physical examination, several diagnostic studies are scheduled. The electrocardiogram is normal. The cholesterol level is 246 mg/dL. (The desired level is < 200 mg/dL.) Triglycerides were slightly elevated as well. Her health care provider prescribes propranolol [Inderal] and suggests some lifestyle changes including a low-salt, reduced-fat diet, daily exercise, and stress reduction strategies. She is scheduled to return within 2 weeks for blood pressure monitoring. Diuretic therapy may be added later, if needed.

You provide her with dietary pamphlets and reinforce the instructions for propranolol therapy.

★ The Pharmacist's Response

Nancy Garretson, age 56. Diagnosed with palpitations. Medications: Inderal (propranolol) and Estrace (estradiol).

Action

Beta-blockers (propranolol/Inderal) can be used for many nervous system disorders: hypertension, angina, arrhythmias, situational anxiety, migraines, and even the prevention of future myocardial infarctions. Careful monitoring of the patient's condition is very important. These medications have frequent side effects. Many disease states are negatively affected with beta-blocker therapy. Diabetics can experience hypoglycemia, but its symptoms may be masked by beta blockers. Patients with

bronchospastic diseases can have aggravations of their conditions by the blockade of beta-$_2$ receptors in the lungs.

Critical Thinking Questions

1. Propranolol [Inderal] is the prototype drug for the beta-adrenergic antagonists (beta blockers). Because of its nonselective beta activity, why would it be inappropriate for a person with asthma?

2. How is propranolol effective in the treatment of cardiac arrhythmias? What effect does it have on angina? What effect does it have on migraine headaches?

3. Develop a teaching plan for Nancy to follow while taking propranolol. What side effects would you include for her to be aware of? Identify three potential side effects that would negatively affect her compliance with the drug regimen.

4. Develop a weekly diet plan that would be helpful in managing Nancy's hypertension.

5. She questions you regarding the rationale for adding a diuretic. What information would you give her?

6. What are the potential side effects or toxic reactions to long-term estrogen therapy? What information would you include in a teaching plan for Nancy about hormonal replacement therapy?

TABLE 21-6 Medication Interactions and Nursing Interventions

Interacting Drugs	Interaction	Interventions
Calcium-channel blockers, hydralazine, loop diuretics, MAO inhibitors, quinidine, & ciprofloxacin	All *increase* levels of the beta-blockers; hypotension	Close monitoring of exaggerated side effects is warranted
Haloperidol & phenothiazines	Synergistic action causes *increased levels* of these drugs and beta-blockers	Stagger times between administration of drugs
Anticoagulants, acetaminophen, clonidine, benzodiazepines, epinephrine, ergot alkaloids, & systemic lidocaine	Levels of these drugs are *increased* in presence of beta-blockers	

Case Study 7 Vignette

Jim Whitman, a 30-year-old artist, has been admitted for a craniotomy to remove a large tumor in the cerebellar area. His symptoms include visual impairment, nystagmus (involuntary eye movements), dizziness, gait changes (staggering), ataxia, and occasional falls. Several diagnostic tests have been done. He admits that each test brings renewed apprehension regarding his prognosis.

Surgery was successful in removing the benign tumor. However, he is at risk of postoperative seizure activity due to edema, bleeding, increased intracranial pressure (ICP), fluid/electrolyte imbalances, or anoxia. Since the risk continues throughout the first year, a prophylactic regime of phenytoin [Dilantin] and diazepam [Valium] will be closely monitored. Drugs frequently ordered in the immediate postoperative period to counteract ICP include: steroids, eg, dexamethasone [Decadron] for antiinflammatory effect, osmotic diuretics to reduce edema, and oxygen for hypoxia. These drugs were ordered for the immediate postoperative period. Mr. Whitman is also at risk for infection due to dexamethasone therapy and should be closely observed.

 ## The The Pharmacist's Response

Jim Whitman, age 30. Craniotomy surgery for tumor.

Action

Multiple drug therapy is normal for seizure therapy. Many seizure disorders are not controlled adequately with one medication. Dilantin and barbituates increase metabolism of corticosteroids and higher doses may be required. Dilantin (phenytoin) drug interactions are many. Consult a drug guide. Adding Valium (diazepam) to seizure therapy may increase phenytoin levels. Barbituates are enzyme inducers; therefore, an established phenytoin dose will need to be increased following barbituate therapy.

 ## Critical Thinking Questions

1. When a person is unable to swallow a whole tablet of phenytoin [Dilantin], how could it be prepared? What effect would its strongly alkaline composition have on the esophagus? What effect would gastric secretions have on the drug?

2. Because of the narrow margin between the therapeutic and toxic serum levels of phenytoin, what neurologic symptoms require close monitoring?

3. What would you include in the client/family education program on phenytoin regarding: urine changes, symptoms of liver dysfunction, consequences of abrupt withdrawal, changes in brands of phenytoin, and flu immunizations?

4. What specific vitamin/mineral/electrolyte deficiencies occur as result of prolonged phenytoin therapy? What is gingival hyperplasia? What prophylactic measures help prevent this side effect?

5. What instructions would you give to a person about concurrent use of OTC medications and diazepam [Valium]? What effects does smoking have on diazepam drug action?

6. Categorize adverse side effects of steroidal antiinflammatory drugs as they relate to the three Master Systems. (Example: stress ulcers/neurologic system.)

7. Why would Mr. Whitman be more susceptible to infection when taking dexamethasone [Decadron]?

Case Study 8 Vignette

Jeanne West, age 50, took early retirement from her teaching career because of debilitating effects and pain from rheumatoid arthritis. Her problems include enlarged and deformed joints of her fingers, wrists, and right knee. Aspiration of fluid from the knee joint and instillation of hydrocortisone acetate last month provided some relief. She takes naproxen [Naprosyn], an NSAID (nonsteroidal antiinflammatory drug), daily. She states that she has trouble sleeping because of pain and she is depressed about her limited ability to perform simple tasks. At times she uses Tylenol with codeine No. 2 tablet at night to relieve the pain.

She lives with her sister, Dorothy, who works part-time as a reference librarian. At times, Jeanne senses that Dorothy resents helping her. She has come to the clinic to seek advice about trying a "second line" drug approach of chloroquine [Aralen], an antimalarial drug, that her doctor suggested to her earlier. She had tried a course of sulfasalazine, but it caused nausea and vomiting.

★ The The Pharmacist's Response

Jeanne West, age 50. Diagnosed with rheumatoid arthritis. Medications include Naprosyn (naproxin), Tylenol No. 2, chloroquine [Aralen].

Action

Nonsteroidal antiinflammatory drugs (NSAIDs) are also used for their analgesic and antipyretic properties. NSAIDs are metabolized by the liver and extensively excreted by the kidneys; therefore, decreased function of these organs will affect drug effects. Aralen (cloroquine) and other antimalarials have also been found to be effective as second-line therapy for treatment of arthritis. Therapeutic effects do not generally occur until several weeks after initiation of therapy. Caution patient regarding common side effects of dizziness, hypotension, photophobia, pruritis, and gastrointestinal disturbances.

Critical Thinking Questions

1. What are the similar side effects of sulfasalazine and chloroquine [Aralen]?

2. What is the rationale for using anti-infective drugs for rheumatoid arthritis?

3. Jeanne takes 500 mg of naproxen [Naprosyn] twice daily and frequently takes one Tylenol with codeine No. 2 tablet at 8:00 PM and one tablet at 12:00 AM. What concerns would you have regarding the effects on her neurologic system?

4. Would this combination of Tylenol with codeine and Naprosyn have any adverse effects on her endocrine and immune systems?

5. What changes would you expect to see in her responses to drugs due to the aging process when she is 65?

6. What instructions would you give to Miss West regarding potential side effects of naproxen related to the neurologic system? To the endocrine system? To the immune system?

TABLE 21-7 Medication Interactions and Nursing Interventions

Interacting Drugs	Interaction	Interventions
Phyentoin, digoxin, lithium	*Increased* blood levels when combined with NSAIDs	Monitor levels of these drugs.
Loop diuretics, ACE inhibitors, beta-blockers and thiazides	All drug levels will be *decreased* with NSAIDs	
Cyclosporine, anticoagulants	NSAIDs *increase* the levels of these drugs (synergistic action with anticoagulants)	Close monitoring for patients on anticoagulants and NSAID therapy

 # Case Study 9 Vignette

Neal Simpson, a 63-year-old mathematics professor, was recently diagnosed with prostatitis. His initial symptoms included fever, chills, urgency, difficulty in initiating a urinary stream, frequent voidings, dysuria, and dull low-back and perineal pain. During the past 10 days, he limited his fluid intake after 5:00 PM to avoid frequent episodes of nocturia. At his wife's insistence, he made an appointment with his primary physician. The ex-

amination revealed a very tender and swollen prostate. A urinalysis including culture and sensitivity was done. Dr. Nelson prescribed ciprofloxacin [Cipro], a broad spectrum anti-infective, and advised Mr. Simpson to drink at least 2–3 L of fluid daily. Additional laboratory testing included a complete blood count and prostate-specific-antigen (PSA) level. His PSA level was 6.5ng/mL. (Normal is 0–4.0 ng/mL for men over 40 years of age.) He was subsequently referred to a urologist, who performed a needle biopsy confirming the diagnosis of prostate cancer.

Dr. Allen explained the several options available and suggested that a cystoscopy and possible transurethral resection of the prostate (TURP) be done. Following the procedure Mr. Simpson will receive hormonal therapy of leuprolide acetate [Lupron], an injectable drug given once a month, and daily oral doses of flutamide [Eulexin] for approximately 1 year. The urologist explained that the newer hormonal medications have fewer adverse side effects than previously prescribed drugs, eg, diethylstilbestrol (DES). Mr. Simpson has been taking Sudafed, an OTC decongestant. He also takes an 80 mg tablet of aspirin daily, as a prophylactic against thromboembolism.

★ The Pharmacist's Response

Neal Simpson, age 63. Diagnosed with prostatitis and cancer of prostate. Medications include Cipro (ciprofloxin), Lupron (leuprolide), Eulexin (flutamide).

Action

Ciprofloxacin is classified in the category of fluoroquinolone antiinfectives, which are active against many gram-negative and gram-positive bacteria. Most often, Cipro is reserved for more serious infections of the lower respiratory tract, skin structure, bone, urinary tract infections, and infectious diarrhea from international travel.

 Critical Thinking Questions

1. What potential side effects would Sudafed have on Mr. Simpson's urinary problems?

2. What potential synergistic effects would there be between leuprolide [Lupron], flutamide [Eulexin], and Sudafed?

3. What is the rationale for using gonadotropin-releasing hormone therapy, such as leuprolide, for treatment of prostate cancer?

4. What effect would Mr. Simpson's hormonal therapy have on his libido and self image?

5. What is the rationale for performing culture and sensitivity testing prior to initiating antimicrobrial therapy?

6. How would you instruct Mr. Simpson regarding the use of antacids while he is taking ciprofloxacin [Cipro]? Why is it necessary for him to be well hydrated when taking ciprofloxacin?

7. How would aspirin affect diagnostic test results related to bleeding time, uric acid levels, liver function, and serum cholesterol?

8. As you instruct Mr. Simpson to self-administer the leuprolide, what precautions would you provide regarding the type of syringe? What precautions about probable symptoms he may experience? What symptons he should report to his physician?

TABLE 21-8 Medication Interactions and Nursing Interventions

Interacting Drugs	Interaction	Interventions
Nervous system drugs—phenytoin	Cipro *decreases* phenytoin levels	Monitor serum levels
Digoxin	Cipro *increases* digoxin levels	Space dosage times
Cimetidine	Cimetidine *increases* Cipro levels	
Endocrine system drug—probenecid	*Increases* Cipro levels by 50%	
Immune system drugs—antineoplastics	*Decreases* Cipro levels	
Cyclosporin, anticoagulants, theophylline	Cipro *increases* drug levels of these drugs	
Alimentary canal drugs—antacids, bismuth, iron salts, zinc salts, & sucralfate (Carafate)	These drugs *decrease* GI absorption of fluoroquinolones	Space dose of both medications at least 2–4 hours apart

Case Study 10 Vignette

Laura Hamilton, a 29-year-old woman in the third trimester of her second pregnancy, entered the clinic for treatment of a persistent cough, sore throat, shortness of breath, and "overwhelming" fatigue. Owing to financial constraints and lack of insurance coverage, she has delayed prenatal health care until today. Yesterday, she awakened to increased throat pain and severe difficulty in swallowing. Neither gargling with warm salt water nor frequent use of cough syrup seemed to help. She has not eaten within the past 24 hours, and has drunk only sips of ginger ale and sucked on ice chips. She says, "I guess I've taken about three bottles of Robitussin (dextromethorphan hydrobromide, OTC preparation) in the last month. I feel rotten and I'm exhausted! I sure hope you can give me something to make me feel better. I can't afford to lose my cashier job at the supermarket."

During the history assessment, she confides that her second husband, Tony, is serving a sentence for armed robbery committed to support his intravenous drug habit. According to a pamphlet she received at a local health fair last year, she could be at increased risk for contracting diseases such as HIV/AIDS and hepatitis B. This information prompted her to have a blood (ELISA) test shortly after she became pregnant. She was very relieved when the test results were negative. However, her recent symptoms are similar to those of HIV/AIDS described in the pamphlet. She is very concerned about herself and the baby. She is also worried about Tony's reaction and what the consequences will be for their family when he is released.

Laura reports that she has frequently used camomile (chamomile) tea to relax, OTC preparation of loperamide [Imodium] for occasional diarrhea, and miconazole nitrate [Monistat] for recurrent vaginal yeast infections during this pregnancy. For sporadic cold sores, she uses allantoin [Herpilyn] ointment.

Laura agrees to diagnostic testing. The ELISA test is positive and is confirmed by a positive Western blot test. The clinic physician prescribes zidovudine [ZDV, Retrovir] and assures Laura that it is highly effective in reducing transmission of HIV to the fetus. The medication will be continued after her delivery if her blood count is low (CD4+ count less than 500), or if she has symptoms of opportunistic infections. She is instructed not to breastfeed the infant and is told that close monitoring of the infant will be necessary for several months. An oral suspension of nystatin [Mycostatin] is ordered as "swish and swallow" four times daily (after meals and at night) for her oral/pharyngeal candidiasis infection. She receives a prescription for nystatin vaginal tablets and is instructed to use them, if needed, until up to 6 weeks before delivery to prevent thrush in her newborn infant. She is referred to Social Services for additional help and counseling.

The Pharmacist's Response

Laura Hamilton (pregnant woman diagnosed with HIV). Medications include Retrovir (zidovudine), Mycostatin (nystation). She also had taken Robitussin, chamomile tea and Immodium.

Action

The first drug passed by the FDA for treatment of HIV was Retrovir (zidovudine or AZT). Since then, Retrovir has been extensively studied for drug interactions. Most HIV patients begin therapy with two or three antiviral agents, owing to the increased chance for viral resistance to drugs. This combination therapy along with the addition of other agents for opportunistic infections creates the potential for serious drug interactions. HIV affects the immune system greatly and most patients must remain on long-term antibiotic/antifungal therapy. Most of these antiinfectives interact with other AIDS therapies.

TABLE 21-9   Medication Interactions and Nursing Interventions

Interacting Drugs	Interaction	Interventions
Acetaminophen	*Decreases* activity of AZT	Close monitoring of patient symptoms/drug levels
Phenytoin	AZT levels can increase while phenytoin levels fluctuate up or down	
Bone marrow suppressive agents, fluconazole, acyclovir/ganciclovir, interferons alpha-1a and beta-1b	All of these agents commonly used in HIV therapy *increase* AZT levels	Patients beginning these therapies need to have dosage adjustments
Rifanycin	*Decreases* AZT levels	

Critical Thinking Questions

1. What potential effects can Robitussin DM have on the fetus?

2. What instructions would you give Laura regarding the long-term use of OTC Robitussin and loperamide [Imodium]?

3. Are there any potential detrimental effects to Laura or her fetus as a result of the chemical (botanical) components is chamomile?

4. What additional instructions would you provide Laura regarding the use of nystatin?

5. What symptoms would you expect to see as adverse reactions to zidovudine in the neurologic system? In the endocrine system? In the immune system?

6. Loperamide [Imodium] is in the B pregnancy category. What potential adverse effects does that pose for the fetus?

References

Balmer, C. (1996). Basic principles of cancer treatment and cancer chemotherapy. In DiPiro et al. (Eds.), (1997). *Pharmacotherapy: A pathological approach* (3rd ed., pp. 2403–2466). Stamford, CT: Appleton & Lange.

Beckett, B. (1997). Headache disorders. In J. DiPiro et al. (Eds.), *Pharmacotherapy: A pathophysiologic approach* (3rd ed., pp: 1279–1291). Stamford, CT: Appleton & Lange.

Cavenee, W. (1995). The genetic basis of cancer. *Scientific American, March.*

Clark, J., Queener, S., & Karb, V. (1997). *Pharmacologic basis of nursing practice.* St. Louis: Mosby.

DiPiro, J., Talbert, R., Yee, G., Matzke, G., Wells, B., & Posey, L. (Eds.). (1997). *Pharmacotherapy: A pathophysiologic approach* (3rd ed.). Stamford, CT: Appleton & Lange.

Dripps, R., Eckenhoff, J., & Vandam, L. (1997). Introduction to anesthesia (9th ed.). Philadelphia: Saunders.

Edwards, J. (1997). Guarding against adverse drug events. *American Journal of Nursing, 97* (5), 26–31.

Ewald, P. (1993). Evolution of virulence. *Scientific American,* April, pp. 86–93.

Gaiser, R. (1997). Pharmacology of local anesthetics. In Dripps, R., Eckenhoff, J., & Vandam, L. (Eds.), *Introduction to anesthesia* (9th ed., pp. 201–215). Philadelphia: Saunders.

Guyton, A. (1996). *Textbook of medical physiology* (8th ed.). Philadelphia: Saunders.

Hickey (1994). *Nursing 94, October,* 34–41.

Kee LeFever, J., & Hayes, E. (1997). *Pharmacology: A nursing process approach* (2nd ed.). Philadelphia: Saunders.

Kelly, H. W., & Kamada, A. (1997). Asthma. In J. DiPiro et al. (Eds.), *Pharmacotherapy: A pathophysiologic approach* (3rd ed., p. 581). Stamford, CT: Appleton & Lange.

Kety, S. (1983). UCSD Medical school presentation, San Diego, CA.

Levine, A. (1992). *Viruses.* New York: Scientific American Library.

McCloskey, J., & Bulechek, G. (Eds.). (1996). *Nursing interventions classifications* (*NIC*). St. Louis: Mosby.

Oldstone, M. (1989). Viral alteration of cell function. *Scientific American.* (August, 42–48).

Rosenberg, S. (1992). *The transformed cell: Unlocking the mysteries of cancer.* New York: Putnam.

Sneader, W. (1985). *Drug discovery: The evolution of modern medicine.* New York: Wiley.

Snyder (1986). *Drugs and the brain.* New York: Scientific American Book Inc.

Stolte, K. (1997). Wellness nursing diagnoses: Accenting the positive. *American Journal of Nursing, 97* (7), 16B–16N.

Theesen, K.A., & Dopheide, J.A. (1997). In J. DiPiro et al. (Eds.) *Pharmacotherapy: A pathophysiologic approach* (3rd ed, pp. 1301–1301). Stamford CT: Appleton & Lange.

Bibliography

Abrams, A. (1995). *Clinical drug therapy: Rationales for nursing practice* (4th ed.). Philadelphia: Lippincott.

Ahrens, S. (1995). Managing heart failure: a blueprint for success. *Nursing95, 25* (12), 26–31.

Altura, B., & Altura, B. (1995). Magnesium in cardiovascular biology. *Scientific American Science & Medicine, 2* (3), 28–37.

Anderson, P., & Knoben, J. (1997). *Handbook of clinical drug data.* Stamford, CT: Appleton & Lange.

Angelucci, P. (1995). Caring for patients with hypothyroidism. *Nursing95, 25* (5), 60–61.

Antipsychotic olanzapine approved. November 1996. *Medical Sciences Bulletin.* VirSci Corporation. http://pharminfo.com

Aricept (donepezil hydrochloride tablets). (1998). Pfizer Inc.— Aricept Product Information. file:///Al/ARICEPTP.HTM

Arky, R., & Davidson, C. (1998). *Physician's desk reference.* Montvale, NJ: Medical Economics Inc.

Balmer (1996)

Balmer, C., & Valley, A. (1997). Basic principles of cancer treatment and cancer chemotherapy. In J. Dipiro et al. (Eds.), *Pharmacotherapy: A pathophysiologic approach* (3rd ed., pp. 1675–1688). Stamford, CT: Appleton & Lange.

Barry III, C. (1996). Penetrating the secrets of tuberculosis. *Science News, 149,* 375.

Borton, D. (1996). WBC count and differential: Reviewing the defensive roster. *Nursing96, 26* (9), 26–30.

Chiocca, E., & Russo, L. (1997). Acute asthma attack. *Nursing97, 27* (7), 43.

Copaxone (glatiramer acetate for injection) Nov. 1997. TEVA Pharmaceutical Industries, Israel.

Cuddy, R. (1995). Hypertension: keeping dangerous blood pressure down. *Nursing95, 25* (8), 34–41.

Davies, P. (1996). Caring for patients with diabetes insipidus. *Nursing96, 26* (5), 62–63.

De Fonseca, R. (1997). Marijuana's effects tracked in rat brains. *Science News, 151,* 397.

De Groot-Kosolcharoen, J. (1996). Culture and sensitivity testing. *Nursing96, 26* (9), 33–38.

DiPiro, I., & Stafford, C. (1997). Allergic and pseudoallergic drug reactions. In J. Dipiro et al. (Eds.), *Pharmacotherapy: A pathophysiologic approach* (3rd ed., pp. 1675–1688). Stamford, CT: Appleton & Lange.

Drass, J. (1996). Caring for patients with insulin-dependent diabetes mellitus. *Nursing96, 26:* 46–47

Eisenberg, M. (1998). Defibrillation: The spark of life. *Scientific American,* June, pp. 86–90.

Fackelmann, K. (1996). Antibiotic-eating germ alarms doctors. *Science News, 150,* 397.

Fackelmann, K. (1997). Drug combo routs HIV from blood and tissue. *Science News, 151,* 285.

Finlay, B. (1995). Bacterial virulence factors. *Scientific American Science & Medicine, 2* (3), 16–25.

Flomax (tamsulosin HCl) (1997). Vir-Sci Corporation. http://www.pharminfo.com/pubs/msb/tam240.html/

Goodwin, S., & Fish, D. (1997). Infections in immunocompromised patients. In J. Dipiro et al. (Eds.), *Pharmacotherapy: A pathophysiologic approach* (3rd ed., pp. 1675–1688). Stamford, CT: Appleton & Lange.

Guyton, A. (1996). *Textbook of medical physiology* (8th ed.). Philadelphia: Saunders.

Harwood, S. (1997). Anaphylaxis. *Nursing97, 27* (2), 33.

Hawkins, D., Bussey, H., & Prisant, L. (1997). In J. DiPiro et al. (Eds.), *Pharmacotherapy: A pathophysiologic approach* (3rd ed., pp. 197–218) Stamford, CT: Appleton & Lange.

Hayes, D. (1997). Bradycardia: Keeping the current flowing. *Nursing97, 27* (6), 50–55.

Held, J. (1995). Caring for a patient with lung cancer. *Nursing95, 25* (10), 34–43.

Heslin, J. (1997). Peptic ulcer disease: Making a case against the prime suspect. *Nursing97, 27* (1), 34–38.

Hoffman, S. (1997). Hitting malaria parasites early and hard. *Science News, 151* (23).

Holcomb, S. (1997). Understanding the ins and outs of diuretic therapy. *Nursing97, 27* (2), 34–40.

Hussar, D. (1996). Essential information on eight new drugs. *Nursing96, 26* (5), 52–56.

Hussar, D. (1997). New drugs. *Nursing97, 27* (1), 41–46.

Hussar, D. (1997). New Drugs. Part II. *Nursing97, 27* (6), 34–39.

Hussar, D. (1997). New Drugs. Part III. *Nursing97, 27* (7), 56–91.

Johnson, J., & Lalonde, R, (1997). Congestive heart failure. In J. DiPiro et al. (Eds.), *Pharmacotherapy: A pathophysiologic approach* (3rd ed., pp. 219–256) Stamford, CT: Appleton & Lange.

Joseph, R. (1996). *Neuropsychiatry, neuropsychology, and clinical neuroscience* (2nd ed.), Baltimore: Williams & Wilkins.

Kaplan, D. (1997). HIV may spare cells—for a short time. *Science News, 151,* 371.

Karch, A. (1996). *Lippincott's nursing drug guide.* Philadelphia: Lippincott.

Kelly, H. W., & Kamada, A. (1997). Asthma. In J. DiPiro et al. (Eds.), *Pharmacotherapy: A pathophysiologic approach* (p. 581). Stamford, CT: Appleton & Lange.

Kenny, P. (1996). Managing HIV infection: how to bolster your patient's fragile health. *Nursing96, 26,* 26–34.

Kim, M., McFarland, G., & McLane, A. (1993). *Pocket guide to nursing diagnoses* (5th ed). St. Louis: Mosby.

Kuncl, N., & Nelson, K. (1997). Antihypertensive drugs: balancing risks and benefits. *Nursing97, 27* (8), 46–49.

LeFever Kee, J. (1991). *Laboratory and diagnostic tests with nursing implications* (3rd ed.). Norwalk, CT: Appleton & Lange.

Loprowski, H. (1995). Visit to an ancient curse. *Scientific American Science & Medicine, 2* (3), 48–57.

Lacy, C., Armstrong, L., Ingrim, N., & Lance, L. (1997). *Drug information handbook* (5th ed.). Cleveland: Lexi-Comp.

Landry, D. (1997). Immunotherapy for cocaine addiction. *Scientific American, 276* (2), 42–45.

Lerner-Durjava, L. (1997). How to stop the pox. *Nursing97,* April, 20.

Levine, A. (1992). *Viruses.* New York: Scientific American Library.

Losick, R., & Kaiser D. (1997). Why and how bacteria communicate. *Scientific American, 276* (2), 68–73.

Majoros, K., & Moccia, J. (1995). Pulmonary embolism: Targeting an elusive enemy. *Nursing96, 26* (4), 26–31.

Mancano, M. (1998). New drugs of 1997. *Pharmacy Times,* March, 88–101.

Marten, P., & Schneiderhan, M. (1996). Assessment of psychiatric illness. In Dipiro et al. (Eds.), *Pharmacotherapy: A pathophysiologic approach* (3rd ed., pp. 1293–1300) Stamford, CT: Appleton & Lange.

Martin, E. (Ed.). (1996). *Intrapartum management modules* (2nd ed.). Philadelphia: Williams & Wilkins.

May, J., Feger, T., & Guill, M. (1997). Allergic rhinitis. In J. Dipiro et al. (Eds.), *Pharmacotherapy: A pathophysiologic approach* (3rd ed., pp. 1675–1688). Stamford, CT: Appleton & Lange.

McFarland, G., & McFarlane, E. (1996). *Nursing diagnosis and intervention.* St. Louis: Mosby.

Meissner, J. (1995). Caring for patients with meningitis. *Nursing95, 25* (7), 50–51.

Meridia (sibutramine hydrochloride monohydrate) capsules, Nov. (1997). North Mount Olive, NJ: Knoll Pharmaceutical Company.

Mower, D. (1997). Brain attack: Treating acute ischemic CVA. *Nursing97, 27* (3), 34–39.

Nemeroff, C. (1998). The neurobiology of depression. *Scientific American,* June *278,* 42–49.

Prandin (repaglinide) (1998). Novo Nordisk Pharmaceuticals, Inc. 100 Overlook Center, Suite 200, Princeton, NJ.

Oldstone, M. (1989). Viral alteration of cell function. *Scientific American,* August, 42.

Olopatadine for itching from allergic conjunctivitis. (1997). March/April. *Medical Sciences Bulletin* http://WWW.pharminfo.com/pubs/msb/olopat237.html.

Opioid analgesic remifentanil approved Sept. (1996). Medical Sciences Bulletin. VirSci Corporation. http://pharminfo.com.

Owen, A. (1995). Tracking the rise and fall of cardiac enzymes. *Nursing95, 25* (5), 34–38.

Pennisi, E. (1994). Bad brakes in cell cycle linked to cancers. *Science News, 145,* 262.

Peterson, I. (1996). Laser beam triggers a membrane breach. *Science News, 150,* 389.

Pettinicihi, T. (1996). Hypertensive crisis. *Nursing96, 26,* 25.

Pharmacia & Upjohn (1998). Mirapex (pramipexole dihydrochloride). Pharmacia & Upjohn Co., Kalamazoo, MI.

Physician's Desk Reference (51st ed.). (1997). Oradell, NJ: Medical Economics.

Polaski, A., & Tatro, S. (1996). *Luckmann's core principles and practice of medical-surgical nursing.* Philadelphia: Saunders.

Posey, L. (1998). Sildenafil approved for male impotence. PNN pharmacotherapy line. Pharmacotherapy News Network. March 30–April 15. PharmInfoNet. http://pharminfo.com.

Pramipexole cleared for marketing. (1997). *Medical Sciences Bulletin,* No. 239. VirSci Corporation. http://pharminfo.com.

Prescribing information Topamax (topiramate) tablets. PharmInfoNet (Mar. 1997). VirSci Corporation. http://pharminfo.com.

Product insert for ProAmatine (midodrine hydrochloride) tablets, (Jan. 1997). Roberts Pharmaceutical Corporation. file:///A|PROAMATI.HTM.

Propecia (finasteride) Dec. (1997). Merck & Co. file:///F|TEMPFILE

Quetiapine approved for management of psychotic disorders. (Nov. 1997). *Medical Sciences Bulletin,* No. 241. VirSci Corporation. htt://pharminfo.com.

Raimer, F. (1995). Clot stoppers: Using anticoagulants safely and effectively. *Nursing95, 25* (3), 34–43.

Raloff, J. (1994). Better leukemia survivial. *Science News, 146,* 230.

Repaglinide approved for mealtime therapy of DM. (Dec. 1997). Novo Nordisk. http://www.pharminfor.com/pubs/pnn20.html#6.

Resler, M., & Tumulty, G. (1983). Glaucoma update. *American Journal of Nursing, 93*(5), 752–756.

Robb-Nicholson, C. (1997). New asthma drugs. *Harvard Women's Health Watch,* January, 7.

Robb-Nicholson, C. (1996). HRT alternatives. *Harvard Women's Health Watch, III* (9), 2–3.

Robb-Nicholson, C. (1996). The importance of folate. *Harvard Women's Health Watch, III* (9), 1.

Robb-Nicholson, C. (1996). Designer estrogens. *Harvard Women's Health Watch, IV* (1), 7.

Ropinirole for Parkinson's disease. (Nov. 1997). *Medical Sciences Bulletin,* No. 241. http://www.pharminfo.com/pubs/msb/ropinirole241.htm1.

Rosenberg, S. (1992). *The transformed cell: Unlocking the mysteries of cancer.* New York: Putnam.

Sandoz Pharma, Ltd. (1998). 1. Zanaflex (tizanidine hydrochloride). San Francisco: Athena Neurosciences, Inc. 1–12. file:///A|/ZANAFLEX.HTM.

Segbefia, I., & Mallet, L. (1997). Are your patients taking their medications correctly? *Nursing97, 27* (41), 58–60.

Selected Articles. (Dec. 1997). PNN Pharmacotherapy Line. Pharmacotherapy News Network. http://www.pharminfo.com/pubs/pnn/pnn20.htm6

Seppa, N. (1997). New cold sore cream on the market. Science News, 151: 337.

Shannon, M., Wilson, B., & Stang, C. (1995). *Govoni & Hayes: drugs and nursing implications* (8th ed.). Stamford, CT: Appleton & Lange.

Smeltzer, S., & Bare, B. (1996). *Brunner and Suddarth's textbook of medical-surgical nursing* (8th ed.). Philadelphia: Lippincott–Raven.

Sneader, W. (1985). *Drug discovery: the evolution of modern medicines.* New York: Wiley.

Specht, D. (1995). Cerebral edema: bringing the brain back down to size. *Nursing95, 25,* 11: 34–38.

Spratto, G., & Woods, A. (1998). *Delmar's therapeutic class drug guide for nurses 1998.* Albany, NY: Delmar.

Sternberg, S. (1996). Bold aim in stroke: spare the brain. *Science News, 150,* 388.

Stolley, J. (1994). When your patient has Alzheimer's disease. *American Journal of Nursing, 94*(8), 34–40.

Talbert, R. (1997). Hyperlipidemia. In J. Dipiro et al. (Eds.), *Pharmacotherapy: A pathophysiologic approach* (3rd ed., pp. 459–489). Stamford, CT: Appleton & Lange.

Travis, J. (1996). Measles virus reveals its killing ways. *Science News, 150,* 20.

Travis, J. (1996). Estrogen eases Alzheimer's symptoms. *Science News, 150,* 399.

Travis, J. (1997). Microbial trigger for autoimmunity? *Science News, 151,* 380.

U.S. Prescribing Information Aricept (donepezil hydrochloride tablets). (April 1998). Pfizer Inc. file:///Al/ARICEPTP.HTM.

U.S. Prescribing Information for Requip (Sept. 1997). SmithKline Beecham. http://www.sb.com/prescribing_information/2000b.cgi?drug=rq.

USPI Update. (1997). United States Pharmacology Convention, Inc.

Vallee, B. (1998). Alcohol in the western world. *Scientific American,* June. 80–85.

Viagra (sildenafil citrate) tablets. (March 1998). Pfizer Inc. file:///Al/VIAGRAPI.HTM.

Wagner, C. R. (1997). AZT shows promise as breast cancer fighter. *Science News, 151,* 397.

Warmkessel, J. (1997). Caring for a patient with colon cancer. *Nursing97, 27* (4), 34–38.

Warmkessel, J. (1997). Caring for patients with non-Hodgkin's lymphoma. *Nursing97, 27* (6), 48–49.

Wells, B., Mandos, L., & Hayes, P. (1997). In J. Dipiro et al. (Eds.), *Pharmacotherapy: A pathophysiologic approach* (3rd ed., pp. 1395–1417). Stamford, CT: Appleton & Lange.

Wilkinson, J. (1996). *Nursing process: A critical thinking approach.* Menlo Park, CA: Addison-Wesley.

Wilson, B., Shannon, M., & Stang, C. (1999). *Nurses drug guide.* Stamford, CT: Appleton & Lange.

Zyprexa (olanzapine) (1997). Eli Lilly and Co., Indianapolis, IN.

Abbreviations
----

ac: (ante cibum) before meal

ACE: angiotensin-converting enzyme

ACT: activated clotting time

ACTH: adrenocorticotropic hormone

ADH: antidiuretic hormone

AIDS: acquired immunodeficiency syndrome

ALT: alanine aminotransferase; an enzyme found in serum and tissue, especially the liver and released during tissue injury; elevations may indicate acute liver damage (formerly SGPT)

ARC: AIDS-related complex

AST: (1) angiotensin sensitivity test. (2) aspartate amino-transferase: An enzyme present in body serum and tissue, especially heart and liver; released into the serum following tissue injury; may indicate liver damage or myocardial infarction (formerly SGOT)

AV: atrioventricular

BBB: blood–brain barrier

BC: birth control.

bid: (*bis in die*) twice a day

BP: blood pressure

BUN: blood urea nitrogen; a measure of kidney function; elevated levels indicate diabetes mellitus, GI bleeding, kidney failure, shock, and some tumors; decreased levels seen in liver disease, malnutrition, and pregnancy

C: centigrade, Celsius

CAD: coronary artery disease; most commonly refers to coronary atherosclerosis, but includes coronary artritis and fibromuscular hyperplasia, and may manifest as angina pectoris and cardiomyopathy

cAMP: cyclic 3′,5′-adenosine monophosphate. cAMP is a second messenger in the cell, formed by the enzyme adenylate cyclase; in the cell cAMP can trigger various intracellular actions, depending on the specific function of the cell.

CBC: complete blood count

C$_{cr}$: creatinine clearance, a measurement of glomerular filtration

cGMP: cyclic 3′,5′-guanosine monophosphate

CHF: congestive heart failure

CNS: central nervous system

COPD: chronic obstructive pulmonary disease

CPR: cardiopulmonary resuscitation

creatinine: A by-product of skeletal muscle metabolism

CSF: cerebrospinal fluid

CTZ: chemoreceptor trigger zone

CVA: cerebrovascular accident; the cause may be obstruction by a clot, or rupture of a blood vessel

d: day

DC: discontinue

DIC: disseminated intravascular coagulation

dL: deciliter (100 mL)

DNA: deoxyribonucleic acid; the carrier of genetic information found in the nucleus and mitochondria of cells

DPT: diphtheria-tetanus-pertussis; a combined vaccine

DS: double strength

DVT: deep vein thrombosis

ECG: electrocardiogram; sometimes abbreviated as EKG

ECT: electroconvulsive therapy; a psychiatric procedure that causes a brief convulsion; used for acute depression not responsive to antidepressants

EEG: electroencephalogram

FBS: fasting blood sugar

ENT: ear/nose/throat

EPS: extrapyramidal symptoms

FSH: follicle-stimulating hormone

g: gram

GABA: gamma-aminobutyric acid; a neurotransmitter involved in inhibiting neuronal conduction

GERD: gastroesophageal reflux disease

GI: gastrointestinal

gtt: drops

GU: genitourinary

h: hour

Hb: hemoglobin.

Hct: hematocrit

HDL: high-density lipoproteins; they transport cholesterol to the liver and help protect against atherosclerosis

Hg: mercury

Hib: *Hemophilus influenzae* type b

HIV: human immunodeficiency virus

hs: at bedtime (*hora somni:* at the hour of sleep)

5-HT: 5-hydroxytryptamine (serotonin)

I&O: intake and output

intrathecal: within the theca, or sheath, of the dura mater that encloses the spinal cord

IOP: intraocular pressure

IPPB: intermittent (or inspiratory) positive-pressure breathing

IV: intravenous

IVFE: intravenous fat emulsion

kg: kilogram

L: liter

lb: pound

LDH: lactic dehydrogenase; a serum indicator of myocardial infarction and muscular dystrophies; LDH levels rise 12–18 h after myocardial cell death

LDL: low-density lipoproteins; these are intermediate-density lipoproteins containing almost no triglycerides, but high concentrations of cholesterol and phospholipids

LE: lupus erythematosus; an immune system disease that results in inflammation and destruction of tissues of the vascular system, kidneys, or skin and nervous system; the cause is still being researched; it may be the result of a viral infection or a dysfunction of the immune system; some drugs may cause a lupus-like reaction

LE Prep: the laboratory test for lupus erythematosus in which the patient's serum specimen is incubated with normal neutrophils; the disease is indicated if the neutrophils become phagocytized

LH: luteinizing hormone

LH-RH: luteinizing hormone-releasing hormone

m: meter

MDI: metered-dose inhaler

MOA: monoamine oxidase; an enzyme that breaks down or oxidizes amines; part of the recycling process of amine neurotransmitters

MOAI: monoamine oxidase inhibitor

μg: microgram

mg: milligram

MI: myocardial infarction

min: minute

mL: milliliter

mo: month

NE: norepinephrine

NMS: neuroleptic malignant syndrome; a potentially deadly adverse response to certain anesthetics or neuroleptics due to defective or overwhelmed intracellular mechanisms for uptake of calcium; leads to a hypermetabolic condition in the muscles, manifested by increased CO_2 production, increased cardiac output, tachycardia, and elevated temperature

NPO: nothing by mouth (*nihil per os*)

NS: normal saline

NSAID: nonsteroidal antiinflammatory drug

NSR: normal sinus rhythm

OTC: over the counter; refers to legal drugs available without prescription

P: pulse

p̄: after

PAT: paroxysmal atrial tachycardia

PBI: protein-bound iodine; a serum measurement of thyroxine (T_4); the normal range is 4–8 μ/mL of serum

pc: after meal (*post cibum*).

PG: prostaglandin; a class of locally produced hormones released by cells to trigger a variety of responses in tissues

pH: hydrogen ion concentration

PO: orally, by mouth (*per os*)

PR: rectally

prn: as needed (*pro re nata*)

PSVT: paroxysmal supraventricular tachycardia

PT: prothrombin time; a test for deficiency of factors V, VII, or X in clotting; a prolonged PT indicates deficiency of one of the factors, indicating possible liver or vitamin K deficiency; PT is used in conjunction with anticoagulation therapy with warfarin

PTT: A test for the length of time the patient's plasma takes to form a clot when thromboplastin and calcium are added; a simultaneous test is done with a normal sample as a control; the normal PTT is 60–85 s after the addition of partial thromboplastin reagent and ionized calcium to the plasma

PVC: premature ventricular contraction

q: each, every (*quaque*)

qd: every day

qh: every hour

qid: four times a day (*quater in die*)

qod: every other day

R: rate

RA: rheumatoid arthritis

RBC: red blood cell

RDA: recommended daily (dietary) allowance

RNA: ribonucleic acid; a cellular messenger to transmit genetic information from the cell's nucleus to the cytoplasm

SA: sinoatrial

SC: subcutaneous

s: second.

SGOT: serum glutamic–oxaloacetic transaminase (see AST)

SGPT: serum glutamic–pyruvic transaminase (see ALT)

SIADH: syndrome of inappropriate antidiuretic hormone

SL: sublingual

SLE: systemic lupus erythematosus (see LE)

SOB: shortness of breath

SR: sustained release

SRSA: slow-reacting substance of anaphylaxis; a mixture of toxic leukotrienes released from mast cells or basophils as part of the immune response

SSRI: selective serotonin reuptake inhibitor

Stevens–Johnson syndrome: An inflammatory disease that is potentially fatal; the symptoms include fever, bullae, mucous membrane ulcers, possibility of pneumonia, joint pain, prostration; possible causes include drug reaction, pregnancy, infections, including herpes virus I.

T: temperature

T$_3$: triiodothyronine; a thyroid hormone that helps control metabolism and temperature

TB: tuberculosis

TCA: tricyclic antidepressant

TSH: thyroid stimulating hormone

TIA: transient ischemic attack

tid: three times a day (*ter in die*)

TSH: thyroid-stimulating hormone

U: units

URI: upper respiratory infection

UTI: urinary tract infection

VLDL: very-low-density lipoprotein; a transporter plasma protein that carries triglycerides from the liver to peripheral sites for use or storage

WBC: white blood cell

wk: week

y: year

Index